Preclinical Evaluation of Lipid-Based Nanosystems

Preclinical Evaluation of Lipid-Based Nanosystems

Editors

Ana Catarina Silva
José Manuel Sousa Lobo

MDPI • Basel • Beijing • Wuhan • Barcelona • Belgrade • Manchester • Tokyo • Cluj • Tianjin

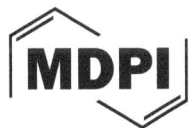

Editors
Ana Catarina Silva
University of Porto
Portugal

José Manuel Sousa Lobo
University of Porto
Portugal

Editorial Office
MDPI
St. Alban-Anlage 66
4052 Basel, Switzerland

This is a reprint of articles from the Special Issue published online in the open access journal *Pharmaceutics* (ISSN 1999-4923) (available at: https://www.mdpi.com/journal/pharmaceutics/special_issues/preclinical_lipid_nano).

For citation purposes, cite each article independently as indicated on the article page online and as indicated below:

LastName, A.A.; LastName, B.B.; LastName, C.C. Article Title. *Journal Name* **Year**, *Volume Number*, Page Range.

ISBN 978-3-0365-1550-2 (Hbk)
ISBN 978-3-0365-1549-6 (PDF)

© 2021 by the authors. Articles in this book are Open Access and distributed under the Creative Commons Attribution (CC BY) license, which allows users to download, copy and build upon published articles, as long as the author and publisher are properly credited, which ensures maximum dissemination and a wider impact of our publications.

The book as a whole is distributed by MDPI under the terms and conditions of the Creative Commons license CC BY-NC-ND.

Contents

Ana Catarina Silva and José Manuel Sousa Lobo
Preclinical Evaluation of Lipid-Based Nanosystems
Reprinted from: *Pharmaceutics* **2021**, *13*, 708, doi:pharmaceutics13050708 1

Eloy Pena-Rodríguez, Maria Lajarin-Reinares, Aida Mata-Ventosa, Sandra Pérez-Torras and Francisco Fernández-Campos
Dexamethasone-Loaded Lipomers: Development, Characterization, and Skin Biodistribution Studies
Reprinted from: *Pharmaceutics* **2021**, *13*, 533, doi:pharmaceutics13040533 7

Anroop B. Nair, Jigar Shah, Bandar E. Al-Dhubiab, Shery Jacob, Snehal S. Patel, Katharigatta N. Venugopala, Mohamed A. Morsy, Sumeet Gupta, Mahesh Attimarad, Nagaraja Sreeharsha and Pottathil Shinu
Clarithromycin Solid Lipid Nanoparticles for Topical Ocular Therapy: Optimization, Evaluation and In Vivo Studies
Reprinted from: *Pharmaceutics* **2021**, *13*, 523, doi:pharmaceutics13040523 27

Jana Kubackova, Ondrej Holas, Jarmila Zbytovska, Barbora Vranikova, Guanghong Zeng, Petr Pavek and Anette Mullertz
Oligonucleotide Delivery across the Caco-2 Monolayer: The Design and Evaluation of Self-Emulsifying Drug Delivery Systems (SEDDS)
Reprinted from: *Pharmaceutics* **2021**, *13*, 459, doi:pharmaceutics13040459 51

Antonio José Guillot, Enrique Jornet-Mollá, Natalia Landsberg, Carmen Milián-Guimerá, M. Carmen Montesinos, Teresa M. Garrigues and Ana Melero
Cyanocobalamin Ultraflexible Lipid Vesicles: Characterization and In Vitro Evaluation of Drug-Skin Depth Profiles
Reprinted from: *Pharmaceutics* **2021**, *13*, 418, doi: 79

Simone A.G. Langeveld, Inés Beekers, Gonzalo Collado-Lara, Antonius F. W. van der Steen, Nico de Jong and Klazina Kooiman
The Impact of Lipid Handling and Phase Distribution on the Acoustic Behavior of Microbubbles
Reprinted from: *Pharmaceutics* **2021**, *13*, 119, doi:pharmaceutics13010119 101

Lourdes Valdivia, Lorena García-Hevia, Manuel Bañobre-López, Juan Gallo, Rafael Valiente and Mónica López Fanarraga
Solid Lipid Particles for Lung Metastasis Treatment
Reprinted from: *Pharmaceutics* **2021**, *13*, 93, doi:pharmaceutics13010093 123

Hala M. Alkhalidi, Khaled M. Hosny and Waleed Y. Rizg
Oral Gel Loaded by Fluconazole–Sesame Oil Nanotransfersomes: Development, Optimization, and Assessment of Antifungal Activity
Reprinted from: *Pharmaceutics* **2020**, *13*, 27, doi:pharmaceutics13010027 137

Sara Hernando, Enara Herran, Rosa Maria Hernandez and Manoli Igartua
Nanostructured Lipid Carriers Made of Ω-3 Polyunsaturated Fatty Acids: In Vitro Evaluation of Emerging Nanocarriers to Treat Neurodegenerative Diseases
Reprinted from: *Pharmaceutics* **2020**, *12*, 928, doi:pharmaceutics12100928 161

Priveledge Mazonde, Sandile M. M. Khamanga and Roderick B. Walker
Design, Optimization, Manufacture and Characterization of Efavirenz-Loaded Flaxseed Oil Nanoemulsions
Reprinted from: *Pharmaceutics* **2020**, *12*, 797, doi:pharmaceutics12090797 183

Maryam Farzan, Gabriela Québatte, Katrin Strittmatter, Florentine Marianne Hilty, Joachim Schoelkopf, Jörg Huwyler and Maxim Puchkov
Spontaneous In Situ Formation of Liposomes from Inert Porous Microparticles for Oral Drug Delivery
Reprinted from: *Pharmaceutics* **2020**, *12*, 777, doi:pharmaceutics12080777 205

Otto K. Kari, Shirin Tavakoli, Petteri Parkkila, Simone Baan, Roosa Savolainen, Teemu Ruoslahti, Niklas G. Johansson, Joseph Ndika, Harri Alenius, Tapani Viitala, Arto Urtti and Tatu Lajunen
Light-Activated Liposomes Coated with Hyaluronic Acid as a Potential Drug Delivery System
Reprinted from: *Pharmaceutics* **2020**, *12*, 763, doi:pharmaceutics12080763 223

Ruba Almasri, Paul Joyce, Hayley B. Schultz, Nicky Thomas, Kristen E. Bremmell and Clive A. Prestidge
Porous Nanostructure, Lipid Composition, and Degree of Drug Supersaturation Modulate In Vitro Fenofibrate Solubilization in Silica-Lipid Hybrids
Reprinted from: *Pharmaceutics* **2020**, *12*, 687, doi:pharmaceutics12070687 247

Maria Principia Scavo, Annalisa Cutrignelli, Nicoletta Depalo, Elisabetta Fanizza, Valentino Laquintana, Giampietro Gasparini, Gianluigi Giannelli and Nunzio Denora
Effectiveness of a Controlled 5-FU Delivery Based on FZD10 Antibody-Conjugated Liposomes in Colorectal Cancer In vitro Models
Reprinted from: *Pharmaceutics* **2020**, *12*, 650, doi: 269

Lisa Belfiore, Darren N. Saunders, Marie Ranson and Kara L. Vine
N-Alkylisatin-Loaded Liposomes Target the Urokinase Plasminogen Activator System in Breast Cancer
Reprinted from: *Pharmaceutics* **2020**, *12*, 641, doi:pharmaceutics12070641 289

Sara Cunha, Cláudia Pina Costa, Joana A. Loureiro, Jorge Alves, Andreia F. Peixoto, Ben Forbes, José Manuel Sousa Lobo and Ana Catarina Silva
Double Optimization of Rivastigmine-Loaded Nanostructured Lipid Carriers (NLC) for Nose-to-Brain Delivery Using the Quality by Design (QbD) Approach: Formulation Variables and Instrumental Parameters
Reprinted from: *Pharmaceutics* **2020**, *12*, 599, doi:pharmaceutics12070599 307

Kevin Hart, Martyn Harvey, Mingtan Tang, Zimei Wu and Grant Cave
Liposomes to Augment Dialysis in Preclinical Models: A Structured Review
Reprinted from: *Pharmaceutics* **2021**, *13*, 395, doi:pharmaceutics13030395 333

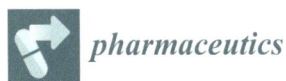

Editorial

Preclinical Evaluation of Lipid-Based Nanosystems

Ana Catarina Silva and José Manuel Sousa Lobo

1 UCIBIO/REQUIMTE, MEDTECH, Laboratory of Pharmaceutical Technology, Department of Drug Sciences, Faculty of Pharmacy, University of Porto, 4050-313 Porto, Portugal; slobo@ff.up.pt
2 FP-ENAS (UFP Energy, Environment and Health Research Unit), CEBIMED (Biomedical Research Centre), Faculty of Health Sciences, University Fernando Pessoa, 4249-004 Porto, Portugal
* Correspondence: ana.silva@ff.up.pt

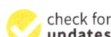

Citation: Silva, A.C.; Sousa Lobo, J.M. Preclinical Evaluation of Lipid-Based Nanosystems. *Pharmaceutics* **2021**, *13*, 708. https://doi.org/10.3390/pharmaceutics13050708

Received: 10 May 2021
Accepted: 11 May 2021
Published: 12 May 2021

Publisher's Note: MDPI stays neutral with regard to jurisdictional claims in published maps and institutional affiliations.

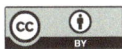

Copyright: © 2021 by the authors. Licensee MDPI, Basel, Switzerland. This article is an open access article distributed under the terms and conditions of the Creative Commons Attribution (CC BY) license (https://creativecommons.org/licenses/by/4.0/).

The use of lipid-based nanosystems, including lipid nanoparticles (solid lipid nanoparticles—SLN, and nanostructured lipid carriers—NLC), nanoemulsions, and liposomes, among others, is widespread. Several researchers have described advantages of the different applications of these nanosystems. For instance, they can increase the targeting and bioavailability of drugs, improving the therapeutic effect. Their use in the cosmetic field is also promising, owing to their moisturizing properties and ability to protect labile cosmetic actives. Thus, it is surprising that only few lipid-based nanosystems have reached the market. This can be explained by the strict regulatory requirements of medicines and the occurrence of unexpected in vivo failure, which highlights the need to conduct more preclinical studies.

Current research is focused on testing the in vitro, ex vivo and in vivo efficacy of lipid-based nanosystems to predict their clinical performance. However, there is a lack of method validation, which compromises the comparison between different studies.

This Special Issue brings together the latest research and reviews that report preclinical studies in vitro, ex vivo and in vivo using lipid-based nanosystems. Readers will find up-to-date information on the most common experiments performed to predict the clinical behavior of lipid-based nanosystems. A series of 15 research articles and a review are presented, with authors from 15 different countries, which demonstrates the universality of the investigations that have been carried out in this area.

F. Fernández-Campos et al. [1] developed lipomers (i.e., lipid core polymeric nanocapsules) loaded with dexamethasone and studied their potential to improve the topical treatment of alopecia areata and other hair-follicle inflammatory diseases. The occurrence of follicular targeting of lipomers suggests that it is possible to have a drug deposition effect within the pilosebaceous unit, which reduces the frequency of administrations, although the safety and efficacy profiles of these lipomers must first be confirmed in clinical trials.

A.B. Nair et al. [2] evaluated the potential of optimized clarithromycin-loaded SLN to improve the ocular permeation of this drug, increasing its therapeutic potential. A 32 full factorial design showed a significant influence of the sonication time and the amount of lipid on the clarithromycin-loaded SLN particle size, entrapment efficiency and drug loading. In addition, the results of the ex vivo permeation studies and in vivo pharmacokinetics studies showed a greater efficacy of the optimized clarithromycin-loaded SLN compared to a drug solution, suggesting that the developed formulation may be a viable drug delivery approach for treating endophthalmitis.

O. Holas et al. [3] investigated the ability of oligonucleotide-loaded self-emulsifying drug delivery systems (SEDDS) to cross intestinal Caco-2 cells. In this study, oligonucleotides were first complexed with cationic lipids to improve lipophilicity and later formulated in SEDDS with negative charge and neutral charge. From the results of their work, the authors suggested the use of SEDDS to improve the oral delivery of oligonucleotides, overcoming difficulties of permeation and stability. However, in vivo testing of oligonucleotide-loaded SEDDS is necessary to obtain more detailed knowledge of this potential for local delivery.

A. Melero et al. [4] developed cyanocobalamin (vitamin B12)-loaded ultraflexible lipid vesicles (liposomes, transfersomes, and ethosomes) with enhanced skin penetration ability, which can be used as a promising alternative to improve the treatment of skin diseases, such as atopic dermatitis and psoriasis. Although vitamin B12 is effective as a nitric oxide scavenger, the hydrophilic character and weight of this molecule limit its diffusion through the skin. In this study, the authors identified the key factors for the efficient production of vitamin B12-loaded lipid vesicles, including size, stability and purification method. In addition, it was observed that the developed lipid vesicles efficiently release vitamin B12 to the deeper layers of the skin, 6 h after the application.

S.A.G. Langeveld et al. [5] studied the use of phospholipid-coated microbubbles as contrast agents for ultrasound molecular imaging and for drug delivery. The authors investigated how lipid handling and phase distribution affect the acoustic behavior of these microbubbles. Varying concentrations of cholesterol were used to modify the lateral molecular packing of 1,2-distearoyl-sn-glycero-3-phosphocholine (DSPC)-based microbubbles, which were produced by a direct method and by an indirect method. The results showed that indirect-produced DSPC microbubbles had a more uniform response to ultrasound than direct-produced DSPC and indirect-produced DSPC-cholesterol microbubbles. Besides, the difference in lipid handling between direct-produced and indirect-produced DSPC microbubbles significantly affected the acoustic behavior, with the latter being the most promising for ultrasound molecular imaging and drug delivery. From these results, the authors concluded that the phase distribution and lipid handling prior to microbubble production significantly affected the acoustic behavior of microbubbles.

M.L. Fanarraga et al. [6] developed doxorubicin-loaded lipid particles (SLPs) (also known as SLN) for the treatment of lung metastatic malignant melanoma. In this study, the authors conducted comparative in vivo experiments in mice, with intravenous doxorubicin-loaded SLPs and intravenous free drug, and observed that the former significantly reduced the number of pulmonary metastatic foci. In addition, prolonged in vitro drug release was observed over 40 days, which suggests the possibility of reaching constant drug levels in situ to inhibit metastatic growth, increasing local drug efficacy, reducing side effects and improving overall survival. Based on these findings, the authors suggested the use of doxorubicin-loaded SLPs as an adjuvant treatment for different types of cancer.

W.Y. Rizg et al. [7] developed fluconazole-loaded sesame oil containing nanotransfersomes to improve the local treatment of oral candidiasis. The Box-Behnken design was used to evaluate the parameters of the production method that interfere with size, entrapment efficiency, zone of inhibition and ulcer index. The optimized formulation of fluconazole-loaded nanotransfersomes was included in a hyaluronic acid-based hydrogel and characterized to assess its suitability for local application in the oral cavity. Finally, ex vivo and in vivo studies confirmed the superior antifungal efficacy of the developed fluconazole-loaded nanotransfersomes, when compared to fluconazole suspension and to hyaluronic acid hydrogel. The authors suggested that the improved antifungal efficacy of the developed formulation could be related to the synergistic effect of its components, such as hyaluronic acid, sesame oil and fluconazole.

M. Igartua an R.M. Hernandez et al. [8] prepared NLC composed of polyunsaturated fatty acids and evaluated their protective and anti-inflammatory effects aiming to produce a new functional nanocarrier to entrap different therapeutic molecules, acting as a synergistic therapy. In their studies, researchers observed that the developed NLC are biocompatible with both dopaminergic and microglia cells and exhibited neuroprotective effects in dopaminergic neuron cells, after exposition to 6-hydroxydopamine hydrochloride (6-OHDA) neurotoxin, and decreased the proinflammatory cytokine levels in microglia cells, after lipopolysaccharide (LPS) stimuli. From these results, it was concluded that the combination of these new NLC with different therapeutic molecules could be an effective tool for the synergistic treatment of neurogenerative diseases.

R.B. Walker et al. [9] developed and characterized efavirenz-loaded flaxseed oil nanoemulsions. The studies consisted of using a D-optimal design to obtain the surfactant mixture that originates kinetically stable low energy nanoemulsions. The authors proposed the use of flaxseed oil nanoemulsions in oral efavirenz formulations due to the health benefits for patients associated with the use of polyunsaturated fatty acids. In addition, it was also mentioned that flaxseed oil is a renewable inexpensive raw material that can be exploited in the preparation of pharmaceutical dosage forms.

M. Puchkov et al. [10] investigated the in situ formation of liposomes from inert porous calcium carbonate microparticles, called dry powder proliposomal formulations. In the experiments, nifedipine was used as a model of a poorly water-soluble oral drug, and the factors that affect liposome formation and drug encapsulation were studied in different simulated gastrointestinal fluids. From the results, the authors proposed the use of a single-step loading of phospholipids and drugs as a simple and effective method for the production of proliposomal formulations, which is suitable for scale-up.

T. Lajunen et al. [11] developed and characterized light-activated liposomes coated with hyaluronic acid for ocular delivery. In their experiments, the researchers observed that, when compared to liposomes coated with polyethylene glycol (PEG), liposomes coated with hyaluronic acid showed improved plasma stability and greater binding to vitreous humor proteins and collagen-related proteins, which is probably related to the reduced vitreal mobility. From these findings, the authors concluded that the hyaluronic acid-coated light-activated liposomes are a promising alternative for intravenous and ocular drug delivery.

C.A. Prestidge et al. [12] studied the impact of the main characteristics of a nanostructured matrix obtained by silica–lipid hybrids in the construction of optimized solid-state lipid-based formulations for the oral delivery of poorly water-soluble drugs. For the experiments, fenofibrate was used as a drug model and the impact of drug loading, type of lipid and type of silica nanostructure on the in vitro dissolution, solubilization, and solid-state stability of fenofibrate was investigated. Based on their research, the authors proposed that the study of the key characteristics of nanostructured matrix silica–lipid hybrids allows the preparation of tailor-made formulations with regard to the release profile or the desired therapeutic result.

M.P. Scavo et al. [13] evaluated the antitumor effect of immuno-liposomes loaded with 5-fluorouracil and surface-coated with an antibody against the Frizzled 10 protein, which is an overexpressed receptor on the surface of colorectal cancer cells. The experiments were conducted in vitro on two different colorectal cell lines, where the Frizzled 10 protein is overexpressed, called metastatic CoLo-205 and non-metastatic CaCo-2 cells. In addition, several characterization studies were performed on the developed immuno-liposomes and their therapeutic efficacy was evaluated in vitro. The overall results of these studies showed that the cytotoxic activity of 5-fluorouracil increased when it was encapsulated in the immuno-liposomes compared to the free compound. Therefore, the authors suggested the use of these immuno-liposomes for the selective treatment of colorectal cancer, although more studies are needed to investigate the specific mechanisms of cell uptake. Moreover, the potential of these liposomes for inclusion in conventional pharmaceutical dosage forms, such as gastro-resistant capsules or suppositories, was proposed.

K.L. Vine et al. [14] tested the in vitro and in vivo uptake of anti-mitotic N-alkylisatin-loaded liposomes functionalized with plasminogen activator inhibitor type 2 to target the urokinase plasminogen activator and its receptor. Receptor-dependent cytotoxicity and uptake of functionalized liposomes were observed in vitro, which was greater for the plasminogen activator urokinase and its receptor overexpressed in breast cancer cells MDA-MB-231 compared to the low expression of MCF-7 breast cancer cells. The targeting ability of the tested functionalized liposomes was observed in vivo, where there was an increase in accumulation at the site of the primary tumor in an animal model of disease compared to non-functionalized liposomes. Based on these findings, the authors proposed the use of functionalized liposomes to target the plasminogen activator urokinase and its receptor-positive breast cancer cells, improving the treatment of triple-negative breast cancer. In addition, the authors suggested the use of these liposomes to target heterogeneous tumor cells, where the plasminogen activator urokinase and its receptor play a key role in the development of metastases.

A.C. Silva et al. [15] applied the quality by design (QbD) approach to perform a double optimization of rivastigmine-loaded NLC, in which quality target product profile (QTPP) was the requirement of nose-to-brain delivery. The first optimization was related to the selection of critical material attributes (CMAs), including ratios of drug, lipids and surfactants, using a central composite design. Afterwards, the formulation with the best critical quality attributes (CQAs) of particle size, polydispersity index, zeta potential, and encapsulation efficiency was selected for the second optimization, which was related to the production methods (ultrasound technique and high-pressure homogenization). Here, the Box–Behnken design was used to evaluate the same CQAs of the first optimization, with high-pressure homogenization selected as the most suitable production method, although the ultrasound technique has also shown effectiveness. From these results, the authors concluded that QbD is a useful approach for the optimization of NLC formulations with specific requirements.

K. Hart et al. [16] reviewed the literature on the use of liposomes to augment dialysis in preclinical models for both endogenous toxins and intoxicants, in particular, on repurposing the use of liposomes in areas of unmet clinical needs. From their investigations, the authors concluded that the use of pH-gradient liposomes with acidic centers in peritoneal dialysis to increase the extraction of ammonia in hepatic failure is the most studied area, which is under phase 1 of clinical trials. In addition, the use of liposomes to remove exogenous intoxicants and protein-bound uremic and hepatic toxins and the use of liposome-supported enzymatic dialysis have also been studied. In conclusion, the authors believe that the use of liposomes for clinical indications other than drug transport will emerge in the next decade.

We would like to thank all the authors of this Special Issue for contributing with high quality works. We also acknowledge all the reviewers who critically evaluated the articles. In addition, we would like to thank the Assistant Editor, Ms. Claudia Li, for her kind help.

Funding: The Applied Molecular Biosciences Unit—UCIBIO, which is financed by national funds from FCT (UIDP/04378/2020 and UIDB/04378/2020), supported this work.

Conflicts of Interest: The authors declare no conflict of interest.

References

1. Pena-Rodríguez, E.; Lajarin-Reinares, M.; Mata-Ventosa, A.; Pérez-Torras, S.; Fernández-Campos, F. Dexamethasone-Loaded Lipomers: Development, Characterization, and Skin Biodistribution Studies. *Pharmaceutics* **2021**, *13*, 533. [CrossRef] [PubMed]
2. Nair, A.B.; Shah, J.; Al-Dhubiab, B.E.; Jacob, S.; Patel, S.S.; Venugopala, K.N.; Morsy, M.A.; Gupta, S.; Attimarad, M.; Sreeharsha, N.; et al. Clarithromycin Solid Lipid Nanoparticles for Topical Ocular Therapy: Optimization, Evaluation and In Vivo Studies. *Pharmaceutics* **2021**, *13*, 523. [CrossRef] [PubMed]
3. Kubackova, J.; Holas, O.; Zbytovska, J.; Vranikova, B.; Zeng, G.; Pavek, P.; Mullertz, A. Oligonucleotide Delivery across the Caco-2 Monolayer: The Design and Evaluation of Self-Emulsifying Drug Delivery Systems (SEDDS). *Pharmaceutics* **2021**, *13*, 459. [CrossRef] [PubMed]
4. Guillot, A.J.; Jornet-Mollá, E.; Landsberg, N.; Milián-Guimerá, C.; Montesinos, M.C.; Garrigues, T.M.; Melero, A. Cyanocobalamin Ultraflexible Lipid Vesicles: Characterization and In Vitro Evaluation of Drug-Skin Depth Profiles. *Pharmaceutics* **2021**, *13*, 418. [CrossRef] [PubMed]
5. Langeveld, S.A.G.; Beekers, I.; Collado-Lara, G.; van der Steen, A.F.W.; de Jong, N.; Kooiman, K. The Impact of Lipid Handling and Phase Distribution on the Acoustic Behavior of Microbubbles. *Pharmaceutics* **2021**, *13*, 119. [CrossRef] [PubMed]
6. Valdivia, L.; García-Hevia, L.; Bañobre-López, M.; Gallo, J.; Valiente, R.; López Fanarraga, M. Solid Lipid Particles for Lung Metastasis Treatment. *Pharmaceutics* **2021**, *13*, 93. [CrossRef] [PubMed]
7. Alkhalidi, H.M.; Hosny, K.M.; Rizg, W.Y. Oral Gel Loaded by Fluconazole-Sesame Oil Nanotransfersomes: Development, Optimization, and Assessment of Antifungal Activity. *Pharmaceutics* **2021**, *13*, 27. [CrossRef] [PubMed]
8. Hernando, S.; Herran, E.; Hernandez, R.M.; Igartua, M. Nanostructured Lipid Carriers Made of Ω-3 Polyunsaturated Fatty Acids: In Vitro Evaluation of Emerging Nanocarriers to Treat Neurodegenerative Diseases. *Pharmaceutics* **2020**, *12*, 928. [CrossRef] [PubMed]

9. Mazonde, P.; Khamanga, S.M.M.; Walker, R.B. Design, Optimization, Manufacture and Characterization of Efavirenz-Loaded Flaxseed Oil Nanoemulsions. *Pharmaceutics* **2020**, *12*, 797. [CrossRef] [PubMed]
10. Farzan, M.; Québatte, G.; Strittmatter, K.; Hilty, F.M.; Schoelkopf, J.; Huwyler, J.; Puchkov, M. Spontaneous In Situ Formation of Liposomes from Inert Porous Microparticles for Oral Drug Delivery. *Pharmaceutics* **2020**, *12*, 777. [CrossRef] [PubMed]
11. Kari, O.K.; Tavakoli, S.; Parkkila, P.; Baan, S.; Savolainen, R.; Ruoslahti, T.; Johansson, N.G.; Ndika, J.; Alenius, H.; Viitala, T.; et al. Light-Activated Liposomes Coated with Hyaluronic Acid as a Potential Drug Delivery System. *Pharmaceutics* **2020**, *12*, 763. [CrossRef] [PubMed]
12. Almasri, R.; Joyce, P.; Schultz, H.B.; Thomas, N.; Bremmell, K.E.; Prestidge, C.A. Porous Nanostructure, Lipid Composition, and Degree of Drug Supersaturation Modulate In Vitro Fenofibrate Solubilization in Silica-Lipid Hybrids. *Pharmaceutics* **2020**, *12*, 687. [CrossRef] [PubMed]
13. Scavo, M.P.; Cutrignelli, A.; Depalo, N.; Fanizza, E.; Laquintana, V.; Gasparini, G.; Giannelli, G.; Denora, N. Effectiveness of a Controlled 5-FU Delivery Based on FZD10 Antibody-Conjugated Liposomes in Colorectal Cancer In vitro Models. *Pharmaceutics* **2020**, *12*, 650. [CrossRef] [PubMed]
14. Belfiore, L.; Saunders, D.N.; Ranson, M.; Vine, K.L. N-Alkylisatin-Loaded Liposomes Target the Urokinase Plasminogen Activator System in Breast Cancer. *Pharmaceutics* **2020**, *12*, 641. [CrossRef] [PubMed]
15. Cunha, S.; Costa, C.P.; Loureiro, J.A.; Alves, J.; Peixoto, A.F.; Forbes, B.; Lobo, J.M.S.; Silva, A.C. Double Optimization of Rivastigmine-Loaded Nanostructured Lipid Carriers (NLC) for Nose-to-Brain Delivery Using the Quality by Design (QbD) Approach: Formulation Variables and Instrumental Parameters. *Pharmaceutics* **2020**, *12*, 599. [CrossRef] [PubMed]
16. Hart, K.; Harvey, M.; Tang, M.; Wu, Z.; Cave, G. Liposomes to Augment Dialysis in Preclinical Models: A Structured Review. *Pharmaceutics* **2021**, *13*, 395. [CrossRef] [PubMed]

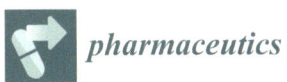

Article

Dexamethasone-Loaded Lipomers: Development, Characterization, and Skin Biodistribution Studies

Eloy Pena-Rodríguez, Maria Lajarin-Reinares, Aida Mata-Ventosa, Sandra Pérez-Torras and Francisco Fernández-Campos

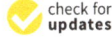

Citation: Pena-Rodríguez, E.; Lajarin-Reinares, M.; Mata-Ventosa, A.; Pérez-Torras, S.; Fernández-Campos, F. Dexamethasone-Loaded Lipomers: Development, Characterization, and Skin Biodistribution Studies. Pharmaceutics 2021, 13, 533. https:// doi.org/10.3390/pharmaceutics13040533

Academic Editor: Ana Catarina Silva

Received: 29 March 2021
Accepted: 8 April 2021
Published: 11 April 2021

Publisher's Note: MDPI stays neutral with regard to jurisdictional claims in published maps and institutional affiliations.

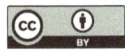

Copyright: © 2021 by the authors. Licensee MDPI, Basel, Switzerland. This article is an open access article distributed under the terms and conditions of the Creative Commons Attribution (CC BY) license (https:// creativecommons.org/licenses/by/ 4.0/).

1   Topical & Oral Development R+D Reig Jofre Laboratories, 08970 Barcelona, Spain; eloy.pena@reigjofre.com (E.P.-R.); mlajarin@reigjofre.com (M.L.-R.)
2   Molecular Pharmacology and Experimental Therapeutics, Department of Biochemistry and Molecular Biomedicine, Institute of Biomedicine (IBUB), University of Barcelona, 08028 Barcelona, Spain; aidamatav@ub.edu (A.M.-V.); s.perez-torras@ub.edu (S.P.-T.)
3   Biomedical Research Networking Center in Hepatic and Digestive Diseases (CIBEREHD), Carlos III Health Institute, 28029 Madrid, Spain
4   Sant Joan de Déu Research Institute (IR SJD-CERCA) Esplugues de Llobregat, 08950 Barcelona, Spain
*   Correspondence: Ffernandez@reigjofre.com; Tel.: +34-935-507-718

Abstract: Follicular targeting has gained more attention in recent decades, due to the possibility of obtaining a depot effect in topical administration and its potential as a tool to treat hair follicle-related diseases. Lipid core ethyl cellulose lipomers were developed and optimized, following which characterization of their physicochemical properties was carried out. Dexamethasone was encapsulated in the lipomers (size, 115 nm; polydispersity, 0.24; zeta-potential (Z-potential), +30 mV) and their in vitro release profiles against dexamethasone in solution were investigated by vertical diffusion Franz cells. The skin biodistribution of the fluorescent-loaded lipomers was observed using confocal microscopy, demonstrating the accumulation of both lipomers and fluorochromes in the hair follicles of pig skin. To confirm this fact, immunofluorescence of the dexamethasone-loaded lipomers was carried out in pig hair follicles. The anti-inflammatory (via TNFα) efficacy of the dexamethasone-loaded lipomers was demonstrated in vitro in an HEK001 human keratinocytes cell culture and the in vitro cytotoxicity of the nanoformulation was investigated.

Keywords: follicular targeting; dexamethasone; alopecia areata; lipomers; lipid polymer hybrid nanocapsules; biodistribution; skin; ethyl cellulose

1. Introduction

Nanoparticles are pharmaceutical forms that are used to improve the efficacy and bioavailability of different poorly water-soluble active ingredients. The physicochemical properties of nanoparticles, such as their high surface-to-volume ratio, the ability to increase permeability through different cell tissues, the possibility of increasing the solubility of active ingredients, or the ability to modulate the release kinetics to achieve depot formulations, make nanoparticles a very attractive approach to improve the therapeutical indices of active ingredients through different routes of administration.

In recent decades, there has been a great deal of research related to modulated targeting and localized release in different parts of the body. The stratum corneum, comprised of a group of low water content corneocytes and a lipid matrix made of ceramides and cholesterol as the main components, acts as a barrier for topical products in a very efficient way [1]. In the past few years, different nanoencapsulation platforms have been developed to transport drugs to the inner layers of the skin. Regarding the transdermal route, it is well-known that flexible particles, such as transfersomes, or micellar systems are capable of increasing permeation [2,3]; however, the loading capacity of these systems is usually low. In recent years, the transfollicular route has gained more attention, as it has been suggested to increase dermal absorption, probably due to accumulation in the pilosebaceous unit.

For example, Lademann et al. demonstrated that, by using nanoparticles made of poly (lactic-co-glycolic acid) (PLGA), it was possible to obtain a depot effect for 10 days in porcine hair follicles, whereas nanoparticles on the skin surface were only detectable for 24 h [4]. Furthermore, nanosystems, such as polymeric nanoparticles or nanostructured lipid carriers, have higher loading capacities [5]. However, there is still a lack of information regarding the accumulation of these systems in the anatomy of the hair follicle.

Lipomers, or lipid core polymeric nanocapsules (LPNCs), are oily vesicles surrounded by a polymeric wall [6]. In polymeric nanospheres, the active is trapped both on the surface of the particle and in its core. They usually have a burst release effect, due to the desorption of the active from the surface, followed by a plateau based on diffusion/erosion mechanisms. Urzula Bazylinska et al. compared the release of a lipophilic active encapsulated in nanospheres and lipid polymer hybrid nanocapsules and verified that the presence of the lipid nucleus increased the encapsulation efficiency and decreased the burst release effect, obtaining a more sustained release [7].

Topical corticosteroids are the most frequently used drugs for the treatment of inflammatory diseases. Dexamethasone (DEX) has been used topically to treat ocular inflammation [8], atopic dermatitis [9], and alopecia areata (AA) [10], among other diseases, with a high benefit-to-risk ratio. In the case of AA, topical corticoids are frequently ineffective and oral or intralesional therapy is required; furthermore, the potential adverse effects and patient discomfort caused by scalp injections must be considered [11]. Some authors have used solutions with a high proportion of ethanol (70%), as a permeation enhancer, to deliver DEX [9]. They found drug accumulation exclusively in the lipid interspaces and did not observe efficient penetration into corneocytes. There exist other topical corticoids in the market, such as mometasone or methylprednisolone, which are also formulated in hydroalcoholic vehicles with a high content of ethanol. Ethanol has been associated with skin irritation or contact dermatitis [12], it could alter the stratum corneum structure [13], and modify the skin microbiota [14], which could be related to skin diseases and inflammatory status. Thus, it is preferable to minimize its use in topical formulations. Other authors encapsulated DEX (hemisuccinate) in liposomes by microfluidics and film hydration techniques [15]. Even though liposomes are very attractive drug delivery systems, the loading capacity is usually low and could be an issue for specific indications that require higher doses. Considering the above, the improvement of topical treatment is still required, to increase patient quality of life and to minimize adverse effects. Lipomers are a promising drug delivery system to improve the therapeutical balance of DEX in AA treatment, due to possible accumulation in the pilosebaceous unit, where the disease takes place, and under the hypothesis that the lipid nucleus increases the loading capacity. This fact leads to a higher drug concentration in the LPNCs, compared with similar particles without the lipidic core, for which the DEX loading capacity was about 1–2% [16].

For this study, DEX-LPNCs were developed and characterized, in terms of their physicochemical properties and drug release. A description of the skin biodistribution and its accumulation on hair follicles is given. Additionally, information about the associated in vitro cytotoxicity and efficacy is shown. It was found that the proposed DEX-loaded LPNCs have potential as a tool for the topical treatment of AA and other inflammatory skin diseases.

2. Materials and Methods

2.1. Materials

DEX (Fagron Ibérica, Barcelona, Spain), ethyl cellulose (EC) (Ashaland Industries Europe GmbH, Rheinweg, Switzerland), Tween 80 and Span 60 (Croda Iberica S.A., Spain), benzalkonium chloride (Sigma Aldrich, Madrid, Spain), medium chain triglycerides (MCT) (Oxi-Med Expres S.A., Barcelona, Spain), ethanol absolute (ET) and ethyl acetate (EA) (Scharlab S.L., Barcelona, Spain), and purified water (Inhouse) were used to formulate the LPNCs. Coumarin 6 (C6) (Sigma Aldrich, St. Louis, MO, USA) and 1,2-dioleoyl-3-[16-N-(lissamine rhodamine B sulfonyl) amino]palmitoyl-sn-glycerol (LRB) (Avanti Polar

Lipids, Alabaster, AL, USA) were used as fluorochromes. Paraformaldehyde (Scharlab S.L., Barcelona, Spain), Sucrose (Acor, Valladolid, Spain), optimal cutting temperature compound (OCT) (Tissue-Tek Sakura Finetek, Torrance, CA, USA), rabbit anti-DEX IgG (Abcam, Cambridge, UK), Alexa Fluor 488 goat anti rabbit (Life Technologies, Carlsbad, CA, USA), Prolong™ Gold Antifade mounting medium (Thermo Fisher Scientific, Barcelona, Spain), and Tween 20 (Sigma-Aldrich, St. Louis, MO, USA) were used to prepare samples for microscopic visualization.

2.2. Synthesis of DEX-Loaded LPNCs, Fluorescent-Loaded LPNCs, and Non-Vesiculated Control Solutions

LPNCs were produced by the Emulsion Solvent Evaporation method invented by Fessi et al. [17]. In this method, an organic phase composed of different ratios of EA and ET, EC (2.33%, w/w), MCT (0.2%, w/w), DEX (1%, w/w), and different concentrations of Span 60, were emulsified in an aqueous phase composed of different concentrations of Tween 80 and benzalkonium chloride (preservative). Emulsification was carried out under probe sonication (amplitude of 40%, 5 min; energy, 7000 W; frequency 23.88 kHz) using a UP400st ultrasonic device (Hielscher Ultrasonics, Germany), to reduce the size of the emulsion droplet. After formation of the emulsion, the system evaporated the organic solvents under vacuum in a rotary evaporator, which led to polymer precipitation and lipomer formation. The whole process was performed at room temperature.

A solution of DEX was prepared in a 1% hydroethanolic solution (90:10 v/v, water:ethanol) for use as a non-encapsulated DEX control (FREE-DEX). LRB- and C6-loaded LPNCs (LRB-C6-LPNCs) were manufactured with the same composition as previously described, but without DEX. LRB was added to the lipid nucleus in a mole-to-mole ratio of MCT:LRB of 1:1000, according to Lymberopoulos et al. [18]. In addition, 0.1% w/w C6 was incorporated into the organic phase (EA:ET), simulating the encapsulation of a hydrophobic active ingredient. Fluorochrome control aqueous solutions used in confocal microscopy were prepared with 3% Tween 80 of LRB and C6, at the same concentration as in the LRB-C6-LPNCs, for use as a control for non-vehicle fluorophores (FREE-LRB-C6).

2.3. Screening of Experimental Variables on Nanoparticle Properties

The properties of the lipomers are influenced by different experimental variables, such as the amount of ingredients and manufacturing conditions. Some preliminary screening trials were performed.

Different batches were produced to fix the % w/w of EC and MCT, in order to maximize the loading capacity of DEX in the LPNCs, while maintaining the hydrodynamic diameter below 150 nm and the polydispersity below 0.3. To select the organic solvent, the viscosity of EC was characterized (Brookfield RDV-III Ultra, Spain. Spindler: SC4-21, speed: 100 rpm; temperature: 25 °C) in EA:ET (1:0, 0:1, 1:1, 1:5, and 5:1 v/v) and the mixture with the lowest viscosity was selected.

The samples were subjected to rotary evaporation in a Heidolph VV1 rotary evaporator (Heidolph Instruments, Germany) with a thermostatized bath at 40 °C for 5, 7, 10, and 15 min. The residual concentration of EA and ET was analyzed by gas chromatography (Agilent A7890 with Headspace AG1888, Santa Clara, CA, USA) following European Pharmacopoeia 7.0, chapter 2.4.24 (Identification and control of residual solvents) [19]. Briefly, carrier gas (Helium) flowed at 1.5 mL/min in a column (DB-WAX, 60 m, 0.25 mm, 0.25 μm; Agilent Technologies, USA) for 30 min. The split ratio was 20, the injector Temperature (T^a) was 250 °C, and the detector T^a was 270 °C. The T^a ramp was increased by 10 °C/min.

In order to obtain stable nanoformulations against aggregation, the influences of the surfactant Tween 80 and co-surfactant Span 60 (Table 1) on the Z-potential (mV), nanoparticle hydrodynamic diameter or Z-average (nm), polydispersity index (PDI), and encapsulation efficiency (%EE) were studied. Statistical analysis of the variables studied were carried out using Minitab 17 statistical software (Minitab, Inc., 2010, State College, PA, USA), with the significance level set as α = 0.05.

Table 1. Levels studied for the surfactants.

Factor	Lower Level	Higher Level
% Tween 80 (w/w)	1.5	2.5
% Span 60 (w/w)	0.16	0.32

2.4. LPNCs Physic-Chemical Characterization

The hydrodynamic size, polydispersity index (PDI), and Z-potential were studied for the LPNCs through Dynamic Light Scattering (DLS) using a Malvern Zetasizer Nano ZS (Malvern Panalytical, Malvern, UK). A dilution of 1:10 in milliQ water was performed to adjust the intensity (attenuator position between 3 and 6).

The LPNCs' morphology, size, and distribution were studied using Transmission Electron Microscopy (TEM). The LPNCs' size was also measured using the particle analysis tool of the Image J software. The TEM grids were coated with formvar of a 1:10 dilution of LPNCs in milliQ water and incubated for 1 min at room temperature. The grids were washed with milliQ water and stained with a 2% w/w uranyl acetate solution (Electron Microscopy Sciences, Hatfield, England) during 1 min at room temperature. They were then dried in a petri dish overnight and observed using a TEM microscope (Jeol JEM 1010 100 kv; Jeol, Tokyo, Japan).

2.5. DEX Quantification

DEX was quantified through HPLC, in terms of encapsulation efficiency (%EE), according to an indirect method (Equation (1)):

$$\%EE = \frac{W_T - W_{NE}}{W_T} \times 100, \quad (1)$$

where W_{NE} is the amount of DEX quantified in the filtrate (DEX not encapsulated) and W_T is the DEX quantified in the total formula. The LPNCs were centrifuged in 100 KDa amicon ultra (Merck Millipore, Barcelona, Spain) at 4500 rpm for 30 min. DEX in the filtrate and in LPNCs (total drug content) were analyzed using a High-Performance Liquid Chromatograph (HPLC) Alliance, with a photodiode array detector (PDA). A C18 column (250 × 4.6 mm, 3 μm) was used with an isocratic mixture of acetonitrile:KH$_2$PO$_4$ 0.05 M buffer (60:40) as the mobile phase, with a flow rate of 1.8 mL/min and an injection volume of 20 μL. The sample and column temperatures were 25 °C.

The amount of total drug entrapped per weight of nanoparticle or loading capacity (%LC) was calculated using the following equation:

$$\%LC = \%EE \times \frac{M_{DEX}}{M_{LPNCs}}, \quad (2)$$

where M_{DEX} is the amount of active ingredient initially added to the formulation and M_{LPNCs} is the mass of the nanoparticle components.

2.6. In Vitro Release Tests of the DEX-Loaded LPNCs

In vitro release of DEX from the LPNCs was studied using vertical Franz cells (Vidrafoc, Barcelona, Spain) with a 12 mL receptor compartment and an effective diffusion area of 1.54 cm^2. A mixture of ethanol and purified water (50:50) was used as receptor medium (RM), at 32 °C and stirred at 500 rpm, to keep the sink conditions throughout the experiment. A total of 0.6 g of LPNCs was applied in the donor compartment, corresponding to 60 mg of DEX. The membrane used was a dialysis membrane (Spectrum Chemical, New Brunswick, NJ, USA) with pore diameter of 12–14 kDa.

Aliquots of 300 μL were taken at certain times (1, 2, 3, 4, 5, 21, 22, 23, and 24 h) and injected into the HPLC with the method described in Section 2.5, to quantify the amount of DEX that had diffused through the membrane.

Kinetic modelling of the release data was studied with the DD-solver [20] Excel Add-on, using a non-linear approach. Model selection was based on the lowest Akaike Information Criteria (AIC), reflecting the lowest deviation of the model with respect to the empirical data [21]. Firstly, the mean release values were adjusted to the model described in Table 2, to obtain the mean population behavior. Then, individual data were adjusted, according to the model selected. The mean and standard deviation of the parameters were reported.

Table 2. Different kinetic models and equations tested.

Kinetic Model	Equation
First Order	$F = F_{max}\left(1 - e^{(-K_1 t)}\right)$
Higuchi	$F = K_H \cdot t^{1/2}$
Korsmeyer–Peppas	$F = K_{KP} \cdot t^n$
Weibull	$F = 1 - e^{\left(\frac{-t}{T_d}\right)\beta}$

In Table 2, F is the fraction of active released at time t, F_{max} is the maximum fraction of active released (i.e., at infinite time), K_1 is the first-order constant, K_H is the Higuchi constant, K_{KP} is the Korsmeyer–Peppas constant (related to the structural and geometric character of the drug release matrix), n is the diffusional exponent indicating the drug-release mechanism (if n is less than 0.43, then a Fickian diffusion release mechanism is implied; if n is between 0.43 and 0.85, then the release mechanism follows an anomalous transport mechanism), T_d represents the time at which 63.2% of the drug is released, and β is the Weibull shape parameter. For values of β lower than 0.75, the release follows a Fickian diffusion, either in Euclidian ($0.69 < \beta < 0.75$) or fractal ($\beta < 0.69$) space. Values of β in the range of 0.75–1.0 indicate a combined mechanism, which is frequently encountered in release studies [22,23].

2.7. Pig Skin Permeation

Pig skin was obtained from a local abattoir (Barcelona, Spain) at the moment of sacrifice. Full thickness skin pieces were defatted (with a scalpel) and frozen at $-20\,^\circ$C until use. On the day of the experiment, skin pieces were mounted on Franz cells with an effective diffusion area of 0.196 cm^2 and around 12 mL of receptor volume capacity (PBS at 32 $^\circ$C and stirred at 500 rpm). TEWL measurements were performed, to check the integrity of the skin samples [12] (TEWL Vapometer SWL4549, Delfin Technologies Ltd., Kuopio, Finland). A solution dose of 76 mg of each of the formulations were given in infinite dose in non-occluded conditions.

2.7.1. Confocal Microscopy Biodistribution of Fluorescent Probes

To study the biodistribution of LPNCs in the skin, confocal fluorescence microscopy was used. For this, C6 was encapsulated in the nanoparticles, to simulate the biodistribution of a hydrophobic small molecule, and LRB was used as fluorophore covalently bound to a lipid (palmitic acid) and included in the lipid core of the LPNCs, in order to track the nanoparticles. The labelled LRB-C6-LPNCs were purified using Visking dialysis tubing with a cut-off of 12,000–14,000 Dalton. The non-encapsulated fraction of both fluorophores was quantified by spectrophotometry (VICTOR Multilabel Plate Reader, Perkinelmer, Massachusetts, USA) and the %EE was calculated following Equation (1).

Full thickness pieces of pig skin were warmed and placed in Franz cells, according to Section 2.7. After 18 h of permeation, the diffusion surface was washed with PBS, cut with a scalpel into pieces of about 0.5 cm^2, and fixed in 4% w/w paraformaldehyde solution for 5 min. Then, the skin samples were incubated in aqueous solutions of increasing sucrose concentration (5%, 15%, and 25% w/w) for 15 min in each solution. They were then placed in plastic molds and dipped in OCT to cut on a cryostat Leica CM 3050 S (Leica Biosystems, Barcelona, Spain) to a 50 µm thickness. The slices were collected on poly-lysine-coated slides and washed with PBS and 0.05% Tween 20 (TPBS) for 5 min, to remove the OCT and permeabilize the samples. On the day of observation, sections were incubated with 15 µL of Hoescht solution (2 µg/mL) for 10 min and washed with TPBS to stain the cell nuclei. The samples were analyzed under a confocal microscope (Leica Microsystems, Wetzlar, Germany). The emission laser wavelengths were 570, 500, and 525 nm and the excitation wavelengths were 561, 488, and 405 nm for LRB, C6, and Hoescht, respectively. About 20 planes were obtained per image, separated by a 3 µm step. Composites of the different planes were created, in terms of the brightest point for each pixel, through the ImageJ tool Z-stack (ImageJ2 v2.35, National Institutes of Health, Bethesda, MD, USA). A skin blank was processed in the same way as the test samples, to quantify skin autofluorescence. The mean intensity was measured with the ImageJ software and was subtracted from the intensity of the red and green channels of the samples.

2.7.2. Immunohistofluorescence Biodistribution

To study the biodistribution of the DEX carried in the LPNCs, immunohistofluorescence (IHF) experiments were carried out. Permeation and skin slices were carried out in the same way as in Section 2.7.1, but the slices were 10 µm thick. Then, 15 µL of a 1/300 dilution of the rabbit polyclonal primary anti-DEX IgG were added, and the samples were left to incubate in a humid environment overnight at 4 °C. Then, the samples were washed with TPBS and incubated with a 1/300 diluted fluorescent secondary goat anti-rabbit IgG Alexa 488 for 2 h under the same incubation conditions. Finally, ProLong Gold Antifade mounting medium was added. The samples were analyzed under a fluorescent field effect microscope. A L5 Leica filter cube was used, and the filters were BP480/40, BS505 for excitation, and BP 527/30 for emission. To study the possible non-specific interactions of the skin, the same process was carried out with non-treated skin samples and processed in the same way as test samples. The resultant intensity was subtracted from the profiles of the samples using the ImageJ software.

2.8. In Vitro Cytotoxicity/Anti-TNFα Efficacy

Cell culture: The HEK001 cell line was obtained from ATCC (Promochem Partnership, Manassas, VA, USA). HEK001 was grown in monolayer on a solid support, at 37 °C in a humidified atmosphere with 5% CO_2 and maintained in keratinocyte serum-free media supplemented with 100 µg/mL epidermal growth factor (EGF) (Life Technologies, Carlsbad, CA, USA), 20 U/mL penicillin, and 20 µg/mL streptomycin (Life Technologies). Mycoplasma-free maintenance was confirmed every two weeks by PCR amplification.

Cell treatments: For the cell viability assays, HEK001 cells were seeded at a density of 5000 cells/well in 96-well culture plates. At 24 h post-seeding, cells were treated with increasing doses of DEX-charged LPNCs, non-charged LPNCs, or the corresponding amount of benzalkonium chloride for 24 h. After 48 h, cell viability was assessed using an MTT (3-[4,5-dimethylthiazol-2-yl]-2,5 diphenyl tetrazolium bromide) colorimetric assay (Sigma-Aldrich, St. Louis, MO, USA). Cell survival for all experiments was expressed as the percentage of viable cells, relative to that in untreated cells (defined as 100%). For the cytokine modulation assays, HEK001 cells were seeded at a density of 700,000 cells/well in 6-well culture plates. At 24 h post-seeding, cells were pre-treated with 10 µg/mL of lipopolysaccharide (LPS) for 1 h and then treated with 0.1 mM of DEX or DEX-loaded LPNCs for 24 h.

RNA isolation and RT-PCR: Total RNA was isolated from cultured cells using the SV Total RNA Isolation System (Promega, Madison, WI, USA), following the manufacturer's instructions. A total of 1 µg of RNA was reverse transcribed to cDNA with M-MLV Reverse Transcriptase (Life Technologies) and random hexamers (Life Technologies). Analyses of the TNFα and GAPDH (endogenous control) mRNA levels were performed by RT-PCR, using commercial TaqMan gene expression assays (Applied Biosystems). Relative quantification of gene expression was assessed using the $\Delta\Delta CT$ method, as described in the TaqMan user manual (User Bulletin no. 2; Applied Biosystems). Gene expression levels for TNFα were normalized to the GAPDH gene. The amounts of mRNA are expressed as arbitrary units.

Statistical analysis: Results from the cell viability and cytokine modulation were statistically analyzed by using GraphPad Prism (8.0.2, 2019, La Jolla, San Diego, CA, USA), with Student's paired t test for cytotoxicity assays and two-way ANOVA for cytokine modulation assays. In all cases, differences were considered significant when the p-value < 0.05.

3. Results and Discussion
3.1. Screening of Experimental Variables on Nanoparticle Properties

The pharmaceutical interest of cellulose derivatives has increased in recent years, due to economic factors (usually due to the low-cost of the excipients, compared with synthetic compounds) and as they originate from renewable resources [24]. EC was selected as the LPNC polymer, as it has been approved by the Food and Drug Administration (FDA) for medical and food applications (i.e., vitamin and mineral tablets), and it has shown good biocompatibility in ocular drug delivery systems [25–27]. Furthermore, EC is cheaper than other commonly used polymers, such as PLGA or polycaprolactone. EC is commonly used in the pharmaceutical industry as a coating material for different drug delivery applications, due to its controlled release properties caused by the porous structure, where the drugs can be trapped and diffuse [24].

The choice of organic phase is a parameter to consider, in terms of toxicity. Chloroform and dichloromethane are organic solvents that are commonly used in the Emulsion Solvent Evaporation method; however, due to their toxicity, it is advisable to avoid them when possible. In this case, ethyl acetate and ethanol were selected, as they have been classified as class III (or low toxic potential) solvents by the European Medicines Agency (EMA) [28]. In the Emulsion Solvent Evaporation method, the viscosity of the organic phase influences the diffusion to the aqueous phase. An organic phase that is too viscous will not diffuse adequately, forming large aggregates that cannot be stabilized in the final formulation. This may be attributed to the increase in viscosity of the dispersed phase, resulting in a reduction of the net shear stress and prompting bigger nanodroplets. The ratio between the continuous and dispersed phases is also an important factor: In the solvent evaporation emulsion method, a high proportion of dispersed phase causes an increase in the size of the nanoparticles, due to the increase in droplet size. Furthermore, due to the hydrophobic nature of DEX, the burst effect would increase, and the encapsulation efficiency would decrease. To avoid this problem, dilutions of EC were made in different binary mixtures of ethanol and ethyl acetate and the viscosities of the different organic phases were characterized. The LPNCs were designed with MCT as the oil core, to increase the %EE and reduce the DEX burst release effect. Benzalkonium chloride was incorporated as a preservative.

Table 3 shows the viscosity results for the different binary mixtures of ethyl acetate (EA) and ethanol (ET) with EC at 2% w/w. The 1:1 and 5:1 ratios were selected as optimal, as they showed the lowest viscosity values. This means a decrease in the viscous forces resisting droplet breakdown and, thus, smaller oil droplets were formed, resulting in a decreased particle size. When LPNCs were produced at the 1:1 ratio, aggregates were observed; so, finally the 5:1 EA:ET ratio was selected as definitive, as it did not show aggregates and obtained low viscosity. To increase the loading capacity of the LPNCs, the EC concentration was increased to the maximum concentration possible to obtain LPNCs with adequate properties, in term of size and PDI [29]. The final EC concentration was fixed at 2.33% w/w in the organic phase (0.35% w/w in the final formulation) and the MCT concentration was set at 0.2% w/w, since at higher concentrations aggregates began to appear.

The stability of LPNCs is directly related to their size, PDI, and Z-potential. Surfactants have an important role in these characteristics and, so, the effect of surfactant concentration on the physicochemical properties of LPNCs was studied. As in any colloidal suspension, lipomers can undergo destabilization processes, such as Ostwald ripening. This process can be avoided by steric stabilization using Tween 80 [30]. Due to its HLB (14.9), Tween 80 acts as a stabilizer of the aqueous phase, coating the surfaces of the LPNCs and preventing their aggregation. Due to the more lipophilic nature of Span 60 (HLB 4.7), it becomes dispersed in the LPNC core when MCT is used [31]. In this case, the percentages of Tween 80 and Span 60 were modified between 1.5% and 2.5% w/w and 0.16% and 0.32% w/w, respectively. As it can be seen from Table 4, four batches were produced and the Z-average, PDI, Z-potential, and %EE were characterized for each of them.

Table 3. Organic phase ethyl cellulose (EC) mixture viscosities.

EA:ET Ratio	Viscosity (cP)
1:1	16
5:1	20.5
1:5	24
1:0	70.5
0:1	25

Table 4. Influence of Span 60 and Tween 80 on the physicochemical parameters.

Batch	% Tween 80	% Span 60	Z-Average (nm)	PDI	Z-Potential (mV)	% EE
LP01	2.5	0.32	117.6 ± 1.2	0.263 ± 0.005	21.7	96.76
LP02	1.5	0.32	130.5 ± 1.1	0.215 ± 0.011	27.2	96.68
LP03	1.5	0.16	114.1 ± 1.1	0.239 ± 0.002	29.1	96.93
LP04	2.5	0.16	125.9 ± 0.5	0.256 ± 0.006	23.5	98.32

A general linear model regression using the Minitab software was performed (with a significance level of $\alpha = 0.05$) to evaluate the effect of the tested experimental variables. The levels of Tween 80 and Span 60 were not significant for the hydrodynamic diameter, the PDI, or for the %EE, but they were significant for the Z-potential ($p = 0.006$ and $p = 0.017$, respectively). In Figure 1, the effects of these surfactants on the surface charge of the LPNCs can be observed. By increasing the amount of surfactant, the positive charge was reduced, as the hydroxyl groups of Tween 80 and Span 60 shielded the positive charge of the nanoparticles.

Thus, formulation LP03 was selected as the final formulation, with lower levels of both surfactants (1.5% w/w of Tween 80 and 0.16% w/w of Span 60). The %LC of batch LP03 was calculated following Equation (2), which resulted in 30.22%, thus confirming the high loading capacity of this type of nanoencapsulation system [5] compared to other drug delivery systems like liposomes, in which Amin et al. reached an LC of 12.6% [16].

Table 5 shows the residual EA and ET found after the evaporation process. EA has a vapor pressure at 25 °C of 1.23 atm, which is higher than the vapor pressure of ethanol at the same temperature (0.08 atm). Due to the higher volatility of EA than ET, after 5 min of rotary evaporation at 40 °C, the residual quantity was already below the limit of quantification (LOQ). Regarding ethanol, with the mildest evaporation conditions, more residues were found, but they were well below the limit established for residual solvents of class 3 (5000 ppm) in the guideline for residual solvents (ICH Q3C) of the European Medicines Agency. Thus, the evaporation conditions were fixed at 5 min and 40 °C.

Table 5. Residual solvents after evaporation at 40 °C.

Evaporation Time (min)	Residual EA (ppm)	Residual ET (ppm)
5	<LOQ	153.0 ± 10.0
7	<LOQ	34.4 ± 4.5
10	<LOQ	12.5 ± 2.3
15	<LOQ	1.5 ± 0.0

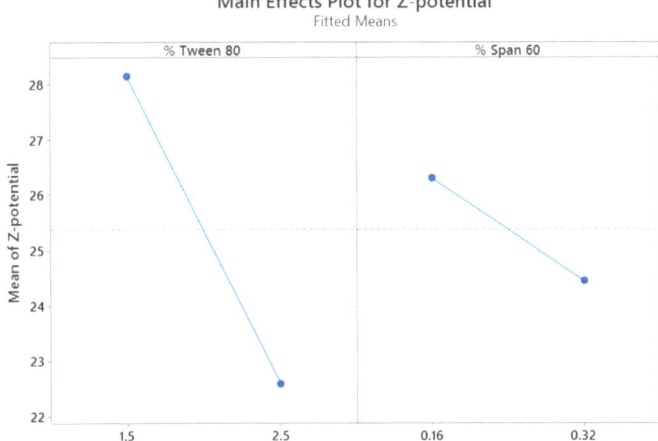

Figure 1. Plots of the main effects of Tween 80 and Span 60 on the Z-potential of the lipid core polymeric nanocapsules (LPNCs).

3.2. Physicochemical Characterization of the LPNCs

Thanks to the high resolution of the TEM images (Figure 2), it is possible to appreciate the lipid nucleus (brighter area) and distinguish it from the polymeric framework (darker area), as can be observed in Figure 2C. Furthermore, the spherical morphology was confirmed. A total of 180 particles were analyzed and a mean size of 126.40 ± 34.93 nm was obtained.

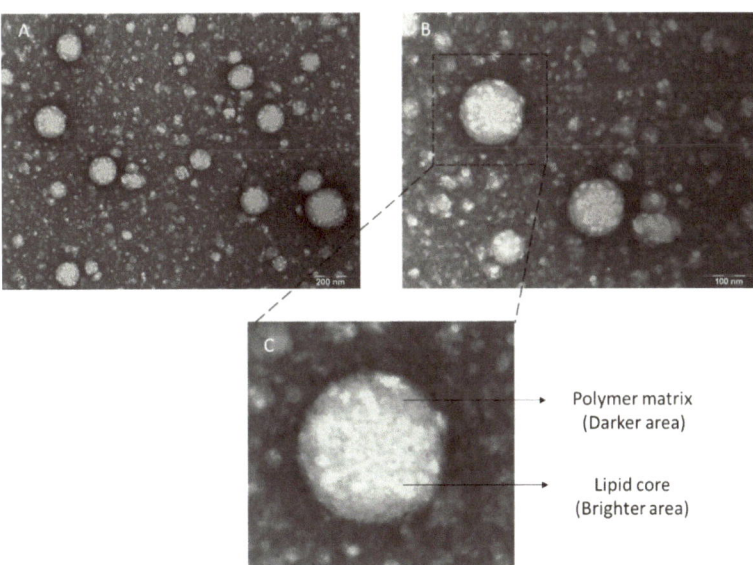

Figure 2. Transmission Electron Microscopy (TEM) images of negative-stained lipid–polymer hybrid LPNCs with 2% uranyl acetate at (**a**) 250,000× magnification; and (**b**) 300,000× magnification. (c) Individual nanoparticle representation zoom.

The diameter distribution of the particles, as measured by TEM, is shown in Figure 3 as a histogram. The average obtained was similar using both TEM and DLS techniques and the %BIAS error for the diameter was 10.78%, which is low.

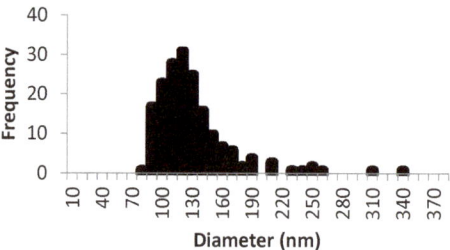

Figure 3. Histogram of lipomers from the measurement of the diameter of the particles (n = 180) using ImageJ software.

3.3. In Vitro Release Test of DEX-Loaded LPNCs and Free DEX

The release data of the free DEX and LPNCs can be seen in Figure 4. After 24 h, the DEX formulated in an ethanolic solution (FREE-DEX) was released at 100%, while the release of DEX loaded in LPNCs (LPNCs-DEX) was more sustained, due to diffusion through the polymeric framework and the affinity of the active for the lipid cores of the particles.

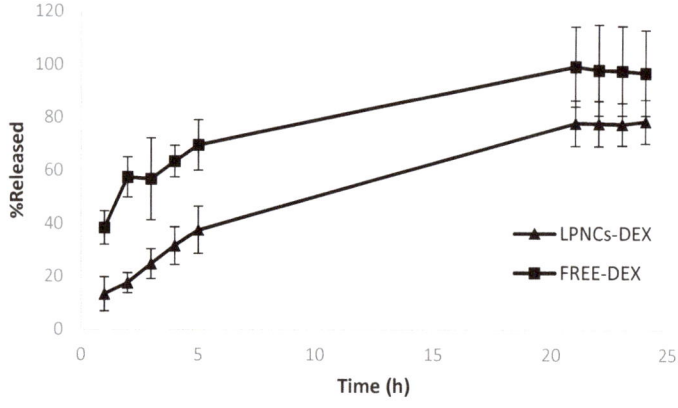

Figure 4. Mean release data obtained from the DEX-loaded LPNCs and from the ethanolic solution of DEX (FREE-DEX) after 24 h of the in vitro release test.

After adjusting the mean release data with the different mathematical models (see Table 6), it was observed that Weibull was the model that best fit (AIC 28.81) the experimental data in the case of LPNCs, and Korsmeyer–Peppas was the model that best fit (AIC 44.86) in the case of DEX formulated in a hydroalcoholic solution.

Once the mean release kinetic behavior was determined, the mean and standard deviation of the individual release data for free DEX and LPNCs-DEX were obtained, as reported in Table 7.

Although the Weibull equation is a non-mechanistic equation, Papadopoulou et al. [22] obtained a relationship between the shape parameter β and the release mechanism, in the same way as the power law equation (Korsmeyer–Peppas equation) does with the exponent n. In the case of LPNCs-DEX, the value of β was between 0.75 and 1, which corresponds to a combined release mechanism; that is, diffusion in a normal Euclidean substrate with the contribution of another release mechanism. This fact was confirmed by the n value (0.573) found for LPNCs reported in Table 6, corresponding to anomalous transport or a combined mechanism. Due to the hybrid nature of these nanoparticles, the active ingredient could be distributed both in the lipid core and the polymeric framework, resulting in an overlap of both release kinetics, such that anomalous transport would be observed. In the case of FREE-DEX, this study was below the limits set in the Korsmeyer–Peppas model (i.e., 0.43). However, Singhvi and Singh [32] reported that, although the value of n obtained was not in the range suggested in Korsmeyer–Peppas model, it also indicates a diffusion-controlled drug release mechanism. This fact could be confirmed by the Weibull model, which had an AIC value close to that of Korsmeyer–Peppas, where the β value for FREE-DEX was 0.698 (i.e., between 0.69 and 0.75), which would indicate the release as a normal diffusion mechanism dominated by the concentration difference without the contribution of other release mechanisms, unlike the case of LPNCs.

Table 6. Model selection and parameter estimation of the LPNCs-DEX and FREE-DEX. Bold type indicates the selected model, based on the lowest AIC.

Formulation	Model	AIC	Parameters	Value
LPNCs-DEX	First order	31.84	k (h^{-1})	0.128
	Higuchi	39.98	k_H (%$h^{-1/2}$)	16.263
	Korsmeyer–Peppas	39.13	k_{KP} (%h^{-n})	7.91
			n	0.573
	Weibull	**28.81**	T_d (h)	**13.49**
			β	**0.79**
FREE-DEX	First-order	68.51	k (h^{-1})	0.192
			Fmax (%)	104.35
	Higuchi	71.60	k_H (%$h^{-1/2}$)	22.475
	Korsmeyer–Peppas	**44.86**	k_{KP} (%h^{-n})	**42.78**
			n	**0.271**
	Weibull	47.43	β	0.698
			Td (h)	3.21

Table 7. Individual modelling and parameters for the LPNCs and FREE DEX release data.

Formulation	Model	Parameters	Value
LPNCs-DEX	Weibull	β	0.82 ± 0.17
		T_d (h)	14.16 ± 4.11
FREE-DEX	Korsmeyer–Peppas	k_{KP} (%h^{-n})	42.39 ± 5.96
		n	0.278 ± 0.034

3.4. Confocal Microscopy Biodistribution of Fluorescent Probes

After the permeation experiment, skin was observed under a confocal microscope, to evaluate the skin distribution of both fluorochromes. The literature has described a high number of fluorochromes that are included in nanoparticles for localization in the skin. Usually, the selection of the tracking compound is based on the aim of the experiment. In this case, C6 was selected as the drug model and LRD to track the nanocapsules. According to the structure of LRD, the hydrocarbon tail would be inside the lipid core and the rhodamine head would likely be located in the polymer shell or in the interphase lipid–polymer in the nanoparticle structure, as with Span 60. To improve visualization, cell nuclei were stained with Hoechst (blue color). The results obtained from the confocal biodistribution study are shown in Figure 5. The autofluorescence value in the red channel (corresponding to LRD) was 5.9 AU and that of the green channel (corresponding to C6) was 0.3 AU. These values were subtracted from the mean intensity of the samples. Using ImageJ software, linear segments were drawn to analyze the intensity profile as a function of depth (in μm). Yellow color corresponds to the co-localization of both fluorochromes.

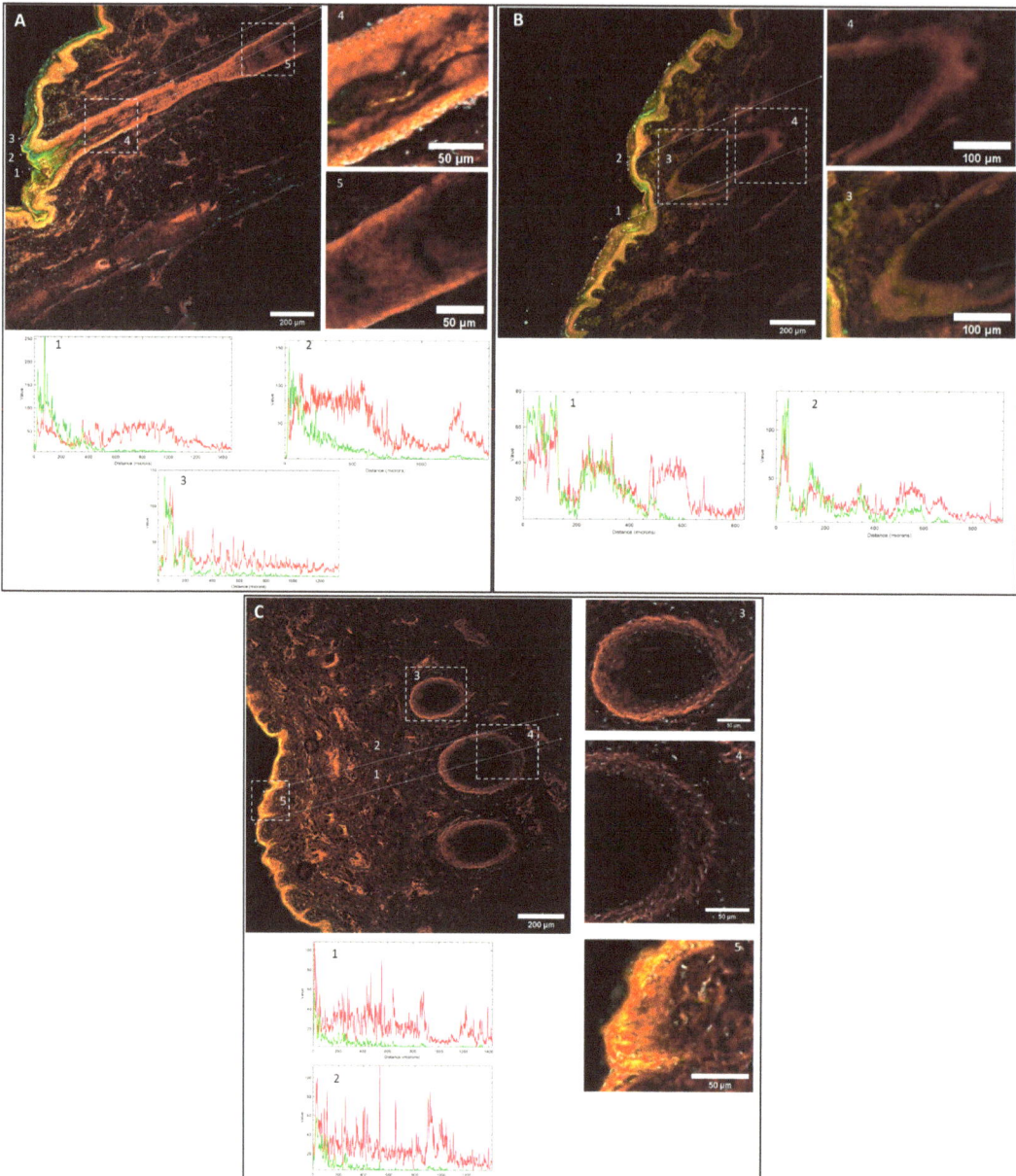

Figure 5. Confocal Microscopy Fluorescence images and plot intensity profiles of pig skin cross-sections. Green color corresponds to C6 and red to LRB fluorescence. Yellow color corresponds to the overlap of C6 and LRB: (**A**,**B**) C6-loaded LRB-labelled LPNCs. (**C**) Free C6 and LRB control solution. Lines numbered 1–3 in Figure 5A; 1–2 in Figure 5B and 1–2 in Figure 5C correspond to Multichannel intensity plot profiles as function of the depth (μm). Dashed squares numbered 4–5 in Figure 5A, 3–4 in Figure 5B and 3–4 in Figure 5C correspond to zoomed in regions. The images were captured using 10× magnification.

Figure 5A,B show the biodistribution patterns of the C6 and LRB fluorophores vehiculated in LPNCs (C6-LRB-LPNCs).

In Figure 5A, three lines are drawn from the stratum corneum to deeper layers of the skin. Line 1 corresponds to the central section of the hair follicle, line 2 corresponds to the follicle edge (outer root sheath area), and line 3 corresponds to a non-follicle section. In the central section (line 1), the intensity of C6 is between 100 and 200 AU in the infundibulum (depth < 100 µm). At depths of 200 µm, the intensity of C6 drops to 50 AU and, as the depth increases, the intensity of the green channel continues to decrease, to about 20 AU at 400 µm (corresponding to the hair follicle isthmus). Beyond 500 µm, in depth (i.e., in the suprabulbar region), the intensity of C6 was low (<10AU), which seems to indicate that C6 does not accumulate in the deeper parts of the follicle. Regarding the intensity in the red color, corresponding to the presence of LRB, a different behavior can be observed. The profile of the center of the follicle (Figure 5A, Line 1) shows an intensity value around 50 AU from the skin surface to 700–800 µm deep. The profile of the border of the follicle (Figure 5A, Line 2) shows a similar profile, with the intensity of the LRB up to 700 µm being around 65 AU. Due to the narrowing of the follicle, the line is outside the follicle, around 1000 µm; however, near the follicle sheath (1200 µm), it can be seen that the intensity of the LRB was around 50 AU. In the non-follicle area (Figure 5A, Line 3), the C6 intensity profile was high to 200 µm in depth, but then decreased quickly, suggesting the accumulation of C6 in the epidermis. It can also be seen that the intensity of LRB outside the follicle at depths greater than 200 µm was clearly lower than that of the follicle lines. In the epidermis, a yellow color can be observed, corresponding to the co-localization of both fluorochromes in this region. In other words, LRB had accumulated throughout the follicle at depths greater than C6.

In Figure 5B, corresponding to another skin section of the permeation with C6-LRB-LPNCs, a section of the hair follicle can be seen. In this case, the section is not longitudinal but a cross-section. The intensity profiles of the different skin annexes and hair follicles followed the same biodistribution for both fluorophores as previously discussed. Accumulation of C6 and LRB was seen up to about 400–500 µm deep. At deeper follicle depths, only LRB accumulation was observed.

Different magnifications were made on sections of the hair follicle, in order to highlight the fluorochrome distribution in the infundibulum (Figure 5A, zoom 4) and in the isthmus area (Figure 5A, zoom 5). In the zooms of Figure 5B, zoom 3 and zoom 4 highlight the transversal hair follicle section with the different fluorochrome distribution previously described.

In Figure 5C, the zoom after permeation of the FREE-C6-LRB control solution can be observed. In this case, the observed biodistribution was different. As they were not delivered in nanoparticles, the fluorophores did not accumulate in the hair follicles. As can be seen in the profiles of lines 1 and 2 of Figure 5C, the intensity of C6 was around 20 AU in the epidermis and decayed at depths greater than 100 µm. The LRB intensity was around 20 AU throughout the entire zoom where you can see the dermis, as well as the hair follicle cross-section.

In addition, when analyzing zooms 3 and 4 of Figure 5C, it can be observed that the intensity of the yellow color in the follicles is almost non-existent, due to the non-accumulation of C6 in the hair follicle. In zoom 5 of Figure 5C, the accumulation of C6 and LRB in the epidermis of a superficial invagination (<100 µm) can be seen.

These results explain the biodistribution of these two hydrophobic fluorophores carried in the LPNCs. The intensity of the green color, corresponding to the accumulation of C6, was greater in the epidermis and in the upper part of the hair follicle, and decreased with increasing depth in the skin. The images obtained by confocal microscopy seem to indicate that the in vitro skin penetration by C6 in the LPNCs accumulated on the epidermis and the hair follicle infundibulum, but did not penetrate into the deepest parts of hair follicles. This fact suggests that C6 is released when it comes into contact with the stratum corneum lipids, due to its hydrophobic nature, leading to greater accumulation in less deep areas.

The intensity in red color, corresponding to LRB, was less than that of C6 in the epidermis but greater than that of C6 when analyzing the profile deeper into the hair follicle. The fact that an accumulation of LRB was observed at these depths suggests that this fluorophore is found in the lipid nucleus of the nanoparticles and travels with them towards the bulb of the follicle. As described in the literature, ethyl cellulose polymer nanoparticles accumulate in skin annexes, due to their geometry and size, and can deliver small molecules to hair follicles through the transfollicular route, limiting distribution to the rest of the skin and to systemic circulation [33].

3.5. Immunohistofluorescence Biodistribution

Confocal laser microscopy is usually employed to study the biodistribution of nanoparticles in different tissues; unfortunately, this is an indirect measurement, as there is no direct tracking of the API. There exist other techniques to study topical biodistribution, such as skin layer separation [34], cyanoacrylate tape-stripping [35], or dermatopharmacokinetics [36]. Techniques such as cyanoacrylate-stripping allow to study hair follicle targeting but usually have a lower spatial resolution than IHF and could have problems, such as analytical interferences, quantification limit issues, lack of complete recovery, or matrix effects. By means of the IHF, it is possible to visualize if there is accumulation in the different anatomical regions of the hair follicle.

Due to this and to confirm the data obtained in the previous section, an IHF experiment was carried out. Rabbit anti-DEX IgG and Alexa Fluor 488 goat anti-rabbit were employed, such that direct visualization of the drug could be performed.

After the IHQ experiment, a different behavior was observed, with respect to the DEX-FREE (Figure 6C,D) and LPNCs-vehiculated DEX (Figure 6A,B). The visualization filter used in ImageJ was Green Fire Blue, where the blue color corresponds to the lowest intensity and the yellow-green color to the highest intensity. Figure 6B shows a longitudinal section of the hair follicle. In panels A, C, and D of Figure 6, cross-sections of the hair follicles are observed. Surface plots were obtained, in order to compare the intensity in a more visual way.

In the same way as in Section 3.6, different lines were drawn to compare the intensity profiles. Line 1 in Figure 6A corresponds to the intensity across the lateral zone of a hair follicle. In this case, an accumulation of DEX was seen (intensity around 140 AU at 500 µM depth). Line 2 corresponds to permeation outside the follicle, for which it was observed that DEX remained restricted to the epidermis and its invaginations, with an intensity of 60 AU. In Figure 6B, three lines are drawn. Lines 1 and 2 correspond to the central zone and the outer sheath of the follicle, respectively. Although the maximum intensity (approximately 100 AU) was observed at around 250 µm, DEX accumulation went to 700 µm, corresponding to the hair follicle bulb (Figure 6B, Zoom 1 and 2). Line 3 corresponds to an area outside the follicle; in this case, the intensity dropped to 25 AU when entering beyond 100 µm and, again, it was observed that DEX remained restricted to the area of the epidermis and stratum corneum. The intensity along the follicle remained around 40 AU—almost double compared to outside the follicle. Surface plots of both images were also made, to obtain a visual image of the accumulation of DEX. It is clear that accumulation in hair follicles has occurred.

Regarding the permeation of FREE-DEX, the behavior was different. Lines 1 and 2 of Figure 6C,D are very similar and show that DEX did not accumulate in hair follicles when it was formulated in this solution. Beyond 50 µm in depth (epidermis), the intensity was low (about 20 AU). This behavior is shown in the surface plots in Figure 6C Zoom 3 and Figure 6D Zoom 3, where FREE-DEX did not accumulate in follicles, only in the stratum corneum and part of the epidermis.

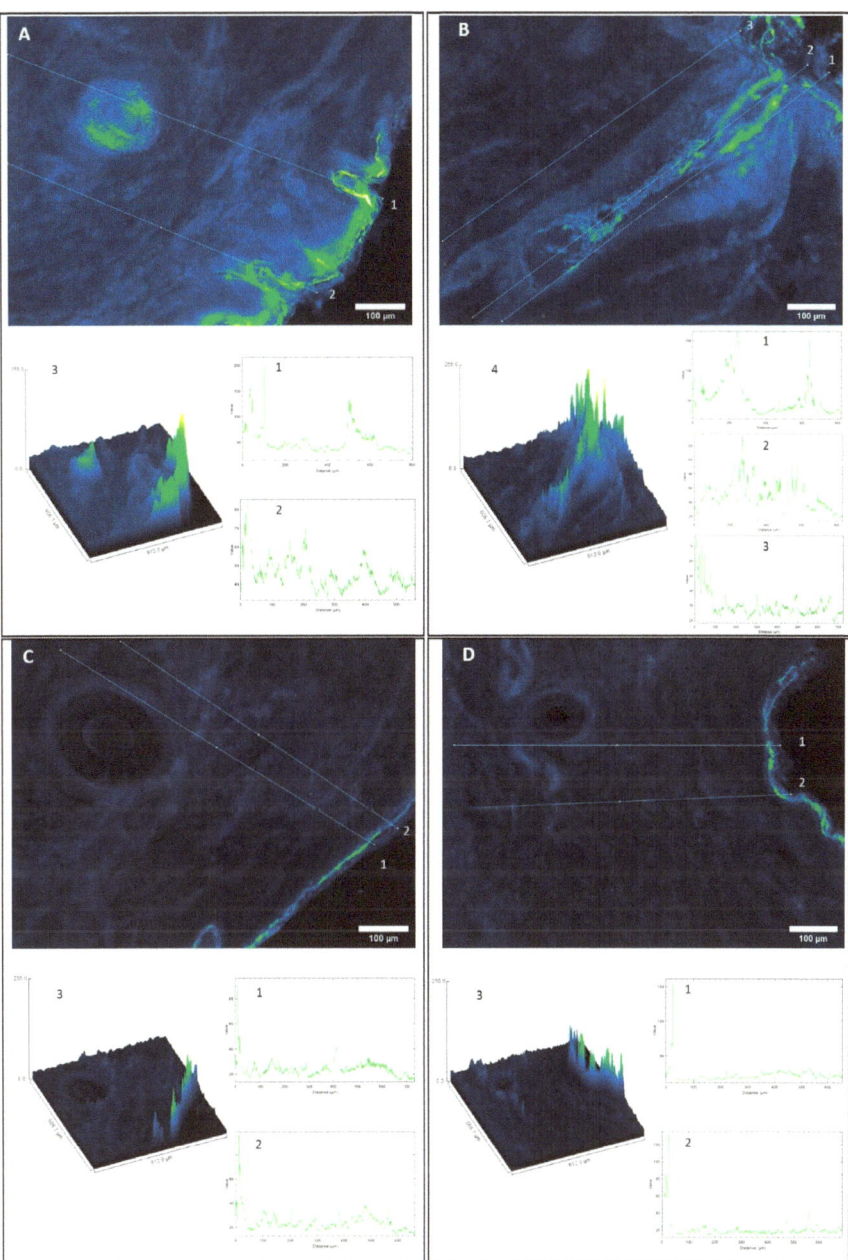

Figure 6. IHF images of a pig skin cross-section. Green color corresponds to high intensity and blue to lower intensity fluorescence of Alexa 488 secondary antibody (Ab)–Primary Ab–DEX complex: (**A**,**B**) DEX-loaded LPNCs; (**C**,**D**) hydroalcoholic DEX control solution. Figure 6A 1–2, Figure 6B 1–3, Figure 6C 1–2 and Figure 6D 1–2 correspond to green intensity plot profiles as function of the depth (µm). Figure 6A 3, Figure 6B 4, Figure 6C 3 and Figure 6D 3 correspond to surface plots. The images were captured using 10× magnifications and the Lookup Table (LUT) used to show the pictures was Green Fire Blue.

When comparing these results with those obtained by confocal microscopy, it can be observed that the biodistribution of DEX was similar to that of LRB, as it accumulated in the deep areas of the follicles (>400 µm). These results corroborate the high encapsulation efficiency results and suggest that it is possible to achieve a controlled and sustained release in the hair follicle by encapsulation in LPNCs. As a result, a depot effect in the pilosebaceous unit is expected. This effect could, on the one hand, reduce the frequency of administration (from the 12 h usually used in topical corticosteroids to 24 h) and then could reduce the associated adverse effects. On the other hand, a depot effect and the release of the drug in the site of action would improve the treatment efficacy and reduce or avoid the systemic or intralesional administration of the drug, reducing the systemic adverse effects (which are usually worse than the adverse effects of topical administration) and patient discomfort caused by injections (in the intralesional therapy). These facts should be evaluated in future clinical trials.

3.6. Cytotoxicity and Anti-TNFα Efficacy

Human-transformed keratinocytes (HEK001 cells) were chosen to assess the DEX-LPNC cytotoxicity (Figure 7A). Non-loaded LPNCs, benzalkonium chloride, and untreated cells were tested as controls. For loaded LPNCs, the inverse dilution factors (5000, 25,000, 50,000, 100,000, and 250,000) corresponded to the respective concentrations of 5, 1, 0.5, 0.25, and 0.1 µM of DEX. For benzalkonium chloride, proper concentrations were 1, 0.2, 0.1, 0.05, and 0.02 µM. The cell viability profiles of the tested compounds exhibited a similar pattern: there was a viability reduction, compared to untreated cells, at higher concentrations of loaded and non-loaded LPNCs. To ascertain the reason for this toxicity, pure benzalkonium chloride was evaluated with the same dilution scheme as the LPNCs, demonstrating that the reason for the viability reduction was caused by the preservative. Although this fact was observed, there exist different commercial products that use the same preservative for the topical route, as described in the FDA inactive ingredients data base [37], demonstrating the suitability of the selected preservative system.

To evaluate the in vitro anti-inflammatory efficacy of the LPNCs, TNFα was selected as a tracker, as it is usually involved in most inflammatory alterations of the skin, particularly in AA [38]. Furthermore, in many cases, it has been identified as a promising target for pharmacological modulation [39]. Figure 7B shows the TNFα expression in HEK001 cells after treatment with DEX-LPNCs and FREE-DEX for 24 h after pre-treatment with 10 µg/mL of LPS to induce inflammation. LPNCs were tested at a DEX level equivalent to 0.1 µM, as the cell viability was not reduced at this concentration level. FREE-DEX at the same concentration level was used as control. A significant reduction in TNFα can be seen in both cases. The lower efficacy of the lipomers, compared with the solution, could be caused by the differential release pattern observed in Figure 4: at 24 h, the amount of DEX released from the lipomers was around 75%, compared with 100% in the solution. Similarly, the difference between the FREE-DEX and lipomers was about 27%, such that the drug release limited the anti-TNFα efficacy. This difference is not expected to appear in real applications, considering that the LPNCs have accumulated in hair follicles and, so, a depot effect would appear (not evaluated in cell culture), such that the slow degradation of the lipomers in the follicle would release the drug into the surrounding and deeper area. After multiple administrations, an increased exposition of DEX would take place, compared with the free drug.

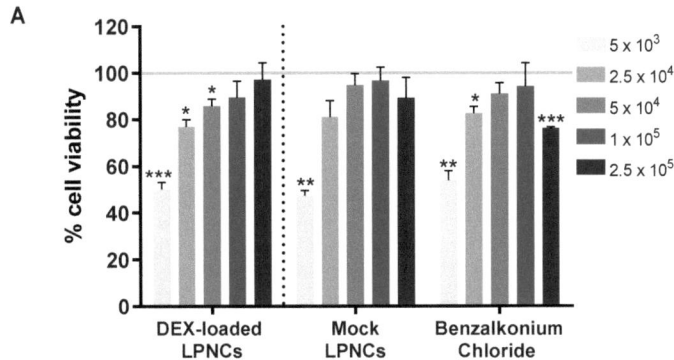

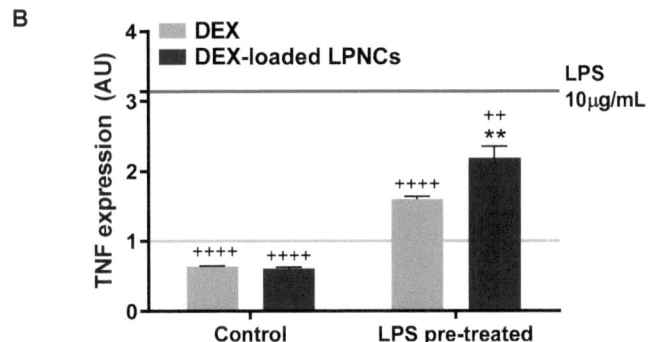

Figure 7. In vitro cell culture studies: (**A**) HEK001 cell viability with MTT assay. The indicated numbers represent the inverse dilution factors, referring to the composition of synthetized LPNCs. For DEX-loaded LPNCs, the dilution factors correspond to the concentrations of 5, 1, 0.5, 0.25, and 0.1 µM of DEX. For benzalkonium chloride, proper concentrations were 1, 0.2, 0.1, 0.05, and 0.02 µM. Data are represented as the mean ± SEM ($n = 3$) of the cell viability percentage, referring to untreated controls (horizontal lane). Statistical significance was assessed by Student's paired t-test; * $p < 0.05$; ** $p < 0.01$; *** $p < 0.005$. (**B**) TNFα mRNA expression was measured after treating cells for 24 h with 0.1 µM of either free dexamethasone (grey) or DEX-loaded LPNCs (dark gray), without (left) or with (right) a 1-h pre-treatment with LPS (10 µg/mL). TNFα expression is represented as the mean ± SEM ($n = 3$); TNFα expression at control and LPS treatment conditions is indicated with horizontal pink and red lanes, respectively. Statistical significance was evaluated by one-way ANOVA compared to the control (*) or LPS (+); ** $p < 0.01$, ++ $p < 0.01$, ++++ $p < 0.001$.

4. Conclusions

LPNCs with a high carrying capacity were successfully developed for the active dexamethasone. When studying the biodistribution of the nanoparticles using confocal microscopy, accumulation in hair follicles and cutaneous annexes was observed, thus proving their ability to achieve follicular targeting. These results were confirmed for DEX biodistribution by immunofluorescence, where DEX-LPNCs demonstrated an increase in accumulation in hair follicles, compared to FREE-DEX. The cytotoxicity of the particles was studied, where toxicity (caused by the preservative, benzalkonium chloride) was observed only at high doses. The anti-inflammatory efficacy of DEX-LPNCs, with TNFα as a tracker, was demonstrated. Its high %LC and %EE, good physicochemical properties (size of 115 nm, low polydispersity, and Z-potential of +30 mV), sustained in vitro release profile, localized release in hair follicles, and anti-inflammatory efficacy make this nanoformulation a very interesting candidate to improve the efficacy and reduce the adverse effects of corticosteroids for diseases in which there is inflammation in the hair follicles, such as alopecia areata. Thanks to the follicular targeting obtained, it could be possible to have a depot effect within the pilosebaceous unit, which could allow us to reduce the frequency of administration compared to classical formulations. The safety and efficacy profiles of the DEX-lipomers should be verified in clinical trials to compare side effects.

Author Contributions: Conceptualization, F.F.-C. and E.P.-R.; methodology, F.F.-C., E.P.-R. and S.P.-T.; software, E.P.-R. and A.M.-V.; validation, E.P.-R., F.F.-C.; formal analysis, E.P.-R., A.M.-V. and M.L.-R.; investigation, E.P.-R. and F.F.-C.; resources, F.F.-C. and S.P.-T.; data curation, E.P.-R., F.F.-C.; writing—original draft preparation, E.P.-R.; writing—review and editing, E.P.-R., F.F.-C., A.M.-V., S.P.-T. and M.L.-R.; visualization E.P.-R., F.F.-C., A.M.-V., S.P.-T. and M.L.-R.; supervision, F.F.-C. and S.P.-T.; project administration, E.P.-R. and F.F.-C.; funding acquisition, F.F.-C., E.P.-R. and S.P.-T. All authors have read and agreed to the published version of the manuscript.

Funding: This research received funding from the Generalitat de Catalunya Industrial Doctorate program of the candidate Eloy Pena Rodíguez, expedient number 2019 DI 1989691.

Institutional Review Board Statement: Ethical review and approval were waived for this study, due to the pig skin used was obtained from an abattoir. No animals were sacrificed specifically to carry out this research.

Informed Consent Statement: Not applicable

Data Availability Statement: The data presented in this study are available on request from the corresponding author. The data are not publicly available due to intellectual property.

Acknowledgments: Assistance provided by Manel Bosch from the University of Barcelona Scientific-Technical service, and by Mari Carmen Moreno from Reig Jofre was greatly appreciated. The authors thank Marçal Pastor Anglada and Carlos Nieto Abad for the guidance and advice provided in this project.

Conflicts of Interest: F.F.-C., E.P.-R. and M.L.R. are employees of Reig Jofre. The authors are not involved in any commercial or marketing activities of the developed product. Other authors declare no conflict of interest. The funders had no role in the design of the study; in the collection, analyses, or interpretation of data; in the writing of the manuscript, or in the decision to publish the results.

References

1. Elias, P.M. Stratum Corneum Defensive Functions: An Integrated View. *J. Investig. Dermatol.* **2005**, *125*, 183–200. [CrossRef]
2. Gupta, M.; Agrawal, U.; Vyas, S.P. Nanocarrier-based topical drug delivery for the treatment of skin diseases. *Expert Opin. Drug Deliv.* **2012**, *9*, 783–804. [CrossRef]
3. Pena-Rodríguez, E.; Moreno, M.C.; Blanco-Fernandez, B.; González, J.; Fernández-Campos, F.; Fernandez, B.-. Epidermal Delivery of Retinyl Palmitate Loaded Transfersomes: Penetration and Biodistribution Studies. *Pharmaceutics* **2020**, *12*, 112. [CrossRef]
4. Lademann, J.; Richter, H.; Teichmann, A.; Otberg, N.; Blume-Peytavi, U.; Luengo, J.; Weiss, B.; Schaefer, U.F.; Lehr, C.-M.; Wepf, R. Nanoparticles—An efficient carrier for drug delivery into the hair follicles. *Eur. J. Pharm. Biopharm.* **2007**, *66*, 159–164. [CrossRef] [PubMed]
5. Shen, S.; Wu, Y.; Liu, Y.; Wu, D. High drug-loading nanomedicines: Progress, current status, and prospects. *Int. J. Nanomed.* **2017**, *12*, 4085–4109. [CrossRef] [PubMed]
6. Venturini, C.G.; Jäger, E.; Oliveira, C.P.; Bernardi, A.; Battastini, A.M.; Guterres, S.S.; Pohlmann, A.R. Formulation of lipid core nanocapsules. *Colloids Surf. A Physicochem. Eng. Asp.* **2011**, *375*, 200–208. [CrossRef]
7. Bazylińska, U.; Lewińska, A.; Lamch, Ł.; Wilk, K.A. Polymeric nanocapsules and nanospheres for encapsulation and long sustained release of hydrophobic cyanine-type photosensitizer. *Colloids Surf. A Physicochem. Eng. Asp.* **2014**, *442*, 42–49. [CrossRef]
8. Saraiya, N.V.; A Goldstein, D. Dexamethasone for ocular inflammation. *Expert Opin. Pharmacother.* **2011**, *12*, 1127–1131. [CrossRef]
9. Yamamoto, K.A.; Klossek, R.; Flesch, F.; Rancan, M.; Weigand, I.; Bykova, M.; Bechtel, S.; Ahlberg, A.; Vogt, U.; Blume-Peytavi, P.; et al. Influence of the skin barrier on the penetration of topical-ly-applied dexamethasone probed by soft X-ray spectromicroscopy. *Eur. J. Pharm. Biopharm.* **2017**, *118*, 30–37. [CrossRef]
10. Leyden, J.L.; Kligman, A.M. Treatment of alopecia areata with steroid solution. *Arch Dermatol.* **1972**, *106*, 924. [CrossRef]
11. Shapiro, J. Current Treatment of Alopecia Areata. *J. Investig. Dermatol. Symp. Proc.* **2013**, *16*, S42–S44. [CrossRef]
12. Lachenmeier, D.W. Safety evaluation of topical applications of ethanol on the skin and inside the oral cavity. *J. Occup. Med. Toxicol.* **2008**, *3*, 26. [CrossRef] [PubMed]
13. Kwak, S.; Brief, E.; Langlais, D.; Kitson, N.; Lafleur, M.; Thewalt, J. Ethanol perturbs lipid organization in models of stratum corneum membranes: An investigation combining differential scanning calorimetry, infrared and 2H NMR spectroscopy. *Biochim. Biophys. Acta Biomembr.* **2012**, *1818*, 1410–1419. [CrossRef] [PubMed]

14. McDonnell, G.; Russell, A.D. Antiseptics and disinfectants: Activity, action, and resistance. *Clin. Microbiol. Rev.* **1999**, *12*, 147–179, Erratum in **2001**, *14*, 227. [CrossRef]
15. Balzus, B.; Sahle, F.F.; Hönzke, S.; Gerecke, C.; Schumacher, F.; Hedtrich, S.; Kleuser, B.; Bodmeier, R. Formulation and ex vivo evaluation of polymeric nanoparticles for controlled delivery of cortico-steroids to the skin and the corneal epithelium. *Eur. J. Pharm. Biopharm.* **2012**, *115*, 122–130. [CrossRef]
16. Al-Amin, M.D.; Bellato, F.; Mastrotto, F.; Garofalo, M.; Malfanti, A.; Salmaso, S.; Caliceti, P. Dexamethasone Loaded Liposomes by Thin-Film Hydration and Microfluidic Procedures: Formulation Challenges. *Int. J. Mol. Sci.* **2020**, *21*, 1611. [CrossRef]
17. Fessi, H.; Puisieux, F.; Devissaguet, J.P.; Ammoury, N.; Benita, S. Nanocapsule formation by interfacial polymer deposition following solvent displacement. *Int. J. Pharm.* **1989**, *55*, R1–R4. [CrossRef]
18. Lymberopoulos, A.; Demopoulou, C.; Kyriazi, M.; Katsarou, M.; Demertzis, N.; Hatziandoniou, S.; Maswadeh, H.; Papaioanou, G.; Demetzos, C.; Maibach, H.; et al. Liposome percutaneous penetration in vivo. *Toxicol. Res. Appl.* **2017**. [CrossRef]
19. European Directorate for the Quality of Medicines & HealthCare, European Pharmacopoeia 7.0, Chapter 2.4.24. Identification and Control of Residual Solvents, 01/2008:20424. Available online: https://www.drugfuture.com/Pharmacopoeia/EP7/DATA/20424E.PDF (accessed on 10 February 2021).
20. Zhang, Y.; Huo, M.; Zhou, J.; Zou, A.; Li, W.; Yao, C.; Xie, S. DDSolver: An Add-In Program for Modeling and Comparison of Drug Dissolution Profiles. *AAPS J.* **2010**, *12*, 263–271. [CrossRef]
21. Monica, L.-L.; Jordi, G.; Francisco, F.-C. In situ bioadhesive film-forming system for topical delivery of mometasone furoate: Characterization and biopharmaceutical properties. *J. Drug Deliv. Sci. Technol.* **2020**, *59*, 101852. [CrossRef]
22. Papadopoulou, V.; Kosmidis, K.; Vlachou, M.; Macheras, P. On the use of the Weibull function for the discernment of drug release mechanisms. *Int. J. Pharm.* **2006**, *309*, 44–50. [CrossRef] [PubMed]
23. Supramaniam, J.; Adnan, R.; Kaus, N.H.M.; Bushra, R. Magnetic nanocellulose alginate hydrogel beads as potential drug delivery system. *Int. J. Biol. Macromol.* **2018**, *118*, 640–648. [CrossRef] [PubMed]
24. Rekhi, G.S.; Jambhekar, S.S. Ethylcellulose—A Polymer Review. *Drug Dev. Ind. Pharm.* **1995**, *21*, 61–77. [CrossRef]
25. Gurtler, F.; Kaltsatos, V.; Boisramé, B.; Gurny, R. Long-acting soluble bioadhesive ophthalmic drug insert (BODI) containing gentamicin for veterinary use: Optimization and clinical investigation. *J. Control. Release* **1995**, *33*, 231–236. [CrossRef]
26. Wasilewska, K.; Winnicka, K. Ethylcellulose—A Pharmaceutical Excipient with Multidirectional Application in Drug Dosage Forms Development. *Materials* **2019**, *12*, 3386. [CrossRef]
27. Kala, S.; Gurudiwan, P.; Juyal, D. Formulation and Evaluation of Besifloxacin Loaded in Situ Gel for Ophthalmic Delivery. *Pharm. Biosci. J.* **2018**, *6*, 36. [CrossRef]
28. Committee for Human Medicinal Products, ICH guideline Q3C (R6) on impurities: Guideline for residual solvents 9 August 2019, EMA/CHMP/ICH/82260/2006. Available online: https://www.ema.europa.eu/en/ich-q3c-r6-residual-solvents (accessed on 18 March 2021).
29. Sharma, N.; Madan, P.; Lin, S. Effect of process and formulation variables on the preparation of parenteral paclitaxel-loaded biodegradable polymeric nanoparticles: A co-surfactant study. *Asian J. Pharm. Sci.* **2016**, *11*, 404–416. [CrossRef]
30. Tan, T.B.; Chu, W.C.; Yussof, N.S.; Abas, F.; Mirhosseini, H.; Cheah, Y.K.; Nehdi, I.A.; Tan, C.P. Physicochemical, morphological and cellular uptake properties of lutein nanodispersions prepared by using surfactants with different stabilizing mechanisms. *Food Funct.* **2016**, *7*, 2043–2051. [CrossRef]
31. Jäger, E.; Venturini, C.G.; Poletto, F.S.; Colomé, L.M.; Pohlmann, J.P.U.; Bernardi, A.; Battastini, A.M.O.; Guterres, S.S.; Pohlmann, A.R. Sustained Release from Lipid-Core Nanocapsules by Varying the Core Viscosity and the Particle Surface Area. *J. Biomed. Nanotechnol.* **2009**, *5*, 130–140. [CrossRef]
32. Singhvi, G.; Singh, M. Review: In vitro drug release characterization models. *Int. J. Pharm. Stud. Res. II* **2011**, 77–84.
33. Morgen, M.; Lu, G.W.; Du, D.; Stehle, R.; Lembke, F.; Cervantes, J.; Ciotti, S.; Haskell, R.; Smithey, D.; Haley, K.; et al. Targeted delivery of a poorly water-soluble compound to hair follicles using polymeric nanoparticle suspensions. *Int. J. Pharm.* **2011**, *416*, 314–322. [CrossRef] [PubMed]
34. Döge, N.; Hönzke, S.; Schumacher, F.; Balzus, B.; Colombo, M.; Hadam, S.; Rancan, F.; Blume-Peytavi, U.; Schäfer-Korting, M.; Schindler, A.; et al. Ethyl cellulose nanocarriers and nanocrystals differentially deliver dexamethasone into intact, tape-stripped or sodium lauryl sulfate-exposed ex vivo human skin—Assessment by intradermal microdialysis and extraction from the different skin layers. *J. Control. Release* **2016**, *242*, 25–34. [CrossRef] [PubMed]
35. Teichmann, A.; Jacobi, U.; Ossadnik, M.; Richter, H.; Koch, S.; Sterry, W.; Lademann, J. Differential Stripping: Determination of the Amount of Topically Applied Substances Penetrated into the Hair Follicles. *J. Investig. Dermatol.* **2005**, *125*, 264–269. [CrossRef] [PubMed]
36. Nicoli, S.; Bunge, A.L.; Delgado-Charro, M.B.; Guy, R.H. Dermatopharmacokinetics: Factors Influencing Drug Clearance from the Stratum Corneum. *Pharm. Res.* **2008**, *26*, 865–871. [CrossRef]
37. FDA Inactive Ingredient Database. Available online: http://www.accessdata.fda.gov/scripts/cder/iig/index.cfm (accessed on 18 March 2021).
38. Kasumagic-Halilovic, E.; Prohic, A.; Cavaljuga, S. Tumor necrosis factor-alpha in patients with alopecia areata. *Indian J. Dermatol.* **2011**, *56*, 494–496. [CrossRef]
39. Tauber, M.; Buche, S.; Reygagne, P.; Berthelot, J.-M.; Aubin, F.; Ghislain, P.-D.; Cohen, J.-D.; Coquerelle, P.; Goujon, E.; Jullien, D.; et al. Alopecia areata occurring during anti-TNF therapy: A national multicenter prospective study. *J. Am. Acad. Dermatol.* **2014**, *70*, 1146–1149. [CrossRef]

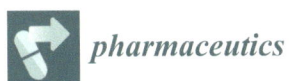

Article

Clarithromycin Solid Lipid Nanoparticles for Topical Ocular Therapy: Optimization, Evaluation and In Vivo Studies

Anroop B. Nair, Jigar Shah, Bandar E. Al-Dhubiab, Shery Jacob, Snehal S. Patel, Katharigatta N. Venugopala, Mohamed A. Morsy, Sumeet Gupta, Mahesh Attimarad, Nagaraja Sreeharsha and Pottathil Shinu

1. Department of Pharmaceutical Sciences, College of Clinical Pharmacy, King Faisal University, Al-Ahsa 31982, Saudi Arabia; baldhubiab@kfu.edu.sa (B.E.A.-D.); kvenugopala@kfu.edu.sa (K.N.V.); momorsy@kfu.edu.sa (M.A.M.); mattimarad@kfu.edu.sa (M.A.); sharsha@kfu.edu.sa (N.S.)
2. Department of Pharmaceutics, Institute of Pharmacy, Nirma University, Ahmedabad 382481, Gujarat, India
3. Department of Pharmaceutical Sciences, College of Pharmacy, Gulf Medical University, Ajman 4184, United Arab Emirates; sheryjacob6876@gmail.com
4. Department of Pharmacology, Institute of Pharmacy, Nirma University, Ahmedabad 382481, Gujarat, India; snehalpharma53@gmail.com
5. Department of Biotechnology and Food Technology, Durban University of Technology, Durban 4000, Natal, South Africa
6. Department of Pharmacology, Faculty of Medicine, Minia University, El-Minia 61511, Egypt
7. Department of Pharmacology, M. M. College of Pharmacy, Maharishi Markandeshwar (Deemed to be University), Mullana 133203, India; sumeetgupta25@gmail.com
8. Department of Pharmaceutics, Vidya Siri College of Pharmacy, Off Sarjapura Road, Bangalore 560035, India
9. Department of Biomedical Sciences, College of Clinical Pharmacy, King Faisal University, Al-Ahsa 31982, Saudi Arabia; spottathail@kfu.edu.sa
* Correspondence: anair@kfu.edu.sa (A.B.N.); jigsh12@gmail.com (J.S.); Tel.: +966-536219868 (A.B.N.); +91-9909007411 (J.S.)

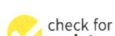

Citation: Nair, A.B.; Shah, J.; Al-Dhubiab, B.E.; Jacob, S.; Patel, S.S.; Venugopala, K.N.; Morsy, M.A.; Gupta, S.; Attimarad, M.; Sreeharsha, N.; et al. Clarithromycin Solid Lipid Nanoparticles for Topical Ocular Therapy: Optimization, Evaluation, and In Vivo Studies. *Pharmaceutics* 2021, 13, 523. https://doi.org/10.3390/pharmaceutics13040523

Academic Editors: Ana Catarina Silva and José Manuel Sousa Lobo

Received: 22 February 2021
Accepted: 6 April 2021
Published: 9 April 2021

Publisher's Note: MDPI stays neutral with regard to jurisdictional claims in published maps and institutional affiliations.

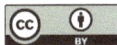

Copyright: © 2021 by the authors. Licensee MDPI, Basel, Switzerland. This article is an open access article distributed under the terms and conditions of the Creative Commons Attribution (CC BY) license (https://creativecommons.org/licenses/by/4.0/).

Abstract: Solid lipid nanoparticles (SLNs) are being extensively exploited as topical ocular carrier systems to enhance the bioavailability of drugs. This study investigated the prospects of drug-loaded SLNs to increase the ocular permeation and improve the therapeutic potential of clarithromycin in topical ocular therapy. SLNs were formulated by high-speed stirring and the ultra-sonication method. Solubility studies were carried out to select stearic acid as lipid former, Tween 80 as surfactant, and Transcutol P as cosurfactant. Clarithromycin-loaded SLN were optimized by fractional factorial screening and 3^2 full factorial designs. Optimized SLNs (CL10) were evaluated for stability, morphology, permeation, irritation, and ocular pharmacokinetics in rabbits. Fractional factorial screening design signifies that the sonication time and amount of lipid affect the SLN formulation. A 3^2 full factorial design established that both factors had significant influences on particle size, percent entrapment efficiency, and percent drug loading of SLNs. The release profile of SLNs (CL9) showed ~80% drug release in 8 h and followed Weibull model kinetics. Optimized SLNs (CL10) showed significantly higher permeation (30.45 µg/cm^2/h; $p < 0.0001$) as compared to control (solution). CL10 showed spherical shape and good stability and was found non-irritant for ocular administration. Pharmacokinetics data demonstrated significant improvement of clarithromycin bioavailability ($p < 0.0001$) from CL10, as evidenced by a 150% increase in C_{max} (~1066 ng/mL) and a 2.8-fold improvement in AUC (5736 ng h/mL) ($p < 0.0001$) as compared to control solution (C_{max}; 655 ng/mL and AUC; 2067 ng h/mL). In summary, the data observed here demonstrate the potential of developed SLNs to improve the ocular permeation and enhance the therapeutic potential of clarithromycin, and hence could be a viable drug delivery approach to treat endophthalmitis.

Keywords: clarithromycin; solid lipid nanoparticles; optimization; permeation; pharmacokinetics

1. Introduction

Ophthalmic drug delivery continues to pose challenges to formulation scientists due to the complex biochemical, anatomical, and physiological ocular barriers. The biological membranes that protects the anterior and posterior segments of the eye, in addition to the unique structure of the cornea, result in poor ocular bioavailability [1]. Topical drug administration to the anterior segment of the eye causes large pre-corneal clearance because of their high tear turn over (0.5–2.2 µL/min) and rapid blinking rate (6–15 times/min) [2]. Consequently, conventional ophthalmic dosage forms must be applied with frequent instillations to attain and/or control targeted drug levels within the anterior segment of the eye. Delivering the drug molecules to the posterior segment of the eye is challenging primarily due to the long diffusion pathway and the cellular characteristics of the vitreous humor [3]. Therefore, alternative techniques are utilized to transport drugs to the posterior vitreous, the uveal tract, retina, or choroid [4]. Endophthalmitis is a severe intraocular inflammatory infection that affects the vitreous and aqueous fluids within the anterior and posterior region of eye [5]. It is the infection generally caused due to organisms such as bacteria, fungi, or parasites that enter the eye through the blood stream, surgery in the eye or other parts near the eye, or sepsis [6]. A literature review indicated that few drug delivery systems have been developed and their efficacy evaluated in animals. In one attempt, the therapeutic effect demonstrated by an intravitreal drug delivery system of voriconazole was superior to intravitreal injection in rabbits [7]. Chitosan nanoparticles containing daptomycin were developed in ocular treatment of bacterial endophthalmitis. It was reported that these nanoparticles had appropriate characteristics to recommend as a non-invasive method for the ocular delivery of daptomycin to the eye [8].

Clarithromycin is a broad spectrum macrolide antibiotic and shows potential action against various organisms, including *Staphylococcus aureus*, *Streptococcus pneumoniae*, *Legionella pneumophila*, *Moraxella catarrhalis*, *Chlamydia trachomatis*, and *Mycobacterium avium* [9]. Clarithromycin is chemically 6-O-methylerythromycin ($C_{38}H_{69}NO_{13}$), with a molecular weight of 747.95 Dalton, pKa value of 8.99, and melting point ranges between 217 and 220 °C [10]. Different solubility studies demonstrated that clarithromycin is soluble in acetone, slightly soluble in methanol, ethanol, and acetonitrile, and practically insoluble in water (0.33 mg/L). Lipophilicity is a major determining factor in a compound's absorption, distribution in the body, penetration across vital membranes and biological barriers, metabolism, and excretion. The pharmacokinetics of clarithromycin in adults showed average oral bioavailability of 53%, plasma concentration between 2.41 and 2.85 µg/L after 500 mg dose, and a half-life of ~4 h [10,11]. Pharmacokinetic and pharmacodynamic investigations suggest that clarithromycin exhibits a similar interaction profile as that of erythromycin [12]. Lipid-based drug delivery system have the potential capacity to entrap both lipophobic and lipophilic drugs, enhance the bioavailability of low aqueous soluble drugs, and protect them against degradation. In the last few decades, liquid nanoemulsions have been increasingly used as drug carriers for lipophilic drugs [13]. However, the feasibility of controlled drug release from nanoemulsions is restricted due to the submicron globule size and the fluid state of the carrier. Alternatively, solid matrices of nanostructured lipid carriers (NLCs) and solid lipid nanoparticles (SLNs) help to improve the stability and safety and provide controlled drug release, and they can incorporate both hydrophilic and hydrophobic molecules and can be used in various routes [14]. The basic difference between NLCs and SLNs is the type of lipids used, where liquid lipids are used in NLCs and solid lipids in SLNs [14].

SLNs are nano-sized (10–1000 nm) particles formed when the solid lipids are dispersed in aqueous media containing surfactants as stabilizers [15]. They widely accepted as a prospective delivery system similar to other colloidal carriers, including liposomes and other polymeric nanoparticles [16,17]. Due to the inclusion of physiologically compatible lipids of either natural or synthetic origin, nonirritant and nontoxic properties in SLNs reduce the potential threats of acute or chronic toxicity [15]. Furthermore, advantages such as sustained and controlled drug release, good physical stability, resistance to degradation of lipids, in vivo acceptability, and ability to increase pre-corneal retention time make SLNs a very adaptive carrier for various drug delivery systems [18]. Indeed, formulations of SLNs can be performed in the absence of organic solvents, can be sterilized, and can also use excipients that are "generally recognized as safe" (GRAS), and hence can be easily scaled-up in industry [19]. The incorporation of lipids in the solid state compared to the liquid form is very effective to obtain controlled drug release, since drug mobility is significantly retarded in solid lipid when compared to liquid oil. Extensive research has been carried in the last two decades to tap the potential of SLNs in delivering drugs through various routes, including the ocular route [19–22]. The literature suggests that SLNs have been widely studied in the treatment of ocular inflammations, infections, glaucoma, cataracts, age related macular degeneration, and as gene therapy carriers [23]. In light of this, the objective of the present study was to design, formulate, and evaluate the potential of drug-loaded SLNs to improve the therapeutic efficacy of clarithromycin in ocular therapy. Fractional factorial design was applied for preliminary screening of various factors utilized in the SLN formulation. A 3^2 full factorial design was employed to evaluate the influence of independent variables on the dependent variables. Selected SLN were assessed for drug permeation using goat cornea and evaluated in vivo in rabbits.

2. Materials and Methods

2.1. Materials

Clarithromycin was provided by Century Pharmaceuticals Ltd., Vadodara, India. Stearic acid, glyceryl monostearate, Tween 20, Tween 80, Span 80, sodium lauryl sulphate, polyethylene glycol 400 (PEG 400), and propylene glycol were commercially procured from Central Drug House, New Delhi, India. Compritol 888ATO, Gelucire 43/01, Precirol ATO5, Geleol, and Transcutol P were procured from Gattefosse India, Mumbai, India. Monegyl T18 and Softemul® were purchased from Mohini Organics, Mumbai, India. Stearylamine was obtained from Hi-Media, Mumbai, India.

2.2. High Performance Liquid Chromatography (HPLC)

Estimation of clarithromycin was done using a Jasco HPLC system (LC–4000, Easton, MD, USA) containing a degasser unit, pump, an automatic injector, as well as an MD–4010 UV–Visible detector and a Phenomenex C-18 column (150 × 4.6 mm, i.d 5 µm). Chromatographic separation of clarithromycin was performed with the help of a mobile phase consisting of acetonitrile: potassium dihydrogen ortho-phosphate (0.02 mM) 40:60 v/v, adjusted to pH 5.5 with phosphoric acid [24]. The temperature in the HPLC column was set at 40 °C, and an isocratic elution of clarithromycin was achieved by allowing the solvent to flow at a fixed rate (1 mL/min) and was monitored at 210 nm. Regression analysis indicated good linearity when clarithromycin concentration was 30–400 ng/mL (r^2 = 0.990).

2.3. Solubility of Drug in Lipids and Surfactants

Preliminary screenings were carried out to evaluate the solubility of clarithromycin in various solid lipids and surfactants according to a method described in the literature [25]. Briefly, a weighed quantity (10 mg) of lipid or surfactant was taken in glass vials and melted above its melting point on a water bath (EIE Instruments, Ahmedabad, India). To the melted solution of lipids or surfactant, 10 mg clarithromycin was added and subsequently vortexed. Then, additional increments of lipid or surfactant were added until the drug was completely solubilized or form a homogenous mixture. The lipid in which clarithromycin showed maximum solubility, and the surfactant where it exhibited minimum solubility were selected for the development of an SLN formulation.

2.4. Formulation of SLN Using Fractional Factorial Screening Design

SLNs containing clarithromycin, lipid, surfactant, and cosurfactant were formulated by high-speed stirring and the ultra-sonication method described in the literature [26]. High speed mixing generally produces an emulsion, which on cooling forms SLNs. Based on the solubility study of drug in lipid, the amounts of lipid used for the screening design were 150 mg and 200 mg, and the concentrations of surfactants selected were 1 and 3%.

Preliminary studies were carried out using different surfactant ratios (surfactant to co-surfactant; 1:9, 3:7, 5:5, 7:3, and 9:1) and evaluated for percent entrapment efficiency and percent drug loading. The selection of the surfactant ratio was based on the target set for percent entrapment efficiency (>85%) and for percent drug loading (>30%).

Screening designs were used to screen the main significant effects from various potential factors that can affect the formulation. Fractional factorial design is one type of screening design. It was applied for screening of all the selected factors utilized for the development of a clarithromycin-loaded SLN formulation. Based on the number of factors, the total number of experimental runs was calculated as sixteen by the equation, 2^{n-1}, where n = number of factors. Selected independent variables included for the screening method were process-related factors, such as homogenization speed and sonication time, in addition to formulation variables like amount of lipid, surfactant concentration, and surfactant ratio. The dependent variables investigated were particle size (R_1), entrapment efficiency (R_2), and drug loading (R_3). The coded and actual values of independent variables for fractional factorial screening design are shown in Table 1.

Table 1. Coded and actual values of independent variables for fractional factorial design.

Independent Variable	Levels	
	+1	−1
A: Homogenization speed (rpm)	12,000	6000
B: Sonication time (min)	10	5
C: Amount of lipid (mg)	200	150
D: Surfactant ratio	3:7	5:5
E: Surfactant concentration (%)	3%	1%

In brief, an accurately weighed quantity of stearic acid and clarithromycin were solubilized in ethanol by heating on a water bath at 65–70 °C, while surfactant and co-surfactant were dissolved in aqueous phase. SLNs were obtained by slowly adding the molten organic phase drop wise into the aqueous phase under continuous stirring using a homogenizer (Remi Motors, Mumbai, India) set at respective speeds for screening design batches, as shown in Table 2. The precipitated SLN-containing dispersions were subjected to further mixing in cold water using a probe sonicator (Brookfield Engineering Laboratories, MA, USA). The SLNs formed were washed with distilled water and filtered. Table 2 shows the coded and actual values for 16 batches of fractional factorial design.

2.5. Evaluation of Screening Design Batches

2.5.1. Particle Size Characterization and Zeta Potential

Particle size analysis, polydispersity index, and zeta potential of the clarithromycin-loaded SLN were determined using a zetasizer (Nanopartica SZ-100, Horiba, Kyoto, Japan). To perform the test, drops (2–3) of test samples placed in the disposable cuvette were exposed to the laser beam. The intensity and physical characteristics of scattered light were measured with the detector, and the particle sizes were subsequently determined [27]. The electrophoretic mobility values were measured after suitable dilution with water at 25 °C.

2.5.2. Percent Drug Entrapment Efficiency and Percent Drug Loading

Formulations were filled in vials and centrifuged at 15,000 rpm using an ultracentrifuge (Remi Motors, Mumbai, India) for 25 min to separate the supernatant and pellets. The pellets were dissolved in methanol, and the drug contents were measured using HPLC. Entrapment efficiency and drug loading were calculated using the formula described in the literature [28].

Table 2. Coded and actual values of fractional factorial design batches.

Batch	Coded Value					Actual Values				
	A	B	C	D	E	A	B	C	D	E
1	1	−1	1	−1	1	12,000	5	200	5:5	3
2	−1	1	1	−1	1	6000	10	200	5:5	3
3	1	1	1	1	1	12,000	10	200	3:7	3
4	−1	1	−1	−1	−1	6000	10	150	5:5	1
5	−1	−1	1	1	1	6000	5	200	3:7	3
6	1	−1	−1	−1	−1	12,000	5	150	5:5	1
7	−1	1	1	1	−1	6000	10	200	3:7	1
8	1	−1	−1	1	1	12,000	5	150	3:7	3
9	1	1	−1	−1	1	12,000	10	150	5:5	3
10	−1	−1	−1	1	−1	6000	5	150	3:7	1
11	−1	−1	−1	−1	1	6000	5	150	5:5	3
12	1	−1	1	1	−1	12,000	5	200	3:7	1
13	−1	−1	1	−1	−1	6000	5	200	5:5	1
14	1	1	1	−1	−1	12,000	10	200	5:5	1
15	−1	1	−1	1	1	6000	10	150	3:7	3
16	1	1	−1	1	−1	12,000	10	150	3:7	1

2.6. Optimization Design

A 3^2 full factorial design was used to assess the influence of independent variables on the dependent variables for the prepared clarithromycin SLNs. Based on the fractional factorial design data, the two factors of amount of lipid (mg) (X1) and sonication time (min) (X2) showed substantial effects on the particle size, drug entrapment efficiency, and drug loading, and hence were applied at 3 levels. In addition, the other three factors, namely homogenization speed, surfactant ratio, and surfactant concentration, were kept constant at 9000 rpm, 5:5, and 3%, respectively, during the experimental run of nine experiments. The dependent variables were Y_1: particle size; Y_2: percent entrapment efficiency; and Y_3: percent drug loading. Table 3 shows coded and actual values of the independent variables of the 3^2 full factorial design.

Table 3. Coded and actual values of independent variables of 3^2 full factorial design.

Independent Variable	Levels		
	+1	0	−1
A: Amount of lipid (mg)	175	150	125
B: Sonication time (min)	8	6	4

The responses Y_1, Y_2, and Y_3 were evaluated using the equation $Y = b_0 + b_1X_1 + b_2X_2 + b_{12}X_1X_2 + b_{11}X_{11} + b_{22}X_{22}$. This equation represents the main factors (X_1 and X_2), interaction factors (X_1X_2), and polynomial factors (X_{11} and X_{22}). The b_0 is the mathematic mean value of total runs, and b_1 and b_2 are the projected coefficients for the factors X_1 and X_2, respectively. For validation of selected statistical design, polynomial equations were generated using Design Expert software, and one-way analysis of variance (ANOVA) was tested. With the help of response surface plots, the correlation between variables and response parameters was established. The method of preparation was the same as per the screening design batches. Table 4 shows the coded and actual values for 9 batches of the 3^2 full factorial design.

Table 4. Coded and actual values for 9 batches of the 3^2 full factorial design.

Batch No.	Coded Value		Actual Value	
	X1	X2		
1	0	+1	150	8
2	−1	+1	125	8
3	+1	+1	175	8
4	+1	0	175	6
5	0	−1	150	4
6	−1	0	125	6
7	−1	−1	125	4
8	+1	−1	175	4
9	0	0	150	6

2.7. Evaluation of Design Batches of SLN

2.7.1. Drug Release

A Franz diffusion cell (Logan Instruments Ltd., Somerset, NJ, USA) having an exposed surface area of 0.79 cm^2, was used to carry out in vitro drug release. In short, a semipermeable membrane (MWCO 12–14 kDa) was held between the donor and receptor compartment. Clarithromycin-loaded SLN dispersion (CL1–CL9, 2.5 mg/mL of drug) or control (drug solution in 10% v/v span 80) was added in the upper compartment. The acceptor compartment (20 mL) contained simulated tear fluid (pH 7.4) with 1% Tween 80 (to maintain sink conditions) [29] and was stirred at 50 rpm. The temperature of the entire assembly was controlled at 37 ± 0.5 °C by means of a thermostatic water bath. At various time intervals, aliquots of samples (1 mL) were drawn and substituted with the equivalent amount of buffer held at the same temperature. A control experiment was performed at the same experimental conditions using a similar strength of clarithromycin solution. The samples were later diluted with mobile phase and quantified for clarithromycin. The data collected were analyzed to calculate regression coefficient (r^2) and interpret various mathematical models [30].

2.7.2. Trans-Corneal Permeation

Ex vivo permeation experiments were performed utilizing the vertical Franz diffusion cell using an isolated goat corneal membrane obtained from a local abattoir (Ahmedabad, India) held between the donor and receptor cell [31]. Testing were done using either optimized formulation (CL10) or control (0.25% drug solution equivalent to 2.5 mg of clarithromycin/mL). The receptor compartment was filled with simulated tear fluid (pH 7.4) with 1% Tween 80 (to maintain sink conditions), and temperature was set at 37 ± 0.5 °C. Suitable volumes of the samples were taken at specific time intervals and similar volumes of fluids at the same temperature. The samples withdrawn from the receptor compartment were appropriately diluted and estimated for clarithromycin by HPLC. The flux was determined as described in the literature [32].

2.7.3. Transmission Electron Microscopy (TEM)

TEM (Holland Technai 20, Phillips, Amsterdam, The Netherlands) with bright field imaging and magnification technique was employed to examine the physical characteristics of SLN, such as particle size, shape, and surface morphology. A drop of the SLN dispersion was allowed to fix to the surface of a carbon coated copper grid, and the excess of dispersion was then wiped off using the tip of a filter paper. A drop of negative staining solution, 1% (w/v) phosphotungstic acid, was applied to the affixed SLNs, and extra stain was removed with a tissue paper [33]. The films were formed on grids by air drying at room temperature, and images were captured at 80 kV by TEM.

2.8. Ocular Compatibility

The biocompatibility of the optimized formulation (CL10) was performed in six albino rabbits (2–3 kg). The experiments were performed in accordance with the guidelines stated by the Committee for the Purpose of Control and Supervision of Experiments on Animals (approval number IP/PCEU/FAC/21/029, dated; 9 June 2017). Eye irritation score was measured according to the guidelines based on the Draize technique [34]. Single topical instillation of 50 µL of product (CL10) was applied on the left eye of each rabbit, whereas the same volume of physiological saline (reference) was applied on the right eye. The sterile formulation was tested two times a day for 21 days. The cornea, iris, and conjunctiva of rabbits were frequently observed during the study period. Similarly, signs of sensitivity reactions, particularly redness, swelling, cloudiness, edema, hemorrhage, discharge, and blindness, were checked [35].

2.9. Pharmacokinetics

The amount of clarithromycin diffused into the aqueous humor of the rabbit eyes after ophthalmic administration was determined to compare the ocular bioavailability between CL10 and control (solution). In vivo pharmacokinetic investigations were performed in New Zealand Albino rabbits (2–3 kg) with two groups ($n = 6$). The experiments were carried out by strictly following the guidelines for animal care at Nirma University (IP/PCEU/FAC/21/029; dated 9 June 2017). Single topical instillation (60 µL of 0.25% w/v drug) of SLN was dropped in one eye of individual rabbit in the first group, while the second eye remained untreated. A similar strength and volume of control solution was instilled into the second group of rabbits. Both eyelids of all rabbits were lightly closed for 2 min to increase the contact of drug with the corneal membrane. Before aqueous humor withdrawal, individual animals were anaesthetized by intramuscular administration of xylazine and ketamine [36]. The aqueous humor was collected using 29-gauge insulin syringe needle [37], and 20 µL of sample was mixed with acetonitrile and centrifuged, and the organic layer was assessed for clarithromycin content by HPLC.

2.10. Stability

An accurately weighed quantity of optimized SLN (CL10) was sealed separately in light resistant glass vials at ambient temperature ($25 \pm 1\ °C$) and under refrigerated conditions ($4 \pm 0.5\ °C$) up to 3 months [38]. The stability of SLN was examined by assessing the drug content, particle size, and drug release during the storage period.

2.11. Statistical Analysis

The software used for Statistical data analysis was GraphPad Prism software (version 6, GraphPad, San Diego, CA, USA). The difference in values at $p < 0.05$ was considered statistically significant.

3. Results and Discussion

3.1. Solubility

The solubility of drug in lipid is necessary for the preparation of SLNs. The solubility of clarithromycin in solid lipids and surfactants was carried out by a modified method [25], as the normal equilibrium solubility method is not realistic for solid lipids. The lipid in which the drug is most soluble was selected, as low drug solubility in lipid can lead to a decrease in encapsulation efficiency and drug loading [14]. In addition, low drug lipid solubility may prevent binding of drug molecules to the lipid, and the drug may remain as free drug and thereby fail to provide sustained release as desired. From the data shown in Figure 1, it was concluded that the least amount of stearic acid was required to solubilize clarithromycin when compared with other lipids tested. In general, stearic acid has been widely used in ophthalmic drug delivery systems, and in particular in formulating SLNs [39]. Similarly, surfactants are also important components in SLNs, as they play a crucial role in the physicochemical properties, dissolution, permeation, and stability of particles [40]. However, the high solubility of the drug in surfactant may cause leaching of the actives out of the solid lipid particles of the prepared formulations [41]. Therefore, a combination of surfactants was selected in such a manner that the drug would have minimum solubility in the surfactants. The applicability of the surfactant and cosurfactant in preparing single phase micro or nanoemulsions was described elsewhere in the literature [42]. Based on solubility criteria, the non-ionic surfactant Tween 80 was selected as the surfactant and Transcutol P as the cosurfactant for the preparation of various SLN formulations. Tween 80 is often used in various conventional ophthalmic formulations since it does not induce ocular sensitivity reactions [43]. Additionally, due to longer hydrocarbon chain length and larger polar head groups, Tweens may expand the zone of the emulsion region [42]. In addition, Transcutol P can enhance the corneal permeability of the drug through different transport mechanisms [44].

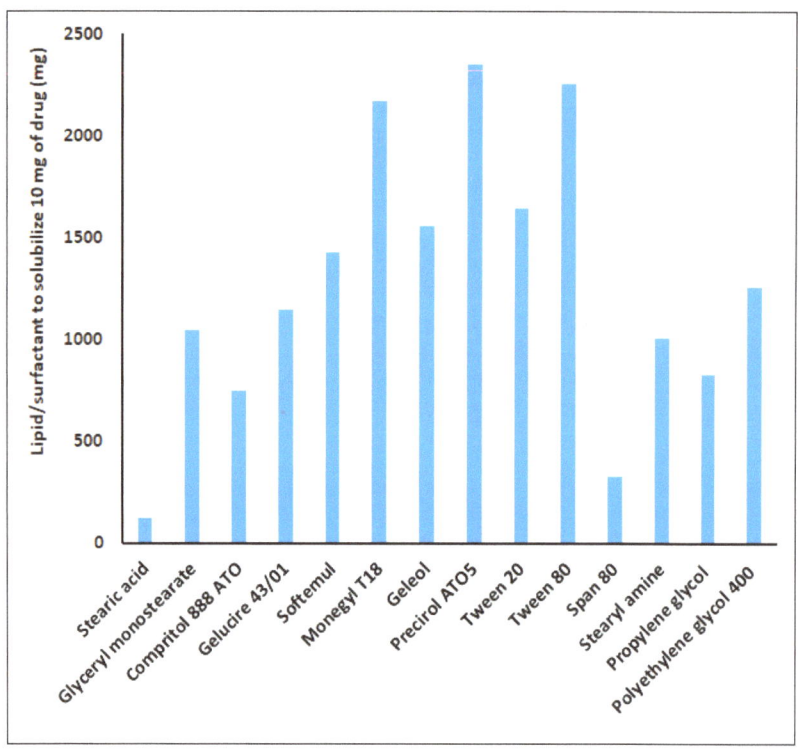

Figure 1. Solubility data showing the amount of lipid/surfactants required to solubilize 10 mg of clarithromycin.

The existence of several colloidal structures such as molecular solubilized emulsifier monomers, mixed micelles, supercooled melts, and drug nanoparticles are important points to consider in SLN formulation. Micelle-forming surfactants are mainly present either on the lipid surface, in micelles or as monomers. The kinetics of drug redistribution between various coexisting colloidal species is very important since the dynamic phenomena are significant for drug stability and drug release [45]. The SLN system can be an efficient carrier system provided that the redistribution of drug between various colloidal forms are prevented. A wide range of drugs with varying lipophilicity has been extensively investigated with respect to their incorporation into SLNs, which signifies the localization of drug within the solid lipid matrix [46]. The log P value of 3.16 for clarithromycin indicates that the drug is mostly located in the lipid matrix. Drug stabilization is a major formulation challenge in colloidal carriers such as SLN due to the enormous surface area and short diffusional pathways. High viscosity provided by lipids actively decreases the diffusion coefficient of the drug inside the carrier system.

3.2. Evaluation of Fractional Factorial Screening Batches of SLN

The evaluation of fractional factorial screening batches of prepared SLN is shown in Table 5. The prepared sixteen batches were evaluated for particle size, percent entrapment efficiency, and percent drug loading.

3.2.1. Effect on Particle Size

The particle size diameter of the SLN dispersions prepared was between 113 nm to 413 nm, as shown in Table 5. From the ANOVA study, it was observed that particle size was significantly ($p < 0.05$) affected by sonication time (min), and it was also confirmed from the Pareto chart (Figure 2a) that t-value of sonication time was above the Bonferroni critical limit, so it had a more significant effect on SLN size. The contour (Figure 2b) and 3D surface plot (Figure 2c) showed that as sonication time decreased from 10 min to 5 min, the size of SLNs also decreased from 413 to 113 nm. This is possible because the sonication can break down the large emulsion drops into tiny particles [25]. On the other hand, the polydispersity index values noticed were in the range of 0.12–0.40 (Table 5).

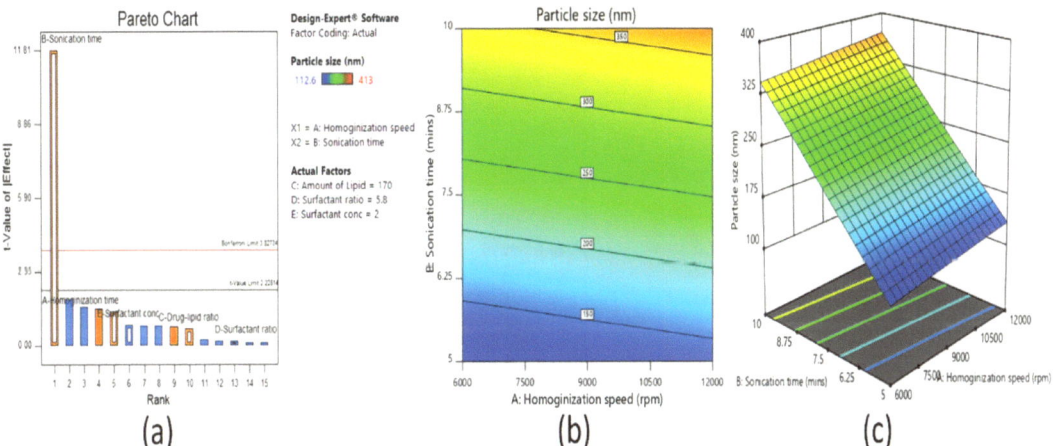

Figure 2. Pareto chart (**a**), contour plot (**b**), and 3D surface plot (**c**) representing the effect on particle size of fractional factorial design.

Table 5. Evaluation of fractional factorial design batches.

Batch No.	Independent Variables with Actual Values					Dependent Variables			
	Homogenization Speed (RPM)	Sonication Time (Min)	Amount of Lipid (mg)	Surfactant Ratio	Surfactant Concentration (%)	Particle Size (nm)	Polydispersity Index	Entrapment Efficiency (%)	Drug Loading (%)
F1	12,000	5	200	5:5	3	115	0.15	84.9	21.2
F2	6000	10	200	5:5	3	357	0.32	69.9	17.5
F3	12,000	10	200	3:7	3	334	0.40	72.4	18.1
F4	6000	10	150	5:5	1	276	0.26	79.1	26.4
F5	6000	5	200	3:7	3	113	0.12	85.8	21.5
F6	12,000	5	150	5:5	1	124	0.18	92.4	30.8
F7	6000	10	200	3:7	3	369	0.31	72.5	18.1
F8	12,000	5	150	3:7	3	113	0.16	87.9	29.3
F9	12,000	10	150	5:5	3	413	0.29	49.9	15.9
F10	6000	5	150	3:7	1	134	0.18	87.3	26.9
F11	6000	5	150	5:5	3	119	0.14	83.7	27.9
F12	12,000	5	200	3:7	1	130	0.14	85.7	21.4
F13	6000	5	200	5:5	1	124	0.12	84.5	21.1
F14	12,000	10	200	5:5	1	397	0.29	75.2	18.9
F15	6000	10	150	3:7	3	284	0.22	77.1	25.7
F16	12,000	10	150	3:7	1	397	0.26	74.9	24.9

3.2.2. Effect on Entrapment Efficiency

Entrapment efficiency refers to the quantity of clarithromycin that was entrapped either within the solid matrix or adsorbed on the surface of nanoparticles. It was quantified by analyzing the amount of drug present in the solid pellets as well as in the aqueous phase of the nanoparticle dispersion. It was concluded from the Pareto chart (Figure 3a) that the sonication time had a substantial influence on the entrapment efficiency. The majority of the formulations possessed high entrapment efficiency of >70%, which also revealed the role of surfactant concentration and ratio, amount of lipid, and homogenization speed on drug incorporation. The selection of suitable stabilizing agents, such as surfactants, and their concentration can have a major impact on the entrapment efficiency of SLN dispersions [45]. Surfactants not only present on the lipid surface but also exists as micelles in the aqueous phase. Micelles and mixed micelles are well known to solubilize the drugs and thus act as an alternate drug localization site. In the current study, sonication likely resulted in more interaction between the particles in lipid and aqueous phases due to the ultrasonic shock waves created by the cavitation forces in the liquid, as described in the literature [47]. These intense forces would have probably caused a rapid transfer of clarithromycin to the core of lipid matrix and subsequently increased entrapment percentage at an optimum sonication time. The contour plot presented in Figure 3b and 3D surface plot in the Figure 3c also confirmed that as sonication time increased (from 5 min to 10 min), the percent entrapment efficiency decreased. This reduction in entrapment efficiency could be due to the extension of sonication time, which in turn would have resulted in greater disintegration of agglomerates, which results in leaking of drug particles from lipid vesicles and thereby decreases the percent entrapment efficiency [48]. However, when the surfactant concentration decreased, a minor improvement in the percent entrapment efficiency was noticed. This could be due to the solubilizing property of surfactant [49] and the existence of an optimum surfactant level, which helped the clarithromycin to stay within the lipid particles and improve the entrapment efficiency of the drug [50].

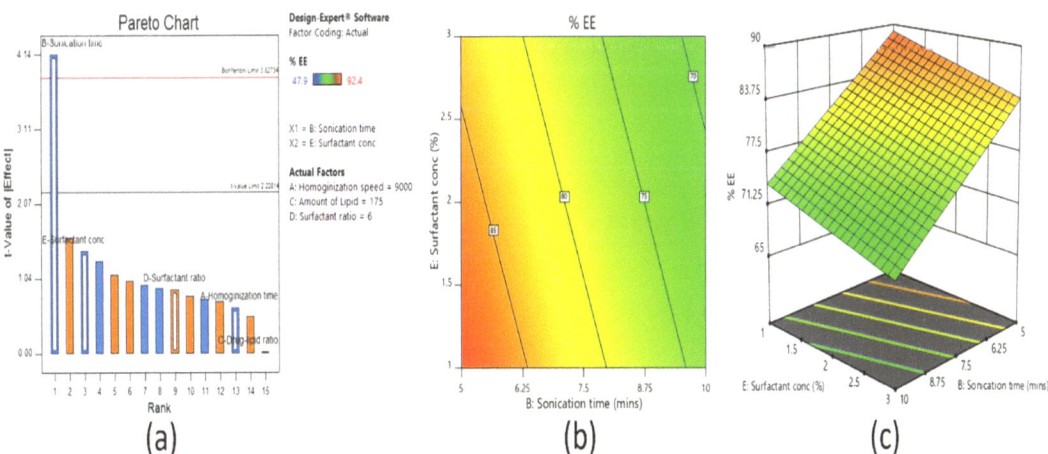

Figure 3. Pareto chart (**a**), contour plot (**b**), and 3D surface plot (**c**) representing the effect on percent entrapment efficiency of fractional factorial design.

3.2.3. Effect on Drug Loading

From the ANOVA study and Pareto chart (Figure 4a), it was observed that the amount of lipid and sonication time had significant effects on percent drug loading, as the t-value was above the limit. The batches with 150 mg of lipid showed good drug entrapment and faster solidification of the nanoparticles. The contour (Figure 4b) and 3D surface response plot (Figure 4c) show that drug loading increased as the sonication time decreased. However, no significant effect in drug loading was noticed with homogenization speed, surfactant concentration, or surfactant ratio.

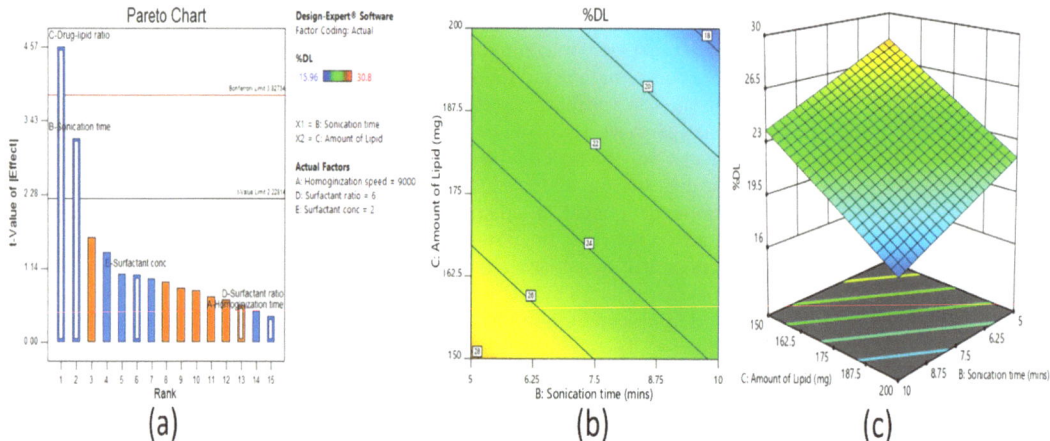

Figure 4. Pareto chart (**a**), contour plot (**b**), and 3D surface plot (**c**) representing the effect on percent drug loading of fractional factorial design.

3.3. The 3^2 Full Factorial Optimization Design

Based on the studies of fractional factorial screening design and data analysis, it was observed that out of five independent variables (including formulation and process variables), two variables (amount of lipid and sonication time) were considered for further optimization. Homogenization speed, surfactant ratio, and surfactant concentration had low or insignificant effects, and hence they were kept constant. A total of nine batches (CL1–CL9) were prepared (Table 6) and were evaluated for particles size, percent entrapment efficiency, and percent drug loading.

Table 6. Evaluation of 3^2 full factorial design batches.

Batch No.	Coded Value		Particle Size (nm)	Polydispersity Index	Entrapment Efficiency (%)	Drug Loading (%)	Zeta Potential (mV)
	Amount of Lipid (mg)	Sonication Time (Min)					
CL1	150	8	339	0.32	70.7	23.6	−21.3
CL2	125	8	404	0.37	74.9	30.0	−16.7
CL3	175	8	316	0.33	65.7	18.8	−21.9
CL4	175	6	163	0.14	79.4	22.7	−29.8
CL5	150	4	236	0.26	80.4	26.9	−18.8
CL6	125	6	173	0.20	76.9	30.8	−25.4
CL7	125	4	274	0.24	79.6	31.8	−21.6
CL8	175	4	245	0.27	81.9	23.4	−23.4
CL9	150	6	154	0.12	87.2	29.1	−18.5

3.4. Evaluation of Design Batches of SLN

3.4.1. Effect on Particle Size

The effect of amount of lipid and sonication time on particle size was studied, and the relevant contour plot and 3D surface response plot are shown in Figure 5a,b, respectively. From the plots, it was observed that as the lipid amount increased from 150 mg to 175 mg, there were increases in particle size (for sonication time 4 and 6 min). This was due to the distribution of sonication energy in the dispersion containing a higher lipid amount dispersion being weaker than in that with the lower lipid amount, which was responsible for more efficient increases in the particle size [25]. However, the same was not observed in the case of 125 mg to 150 mg due to the effect of sonication time. In the case of sonication time, as it increased from 4 to 6 min, particle size decreased, as mentioned earlier, due to more sonication energy reducing the size of the nanoemulsion droplets [25]. However, by further increasing the tie from 6 to 8 min, particle size increased. This was due to more sonication energy, smaller droplet agglomerates, and increases in the size. As per this study, it was observed that a lipid amount of 150 mg and a sonication time of 6 min could be considered as the optimum value. The below polynomial equation (Equation (1)) shows the main, interactive, and polynomial effects of amount of lipid and sonication time on particle size.

$$\text{Particle size} = +150.41 - 21.17 \times X_1 + 50.67 \times X_2 - 14.95 \times X_1 X_2 + 19.13 \times X_{11} + 139.23 \times X_{22} \quad (1)$$

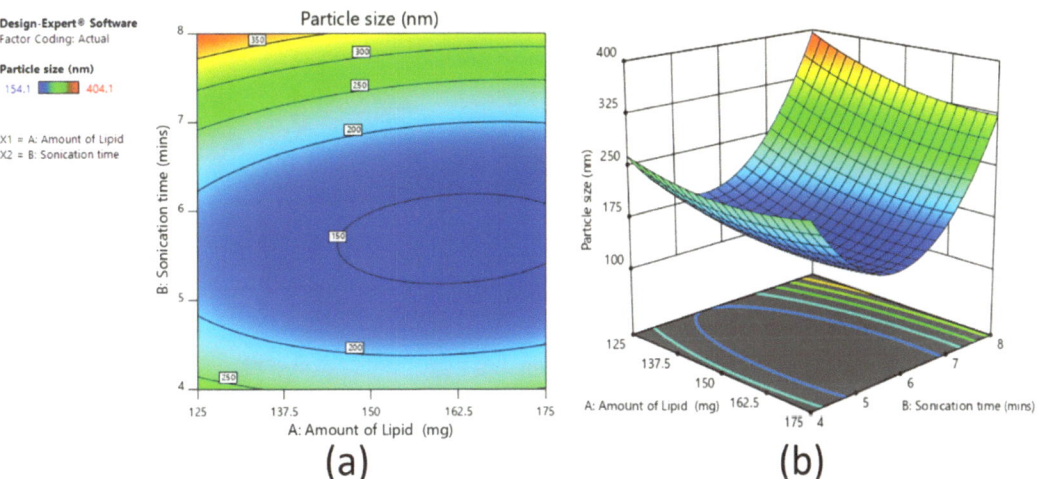

Figure 5. Contour plot (**a**) and 3D surface plot (**b**) representing the effect on particle size for full factorial design batches.

The reduced equation by considering the significant term/s ($p < 0.05$) for particle size can be written as Equation (2):

$$\text{particle size} = +150.41 - 21.17 \times X_1 + 50.67 \times X_2 + 139.23 \times X_{22} \quad (2)$$

On the other hand, the polydispersity index values noticed were in the range of 0.12–0.37 (for sonication times of 4 and 6 min; Table 6), suggesting particles were monodispersed [51], while they were polydispersed when the sonication time was 6 min.

3.4.2. Effect on Entrapment Efficiency

Figure 6a,b shows the contour plot and 3D surface plot on the effect of the amount of lipid and sonication time on percent entrapment efficiency. It was observed that as sonication time increased, percent entrapment efficiency increased up to 6 min and then decreased from 6 min to 8 min. This was due to higher sonication, which increased the mixture viscosity (with increased lipid concentration) and increased drug solubility within the lipid core and thereby increased the entrapment efficiency [52]. In this study, at lower sonication time (4 min), as the lipid amount increased, entrapment efficiency increased from 79.6% to 81.9%. The reverse condition was observed in cases of higher sonication time (8 min); as the lipid amount increased, the percent entrapment efficiency decreased from 74.9% to 65.7%. However, at medium sonication time (6 min), near to a significant difference was observed in the entrapment efficiency, initially increasing from 76.9% to 87.2% and then decreasing to 79.4%, with respect to the lipid amount (150 mg). The batch showed good entrapment efficiency of about 87.2%. In addition, the polynomial equation confirmed that the effect of sonication time was more significant on percent entrapment efficiency than the amount of lipid.

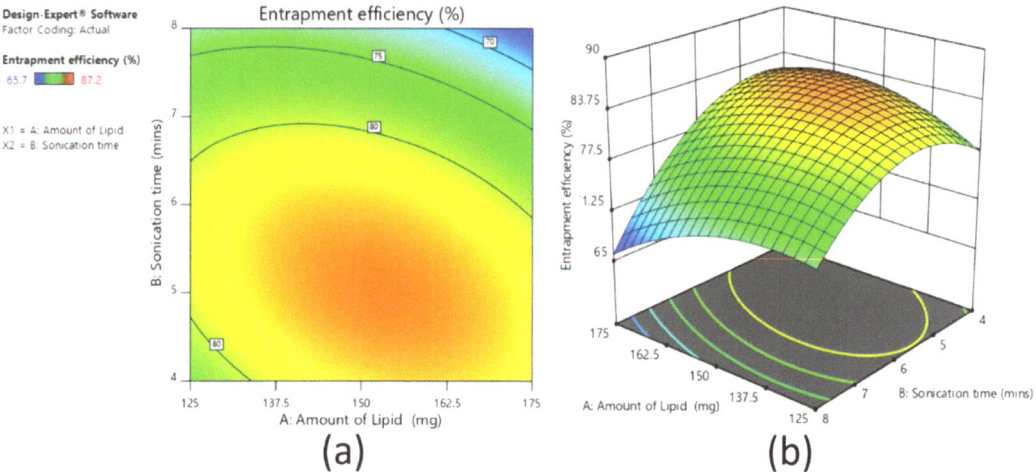

Figure 6. Contour plot (**a**) and 3D surface plot (**b**) representing the effect on percent entrapment efficiency for full factorial design batches.

The polynomial equation (Equation (3)) of percent entrapment efficiency is as follows:

$$\text{Percent entrapment efficiency} = +83.19 - 0.73 \times X_1 - 5.10 \times X_2 - 2.87 \times X_1X_2 - 3.03 \times X_{11} - 5.63 \times X_{22} \quad (3)$$

The reduced equation by considering the significant term ($p < 0.05$) for percent entrapment efficiency can be written as Equation (4):

$$\text{percent entrapment efficiency} = -5.10 \times X_2 \quad (4)$$

3.4.3. Effect on Drug Loading

From Figure 7a,b, it was observed that as the amount of lipid increases, the percent drug loading decreases. This is due to the fixed drug amount in the formulation, as the drug concentration remained the same regardless of the increased lipid concentration that caused a decrease in the drug:lipid ratio with increasing lipid concentration [25]. For sonication time, also as time increased, there was a minor decrease in the percent of drug loading. The polynomial equation showing a negative sign for both variables indicates that the variables have inverse relations with percent drug loading. The polynomial equation (Equation (5)) is as follows:

$$\text{Percent drug loading} = +26.32 - 4.62 \times X_1 - 1.63 \times X_2 \quad (5)$$

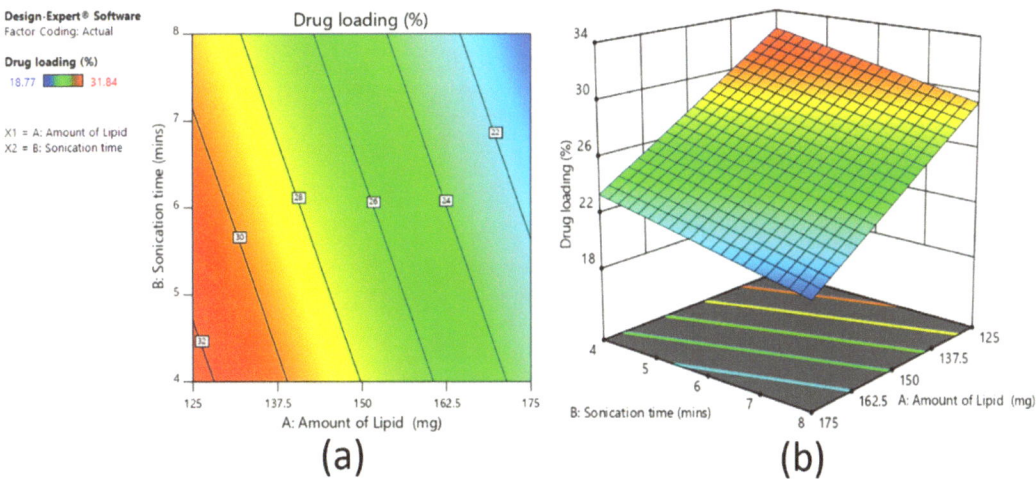

Figure 7. Contour plot (**a**) and 3D surface plot (**b**) representing the effect on percent drug loading for full factorial design batches.

The reduced equation is the same, as both factors significantly affect percent drug loading.

In summary, it can be concluded that for particle size, sonication time is the key variable, and with 6 min of sonication time, the targeted particle size can be achieved. In terms of percent entrapment efficiency, again sonication time of 6 min would be highly effective, while with increases in the amount of lipid beyond a certain limit, there would be no further increase in percent entrapment efficiency. At last, considering the percent drug loading, the amount of lipid with a significant effect was 125 mg and 150 mg on targeted drug loading and sonication time at 4 min to 6 min. Thus, an overall conclusion from the design study is that around 150 mg amount of lipid and 6 min of sonication time would give the required particle size, percent entrapment efficiency, and percent drug loading.

3.5. In Vitro Drug Release

The release of clarithromycin from SLNs was carried out using a dialysis membrane in Franz diffusion cells. Figure 8 shows the cumulative percentage release of clarithromycin SLNs at specified time intervals from CL1 to CL9. Figure 8 signifies that the drug release profiles of various formulations showed similar patterns of initially slow and then progressively increasing over the time and was higher than 70% in 8 h for all SLNs tested. It was reported that SLN can retard the drug release when the chosen drug has a higher melting point compared to the lipid matrix [46]. It was also disclosed that other factors such as interactions between drug–lipid and surfactant–lipid, as well as solubility of drug in the lipid can play a major role in the drug release from SLNs [53]. Thus, one of the possible explanations for the observed drug release profile could be due to the large differences in the melting point of clarithromycin and stearic acid used. In addition, such release is also possible due to the higher lipid viscosity contributed by the drug–lipid interaction combined with slow diffusion of clarithromycin from the waxy matrix. Amongst all the designed formulations, CL9 had the lowest particle size (154 nm), higher entrapment efficiency (87.2%), and good drug loading (29.1%), which were in well-defined ranges targeted for SLN formulation. The CL9 formulation also exhibited higher drug release (~80% in 8 h). However, the release of clarithromycin in solution (control) was quick, and the whole drug was released in 1 h. The mechanism of clarithromycin release kinetics from CL9 batch was studied using standard mathematical models. Goodness of fit models were selected by evaluating the r^2 value, sum of squares of residuals, and Fischer ratio in order to avoid errors in the prediction of the release mechanism [29]. The data indicated higher

r^2 value (0.9736), least squares of residuals value (121.54), and Fischer ratio value (17.36) with Weibull model kinetics. Furthermore, the diffusion exponent value ($n < 0.5$) implied the Fickian diffusion mechanism of clarithromycin from CL9.

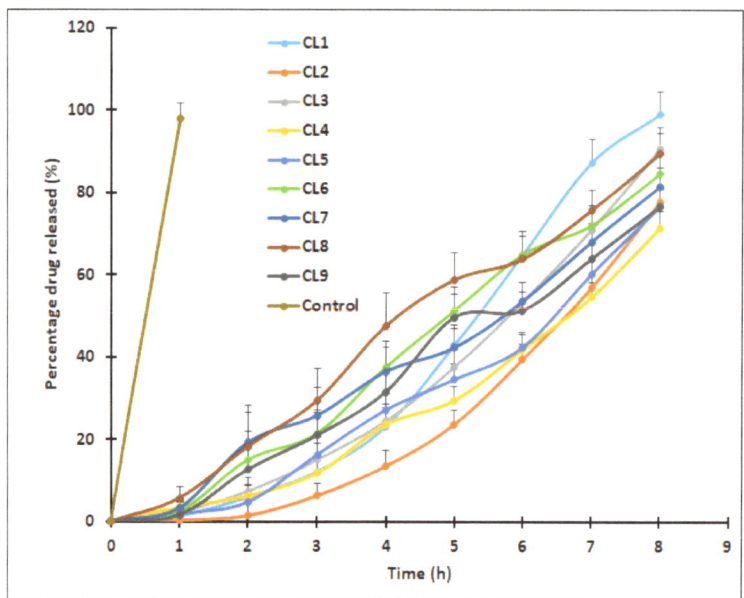

Figure 8. Comparison of percentage of clarithromycin release from solid lipid nanoparticles (CL1–CL9) and drug solution (control). Data represented are mean $\pm$ S.D. (n = 6).

3.6. Design Space

Since it is difficult to predict the influence of SLN composition and preparation technique on the particle size and percent entrapment efficiency, systematic approaches such as quality by design (QbD) were applied to comprehensively analyze and characterize the design space of the formulation. Using design expert software, design space was obtained by selecting the required range for each dependent variable to obtain the optimized batch. The optimized batch was selected by adding flags to the design space at the design point, which showed that the best response was selected as the optimized batch, and it was further evaluated. Figure 9 shows the overlay plot for the optimized SLN batch (CL10) with low particle size (147 nm), higher entrapment efficiency (83.6%), and good drug loading (26.5%), and its corresponding value of X1 (amount of lipid in mg) was 149.64 and X2 (sonication time in min) was 5.8. Based on these values, the optimized batch was prepared (composition in Table 7). The optimized batch was further evaluated, and the comparison of values (overlay plot-predicted and practical-observed) of dependent variables is shown in Table 8. It was revealed that the predicted values and observed values were similar to each other. The representative size distribution curve and zeta potential distribution of CL10 are depicted in Figure 10.

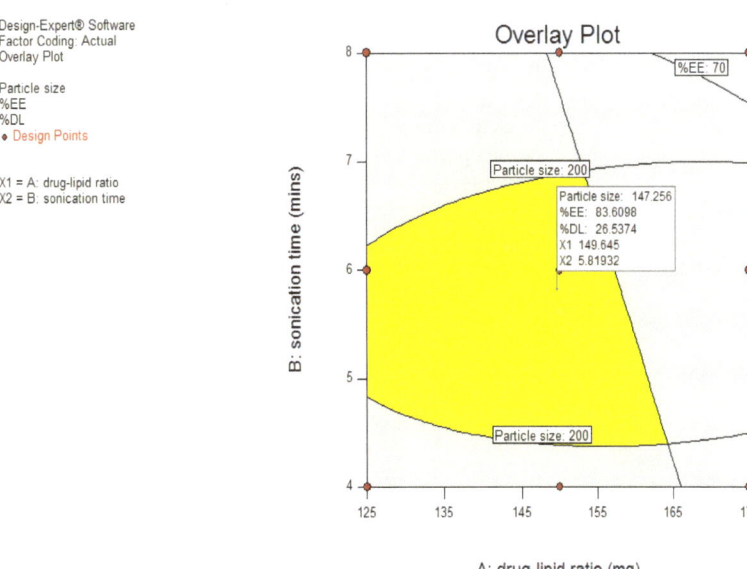

Figure 9. Overlay plot of optimized solid lipid nanoparticle batch using design space.

Table 7. Composition of optimized solid lipid nanoparticle batch (CL10) based on design space.

Ingredients	Quantity
Stearic acid	149.64 mg
Tween 80	0.3 mL
Transcutol P	0.3 mL
Water	20 mL
Ethanol	5 mL
Homogenization speed	9000 rpm
Sonication time	5.8 min

Table 8. Evaluation of optimized solid lipid nanoparticle batch (CL10).

Parameter	Predicted Value	Observed Value *
Entrapment efficiency (%)	83.6	81.3 ± 4.6
Drug loading (%)	26.5	27.1 ± 3.9
Particle size (nm)	147	157 ± 42.4
Polydispersity index	0.12	0.13 ± 0.02
Zeta potential (mV)	−18.4	−17.2 ± 3.1
In vitro drug release (%)	87	89.4 ± 4.5

* All values are expressed as mean ± S.D.; $n = 6$.

3.7. Trans-Corneal Permeation

Goat cornea was used for the ex vivo drug permeation investigations for the optimized SLNs (CL10) and control (solution). Various studies have used the goat membrane as a barrier, as this membrane is multi-layered and mimics the human corneal membrane [54]. It is well known that the physico-chemical characteristics of the drug, physiology of the membrane, and the availability of transport routes can affect the permeation of drug molecules into and through the biological membrane [55,56]. The amount of clarithromycin permeated through the cornea membrane from the formulation and control are depicted in Figure 11. Two distinct permeation profiles were noticed, with greater flux (30.45 µg/cm^2/h; $p < 0.0001$) exhibited by CL10 when compared with control (10.94 µg/cm^2/h). In the case of CL10, permeation was rapid in the initial 3 h (142.2 ± 14.1 µg/cm^2), while it was relatively slow and low with the control (33.7 ± 11.1 µg/cm^2 in 3 h). The greater permeation noticed in the optimized CL10 indicates that the pharmaceutical characteristics of the prepared SLNs (Table 8) are ideal for cornea permeation. Indeed, the higher clarithromycin permeation observed with CL10 suggests that the drug transport could be prominently due to the nanoparticles, as the drug permeation was very low in the control. Moreover, the greater drug concentration above therapeutic levels observed here is also important, as it will avoid microbial resistance. Overall, the observed data here signifies that the SLN could be an ideal carrier for the ocular delivery of clarithromycin.

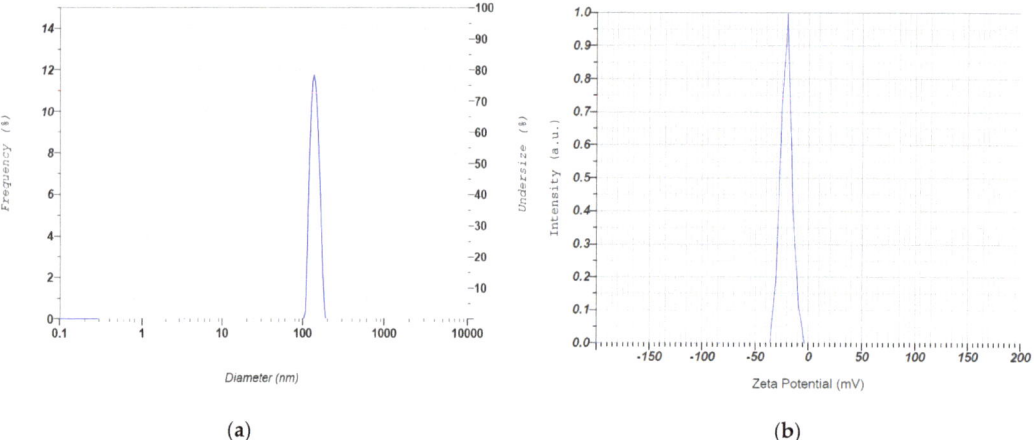

Figure 10. Representative size distribution curve (**a**) and zeta potential distribution (**b**) of optimized clarithromycin solid lipid nanoparticle (CL10).

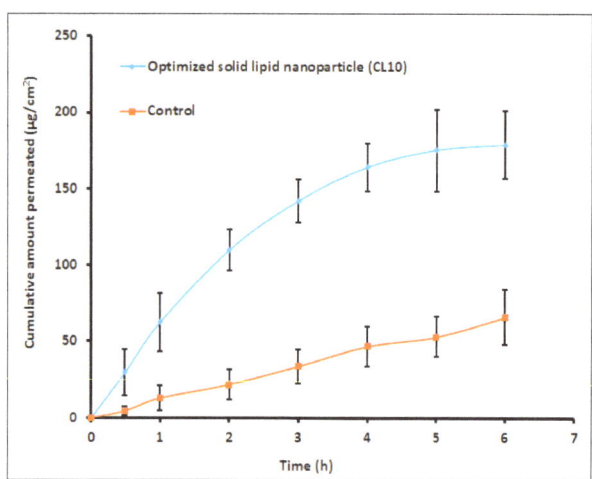

Figure 11. Cumulative amount of clarithromycin permeated through the goat cornea from solid lipid nanoparticles (CL10) and control (solution). Data represented are mean ± S.D. ($n = 6$).

3.8. TEM

A representative TEM micrograph of the optimized SLN (CL10) is shown in Figure 12. The image shows the drug encapsulated in the lipid matrix. It was also observed that the lipid nanoparticles were coarsely spherical in shape and uniformly distributed. The particle size was found to be in the range of 100–200 nm. The particle size range observed in TEM image was in good agreement with the values observed in particle size analysis.

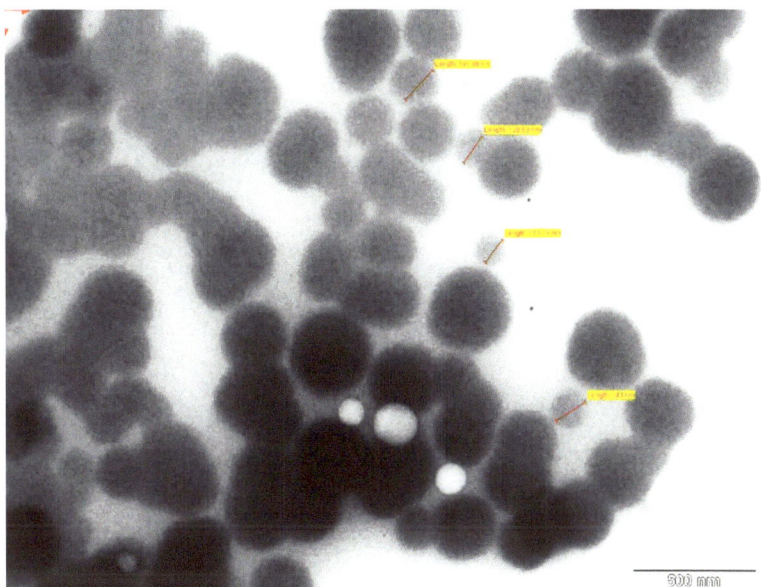

Figure 12. Surface morphology of optimized clarithromycin solid lipid nanoparticles (CL10). Red arrow indicates the diameter of nanoparticle.

3.9. Ocular Compatibility

Eye irritation score from individual rabbits was added to obtain the total irritation score, which was subsequently divided by the total number of eyes used for the ocular irritancy test to obtain the final eye irritation score. The calculated eye irritation score in CL10 was 0.50, while it was 0.17 in the reference. The irritation score observed in CL10 was relatively low and could be classified as practically non-irritant [57]. Further, instillation of CL10 did not cause redness, swelling, or excessive lachrymation in the eye. Overall, the data signified that CL10 is safe and non-irritant for ocular administration.

3.10. Pharmacokinetics

Ocular bioavailability is calculated as the amount of clarithromycin in the aqueous humor of rabbit eyes of first (CL10) and second groups (control) after single dose administration. The efficacy of topical antibiotics relies on the potential of the formulation to permeate across the corneal tissues and deliver an effective antimicrobial level in the target area. Various pharmacokinetic parameters including t_{max}, C_{max}, and AUC were computed from the graph plotted between concentrations (ng/mL) in aqueous humor and time (h) by non-compartment model analysis. Data in Figure 13 signify that the drug aqueous humor level in CL10 and control were significantly different throughout the study period in the current experimental conditions. A certain amount of drug was detected in 0.5 h in both cases. The amount of clarithromycin permeated in control experiments could be related to the drug's lipophilic nature and high partition coefficient. At 1 h, the clarithromycin level increased (881.08 ± 80.96 ng/mL and 654.99 ± 39.53 ng/mL in CL10 and control, respectively), though it was statistically different ($p < 0.0001$). At 2 h, absorption of clarithromycin in CL10 was extended, and the drug level reached ~1000 ng/mL, while the clarithromycin level declined sharply in the control (~500 ng/mL). These data signify that ophthalmic drops were retained in the ocular cavity for a short time because of extensive pre-corneal drug loss through nasolacrimal discharge and tear turnover. Further, the t_{max} value for CL10 was 2 h, while it was 1 h in the control. On the other hand, CL10 showed a 150% increase in C_{max} (~1066 ng/mL) and a 2.8-fold improvement in AUC (5736 ng h/mL) ($p < 0.0001$) as compared to the control solution (C_{max}; 655 ng/mL and AUC; 2067 ng h/mL). Thus, it can be concluded from the available data that intraocular permeation of clarithromycin was significantly improved by the optimized SLNs. This observation is also in agreement with ex vivo permeation data, wherein the flux was considerably higher in CL10 (Figure 11). The ocular pharmacokinetics data observed with CL10 were also significantly higher than the values reported in the literature tested with same concentration of clarithromycin eye drops [58]. Therefore, ocular residence time of CL10 proved extended duration of action in comparison to control. The average drug concentration noticed in Figure 13 in the aqueous humor was more than the minimum effective concentration of clarithromycin in various bacterial endophthalmitis [59].

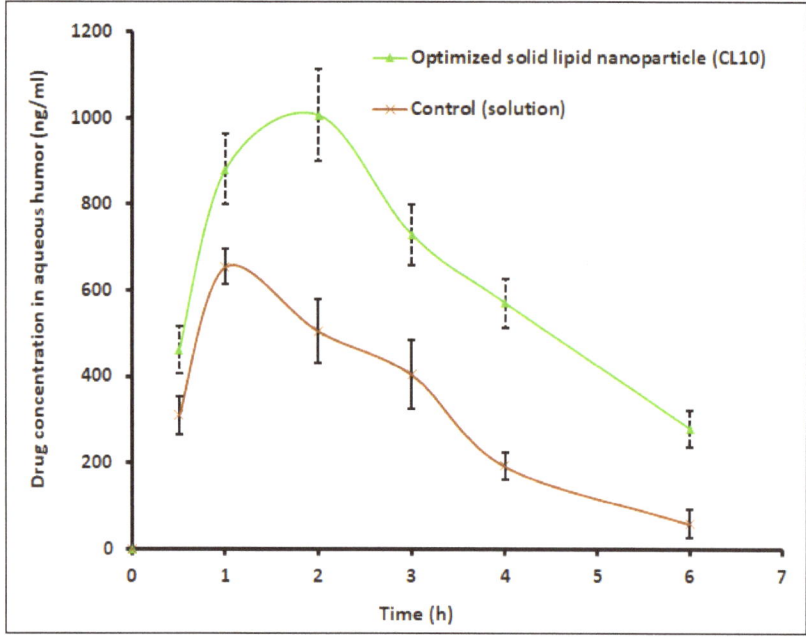

Figure 13. Ocular pharmacokinetics profile of clarithromycin after topical application of solid lipid nanoparticle (CL10) and control (solution) in rabbits. Data represented are mean ± S.D. ($n = 6$).

3.11. Stability

The optimized clarithromycin SLN (CL10) showed no significant variation in the drug content, particle size, or drug release after 3 months in both storage conditions (4 °C and 25 °C), as noticed in Table 9. Therefore, the stability data indicate good physical stability of the prepared SLNs during their storage at 4 °C and 25 °C for 3 months.

Table 9. Stability data of optimized solid lipid nanoparticle batch (CL10) after 3 months.

Parameter	Refrigerated Temperature	Room Temperature
Drug content (%)	97.6 ± 4.9	95.8 ± 4.6
Particle size (nm)	165 ± 54.6	172 ± 61.5
In vitro drug release (%)	88.8 ± 7.1	86.3 ± 5.0

All values are expressed as mean ± S.D.; $n = 6$.

4. Conclusions

The solubility of clarithromycin in various lipid and surfactants was studied, and based on solubility criteria, stearic acid (lipid), Tween 80 (nonionic surfactant), and Transcutol P (cosurfactant) were selected for the preparation of SLNs. Initial fractional factorial design suggests that the sonication time and amount of lipid significantly influence the SLN formulation. Further, 3^2 full factorial design data also confirms that both the factors significantly affect the particle size, drug entrapment efficiency, and drug loading. The drug content and entrapment efficiency of SLNs were enhanced by increasing the concentration of lipid since higher hydrophobicity of the longer chain of stearic acid resulted in a high-loaded clarithromycin. Ex vivo permeation and in vivo pharmacokinetics data signify greater efficacy by the optimized clarithromycin-loaded SLN (CL10). Indeed, the clarithromycin observed in the aqueous humor was significantly higher than the minimum effective concentration of clarithromycin in bacterial endophthalmitis. Further, the topical ocular therapy of clarithromycin could be more advantageous than its oral counterpart because topical administration could minimize the side effects as well as diminish the possibility of producing resistant strains of bacteria. Being a noninvasive approach, topical ocular therapy is more preferred and possesses higher patient compliance in the treatment of various diseases in the anterior segment. Thus, the developed SLN of clarithromycin-loaded nanoparticles has greater potential and can be a promising alternative to conventional therapy for the effective management of bacterial endophthalmitis. Further studies need to be carried out to understand the interaction of SLNs with the biological environment for successful commercialization and regulatory approval.

Author Contributions: Conceptualization, A.B.N., J.S., B.E.A.-D., and S.J.; Data Curation, A.B.N., J.S., S.S.P., M.A.M., S.G., and M.A.; Formal Analysis, A.B.N., J.S., B.E.A.-D., S.J., S.S.P., K.N.V., and M.A.M.; Funding Acquisition, A.B.N., J.S., B.E.A.-D., K.N.V., M.A.M., M.A., and N.S.; Investigation, A.B.N., J.S., B.E.A.-D., S.J., S.S.P., K.N.V., M.A.M., S.G., M.A., N.S., and P.S.; Methodology, A.B.N., J.S., B.E.A.-D., S.J., S.S.P., K.N.V., M.A.M., S.G., M.A., N.S., and P.S.; Writing—Original Draft Preparation, S.S.P., K.N.V., M.A.M., S.G., M.A., N.S., and P.S.; Writing—Review and Editing, A.B.N., J.S., B.E.A.-D., and S.J. All authors have read and agreed to the published version of the manuscript.

Funding: This research was funded by the Deanship of Scientific Research, King Faisal University, grant number 1811021, and the APC was funded by the Deanship of Scientific Research, King Faisal University.

Institutional Review Board Statement: The study was conducted according to the guidelines of the Declaration of Helsinki, and approved by the Institutional Ethics Committee of Nirma University (protocol Number IP/PCEU/FAC/21/029; dated 9 June 2017).

Informed Consent Statement: Not applicable.

Data Availability Statement: The data presented in this study are contained within the article.

Acknowledgments: The authors thank the Deanship of Scientific Research at King Faisal University for the financial support of research project number 1811021.

Conflicts of Interest: The authors declare no conflict of interest.

References

1. Shah, J.; Nair, A.B.; Jacob, S.; Patel, R.K.; Shah, H.; Shehata, T.M.; Morsy, M.A. Nanoemulsion Based Vehicle for Effective Ocular Delivery of Moxifloxacin Using Experimental Design and Pharmacokinetic Study in Rabbits. *Pharmaceutics* **2019**, *11*, 230. [CrossRef]
2. Lin, S.; Ge, C.; Wang, D.; Xie, Q.; Wu, B.; Wang, J.; Nan, K.; Zheng, Q.; Chen, W. Overcoming the Anatomical and Physiological Barriers in Topical Eye Surface Medication Using a Peptide-Decorated Polymeric Micelle. *ACS Appl. Mater. Interfaces* **2019**, *11*, 39603–39612. [CrossRef]
3. Varela-Fernández, R.; Díaz-Tomé, V.; Luaces-Rodríguez, A.; Conde-Penedo, A.; García-Otero, X.; Luzardo-Álvarez, A.; Fernández-Ferreiro, A.; Otero-Espinar, F.J. Drug Delivery to the Posterior Segment of the Eye: Biopharmaceutic and Pharmacokinetic Considerations. *Pharmaceutics* **2020**, *12*, 269. [CrossRef]
4. Shah, J.N.; Shah, H.J.; Groshev, A.; Hirani, A.A.; Pathak, Y.V.; Sutariya, V. Nanoparticulate transscleral ocular drug delivery. *J. Biomol. Res. Ther.* **2014**, *3*, 1–14.
5. Durand, M.L. Endophthalmitis. *Clin. Microbiol. Infect.* **2013**, *19*, 227–234. [CrossRef]
6. Kernt, M.; Kampik, A. Endophthalmitis: Pathogenesis, clinical presentation, management, and perspectives. *Clin. Ophthalmol. Auckl. N.Z.* **2010**, *4*, 121–135. [CrossRef]
7. Yang, L.; Dong, X.; Wu, X.; Xie, L.; Min, X. Intravitreally implantable voriconazole delivery system for experimental fungal endophthalmitis. *Retin. Phila. Pa.* **2011**, *31*, 1791–1800. [CrossRef]
8. Silva, N.C.; Silva, S.; Sarmento, B.; Pintado, M. Chitosan nanoparticles for daptomycin delivery in ocular treatment of bacterial endophthalmitis. *Drug Deliv.* **2015**, *22*, 885–893. [CrossRef] [PubMed]
9. Gutiérrez-Castrellón, P.; Mayorga-Buitron, J.L.; Bosch-Canto, V.; Solomon-Santibañez, G.; de Colsa-Ranero, A. Efficacy and safety of clarithromycin in pediatric patients with upper respiratory infections: A systematic review with meta-analysis. *Rev. Invest. Clin.* **2012**, *64*, 126–135. [PubMed]
10. Anonymous. Clarithromycin. *Tuberculosis* **2008**, *88*, 92–95. [CrossRef]
11. Rodvold, K.A. Clinical pharmacokinetics of clarithromycin. *Clin. Pharmacokinet.* **1999**, *37*, 385–398. [CrossRef]
12. Pai, M.P.; Graci, D.M.; Amsden, G.W. Macrolide drug interactions: An update. *Ann. Pharmacother.* **2000**, *34*, 495–513. [CrossRef]
13. Ali, A.; Ansari, V.A.; Ahmad, U.; Akhtar, J.; Jahan, A. Nanoemulsion: An Advanced Vehicle For Efficient Drug Delivery. *Drug Res.* **2017**, *67*, 617–631. [CrossRef] [PubMed]
14. Duong, V.A.; Nguyen, T.T.; Maeng, H.J. Preparation of Solid Lipid Nanoparticles and Nanostructured Lipid Carriers for Drug Delivery and the Effects of Preparation Parameters of Solvent Injection Method. *Mol. Basel Switz.* **2020**, *25*, 4781. [CrossRef] [PubMed]
15. Borges, A.; Freitas, V.; Mateus, N.; Fernandes, I.; Oliveira, J. Solid Lipid Nanoparticles as Carriers of Natural Phenolic Compounds. *Antioxid. Basel Switz.* **2020**, *9*, 998. [CrossRef] [PubMed]
16. Rajpoot, K. Solid Lipid Nanoparticles: A Promising Nanomaterial in Drug Delivery. *Curr. Pharm. Des.* **2019**, *25*, 3943–3959. [CrossRef] [PubMed]
17. Kamboj, S.; Bala, S.; Nair, A.B. Solid Lipid Nanoparticles: An Effective Lipid Based Technology for Poorly Water Soluble Drugs. *Int. J. Pharm. Sci. Rev. Res.* **2010**, *5*, 78–90.
18. Wissing, S.A.; Kayser, O.; Müller, R.H. Solid lipid nanoparticles for parenteral drug delivery. *Adv. Drug Deliv. Rev.* **2004**, *56*, 1257–1272. [CrossRef]
19. Weber, S.; Zimmer, A.; Pardeike, J. Solid Lipid Nanoparticles (SLN) and Nanostructured Lipid Carriers (NLC) for pulmonary application: A review of the state of the art. *Eur. J. Pharm. Biopharm.* **2014**, *86*, 7–22. [CrossRef] [PubMed]
20. Paliwal, R.; Paliwal, S.R.; Kenwat, R.; Kurmi, B.D.; Sahu, M.K. Solid lipid nanoparticles: A review on recent perspectives and patents. *Expert Opin. Ther. Pat.* **2020**, *30*, 179–194. [CrossRef]
21. Garcês, A.; Amaral, M.H.; Sousa Lobo, J.M.; Silva, A.C. Formulations based on solid lipid nanoparticles (SLN) and nanostructured lipid carriers (NLC) for cutaneous use: A review. *Eur. J. Pharm. Sci. Off. J. Eur. Fed. Pharm. Sci.* **2018**, *112*, 159–167. [CrossRef] [PubMed]
22. Salah, E.; Abouelfetouh, M.M.; Pan, Y.; Chen, D.; Xie, S. Solid lipid nanoparticles for enhanced oral absorption: A review. *Colloids Surf. B Biointerfaces* **2020**, *196*, 111305. [CrossRef]
23. Sánchez-López, E.; Espina, M.; Doktorovova, S.; Souto, E.B.; García, M.L. Lipid nanoparticles (SLN, NLC): Overcoming the anatomical and physiological barriers of the eye—Part II—Ocular drug-loaded lipid nanoparticles. *Eur. J. Pharm. Biopharm.* **2017**, *110*, 58–69. [CrossRef]
24. Lu, Y.; Zhang, Y.; Yang, Z.; Tang, X. Formulation of an intravenous emulsion loaded with a clarithromycin-phospholipid complex and its pharmacokinetics in rats. *Int. J. Pharm.* **2009**, *366*, 160–169. [CrossRef] [PubMed]
25. Das, S.; Ng, W.K.; Kanaujia, P.; Kim, S.; Tan, R.B. Formulation design, preparation and physicochemical characterizations of solid lipid nanoparticles containing a hydrophobic drug: Effects of process variables. *Colloids Surf. B Biointerfaces* **2011**, *88*, 483–489. [CrossRef]
26. Severino, P.; Santana, M.H.A.; Souto, E.B. Optimizing SLN and NLC by 22 full factorial design: Effect of homogenization technique. *Mater. Sci. Eng. C* **2012**, *32*, 1375–1379. [CrossRef]
27. Harsha, S.N.; Aldhubiab, B.E.; Nair, A.B.; Alhaider, I.A.; Attimarad, M.; Venugopala, K.N.; Srinivasan, S.; Gangadhar, N.; Asif, A.H. Nanoparticle formulation by Büchi B-90 Nano Spray Dryer for oral mucoadhesion. *Drug Des. Dev. Ther.* **2015**, *9*, 273–282. [CrossRef]

28. Nair, A.B.; Al-Dhubiab, B.E.; Shah, J.; Attimarad, M.; Harsha, S. Poly (lactic acid-co-glycolic acid) Nanospheres improved the oral delivery of candesartan cilexetil. *Indian J. Pharm. Educ. Res* **2017**, *51*, 571–579. [CrossRef]
29. Öztürk, A.A.; Aygül, A.; Şenel, B. Influence of glyceryl behenate, tripalmitin and stearic acid on the properties of clarithromycin incorporated solid lipid nanoparticles (SLNs): Formulation, characterization, antibacterial activity and cytotoxicity. *J. Drug Deliv. Sci. Technol.* **2019**, *54*, 101240. [CrossRef]
30. Nair, A.; Gupta, R.; Vasanti, S. In vitro controlled release of alfuzosin hydrochloride using HPMC-based matrix tablets and its comparison with marketed product. *Pharm. Dev. Technol.* **2007**, *12*, 621–625. [CrossRef]
31. Nair, A.B.; Shah, J.; Jacob, S.; Al-Dhubiab, B.E.; Sreeharsha, N.; Morsy, M.A.; Gupta, S.; Attimarad, M.; Shinu, P.; Venugopala, K.N. Experimental design, formulation and in vivo evaluation of a novel topical in situ gel system to treat ocular infections. *PLoS ONE* **2021**, *16*, e0248857. [CrossRef]
32. Nair, A.B.; Jacob, S.; Al-Dhubiab, B.E.; Alhumam, R.N. Influence of skin permeation enhancers on the transdermal delivery of palonosetron: An in vitro evaluation. *J. Appl. Biomed.* **2018**, *16*, 192–197. [CrossRef]
33. Shah, J.; Nair, A.B.; Shah, H.; Jacob, S.; Shehata, T.M.; Morsy, M.A. Enhancement in antinociceptive and anti-inflammatory effects of tramadol by transdermal proniosome gel. *Asian J. Pharm. Sci.* **2020**, *15*, 786–796. [CrossRef]
34. Wilhelmus, K.R. The Draize eye test. *Surv. Ophthalmol.* **2001**, *45*, 493–515. [CrossRef]
35. Wilson, S.L.; Ahearne, M.; Hopkinson, A. An overview of current techniques for ocular toxicity testing. *Toxicology* **2015**, *327*, 32–46. [CrossRef]
36. Nair, A.; Morsy, M.A.; Jacob, S. Dose translation between laboratory animals and human in preclinical and clinical phases of drug development. *Drug Dev. Res.* **2018**, *79*, 373–382. [CrossRef] [PubMed]
37. Singh, M.; Guzman-Aranguez, A.; Hussain, A.; Srinivas, C.S.; Kaur, I.P. Solid lipid nanoparticles for ocular delivery of isoniazid: Evaluation, proof of concept and in vivo safety & kinetics. *Nanomed. Lond. Engl.* **2019**, *14*, 465–491. [CrossRef]
38. Nair, A.B.; Sreeharsha, N.; Al-Dhubiab, B.E.; Hiremath, J.G.; Shinu, P.; Attimarad, M.; Venugopala, K.N.; Mutahar, M. HPMC- and PLGA-Based Nanoparticles for the Mucoadhesive Delivery of Sitagliptin: Optimization and In Vivo Evaluation in Rats. *Mater. Basel Switz.* **2019**, *12*, 4239. [CrossRef] [PubMed]
39. Dubald, M.; Bourgeois, S.; Andrieu, V.; Fessi, H. Ophthalmic Drug Delivery Systems for Antibiotherapy—A Review. *Pharmaceutics* **2018**, *10*, 10. [CrossRef] [PubMed]
40. Botto, C.; Mauro, N.; Amore, E.; Martorana, E.; Giammona, G.; Bondì, M.L. Surfactant effect on the physicochemical characteristics of cationic solid lipid nanoparticles. *Int. J. Pharm.* **2017**, *516*, 334–341. [CrossRef] [PubMed]
41. Parhi, R.; Suresh, P. Production of solid lipid nanoparticles-drug loading and release mechanism. *J. Chem. Pharm. Res.* **2010**, *2*, 211–227.
42. Pavoni, L.; Perinelli, D.R.; Bonacucina, G.; Cespi, M.; Palmieri, G.F. An Overview of Micro- and Nanoemulsions as Vehicles for Essential Oils: Formulation, Preparation and Stability. *Nanomater. Basel Switz.* **2020**, *10*, 135. [CrossRef] [PubMed]
43. Jiao, J. Polyoxyethylated nonionic surfactants and their applications in topical ocular drug delivery. *Adv. Drug Deliv. Rev.* **2008**, *60*, 1663–1673. [CrossRef] [PubMed]
44. Moiseev, R.V.; Morrison, P.W.J.; Steele, F.; Khutoryanskiy, V.V. Penetration Enhancers in Ocular Drug Delivery. *Pharmaceutics* **2019**, *11*, 321. [CrossRef] [PubMed]
45. Mehnert, W.; Mäder, K. Solid lipid nanoparticles: Production, characterization and applications. *Adv. Drug Deliv. Rev.* **2001**, *47*, 165–196. [CrossRef]
46. zur Mühlen, A.; Schwarz, C.; Mehnert, W. Solid lipid nanoparticles (SLN) for controlled drug delivery—Drug release and release mechanism. *Eur. J. Pharm. Biopharm. Off. J. Arb. Pharm. Verfahr.* **1998**, *45*, 149–155. [CrossRef]
47. Leong, T.S.H.; Martin, G.J.O.; Ashokkumar, M. Ultrasonic encapsulation—A review. *Ultrason. Sonochem.* **2017**, *35*, 605–614. [CrossRef]
48. Pradhan, S.; Hedberg, J.; Blomberg, E.; Wold, S.; Wallinder, I.O. Effect of sonication on particle dispersion, administered dose and metal release of non-functionalized, non-inert metal nanoparticles. *J. Nanopart. Res.* **2016**, *18*, 1–14. [CrossRef]
49. Sharma, M.; Gupta, N.; Gupta, S. Implications of designing clarithromycin loaded solid lipid nanoparticles on their pharmacokinetics, antibacterial activity and safety. *RSC Adv.* **2016**, *6*, 76621–76631. [CrossRef]
50. Baig, M.S.; Ahad, A.; Aslam, M.; Imam, S.S.; Aqil, M.; Ali, A. Application of Box-Behnken design for preparation of levofloxacin-loaded stearic acid solid lipid nanoparticles for ocular delivery: Optimization, in vitro release, ocular tolerance, and antibacterial activity. *Int. J. Biol. Macromol.* **2016**, *85*, 258–270. [CrossRef]
51. Shah, H.; Nair, A.B.; Shah, J.; Jacob, S.; Bharadia, P.; Haroun, M. Proniosomal vesicles as an effective strategy to optimize naproxen transdermal delivery. *J. Drug Deliv. Sci. Technol.* **2021**, *63*, 102479. [CrossRef]
52. Khames, A.; Khaleel, M.A.; El-Badawy, M.F.; El-Nezhawy, A.O.H. Natamycin solid lipid nanoparticles—Sustained ocular delivery system of higher corneal penetration against deep fungal keratitis: Preparation and optimization. *Int. J. Nanomed.* **2019**, *14*, 2515–2531. [CrossRef] [PubMed]
53. Zur Mühlen, A.; Mehnert, W. Drug incorporation and delivery of prednisolone loaded solid lipid nanoparticles. In Proceedings of the 1st World Meeting APGI/APV, Budapest, Hungary, 9–11 May 1995; pp. 9–11.
54. Ranch, K.M.; Maulvi, F.A.; Naik, M.J.; Koli, A.R.; Parikh, R.K.; Shah, D.O. Optimization of a novel in situ gel for sustained ocular drug delivery using Box-Behnken design: In vitro, ex vivo, in vivo and human studies. *Int. J. Pharm.* **2019**, *554*, 264–275. [CrossRef]

55. Nair, A.B.; Chakraborty, B.; Murthy, S.N. Effect of polyethylene glycols on the trans-ungual delivery of terbinafine. *Curr. Drug Deliv.* **2010**, *7*, 407–414. [CrossRef] [PubMed]
56. Nair, A.B.; Singh, K.; Al-Dhubiab, B.E.; Attimarad, M.; Harsha, S.; Alhaider, I.A. Skin uptake and clearance of ciclopirox following topical application. *Biopharm. Drug Dispos.* **2013**, *34*, 540–549. [CrossRef] [PubMed]
57. Wolska, E.; Sznitowska, M.; Chorążewicz, J.; Szerkus, O.; Radwańska, A.; Markuszewski, M.J.; Kaliszan, R.; Raczyńska, K. Ocular irritation and cyclosporine A distribution in the eye tissues after administration of Solid Lipid Microparticles in the rabbit model. *Eur. J. Pharm. Sci.* **2018**, *121*, 95–105. [CrossRef] [PubMed]
58. Zhang, J.; Wang, L.; Zhou, J.; Zhang, L.; Xia, H.; Zhou, T.; Zhang, H. Ocular penetration and pharmacokinetics of topical clarithromycin eye drops to rabbits. *J. Ocul. Pharmacol. Ther. Off. J. Assoc. Ocul. Pharmacol. Ther.* **2014**, *30*, 42–48. [CrossRef] [PubMed]
59. Brockhaus, L.; Goldblum, D.; Eggenschwiler, L.; Zimmerli, S.; Marzolini, C. Revisiting systemic treatment of bacterial endophthalmitis: A review of intravitreal penetration of systemic antibiotics. *Clin. Microbiol. Infect.* **2019**, *25*, 1364–1369. [CrossRef] [PubMed]

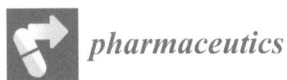

Article

Oligonucleotide Delivery across the Caco-2 Monolayer: The Design and Evaluation of Self-Emulsifying Drug Delivery Systems (SEDDS)

Jana Kubackova, Ondrej Holas, Jarmila Zbytovska, Barbora Vranikova, Guanghong Zeng, Petr Pavek and Anette Mullertz

1. Department of Pharmaceutical Technology, Faculty of Pharmacy in Hradec Kralove, Charles University, Akademika Heyrovskeho 1203, 500 05 Hradec Kralove, Czech Republic; kubackja@faf.cuni.cz (J.K.); Jarmila.Zbytovska@vscht.cz (J.Z.); vranikovab@faf.cuni.cz (B.V.)
2. Faculty of Chemical Technology, University of Chemistry and Technology Prague, Technicka 5, 166 28 Prague, Czech Republic
3. DFM A/S (Danish National Metrology Institute), Kogle Alle 5, 2970 Hørsholm, Denmark; GUZE@novonordisk.com
4. Department of Pharmacology, Faculty of Pharmacy in Hradec Kralove, Charles University, Akademika Heyrovskeho 1203, 500 05 Hradec Kralove, Czech Republic; pavek@faf.cuni.cz
5. Department of Pharmacy, Faculty of Health and Medical Sciences, University of Copenhagen, 2100 Copenhagen, Denmark; anette.mullertz@sund.ku.dk
6. Bioneer: FARMA, Department of Pharmacy, Faculty of Health and Medical Sciences, University of Copenhagen, Universitetsparken 2, 2100 Copenhagen, Denmark
* Correspondence: holao3aa@faf.cuni.cz; Tel.: +420495067412

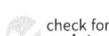

Citation: Kubackova, J.; Holas, O.; Zbytovska, J.; Vranikova, B.; Zeng, G.; Pavek, P.; Mullertz, A. Oligonucleotide Delivery across the Caco-2 Monolayer: The Design and Evaluation of Self-Emulsifying Drug Delivery Systems (SEDDS). *Pharmaceutics* 2021, 13, 459. https://doi.org/10.3390/pharmaceutics13040459

Academic Editor: Ana Catarina Silva

Received: 15 February 2021
Accepted: 24 March 2021
Published: 28 March 2021

Publisher's Note: MDPI stays neutral with regard to jurisdictional claims in published maps and institutional affiliations.

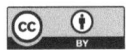

Copyright: © 2021 by the authors. Licensee MDPI, Basel, Switzerland. This article is an open access article distributed under the terms and conditions of the Creative Commons Attribution (CC BY) license (https://creativecommons.org/licenses/by/4.0/).

Abstract: Oligonucleotides (OND) represent a promising therapeutic approach. However, their instability and low intestinal permeability hamper oral bioavailability. Well-established for oral delivery, self-emulsifying drug delivery systems (SEDDS) can overcome the weakness of other delivery systems such as long-term instability of nanoparticles or complicated formulation processes. Therefore, the present study aims to prepare SEDDS for delivery of a nonspecific fluorescently labeled OND across the intestinal Caco-2 monolayer. The hydrophobic ion pairing of an OND and a cationic lipid served as an effective hydrophobization method using either dimethyldioctadecylammonium bromide (DDAB) or 1,2-dioleoyl-3-trimethylammonium propane (DOTAP). This strategy allowed a successful loading of OND-cationic lipid complexes into both negatively charged and neutral SEDDS. Subjecting both complex-loaded SEDDS to a nuclease, the negatively charged SEDDS protected about 16% of the complexed OND in contrast to 58% protected by its neutral counterpart. Furthermore, both SEDDS containing permeation-enhancing excipients facilitated delivery of OND across the intestinal Caco-2 cell monolayer. The negatively charged SEDDS showed a more stable permeability profile over 120 min, with a permeability of about 2×10^{-7} cm/s, unlike neutral SEDDS, which displayed an increasing permeability reaching up to 7×10^{-7} cm/s. In conclusion, these novel SEDDS-based formulations provide a promising tool for OND protection and delivery across the Caco-2 cell monolayer.

Keywords: oligonucleotide; self-emulsifying drug delivery systems; hydrophobic ion pairing; intestinal permeation enhancers; Caco-2 monolayer

1. Introduction

Gene therapy offers highly specific therapeutics without significant side effects. It covers a wide variety of approaches, ranging from the replacement of malfunctioning genetic information, often in the form of a large nonviral plasmid DNA (pDNA), to the currently more investigated oligonucleotide (OND)-based therapy acting on the level of mRNA destabilization or translation [1,2]. As for OND-based therapy, synthetic 20–30-mer nucleotides connected by phosphodiester bonds form a polyanionic backbone that determines the physicochemical properties of this hydrophilic macromolecule independently of the nucleotide sequence [3]. Therefore, there should be versatility in formulating OND for various applications. Nevertheless, the nucleotide structure is unstable in the presence of nucleases. Rapid enzymatic degradation combined with insufficient cellular uptake, often followed by entrapment in endosomes, makes the delivery of OND challenging [4]. Nonviral drug delivery systems, mainly lipid-based nanoformulations, have emerged as a promising option to overcome not only these limitations but, also, to enable oral delivery [5].

Oral delivery is the preferred route of administration—in particular, in the case of local gastrointestinal diseases. Many of these pathologies are defined or accompanied by intestinal inflammation, such as inflammatory bowel disease [6,7]. Novel colloidal drug delivery systems benefit from the enhanced permeation and retention effect of the inflamed tissue, which leads to increased accumulation of nanocarriers (~100–500 nm) within the leaky inflammatory site, which is also accompanied with an altered mucus layer [8,9]. Moreover, the increased accumulation of nanocarriers enables their uptake by phagocytic immune cells invading the area affected by inflammation; their rapid elimination due to diarrhea commonly present is avoided. In addition to the size of carriers, negative surface charge and hydrophilic surface decoration are also strategies utilized for passive targeting to the inflamed intestinal tissue [9–11]. The local delivery of OND has been investigated using many kinds of polymeric nanoparticles [12], lipid nanoparticles [13], microencapsulated nanogel [14], thioketal nanoparticles [15] and nanoparticles-in-microspheres multicompartment systems [16].

Self-emulsifying drug delivery systems (SEDDS) are isotropic mixtures of oils, surfactants, cosurfactants and cosolvents forming oil-in-water nanoemulsions upon gentle dispersion in an aqueous environment, e.g., gastrointestinal fluids [17]. These oral lipid-based drug delivery systems were originally established to improve the bioavailability of small poorly water-soluble molecules [18]. Recently, the delivery of hydrophilic macromolecules in SEDDS has gained increasing attention in order to take advantage of its beneficial properties, such as easy upscaling, nanosize of formed droplets and protection of the loaded substance from chemical and enzymatic degradation [19]. Nevertheless, the hydrophilicity of a potential hydrophilic substance needs to be reduced, usually by hydrophobic ion pairing [19]. The hydrophobic ion pairing of nucleic acids is a method based on replacing the counterions associated with negatively charged phosphate groups with surfactants carrying the positive charge. This method leads to a lipophilicity increase of the resulting ion-paired complexes [20]. For this purpose, positively charged surfactants, such as dimethyldioctadecylammonium bromide (DDAB) and 1,2-dioleoyl-3-trimethylammonium propane (DOTAP), are frequently utilized [21–24]. In addition, these quaternary ammonium salts enhance endosomal escape so the nucleic acid can reach the cytosol [25,26].

ONDs as hydrophilic macromolecules use predominantly paracellular transport through the intestinal monolayer; therefore, their permeability under physiological conditions is very limited [27]. Oral formulations containing intestinal permeation enhancers (PEs) have been widely investigated to enhance oral delivery of hydrophilic macromolecules [28]. PEs based on medium-chain fatty acids (MCFA) have been found to enhance paracellular transport via the opening of tight junctions (TJs) in a reversible manner by interaction with the cytoskeleton [29,30]. In addition, at higher concentrations the action of MCFA might be supported by transcellular permeation as a result of cell membrane alterations [28].

Hauptstein et al. pioneered the delivery of nucleic acids in SEDDS. In their research, several hydrophobic pDNA-cationic lipid complexes were tested. Among the tested cationic lipids, the complexes with cetrimide delivered in SEDDS showed a good transfection efficiency of HEK-293 cells comparable to Lipofectin®, a gold standard transfection reagent [31]. Mahmood et al. improved the transfection efficiency of pDNA-cetrimide in analogical SEDDS by the incorporation of a cell-penetrating peptide and confirmed an internalization of 50-nm nanoemulsions in Caco-2 cells [32]. Both studies focused on the delivery of large pDNA into cells. In contrast to considerably larger pDNA molecules, this study focuses on the delivery of short OND sequences as emerging, highly potent therapeutics.

The aim of this study was to prepare and characterize MCFA-based SEDDS loaded with hydrophobized OND and to investigate the ability of this system to deliver OND across the intestinal Caco-2 monolayer. This formulation approach has a considerable potential to overcome OND low stability and poor permeability. In this study, firstly, hydrophobized complexes of cationic lipids (DDAB or DOTAP) and a model fluorescently labeled 20-mer OND were thoroughly described and subsequently loaded into SEDDS (Figure 1). Dispersed SEDDS (negatively charged or neutral SEDDS) were characterized in terms of size, zeta potential, lipolysis, protective effect against nucleases and OND permeability.

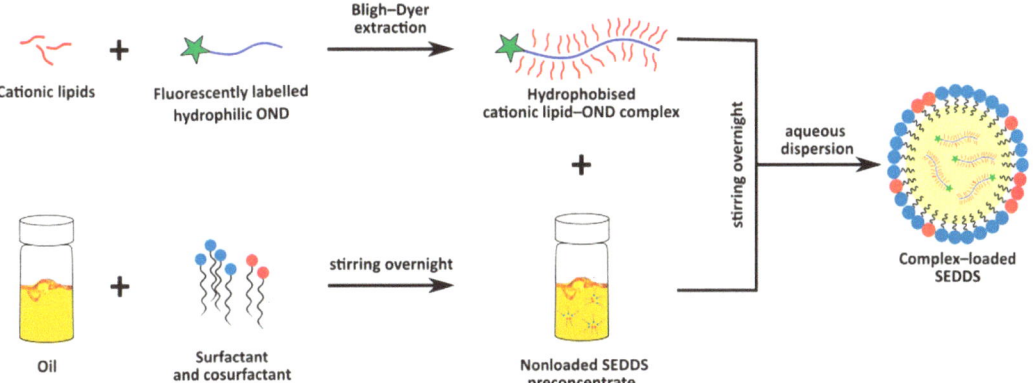

Figure 1. A general scheme showing the formulation of an oligonucleotide (OND) into a self-emulsifying drug delivery system (SEDDS).

2. Materials and Methods

2.1. Materials

The 20-mer model 5′-6-carboxyfluorescein (FAM) labelled OND composed of random DNA nucleotides (molecular weight 6654.5 Da) was purchased from Generi Biotech (Hradec Kralove, Czech Republic). Lipoid S LPC 80® (LPC) (from soybeans, containing 80.8% monoacyl phosphatidylcholine and 13.2% phosphatidylcholine) and phospholipids Lipoid S PC (from soybeans, containing 98.0%phosphatidylcholine) were provided by Lipoid GmbH (Ludwigshafen am Rhein, Germany). Labrasol® (caprylocaproyl macrogol-8 glycerides), Maisine CC® (glyceryl monolinoleate) and Peceol® (glyceryl monooleate) were provided by Gattefossé (Saint-Priest, France). Captex 300® (glyceryl tricaprylate/tricaprate) was provided by Abitec (Columbus, OH, USA) and Citrem® (glycerides of citric acid) by Danisco-DuPont (Grindsted, Denmark). Dimethyldioctadecylammonium bromide (DDAB), bovine bile extract, maleic acid, porcine pancreatic lipase extract, bovine serum albumin (BSA), 2-(N-morpholino)ethansulfonic acid (MES), N-2-hydroxyethylpiperazine-N′-2-ethanesulfonic acid (HEPES) and orlistat were purchased from Sigma-Aldrich (now Merck, Darmstadt, Germany). 1,2-dioleoyl-3-trimethylammonium propane (chloride salt) (DOTAP) was purchased from Avanti Polar Lipids (Alabaster, AL, USA). Gibco® Hanks' Balanced Salt Solution (HBSS) was purchased from Thermo Fisher Scientific (Copenhagen, Denmark). S1 nuclease (Cat. No. EN0321) was purchased from Thermo Fisher Scientific (Waltham, MA, USA). Triethylamine 99.5%, glacial acetic acid 99.99%, and acetonitrile were of HPLC grade. Deionized (DI) water was purified by SG Ultraclear water systems (SG Ultra Clear™ 2002, SG Water GmbH, Barsbüttel, Germany). Hoechst 33342 and propidium iodide (PI) were purchased from Molecular Probes (Eugene, OR, USA). All other chemicals were of analytical grade and commercially available.

2.2. Complex Preparation

The OND and a cationic lipid (DDAB or DOTAP) were dissolved in 1 mL of Bligh–Dyer monophase consisting of chloroform:methanol:water 1:2.2:1, as previously described [33]. The monophase was separated into a two-phase system by the addition of an aliquot of 250 µL of water and chloroform. Subsequently, the mixture was vigorously vortexed for 1 min and centrifuged at $600\times g$ for 5 min to achieve complete phase separation. The chloroform phase containing OND complexed with DDAB and DOTAP was collected, and the solvent was evaporated under nitrogen flow. The amount of complexed OND was quantified indirectly from the amount of noncomplexed OND in the aqueous phase. The fluorescence of FAM-labeled OND was measured in the aqueous phase at the excitation and emission wavelengths of 495 nm and 520 nm, respectively, in a microplate reader (FLUOstar Omega, BMG Labtech, Ortenberg, Germany). Complexation efficiency (CE) was calculated as follows:

$$CE = [(\text{initial amount of OND} - \text{amount of OND present in aq.phase})/(\text{initial amount of OND})] \times 100\% \quad (1)$$

Various charge ratios (+/−) of the cationic ammonium head of a cationic lipid and the anionic phosphate group of the OND backbone were tested in order to achieve efficient CE (>95%), starting at the ratio 1:1 and increasing the amount of cationic lipid. Prepared complexes were stored at −20 °C until further use [22,23].

To evaluate the changes introduced by complexation of a cationic lipid and OND, a physical mixture was prepared at the charge ratio of cationic lipid:OND 3:1. The required amount of a cationic lipid was weighed in a 4 mL screw thread glass vial (Thermo Fisher Scientific (Waltham, MA, USA). It was dissolved in a volume of chloroform sufficient to completely dissolve the lipid. Chloroform was subsequently evaporated under a nitrogen stream. The corresponding amount of OND solution was added into the glass vial, and the solvent was evaporated under the nitrogen stream. Solid lipid and OND were mixed into a physical mixture.

2.3. Effect of SEDDS Lipid Excipients on Complex Stability

Cationic lipid–OND complexes were prepared in the Bligh–Dyer monophase (chloroform:methanol:water 1:2.2:1) and two phases separated with an aliquot of water and chloroform, as described in Section 2.2 [23]. The effect of the lipid excipients (Captex 300, Labrasol, LPC, Citrem, Maisine CC and Peceol) in the SEDDS on the complex stability was studied. A tested SEDDS lipid excipient in the amount relevant to SEDDS composition was dissolved in chloroform and added directly to the chloroform phase containing preformed complexes. As a control, pure chloroform was added. Water:methanol solution (ratio 1:1) was added to the aqueous layer in order to keep the ratio of the top and bottom layer constant. The system was vigorously vortexed for 1 min and subsequently centrifuged at $600\times g$ for 5 min. The amount of OND in the aqueous phase was determined by fluorescence, as described in Section 2.2. The CE of OND was calculated by Equation (1) and is indicated relative to the control (no added lipid).

2.4. Atomic Force Microscopy (AFM)

The morphology of OND and complexes was investigated by AFM imaging. AFM was performed on the Park NX20 (Park Systems, Suwon, South Korea) with tapping mode in the air, using PointProbe®Plus Non-Contact/Tapping Mode - High Resonance Frequency - Reflex Coating (known as PPP-NCHR) probes with a nominal tip radius of 7 nm. Samples deposited on freshly cleaved mica were used. For proper fixation of the nucleic acid, a divalent cation Mg^{2+} (10 mM) to electrostatically bridge the negatively charged surface of mica substrate to the anionic OND backbone was used [34,35]. Therefore, the mica was treated with 10-mM $MgSO_4$ for 5 min before the OND solution was applied.

Ten microliters of 1-nM OND solution was allowed to attach for 5 min, rinsed with DI water and dried under nitrogen flow. Mica surface treatment was not necessary to absorb lipophilic complexes. The samples of the complexes were initially dissolved in chloroform and subsequently diluted in methanol. Ten microliters of 0.01-nM complex solution in methanol were spin-coated on fresh mica at 1000 rpm. Results were analyzed by SPIP (Image Metrology A/S, Hørsholm, Denmark) using the Particle and Pore analysis module, which enables height and volume analyses of the particles.

2.5. Differential Scanning Calorimetry (DSC)

DSC was performed with the DSC 200 F3 Maia instrument (NETZSCH-Gerätebau GmbH, Selb, Germany). The samples, bulk lipids and their respective complexes were prepared as described in Section 2.2, and the physical mixtures of the same ratio between a cationic lipid:OND 3:1, prepared by mixing, were sealed in standard aluminum crucibles. The samples were cooled down to $-50\ °C$ and kept at this temperature under isothermal conditions for 10 min. The analysis was performed at a heating rate 10 K/min in the range from -50 to $150\ °C$. An empty sealed crucible was used as a reference. The obtained thermograms were evaluated by Proteus Software (NETZSCH-Gerätebau GmbH, Selb, Germany).

2.6. Attenuated Total Reflectance-Fourier-Transform Infrared (ATR-FTIR) Spectroscopy

FTIR spectra were recorded with the MB 3000-PH apparatus equipped with the MIRacle ATR sampling kit and the software Horizon MB (ABB MEASUREMENT & ANALYTICS, Zurich, Switzerland). ATR-FTIR measurement was performed on samples in a solid state placed over ZnSe ATR crystal. Typical spectra were accumulated over the spectral range 4000–400 cm^{-1} with the coaddition of 64 scans at a resolution of 16 cm^{-1} in triplicate. Reference spectra were also obtained and subtracted from the raw spectra. Spectra of blank lipids, complexes at different charge ratios, physical mixtures of cationic lipid:OND 3:1 and OND were obtained. In order to observe complex-specific bands, spectra of the respective cationic lipids and OND were subtracted from the spectra of a complex.

2.7. Preparation of SEDDS Formulations

The composition of the utilized SEDDS is depicted in Table 1, as described by Ramakrishnan Venkatasubramanian et al. (data not published, manuscript in preparation).

Table 1. Composition of the self-emulsifying drug delivery systems (SEDDS).

SEDDS	Captex 300 (%w/w)	Labrasol (%w/w)	Lipoid S LPC 80 (%w/w)	Citrem (%w/w)	Maisine CC (%w/w)	Peceol (%w/w)
Citrem (negatively charged)	20	40	20	20	-	-
Standard (neutral)	20	40	20	-	10	10

The structure of utilized SEDDS excipients is shown in Figure 2. All excipients were weighed in a glass vial and homogenized by stirring with a magnetic bar at 37 °C overnight. Two SEDDS were used, each differing in the surface charge: negatively charged Citrem SEDDS and neutral Standard SEDDS. The chosen SEDDS were reported to differ only in the surface charge while maintaining a comparable size suitable for targeting in leaky inflammatory lesions.

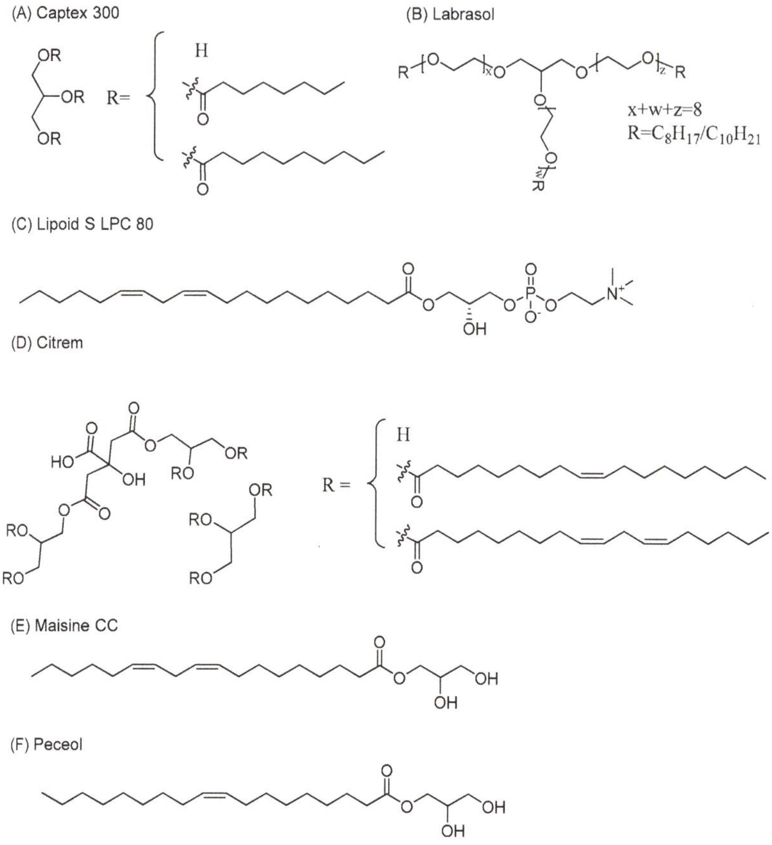

Figure 2. Chemical structures of SEDDS excipients (the structure of Labrasol was adapted from [36], and the structure of Citrem was adapted from [37]).

The SEDDS were loaded with the OND complexed with a cationic lipid, the cationic lipid itself or orlistat. The loaded substance was weighted into a vial. Subsequently, the amount of SEDDS was added to reach the required concentration of 100 nmol of a complex per 1 g of SEDDS, 3.8 mg of DDAB or 4.2 mg of DOTAP per 1 g of SEDDS. Orlistat inhibits the activity of gastrointestinal lipases, and in this study, it was used at a concentration of 0.25% (w/w), prepared as 2.5 mg of orlistat dissolved in 1 g of SEDDS. Loading was achieved by dissolution of the loaded substance in the SEDDS under stirring with a magnetic bar at 37 °C overnight. The loaded substances and their respective concentrations utilized throughout the study are summarized in Table 2. The amount of loaded cationic lipids was equivalent to the amount present in the ion-paired complexes.

Table 2. The loaded self-emulsifying drug delivery systems (SEDDS).

Name of Formulation	Loaded Substance	Concentration of Loaded Substance in SEDDS
DDAB-OND in SEDDS	Complex of DDAB and OND at the charge ratio 3:1	100 nmol of OND/g SEDDS
DOTAP-OND in SEDDS	Complex of DOTAP and OND at the charge ratio 3:1	100 nmol of OND/g SEDDS
DDAB in SEDDS	DDAB	3.8 mg/g SEDDS
DOTAP in SEDDS	DOTAP	4.2 mg/g SEDDS
SEDDS + Orlistat	Orlistat	0.25% (w/w)

DDAB: dimethyldioctadecylammonium bromide, DOTAP: 1,2-dioleoyl-3-trimethylammonium-propane (chloride salt) and OND: oligonucleotide.

2.8. Characterization of Dispersed SEDDS

The dispersions of both Citrem and Standard SEDDS were characterized in terms of size and polydispersity index (PdI) by dynamic light scattering; zeta potential was measured by laser Doppler electrophoresis using Zetasizer Nano ZS (Malvern Instruments, Worcestershire, UK). The dispersions of blank and complex-loaded SEDDS were dispersed 1:100 (w/w) in DI water and 10-mM MES-HBSS buffer (pH 6.5) immediately before the experiment and evaluated at 37 °C. Data were collected in triplicate.

2.9. Dynamic In Vitro Lipolysis of SEDDS

Dynamic one-compartment in vitro lipolysis was carried out under human fasted-state conditions, as previously described [38–40]. Nonloaded Citrem and Standard SEDDS both without and with the addition of orlistat 0.25% (w/w) were tested. The addition of orlistat, a lipase inhibitor, into the SEDDS composition has previously been described to inhibit the digestion of SEDDS [41]. SEDDS (0.5 g) was added into a temperature-controlled vessel containing fasted-state simulated intestinal fluid (FaSSIF) used as the lipolysis medium (2.95-mM bovine bile, 0.26-mM soy phospholipids, 2.0-mM maleic acid, 2.0-mM Tris, 50.0-mM NaCl and 1.4 mM $CaCl_2$, adjusted to pH 6.5). The digestion of the lipids was initiated by the addition of 5 mL of pancreatin solution with a final activity of 500 USP units/mL. The pancreatin solution was prepared by combining the appropriate amount of porcine pancreatin and adding intestinal lipolysis medium. The resulting suspension was vortexed and centrifuged (7 min, 6500× g). pH 6.5 was maintained by an automated pH stat (Metrohm Titrino 744, Tiamo Version 1.3, Herisau, Switzerland), as the released free fatty acids were continuously titrated by 0.4-M NaOH. The lipolysis was performed for 60 min in three independent experiments (n = 3).

2.10. Cryogenic Transmission Electron Microscopy

The structures formed upon the dispersion of the SEDDS 1:100 (w/w) in FaSSIF (Biorelevant, London, UK) at 37 °C were observed by cryogenic transmission electron microscopy (cryo-TEM). Individual samples (3.5 µL) were loaded on freshly glow-discharged TEM grids (Quantifoil, Cu, 200 mesh, R2/1) inside the Thermo Scientific Vitrobot Mark IV (Thermo Fisher Scientific, Waltham, MA, USA) and plunged frozen into liquid ethane. The Vitrobot chamber was kept at 4 °C and 100% relative humidity during the entire process. Each sample was incubated for 30 s on the grid and blotted for 5 s prior to vitrification. The grids were subsequently mounted into the Autogrid cartridge and loaded into the Thermo Scientific Talos Arctica transmission electron microscope (Thermo Fisher Scientific, Waltham, MA, USA). The microscope was operated at 200 kV, and cryo-TEM data was collected on the Thermo Scientific Falcon 3EC direct electron detector operating in charge integration mode. The micrographs were acquired using SerialEM software at magnifications corresponding to the calibrated pixel sizes of 22.16 Å/px and 3.15 Å/px, respectively. Each micrograph collected at 3.15 Å/px comprised an overall dose of 10 e/Å^2.

2.11. Degradation by Nucleases

In order to assess the ability of the SEDDS to protect the encapsulated OND complexes against degradation by nucleases, formulations were incubated with S1 nuclease (100 U/µL), an enzyme that specifically degrades single-stranded nucleic acids. Stability studies were carried out in the following formulations: aqueous solution of naked OND, aqueous dispersion of complexed DDAB-OND in the SEDDS and DOTAP-OND in the SEDDS and dispersion of the nonloaded SEDDS in an aqueous solution of naked OND. The SEDDS were dispersed immediately before the experiment.

The S1 nuclease assay (Thermo Fisher Scientific, Waltham, MA, USA) was performed according to the manufacturer's instructions. Briefly, equivalents containing 1.2 µg of OND were incubated with 12 U of S1 nuclease in the presence of the reaction buffer pH 4.5 at 25 °C. As controls, the same formulations were incubated in an acetate buffer of pH 4.5. The reaction was terminated after 30 min by the addition of 0.5-M EDTA and incubation for 10 min at 70 °C. Nondegraded intact OND was precipitated via ethanol precipitation. From each formulation, 60 µL was taken, and 1.3 µL of 5%NH_4OH, 30 µL of 7.5-M ammonium acetate and 400 µL of 96% ethanol were added into the samples, which were kept at −80 °C for at least one hour. Following this, the samples were centrifuged at 15,000× g for 30 min at 4 °C. Intact OND was pelleted and dissolved in 500 µL of 100-mM triethylammonium acetate (TEAA). The samples were subjected to HPLC analysis. Additionally, 100 µL of supernatant was diluted with 500 µL of 100-mM TEAA.

Thirty microliters of the samples were analyzed using the Waters Symmetry C18 (3.5 µm; 4.6 × 75 mm) HPLC column (Waters Corporation, Milford, MA, USA). The mobile phase consisted of 2 eluents, eluent A of 100-mM TEAA (pH 7.0) and eluent B of acetonitrile, with a linear gradient starting from 1 min at 10% to 30% B in 4 min. Thirty percent B eluent was maintained for 1 min, then decreased to 10% B in 1 min and maintained at this level for 4 min before analysis of the following sample. The flow rate was 1 mL/min. FAM-labeled OND was detected by fluorescent detection excitation/emission 495 nm/520 nm according to the procedure described previously [42]. Each formulation was tested in triplicate. The percentage of intact OND was calculated as a ratio of area under the curve (AUC) of protected OND found in the pellets after incubation with S1 nuclease and pelleted OND recovered from the respective formulations, as described by Equation (2).

$$\text{intact OND} = [\text{AUC of pelleted OND (formualtation + S1 nuclease)}/\text{AUC of pelleted OND (formulation)}] \times 100\% \quad (2)$$

2.12. Caco-2 Cell Monolayer Transport Study

Caco-2 cells, a model of human enterocyte epithelial cells, were obtained from the American Type Culture Collection (ATCC) (Manassas, VA, USA). The cells were seeded on T12 filter inserts (pore size 0.4 mm, 1.13 cm^2 growth area, Corning, Sigma–Aldrich, Copenhagen, Denmark) at a final density of 1 × 10^5 cells/cm^2. The cells were cultured for 20–23 days before the transport study was conducted.

Transport experiments were conducted on a horizontal shaker at 37 °C using a pH gradient mimicking physiological conditions. A volume of 500 µL of 10-mM MES-HBSS buffer (pH 6.5, 0.05% w/v BSA) was used on the apical side and 1000 µL of 10-mM HEPES-HBSS buffer (pH 7.4, 0.05% w/v BSA) on the basolateral one for 120 min. The experiment was initiated by applying 500 µL of a formulation on the apical side. The following formulations were tested: OND solution, DDAB-OND in the SEDDS, DOTAP-OND in the SEDDS, DDAB in the SEDDS dispersed in OND solution, DOTAP in the SEDDS in dispersed OND solution and nonloaded blank SEDDS dispersed in OND solution for both the Citrem and Standard SEDDS. The SEDDS were dispersed 1:100 (w/w) shortly before the experiment in a MES-HBSS-based buffer preheated to 37 °C. All formulations finally contained 1 nmol/mL of OND.

Transepithelial electrical resistance (TEER) was monitored with the EVOM Epithelial Voltohmmeter (World Precision Instruments, East Lyme, CT, USA). Before and after the experiment, the cell culture cup Endohm chamber was used at 25 °C in MES–HBSS and HEPES–HBSS applied apically and basolaterally, respectively. In addition, TEER values were also monitored using chopstick electrodes throughout the experiment at 30, 60, 90 and 120 min at 37 °C.

Samples of 100 µL were taken from the basolateral side at predetermined time points (15, 30, 45, 60, 90 and 120 min) and replaced with the same volume of fresh prewarmed HEPES-HBSS buffer. The withdrawn samples were analyzed for fluorescently labeled OND by measuring fluorescence excitation/emission wavelengths at 495/520 nm in a microplate reader (FLUOstar Omega, BMG Labtech, Ortenberg, Germany). The apparent permeability coefficient (P_{app}), and transported OND accumulated basolaterally across the Caco-2 monolayer were calculated using the following Equations (3) and (4).

$$P_{app} = J/C_0 = Q/(C_0 \times A) \quad (3)$$

$$\text{transported OND} = [Q/(0.5 \times C_0)] \times 100\% \quad (4)$$

where J indicates the flux over a steady-state time period (pmol/s/cm), and C_0 stands for the initial concentration of OND in the apical compartment (pmol/mL). Q is the accumulated mass of OND transported across the monolayer on the basolateral side (pmol) of the area A (cm^2) of membrane filters.

2.13. In Vitro Cytotoxicity Study

Cytotoxicity of the formulations was investigated as the loss of cell membrane integrity accompanied by release of a cytoplasm enzyme lactate dehydrogenase (LDH). The cytotoxicity study was conducted by the Cytotoxicity Detection Kit (LDH) (Roche, France) according to manufacturer's instructions after 120 min of the transport experiment in the Caco-2 cells. Briefly, a 40-µL sample of apical medium was diluted 5-fold by DI water. Fifty microliters of the diluted sample were pipetted into a clear 96-well multiwell plate in duplicates, and 50 µL of LDH reaction mixture was added. The 96-well plate was incubated for 30 min at 37 °C in a horizontal shaker in the dark. Subsequently, the absorbance was measured at 492 nm.

Results are depicted as cell viability (%). Relative cytotoxicity (%) was calculated according to the manufacturer's instructions, and the resulting values were deducted from 100% to obtain cell viability (%).

2.14. Uptake Study

Caco-2 cells were seeded onto confocal dishes (Nunc™ 4-well Rectangular Dishes, Thermo Fisher Scientific, Waltham, MA, USA) at a density of 10^5 cells/cm^2 and were cultured for 7 days until 100% confluence was reached. The experiment was initiated by the addition of 0.5 mL of a test sample. In order to mimic the intestinal environment, the test samples were prepared in 10-mM MES-HBSS buffer (pH 6.5, 0.05% *w/v* BSA). The uptake of OND was evaluated by testing the following samples: OND solution, nonloaded SEDDS dispersed in OND solution, DDAB-OND in SEDDS and DOTAP-OND in SEDDS dispersed in MES-HBSS buffer. The experiment was carried out for both Citrem and Standard SEDDS, and SEDDS were dispersed at 1:1000 (*w/w*). The cells were incubated with the samples for 2 h at 37 °C and 5% CO$_2$ without shaking. Fifteen minutes before the termination of the incubation, cell nuclei were stained by the addition of 10 µL of Hoechst 33342 (1 mg/mL). At the same timepoint, 10 µL of propidium iodide (PI) (0.1 mg/mL) was added to detect dead cells.

Immediately after incubation, cells were washed twice with prewarmed Opti-MEM® medium (Thermo Fisher Scientific, Waltham, MA, USA). Images were acquired with the Nikon Ti-E (Nikon, Minato, Japan) epifluorescence microscope equipped with a cooled scientific CMOS camera (AndorZyla 5.5; Andor Technology, Belfast, UK) and LED fluorescence source (CoolLED pE-300; CoolLED, Andover, UK). DAPI, FITC and Cy3 filter sets were used for image Hoechst, FAM-labeled OND and PI, respectively. Three representative images of each sample were taken using NIS Elements AR 4.20 software (Laboratory Imaging, Prague, Czech Republic).

2.15. Statistical Analysis

Statistical analysis was performed using Graph Prism 8 (GraphPad Software, San Diego, CA, USA). One-way ANOVA followed by Tukey's post-hoc test was carried out for the evaluation of size and zeta potential of the dispersed SEDDS. Two-way ANOVA followed by Tukey's test was performed to evaluate lipolysis data and in vitro data. One-way ANOVA followed by Dunnett's post-hoc test was used, as the impact of the other lipids on the complex stability was evaluated as well, as in the case of the in vitro data. Data are presented as mean ± standard deviation (SD). Significant difference was considered at $p < 0.05$.

3. Results

3.1. Complex Preparation

First, complexes of a cationic lipid and 20-mer fluorescently labeled OND were prepared using the Bligh–Dyer method [23,33]. Various charge ratios between a quaternary ammonium head group of a cationic lipid (N^+) and a nucleotide phosphate group in the backbone of 20-mer OND (PO_2^-) were investigated. Upon complexation, no visible precipitated material in the aqueous phase nor at the interface was observed. The CE of DDAB-OND and DOTAP-OND are depicted in Table 3. Efficient CE (>95%) was achieved for the charge ratio of cationic lipid:OND 3:1, which equals the molar ratio 60:1. Moreover, at this charge ratio, there was no significant difference in CE between DDAB and DOTAP. It is noteworthy that DOTAP also enables a more efficient hydrophobization of OND at a lower charge ratio than DDAB.

Table 3. Complexation efficiency (CE, %) of OND with a cationic lipid (DDAB or DOTAP) using the Bligh–Dyer method. Various charge ratios between a quaternary ammonium head group of a cationic lipid (N+) and a nucleotide phosphate group in the backbone of 20-mer OND (PO_2^-) were tested.

Charge Ratio N^+: PO_2^-	Molar Ratio Cationic Lipid: OND	CE (%)	
		DDAB	DOTAP
1:1	20:1	58.3 ± 0.7	84.6 ± 1.4
2:1	40:1	84.0 ± 2.8	100.1 ± 0.1
3:1	60:1	96.5 ± 2.0	100.4 ± 0.1

Results are presented as mean ± SD ($n = 3$).

3.2. Effect of SEDDS Lipid Excipents on Complex Stability

Next, the impact of the SEDDS excipients on the destabilization of the complexes was tested. The tested excipients included anionic Citrem, zwitterionic LPC and neutral Captex 300, Labrasol, Maisine CC and Peceol. The results from the combination of LPC and DOTAP-OND could not be determined as emulsification occurred, disabling phase separation under the method's conditions.

Only anionic Citrem had a negative impact on the stability of both DDAB-OND and DOTAP-OND ($p < 0.001$) (Table 4). Zwitterionic LPC and neutral excipients had no impact on the complex stability. These results are in accordance with the observations by Wong et al. [23].

Table 4. Effect of SEDDS excipients on the complex stability. The complexation efficiency (CE %) after interactions with a SEDDS excipient is reported relative to the control where no SEDDS excipient was added (CE = 100%).

SEDDS Excipient	CE (%)	
	DDAB-OND	DOTAP-OND
Citrem	97.3 ± 0.2 ***	97.7 ± 0.2 ***
LPC	100.0 ± 0.2	n.d.
Captex 300	100.3 ± 0.1	100.1 ± 0.1
Labrasol	100.5 ± 0.2	100.2 ± 0.1
Maisine CC	100.8 ± 0.1	100.4 ± 0.1
Peceol	100.2 ± 0.4	100.3 ± 0.1

*** statistically significant difference relative to a control with added lipid. Results are presented as mean ± SD (n = 3). n.d. = not determined.

3.3. Atomic Force Microscopy (AFM)

OND and the cationic lipid-OND complexes were imaged by AFM in order to compare their size and morphology. It is important to note that AFM imaging only provides information on surface immobilized structures, and the absolute accuracy is limited by the physical convolution between the tip (radius around 7 nm) and the sample. Nevertheless, AFM topography images are useful for comparing the sizes and for providing a direct observation of the morphology of the OND and complexes on the surfaces.

Figure 3A shows a topographic image of OND molecules dispersed on mica. The molecules were compacted instead of stretched out over the mica substrate, suggesting a potential effect of Mg^{2+} (a bridging agent used for deposition on the mica substrate) on the molecular conformation [34]. An analysis of height cross-sections indicates a step height of around 1 nm, which is in agreement with the size of a single strand DNA OND, as a double helix of DNA has a diameter of 20 Å (=2 nm) [43,44].

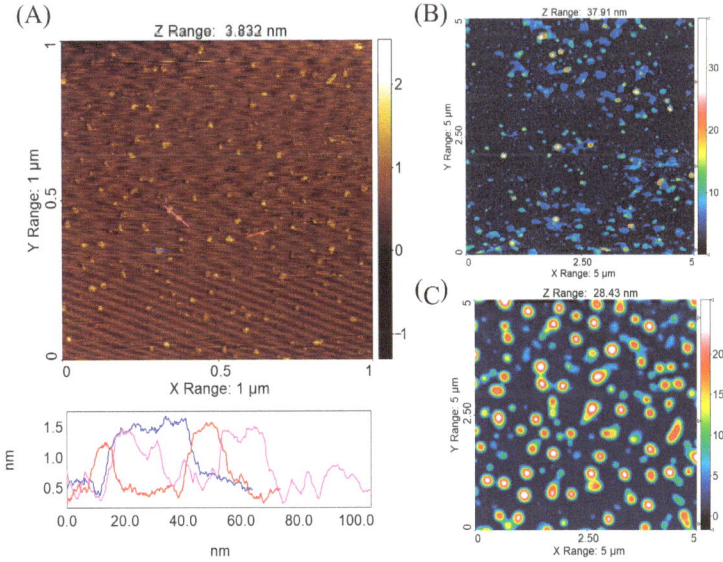

Figure 3. Atomic force microscopy (AFM) topography images of structures absorbed in air on mica: (**A**) OND—the height profile corresponds to three colored sections in the graph below the image, (**B**) dimethyldioctadecylammonium bromide (DDAB)-OND complex and (**C**) 1,2-dioleoyl-3-trimethylammonium propane (DOTAP)-OND complex, with both complexes prepared at a charge ratio 3:1 (cationic lipid:OND).

The AFM topographic image of DDAB-OND complexes (Figure 3B) reveals a mixture of nanoparticulate complexes and membrane patches which are presumably the result of collapsed lipid capsules during sample drying. The height of the membrane patches is 4 to 5 nm. In contrast, the topographic image of the DOTAP-OND complexes (Figure 3C) shows mostly homogenous and intact particles. Average height of the particles was 15.1 ± 6.3 nm ($n = 167$) and 20.9 ± 3.5 nm ($n = 70$) for DDAB-OND and DOTAP-OND, respectively. The actual height of both complexes in solution should be higher, as significant deformation is expected during drying and immobilization on the substrate during sample preparation. The spherical lipid capsule collapsed into a shape of a flattened disc, having maintained its volume. Using the reported particle volume from SPIP software, the diameter of the particles was calculated for the original thermodynamically favoured spherical shape. The expected diameters of the spherical complexes are in the range of 31.6–63.4 nm for the DDAB-OND complexes and 75.4–128.2 nm for the DOTAP-OND complexes.

3.4. Differential Scanning Calorimetry (DSC)

Figure 4 depicts thermograms of the bulk lipids (DDAB/DOTAP), physical mixtures (mix DDAB/DOTAP+OND) and complexes (DDAB/DOTAP-OND), both at the charge ratio 3:1. The bulk lipids showed melting peaks at 88.5 °C and 6.3 °C, respectively, for DDAB and DOTAP. This difference is a function of the chemical structure of the cationic lipids. Double bonds in DOTAP's aliphatic C18 chains lead to more loose packing, which provide more fluidity, resulting in a lower melting point [45].

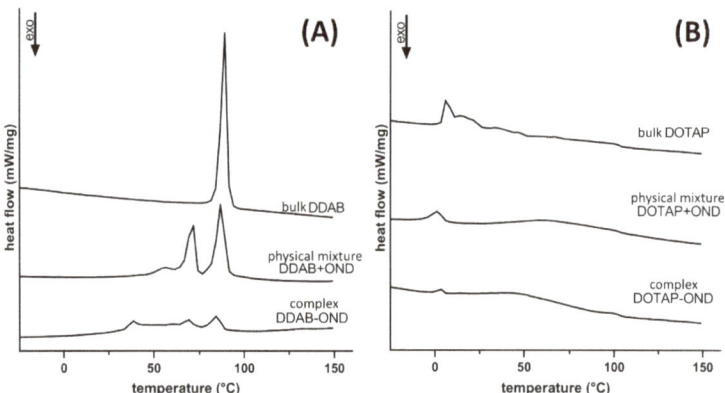

Figure 4. Differential scanning calorimetry of the bulk lipids, physical mixtures and complexes of (**A**) DDAB and (**B**) DOTAP. Thermograms were recorded from -50 up to 150 °C at the heating rate 10 °C/min.

For DDAB, both the physical mixture and the complex revealed several melting peaks, and they melted at lower temperatures (Figure 4A). The melting peaks were found at 56.5, 71.6 and 86.7 °C for the physical mixture and at 39.0, 68.3 and 85.0 °C for DDAB-OND. Evidently, the complex shows different thermotropic behavior compared to the physical mixture.

Upon mixing and complexing DOTAP with OND, the melting temperature decreased to 1.3 and 3.5 °C, respectively (Figure 4B).

3.5. ATR-FTIR Spectroscopy

In the region of the FTIR spectra depicting changes in base pairing (1800–1500 cm^{-1}), OND bands of 1643 cm^{-1} and 1605 cm^{-1} were observed (Figure 5A,B). Upon complex formation, these bands moved to the higher wavenumbers of 1659 cm^{-1} and 1697 cm^{-1}. The positive shift in this FTIR region suggests the disintegration of the hydrogen bonding network involved in base pairing [24,46]. Although the model OND is single-stranded, partial base pairing could arise.

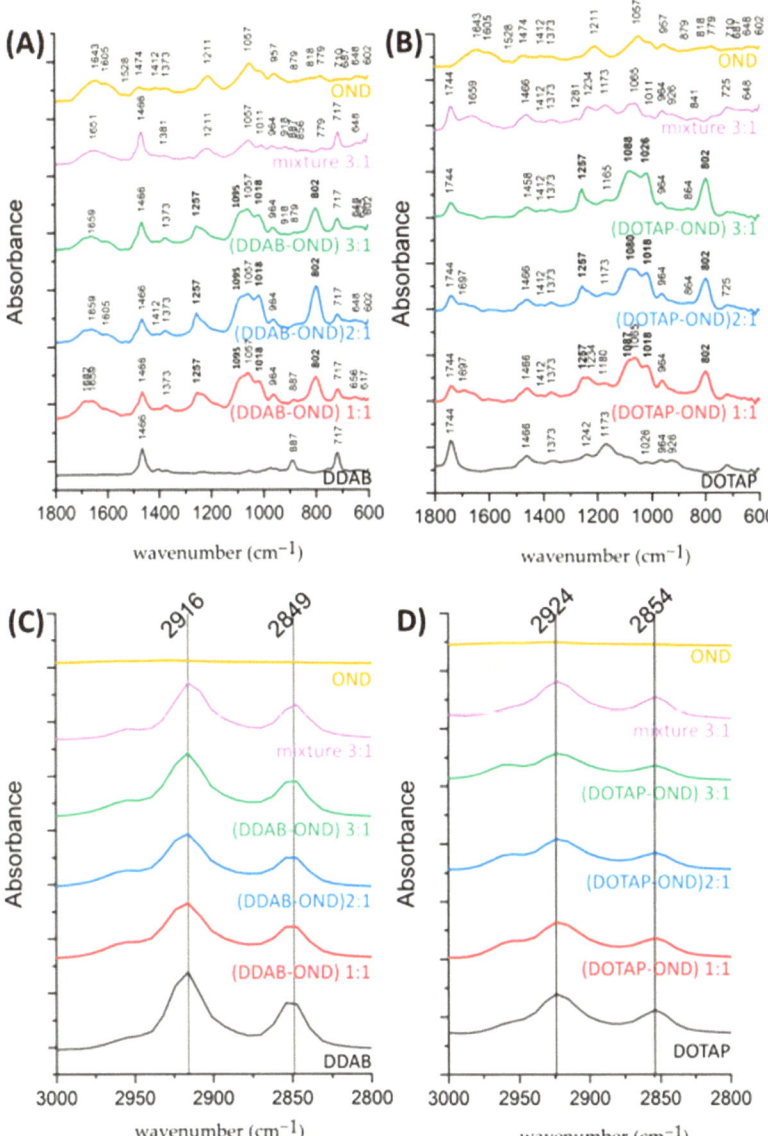

Figure 5. Attenuated total reflectance-Fourier-transform infrared (ATR-FTIR) absorbance spectra of OND, cationic lipid-OND complexes at various ratios, a cationic lipid-OND physical mixture at the ratio 3:1 and a bulk cationic lipid. Spectra of the OND-specific region (1800–600 cm^{-1}) of DDAB-OND (**A**) and DOTAP-OND (**B**), and the spectra of the lipid CH2 stretching vibrations (3000–2800 cm^{-1}) of DDAB-OND (**C**) and DOTAP-OND (**D**).

The list of complex-specific bands is summarized in Table 5. The OND peak at 1211 cm^{-1} shifted positively to 1257 cm^{-1} in both complexes but remained at the same position (1211 cm^{-1}) in the mixture. A new band appeared at 1095 cm^{-1} and 1088–1080 cm^{-1} in

DDAB-OND and DOTAP-OND, respectively. These bands characterize P=O vibrations. The peak at 1018 cm^{-1}, typical for the P-O-C bond, gained more intensity upon complexation. This suggests an increase in the vibrational frequencies of anionic PO$_2$ in the OND backbone as a result of an interaction with the cationic head of a lipid.

An intense peak at 802 cm^{-1} was observed in all complexes, suggesting a change in the conformation of deoxyribose (Figure 5A,B). Together with this intense peak, a broader peak at 864 cm^{-1} in the case of DOTAP-OND suggests an N-type (C3'-endo) sugar puckering mode [46]. For DDAB-OND, no other markers of the N-type puckering mode existed. This could be due to the DDAB peak occurring at a similar wavelength (887 cm^{-1}), resulting in an interference with other N-type marker bands. In the physical mixtures, there were less intensive and broader peaks at 879–887 cm^{-1} and 840 cm^{-1} in DDAB-OND and DOTAP-OND, respectively. These bands are characteristic of S-type sugars [46]. In contrast, the bands found in OND showed a rather broad shoulder peak at 818 cm^{-1}. The position of this broad shoulder peak is unspecific and might suggest the presence of both sugar puckering modes.

The spectra of the cationic lipids carried several specific bands (Figure 5C,D). The ester group of DOTAP gave rise to a peak at 1744 cm^{-1} [47,48] that also remains in the same position after complexation with OND. A weak band of around 1489 cm^{-1} characteristic of the trimethylammonium headgroups [47] was not observed in any of the cationic lipids. This weak band is likely overlapped by the CH$_2$ scissoring deformation at 1466 cm^{-1} seen in both lipids. In the formed complexes, this peak did not change its position, which correlates with the behavior of lipid peaks at higher wavelengths in the C-H stretching region. In DDAB, the symmetric (2849 cm^{-1}) and asymmetric (2916 cm^{-1}) CH$_2$ vibrations and, similarly, the symmetric (2854 cm^{-1}) and asymmetric (2924 cm^{-1}) CH$_2$ vibrations of DOTAP remained at the same vibrational frequency upon complexation at all tested ratios [47], which indicated no changes in the lipid chain arrangement.

Table 5. Bands specific to the complexes of both cationic lipids and OND. Fourier-transform infrared (FTIR) spectra of the respective cationic lipid and OND were subtracted from the FTIR spectra of the complexes to obtain complex-specific bands. Bands were observed in the complexes at all ratios if not otherwise specified.

Complex-Specific Bands (cm^{-1})	Marker Bands Characteristic of	Assignment	Reference
1257	Phosphate-deoxyribose backbone	Organic phosphate P=O, vibrational asymmetric band	[24,46,48,49]
1095 DDAB-OND 1088-1080 DOTAP-OND	Phosphate-deoxyribose backbone	Organic phosphate P=O, vibrational symmetric band	[24,46,49]
1018	Phosphate-deoxyribose backbone	P-O-C aliphatic phosphate	[48]
802	Deoxyribose conformation	N-type (C3'-endo) puckering mode	[46]

3.6. Characterization of Dispersed SEDDS

Both Citrem and Standard SEDDS preconcentrates were clear oily formulations that immediately dispersed into milky emulsions both in DI water and MES-HBSS buffer (pH 6.5). The dispersion in DI water was evaluated in order to assess properties of the formulations and in MES-HBSS to mimic the pH, as well as a more complex environment of in vitro testing media, as shown in Table 6.

Table 6. Size and zeta potential of Citrem and Standard SEDDS. The parameters were tested in deionized (DI) water and in 2-(N-morpholino)ethansulfonic acid-Hanks' Balanced Salt Solution (MES-HBSS) (pH 6.5). PdI: polydispersity index.

SEDDS	Loaded Substance	Size (nm)		PdI		Zeta Potential (mV)	
		DI Water	MES-HBSS	DI Water	MES-HBSS	DI Water	MES-HBSS
Citrem	nonloaded	201 ± 11	207 ± 16	0.36	0.27	−35.5 ± 0.6	−10.9 ± 0.7
	DDAB-OND	209 ± 14	237 ± 11	0.30	0.23	−24.1 ± 0.8 ###	−9.9 ± 0.7
	DOTAP-OND	195 ± 19	213 ± 5	0.30	0.22	−26.5 ± 1.2 ###	−9.4 ± 0.5
Standard	nonloaded	223 ± 10	213 ± 44	0.17	0.22	−5.2 ± 2.1	−1.2 ± 0.5
	DDAB-OND	256 ± 22	267 ± 10 ***	0.28	0.12	13.0 ± 1.3 ###	0.2 ± 0.5
	DOTAP-OND	240 ± 9 *	183 ± 27	0.23	0.25	14.0 ± 0.9 ###	0.3 ± 0.3

* $p < 0.05$ statistical difference relative to nonloaded Standard SEDDS in DI water, *** $p < 0.001$ statistical difference relative to nonloaded Standard SEDDS in MES-HBSS buffer and ### $p < 0.001$ statistical difference relative to the respective nonloaded SEDDS. Results are presented as mean ± SD ($n = 3$).

The size (z-average) was found between 180 and 270 nm for both SEDDS in both investigated media, with the PdI ranging from 0.125 to 0.360. In the case of the Citrem SEDDS, there was no significant difference in size across the formulations and media. The Standard SEDDS loaded with DOTAP-OND formed significantly larger nanostructures in the DI water than nonloaded Standard SEDDS (* $p < 0.05$). In MES-HBSS buffer, a similar phenomenon was observed; in this case, the DDAB-OND-loaded Standard SEDDS created larger structures than the nonloaded formulation (*** $p < 0.001$).

The zeta potential was significantly influenced by the composition of SEDDS and the dispersing media. In DI water, both nonloaded SEDDS showed a negative surface charge: −35.5 ± 0.6 and −5.2 ± 2.1 mV for Citrem and Standard SEDDS, respectively. After loading, the surface charge of the Citrem SEDDS increased to about −25 mV (### $p < 0.001$) and turned positive in the loaded Standard SEDDS to about 13 mV (### $p < 0.001$). Both complexes increased the zeta potential of the nonloaded Citrem and Standard SEDDS to the same extent. The Citrem and Standard SEDDS in MES-HBSS buffer (pH 6.5) showed no significant differences within the same kind of SEDDS among the nonloaded and loaded SEDDS; about −9.5 and 0 mV for Citrem and Standard SEDDS, respectively.

3.7. Dynamic In Vitro Lipolysis of SEDDS

Human intestinal digestion of SEDDS under fasted-state conditions was simulated by dynamic in vitro lipolysis. Lipolysis of the SEDDS was performed with the nonloaded Citrem and Standard SEDDS, as well as both SEDDS with orlistat, in order to evaluate the degree of digestion (Figure 6). The amount of released free fatty acids was the same for both SEDDS. The addition of orlistat significantly decreased lipolysis to ~10% of the formulations with no orlistat (*** $p < 0.001$). No significant difference was observed between the Citrem and Standard SEDDS upon the addition of orlistat. Moreover, lipolysis of DDAB in SEDDS and DOTAP in SEDDS was performed. None of cationic lipids had any impact on the digestion process (data not shown).

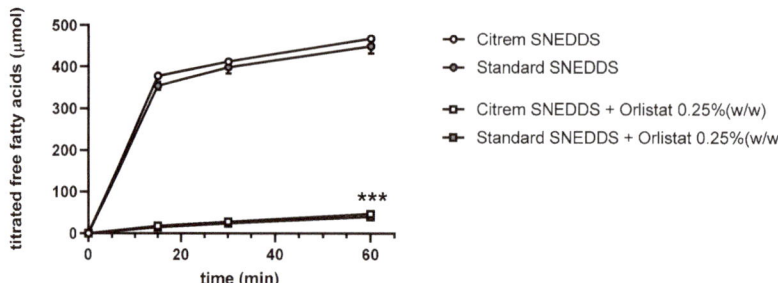

Figure 6. In vitro profile of digestion of SEDDS in fasted-state simulated intestinal fluid presented as the amount of free fatty acids titrated by sodium hydroxide over 60 min. Data are presented as mean ± SD ($n = 3$). *** $p < 0.001$—significant effect of orlistat on SEDDS lipolysis.

3.8. Cryo-TEM

SEDDS were dispersed in FaSSIF at 37 °C in the ratio 1:100 (v/v). The final concentration of OND in dispersion of loaded SEDDS was 1 nmol/mL. In total, 69 images were evaluated, with one representative image per formulation presented in Figure 7. Figure 7A–C depicts the dispersed Citrem SEDDS, nonloaded, DDAB-OND and DOTAP-OND-loaded, respectively. Figure 7D–F shows the Standard SEDDS, nonloaded, DDAB-OND and DOTAP-OND-loaded, respectively.

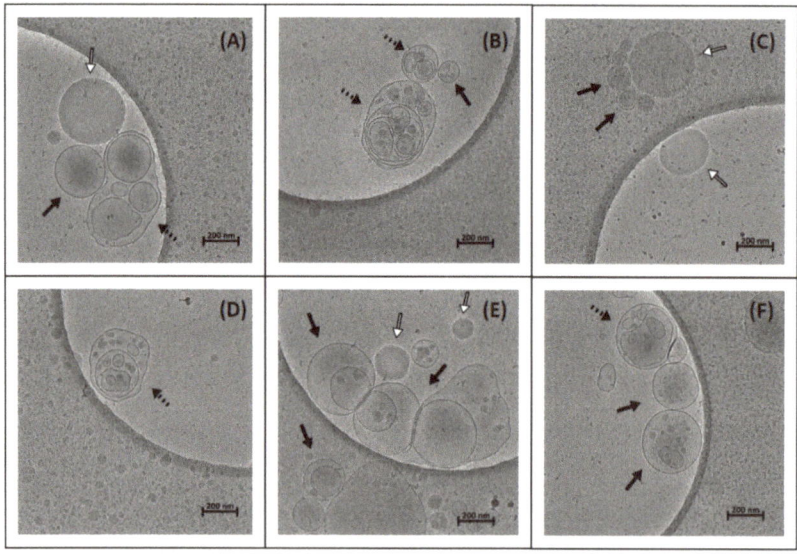

Figure 7. Cryo-TEM images of SEDDS, dilution 1:100 (v/v) in fasted-state simulated intestinal fluid (FaSSIF). (**A**) Nonloaded Citrem SEDDS, (**B**) DDAB-OND-loaded Citrem SEDDS (100 nmol/g), (**C**) DOTAP-OND-loaded Citrem SEDDS (100 nmol/g), (**D**) nonloaded Standard SEDDS, (**E**) DDAB-OND-loaded Standard SEDDS (100 nmol/g) and (**F**) DOTAP-OND-loaded Citrem SEDDS (100 nmol/g). Full arrows indicate uni- and multilamellar vesicles, dashed arrows indicate more complex vesicular structures and open arrows indicate oil droplets.

All formulations dispersed into nanosized structures. Predominantly, spherical uni- and multilamellar vesicles (darker and more pronounced borders) were observed, while oil droplets occurred less frequently (darker spheres with brighter borders). Wu et al. described similar differences between vesicles and oil droplets in a soybean oil-in-water emulsion stabilized by egg yolk lecithin [50]. The nanostructures varied in size from 100 to 300 nm. In addition, cryo-TEM detected more complex spherical and elongated vesicular structures (such as in Figure 5A,B,D), usually of larger sizes (>300 nm). No apparent differences between the six different SEDDS could be observed.

3.9. Protection Against Nuclease Degradation

The S1 nuclease completely degraded OND in an aqueous solution of naked OND (data not shown). Dispersions of both nonloaded SEDDS in the aqueous solution of naked OND showed the same pattern. This confirmed that neither the composition of Citrem SEDDS nor Standard SEDDS interfered with the activity of the enzyme.

If OND becomes cleaved by a nuclease, short OND fragments are detected in the supernatant that do not precipitate into pellets. The amount of OND that remain intact upon contact with the S1 nuclease was detected in the pellets and is shown in Table 7. There was a significant difference in the amount of OND protected by the Citrem and Standard SEDDS, as the Standard SEDDS showed about 3.5-fold higher protection ($p < 0.001$). On the other hand, no difference was observed between DDAB-OND and DOTAP-OND in any of the SEDDS.

Table 7. Percentage of OND protected from degradation after 30 min of incubation in the presence of the S1 nuclease.

SEDDS	Intact OND (%)	
	DDAB-OND in SEDDS	DOTAP-OND in SEDDS
Citrem	16.0 ± 1.5	15.7 ± 1.0
Standard	59.9 ± 3.4 ***	57.1 ± 3.0 ***

*** $p < 0.001$ is the statistically significant difference between Citrem and Standard SEDDS. Data are presented as mean ± SD ($n = 3$).

3.10. Caco-2 Cell Monolayer Transport Study

Several parameters of the prepared formulations were investigated in vitro in the Caco-2 monolayer. As an indicator of permeation enhancement, the TEER values were determined by an Endohm chamber at 25 °C before and after the experiment. After 120 min, the TEER decreased significantly if incubated with the Citrem or Standard SEDDS. No changes occurred after incubation with OND solution or the MES-HBSS buffer serving as the control. There were no significant changes among the formulations based on the Citrem SEDDS nor Standard SEDDS, indicating that the TEER changes can be attributed to the two SEDDS. Nevertheless, the extent to which the two SEDDS decreased the TEER differed significantly. The final TEER at 120 min of the Citrem SEDDS and Standard SEDDS-treated wells represented 66% ± 10% and 28% ± 4% of the initial TEER values, respectively ($p < 0.01$) (Figure 8A). In addition, the TEER values seem to be influenced differently by the Citrem and the Standard SEDDS.

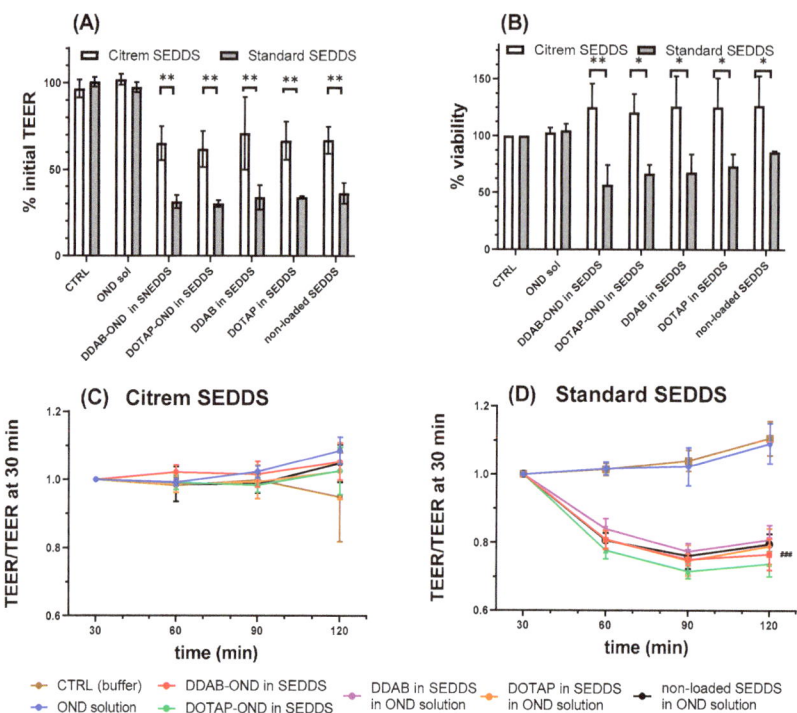

Figure 8. (**A**) Percent of initial transepithelial electrical resistance (TEER) measured by Endohm chamber after 120 min of incubation in both Citrem and Standard SEDDS. ** denotes a significant difference of TEER decline ($p < 0.01$) between the Citrem and Standard SEDDS. All SEDDS-incubated cells showed significantly lower TEER relative to the respective CTRL (buffer) and OND solution. (**B**) Percent of viability by lactate dehydrogenase (LDH) assay after 120 min of incubation with Citrem and Standard SEDDS. * and ** denote significant differences in the viability between different SEDDS (* $p < 0.05$ and ** $p < 0.01$). (**C**,**D**) Relative TEER values measured by chopstick electrodes at 37 °C for Citrem SEDDS (**C**) and Standard SEDDS (**D**). (**D**) ### represents a significant difference of the relative TEER values of SEDDS-treated cells relative to the CTRL and OND solution ($p < 0.001$). Results are presented as mean ± SD ($n = 5$ to 6).

This aspect was further evaluated by chopstick electrodes throughout the experiment at 37 °C starting from 30 min of the experiment and related to this time point. The cells incubated with the Citrem SEDDS had already reached the final TEER values by this time point, with the values remaining unchanged until the end of the experiment. This contrasts with the Standard SEDDS, in which TEER after 60 min reached a plateau at 80% of the TEER at 30 min (Figure 8C,D).

Figure 9A,B shows the cumulative OND transport into the basolateral compartment. At 120 min, both SEDDS displayed a significant increase of transported OND compared to the OND solution (Citrem SEDDS # $p < 0.05$ and Standard SEDDS ## $p < 0.01$ and ### $p < 0.001$). In the case of Citrem SEDDS (Figure 9A), no difference was observed between the two complexes. For the Standard SEDDS (Figure 9B), DDAB and DOTAP in the SEDDS and, also, the nonloaded SEDDS enabled the transport of higher amounts of OND than DDAB-OND and DOTAP-OND in SEDDS over 120 min (* $p < 0.05$). The total transported mass of OND after 120 min is summarized in Table 8.

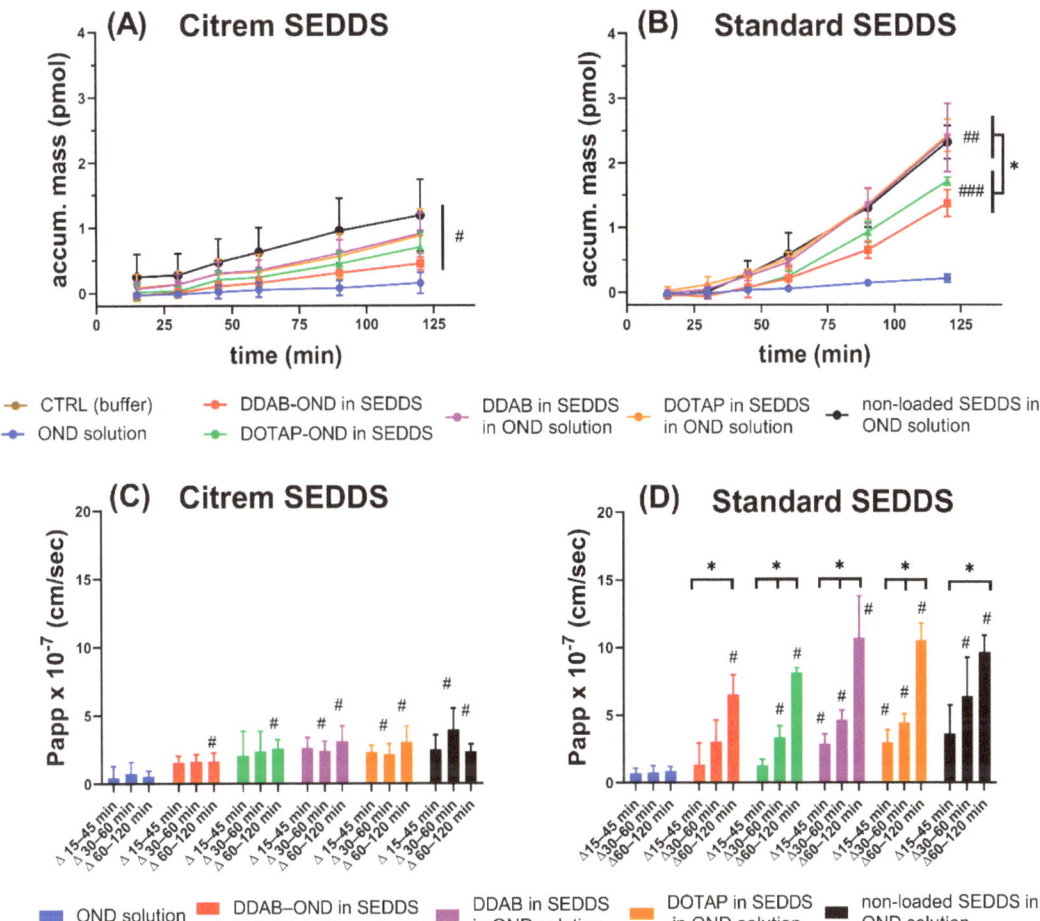

Figure 9. The transported OND accumulated in the basolateral compartment for Citrem SEDDS (**A**) and Standard SEDDS (**B**). The apparent permeability coefficient (P_{app}) values for specified time intervals in the Citrem SEDDS (**C**) and Standard SEDDS (**D**). (**A,B**) #, ## and ### represent significant differences of the flux curves of SEDDS-treated cells relative to the OND solution (# $p < 0.05$, ## $p < 0.01$ and ### $p < 0.001$). (**B**) * represents a significant difference between complex-loaded Standard SEDDS and a group of other Standard SEDDS formulations (* $p < 0.05$). (**C,D**) Bars marked by # showed a significant difference in the P_{app} relative to the respective bars of the OND solution ($p < 0.05$). (**D**) The significant differences between the time intervals in the Standard SEDDS is denoted as * $p < 0.05$. The results are presented as mean ± SD (n = 5 to 6).

Table 8. Transported OND accumulated in the basolateral compartment after 120 min presented as the total mass (pmol) and % of the initial apical mass.

Formulation	Citrem SEDDS		Standard SEDDS	
	Transported OND Accumulated Basolaterally at 120 min		Transported OND Accumulated Basolaterally at 120 min	
	pmol	%	pmol	%
OND solution	0.15 ± 0.16	0.03	0.21 ± 0.06	0.04
DDAB-OND in SEDDS	0.45 ± 0.10 *	0.09	1.37 ± 0.21 **	0.28
DOTAP-OND in SEDDS	0.70 ± 0.23 ***	0.14	1.72 ± 0.06 ***	0.34
DDAB in SEDDS	0.91 ± 0.31 **	0.18	2.40 ± 0.53 **	0.48
DOTAP in SEDDS	0.88 ± 0.41 **	0.17	2.43 ± 0.25 ***	0.49
Nonloaded SEDDS	1.19 ± 0.55 **	0.24	2.32 ± 0.26 ***	0.46

Results are presented as mean ± SD (n = 5 to 6). * $p < 0.05$, ** $p < 0.01$ and *** $p < 0.001$ = statistically significant differences in transported OND formulated into SEDDS in comparison to the OND solution.

A linear steady state of the flux curves was taken as the basis for the calculation of P_{app}. In order to investigate in detail changes in permeability across the Caco-2 monolayer during 120 min, the time frame of the experiment was divided into three intervals, i.e., Δ15–45 min, Δ30–60 min and Δ60–120 min, with the P_{app} values calculated for each interval. As can be seen in Figure 9C, the P_{app} was stable for all Citrem SEDDS formulations at all time intervals. OND solutions containing dispersions of the Citrem SEDDS with or without DDAB or DOTAP already showed a significant increase at the interval of Δ30–60 min relative to the OND solution. At the final interval of Δ60–120 min, all Citrem SEDDS significantly improved the permeability of OND relative to the respective time intervals of the OND solution ($p < 0.05$). In contrast, for the Standard SEDDS, the P_{app} increased over time for all formulations ($p < 0.05$) (Figure 9D). Only the OND solution with dispersions of DDAB and DOTAP in the Standard SEDDS already increased the P_{app} at the initial time interval Δ15–45 min. At the following interval of Δ30–60 min, the P_{app} of DOTAP-OND in the Standard SEDDS and the nonloaded Standard SEDDS was also enhanced significantly. Finally, at the interval of Δ60–120 min, all formulations of the Standard SEDDS showed an increase in P_{app} relative to the OND solution.

3.11. In Vitro Toxicity Study

The viability of the Caco-2 cells was evaluated by an LDH assay after 120 min of treatment with all SEDDS (Figure 8B). The OND solution was confirmed to be nontoxic. For both the Citrem and Standard SEDDS, there were no significant differences between the applied SEDDS formulations, which suggests that the main contribution to the cytotoxicity is from the surfactants in SEDDS and not the cationic lipids or the complexes. All Citrem SEDDS had viability values close to 100%, while the Standard SEDDS had a decreased viability to about 70% (* $p < 0.05$ and ** $p < 0.01$). These data might indicate increased cell stress due to compromised integrity of the cell membrane.

3.12. Uptake Study

The uptake of the fluorescently labeled OND formulated into SEDDS was examined in confluent Caco-2 cells using fluorescent microscopy. Figure 10 shows merged images: blue Hoechst staining cell nuclei, red PI staining dead cells and green FAM-labeled OND. Images depicting staining with a single dye can be found in the Supplementary Materials (Figure S1).

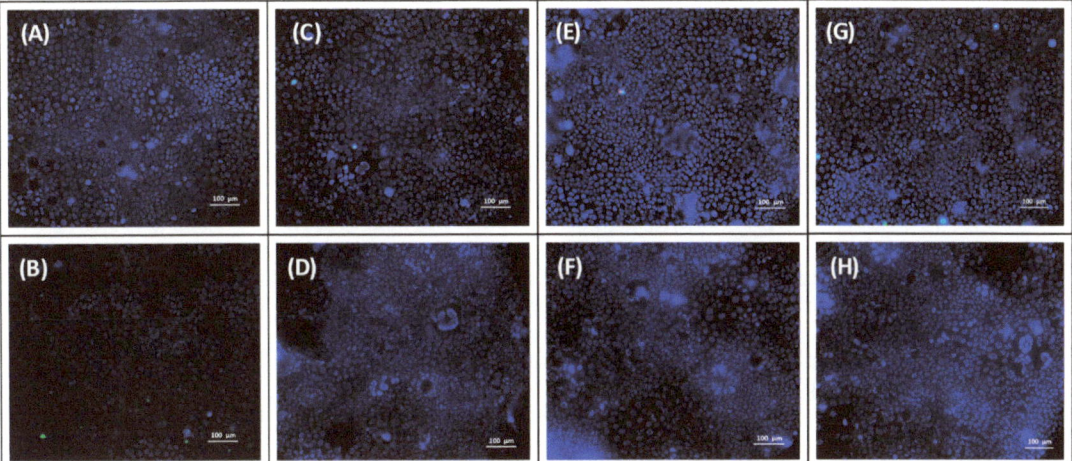

Figure 10. Fluorescence microscope images of fluorescently labeled oligonucleotide (OND) (**A**) MES-HBSS buffer, (**B**) OND solution in MES-HBSS buffer, (**C**,**D**) nonloaded Citrem and Standard SEDDS dispersed in OND solution, respectively, (**E**,**F**) DDAB-OND loaded in Citrem and Standard SEDDS, respectively, and (**G**,**H**) DOTAP-OND loaded in Citrem and Standard SEDDS, respectively. The size bar represents 100 µm. Blue represents the cell nuclei of living cells stained by Hoechst dye, red represents dead cells stained by propidium iodide and green represents fluorescently labeled OND.

Similar to the OND solution (Figure 10B), no OND was observed in living Caco-2 cells upon incubation with the Citrem or Standard SEDDS or when OND was administrated in the aqueous phase (nonloaded SEDDS; Figure 10C,D) or complexed inside the SEDDS (DDAB-OND and DOTAP-OND; Figure 10E,F and Figure 10G,H, respectively). The green signal of FAM-labeled OND was observed only in combination with the red signal indicating that OND was localized only inside dead Caco-2 cells.

4. Discussion

4.1. Preparation of Cationic Lipid-OND Complexes

Cationic lipid-DNA complexes have been shown to be a less immunogenic but, also, a less efficient alternative to viral vectors for the delivery of nucleic acids [4]. These macromolecules are often formulated as lipoplexes with preformed liposomes to enhance the cell transfection of large DNA molecules (several kb) [51], as well as shorter siRNA (tenths of bp) [52], for parenteral delivery to the systemic circulation. In this study, we prepared hydrophobic complexes consisting of cationic lipids and OND in order to load them into SEDDS, a well-established lipid-based oral delivery system. The presented experiments were conducted with a model nonspecific fluorescently labeled OND. Nevertheless, the structural features involved in the key procedures, such as the preparation of ion pairs with cationic lipids and, thus, hydrophilicity reduction, are applicable for potential therapeutic OND sequences. Therefore, the easily detectable fluorescently labeled model OND was used to investigate this innovative formulation process.

Monovalent cationic lipids with two lipophilic chains, DDAB and DOTAP, are known to be less toxic than their single-tailed counterparts [53]. Both aliphatic chains of DDAB are saturated, unlike the chains of DOTAP, which have a double bond in the C9 position. This influences their physicochemical properties; DDAB exists in the gel state and DOTAP in the liquid crystalline state at room temperature [54]. In the present study, it was found that the more flexible DOTAP chains seem to be more easily assembled around the OND core, leading to CE > 95% already at the charge ratio 2:1 ($N^+:PO_2^-$). At the ratio 3:1 ($N^+:PO_2^-$), there was no significant difference between the CE of the cationic lipids (Table 3). At all employed ratios, no lipid was observed at the interface during the Bligh–Dyer extraction, suggesting that most of the lipid contributed to the complexation. The ability of DDAB to create a more ordered structure was shown also by DSC, as several melting peaks of crystalline assembles were observed (Figure 4). The more ordered structure and, consequently, tighter molecular packing could explain the smaller size of the DDAB-OND complexes, as detected by AFM (Figure 3).

The formation of complexes between a cationic lipid added as a monomer or in micellar form and plasmid DNA (pDNA) has already been described and well-characterized [23,55]. In both published preparation methods, a sufficient recovery of pDNA was reported at the charge ratio 1:1. The recovery process was more efficient (>90%) if a lipid was added in excess of 1.5:1 (N^+:PO_2^-) [55]. For shorter siRNA, the need of higher lipid/OND ratio was reported [52,56]. It is widely accepted that the mechanism of complex formation is common for any type of nucleic acid and cationic lipid [57]. In other words, both components of the complex self-assemble into a core–shell structure based on the ion pairing—more specifically, primarily on electrostatic interactions between the cationic headgroup of a lipid and anionic phosphate of the nucleic acid backbone.

The ATR-FTIR analysis (Figure 5 and Table 5) showed complex-specific bands that occurred mostly in the region characteristic of changes in the phosphate-deoxyribose backbone and confirmed the interactions with the OND backbone in the complex formation process. These interactions could not be observed in physical mixtures prepared with the same cationic lipid:OND ratio. Previous studies showed that electrostatic interactions help to form inverted micelles, encapsulating the nucleic acid in the core surrounded by the shell of the cationic lipid [23]. This is in agreement with the AFM topography images showing collapsed lipid shells around the cores, as observed in both the DDAB and DOTAP complexes (Figure 3).

4.2. Loading the Complexes into Citrem and Standard SEDDS and Evaluation of the Formulations

Both nonloaded and complex-loaded SEDDS were characterized in terms of size and zeta potential in DI water and MES-HBSS buffer (pH 6.5). The Citrem SEDDS created more uniform nanostructures in terms of size, irrespective of the investigated loading and media. Dispersion of the Standard SEDDS seemed to be more influenced by a loaded substance, as a significant difference in size among the Standard SEDDS formulations was observed (Table 6). However, all SEDDS remained in the range suitable to trigger phagocytosis by macrophages, which are highly active in inflamed intestinal tissue [11,58]. Moreover, in the affected area, positively charged proteins are overexpressed [9]. Thus, negatively charged formulations such as Citrem SEDDS present an attractive approach for local targeting to the diseased tissue.

In DI water, a significant difference in zeta potential between nonloaded and complex-loaded SEDDS was observed for both the Citrem and Standard SEDDS. After complex loading, the zeta potential becomes more positive, suggesting the interference of both cationic lipids from the complexes with the surface charge. Given that OND was complexed with cationic lipids in excess, the shift of zeta potential towards more positive values can be expected. Nevertheless, these differences were not observed in the MES-HBSS buffer (pH 6.5). An interplay between ions present in the buffer and decreased pH seemed to mitigate the differences in zeta potential for individual SEDDS.

The Citrem and Standard SEDDS dispersed in FaSSIF were imaged by cryo-TEM (Figure 7). Previous studies imaging dispersed SEDDS by Tran et al. [59] and Fatouros et al. [60] showed oil droplets after SEDDS dispersion, unlike the Citrem and Standard SEDDS, for which vesicular nanostructures prevailed over oil droplets. In comparison to SEDDS characterized in the previous cryo-TEM studies, Citrem and Standard SEDDS contain a higher percentage of lipophilic surfactants. High concentration of lipophilic surface-active molecules can lead to the formation of vesicles, as well as higher complexity and diversity of the vesicular structures.

The majority of the observed nanostructures were between 100 and 300 nm. This range correlates with the size measured by dynamic light scattering (Table 6).

As the impact of the SEDDS excipients on the complex stability was evaluated, a slight but significant decrease in complex stability induced by anionic Citrem was observed (Table 4). However, this slight decrease seems to have translated into a low ability of the Citrem SEDDS to protect OND. In the presence of the S1 nuclease, only 16% of the loaded OND amount was protected against hydrolysis (Table 7). The Standard SEDDS excipients showed no interference with the complex stability, which improved the protection of the loaded OND 3.5-fold (up to 58% of the loaded OND amount). This suggests that there are also other factors in addition to the negatively charged Citrem that lead to complex destabilization.

Both the Citrem and Standard SEDDS disperse into nanodroplets and vesicular structures (Figure 7). Complexed OND is likely to remain inside the nanodroplets; the vesicle formation, however, could impair the complex stability. It would require further examination to track the complex inside the vesicles and to evaluate the impact of vesicular structures on the stability of the complexes. Thus, OND protection could be further improved by optimization of the SEDDS composition.

Upon oral administration, SEDDS excipients undergo digestion by lipases present in the gastrointestinal tract. The impact of gastric lipases, together with low gastric pH, can be circumvented by administering SEDDS preconcentrates in enteric-coated capsules. In the small intestine, the majority of triglycerides are digested by lipases [61]. In order to maintain the dispersed colloidal structures intact and, thus, to prolong the protection of OND, a lipase inhibitor, orlistat, was added to the SEDDS. Only 0.25% (w/w) of orlistat sufficed to decrease the level of lipolysis in the tested SEDDS to about 10% (Figure 6). This indicates that orlistat incorporation is a potentially useful approach to inhibit SEDDS digestion and to enable the delivery of well-protected OND. Previous studies have shown that the inhibition of lipolysis of a MCFA-based delivery system did not interfere with its permeation-enhancing effect [62,63].

4.3. In Vitro Performance of the Formulations

The ability of the Citrem and Standard SEDDS to enhance the permeation of OND was investigated in a transport study across the Caco-2 cell monolayer. A significant increase in OND in the basolateral compartment of the SEDDS-treated cells correlated with a decrease in TEER. No changes in TEER after 30 min in the Citrem SEDDS treated samples led to a stable P_{app}. The TJs opening by the Standard SEDDS plateaued after 60 min, and the final TEER was reached (Figure 8C,D). This resulted in a significantly enhanced permeation for the Standard SEDDS formulations compared to the respective Citrem SEDDS formulations. Finally, all SEDDS formulations enabled a significantly higher amount of transported OND to the basolateral compartment relative to the OND solution (Figure 9). For the Citrem SEDDS, there was no significant difference among the formulations, while the DDAB, DOTAP-loaded and nonloaded Standard SEDDS dispersed in OND solution showed a superior permeation of OND compared to the complex-loaded Standard SEDDS. Due to the complexation, OND is associated within the dispersed SEDDS and, thus, is not readily available for permeation, unlike the case of the noncomplexed OND dissolved in the dispersion medium. Nevertheless, loading OND complexed with a cationic lipid into SEDDS enables the crucial codelivery with PEs into the site of the action [64]. In addition, specific delivery through the intestinal monolayer provided by the Citrem and Standard SEDDS was confirmed, as no fluorescently labeled OND was localized inside the Caco-2 cells after the two-hour-long uptake study (Figure 10). This observation is in accordance with Li et al., who reported only intercellular localization of a macromolecular loading when it was delivered in MCFA-based formulations. In contrast, the loading was observed perinuclearly when employing a formulation based on long-chain fatty acids [65].

The performed experiments did not offer a conclusive answer regarding the choice of a cationic lipid for OND complexation. Although differing in the minimal amount of lipid needed for the complexation (Table 3), as well as the size of the complexes (Figure 3), no differences in the ability to protect OND (Table 7) and in the in vitro performance were observed (Figure 9).

Utilized SEDDS excipients are generally recognized as safe (GRAS) and/or approved by the European and US Pharmacopeia [37,66,67]. All SEDDS disperse into nanoparticles of a comparable size of about 200 nm, but they differ in zeta potential. The addition of Citrem into SEDDS decreases the surface charge of the formed colloidal nanostructures. The negative surface charge diminishes the interactions between SEDDS droplets and the negatively charged cell membranes of the Caco-2 cell monolayer. Due to the lack of this kind of repulsion between the cell surface and Standard SEDDS, there will be more frequent interactions between the Standard SEDDS and the cell membrane, resulting in membrane disturbance and LDH release (Figure 8B). Simultaneously, the opening of TJs by Citrem SEDDS occurs in a less intense manner. Nevertheless, it is noteworthy that McCartney et al. showed the reversible nature of Labrasol-induced reduction in TEER. The same study also reported that a static system such as the Caco-2 monolayer has a limited repair capacity compared to rat colonic mucosae [62].

Medium-chain triglyceride-based SEDDS confirmed their potential in vivo as they outperformed SEDDS based on long-chain triglycerides for the delivery of insulin [63]. However, generally, the SEDDS in vitro–in vivo correlation is known to not always be satisfactory [19], mainly due to the dynamic in vivo environment of complex intestinal fluids of both endogenous and dietary origin and the challenging crossing of the mucus layer [28]. Pathophysiological inflammatory changes, such as the overexpression of positively charged proteins and highly active phagocytes, create conditions for passive targeting. These changes specific to the inflammatory site might favor the negatively charged SEDDS in terms of enhanced effectivity at the target tissue. On the other hand, the permeation enhancement effect of the neutral Standard SEDDS was shown to be more pronounced in the Caco-2 monolayer. The preferential uptake of negatively charged particles by phagocytic cells [68] might limit the ability of the neutral SEDDS to deliver OND into targeted phagocytes.

5. Conclusions

The SEDDS based on MCFA was proven to be a viable delivery system across the Caco-2 monolayer for OND drugs. Hydrophobic ion pairing of OND with a cationic lipid, either DDAB or DOTAP, led to the formation of specific complexes, as confirmed by AFM and FTIR. Complexation reduced the hydrophilicity of OND and increased its solubility in lipids. The resulting ion-paired complexes subsequently allowed for their formulation into SEDDS: negatively charged or neutral SEDDS. A morphological evaluation of these SEDDS using cryo-TEM showed the presence of both nanosized oil droplets and vesicular structures. Negatively charged SEDDS did not significantly affect the Caco-2 viability. Additionally, neutral SEDDS enabled a higher OND permeability across the Caco-2 monolayer into the lamina propria, as well as better OND protection against hydrolytic decomposition in comparison to its charged counterpart. The lipolysis of both SEDDS was inhibited with the addition of orlistat, enabling the prolonged protection of OND in the gastrointestinal tract. The evaluation of further properties of the tested formulations, e.g., passive targeting and their effect on intestinal histology, in an appropriate in vivo model could reveal more details of this potent delivery system for local OND delivery.

Supplementary Materials: The following are available online at https://www.mdpi.com/article/pharmaceutics13040459/s1: Figure S1: Fluorescence microscope images.

Author Contributions: Conceptualization, P.P., O.H. and A.M.; methodology, J.K. and G.Z.; validation, J.K., O.H. and A.M.; formal analysis, J.K., J.Z. and O.H.; investigation, J.K. and G.Z.; resources, A.M. and P.P.; data curation, J.K.; writing—original draft preparation, J.K.; writing—review and editing, O.H., P.P., B.V. and A.M.; visualization, J.K. and B.V.; supervision, O.H., J.Z. and A.M.; project administration, A.M. and P.P. and funding acquisition, P.P. All authors have read and agreed to the published version of the manuscript.

Funding: This research was supported by the EFSA-CDN project (Reg. No. CZ.02.1.01/0.0/0.0/16 _019/0000841) co-funded by the European Union. This work was supported by the Czech Ministry of Education and Sports, project no. SVV 260 401. Jana Kubackova is grateful for the financial support from the Mobility Fund of Charles University (FM/c/2029-1-011), European Network on Understanding Gastrointestinal Absorption-related Processes (UNGAP) Cost action project (CA16205) and Erasmus+.

Institutional Review Board Statement: Not applicable.

Informed Consent Statement: Not applicable.

Data Availability Statement: The data is available on reasonable request from the corresponding author.

Acknowledgments: CIISB: the Instruct-CZ Centre of the Instruct-ERIC EU consortium, funded by the MEYS CR infrastructure project LM2018127, is gratefully acknowledged for the financial support of the measurements at the CF Cryo-EM. Authors are grateful to Jan Dusek and Miloslav Machacek for their assistance with cell culture experiments.

Conflicts of Interest: The authors declare no conflict of interest.

References

1. Gao, X.; Kim, K.; Liu, D. Nonviral gene delivery: What we know and what is next. *AAPS J.* **2007**, *9*, E92–E104. [CrossRef]
2. Lam, J.K.W.; Chow, M.Y.T.; Zhang, Y.; Leung, S.W.S. siRNA Versus miRNA as Therapeutics for Gene Silencing. *Mol. Ther. Nucleic Acids* **2015**, *4*, 1–20. [CrossRef] [PubMed]
3. Andersson, S.; Antonsson, M.; Elebring, M.; Jansson-Löfmark, R.; Weidolf, L. Drug metabolism and pharmacokinetic strategies for oligonucleotide- and mRNA-based drug development. *Drug Discov. Today* **2018**, *23*, 1733–1745. [CrossRef] [PubMed]
4. Roth, C.M. Delivery of genes and oligonucleotides. In *Drug Delivery: Principles and Applications*; John Wiley & Sons, Inc.: Hoboken, NJ, USA, 2016; pp. 655–673.
5. O'Driscoll, C.M.; Bernkop-Schnürch, A.; Friedl, J.D.; Préat, V.; Jannin, V. Oral delivery of non-viral nucleic acid-based therapeutics-do we have the guts for this? *Eur. J. Pharm. Sci.* **2019**, *93*, 206–220. [CrossRef] [PubMed]
6. Podolasky, D.K. Inflammatory bowel disease. *N. Engl. J. Med.* **2002**, *347*, 417–429. [CrossRef]
7. Zhang, Y.Z.; Li, Y.Y. Inflammatory bowel disease: Pathogenesis. *World J. Gastroenterol.* **2014**, *20*, 91–99. [CrossRef]
8. Eisenstein, M. Biology: A slow-motion epidemic. *Nature* **2016**, *540*, S98–S99. [CrossRef]
9. Hua, S.; Marks, E.; Schneider, J.J.; Keely, S. Advances in oral nano-delivery systems for colon targeted drug delivery in inflammatory bowel disease: Selective targeting to diseased versus healthy tissue. *Nanomed. Nanotechnol. Biol. Med.* **2015**, *11*, 1117–1132. [CrossRef]
10. Youshia, J.; Lamprecht, A. Size-dependent nanoparticulate drug delivery in inflammatory bowel diseases. *Expert Opin. Drug Deliv.* **2016**, *13*, 281–294. [CrossRef]
11. Collnot, E.M.; Ali, H.; Lehr, C.M. Nano- and microparticulate drug carriers for targeting of the inflamed intestinal mucosa. *J. Control. Release* **2012**, *161*, 235–246. [CrossRef] [PubMed]
12. Guo, J.; Jiang, X.; Gui, S. RNA interference-based nanosystems for inflammatory bowel disease therapy. *Int. J. Nanomed.* **2016**, *11*, 5287–5310. [CrossRef]
13. Ball, R.L.; Bajaj, P.; Whitehead, K.A. Oral delivery of siRNA lipid nanoparticles: Fate in the GI tract. *Sci. Rep.* **2018**, *8*, 2178. [CrossRef]
14. Knipe, J.M.; Strong, L.E.; Peppas, N.A. Enzyme- and pH-Responsive Microencapsulated Nanogels for Oral Delivery of siRNA to Induce TNF-α Knockdown in the Intestine. *Biomacromolecules* **2016**, *17*, 788–797. [CrossRef] [PubMed]
15. Wilson, D.S.; Dalmasso, G.; Wang, L.; Sitaraman, S.V.; Merlin, D.; Murthy, N. Orally delivered thioketal nanoparticles loaded with TNF-α-siRNA target inflammation and inhibit gene expression in the intestines. *Nat. Mater.* **2010**, *9*, 923–928. [CrossRef]
16. Attarwala, H.; Han, M.; Kim, J.; Amiji, M. Oral nucleic acid therapy using multicompartmental delivery systems. *Wiley Interdiscip. Rev. Nanomed. Nanobiotechnol.* **2018**, *10*, e1478. [CrossRef] [PubMed]
17. Müllertz, A.; Ogbonna, A.; Ren, S.; Rades, T. New perspectives on lipid and surfactant based drug delivery systems for oral delivery of poorly soluble drugs. *J. Pharm. Pharmacol.* **2010**, *62*, 1622–1636. [CrossRef]
18. Gursoy, R.N.; Benita, S. Self-emulsifying drug delivery systems (SEDDS) for improved oral delivery of lipophilic drugs. *Biomed. Pharmacother.* **2004**, *58*, 173–182. [CrossRef]
19. Mahmood, A.; Bernkop-Schnürch, A. SEDDS: A game changing approach for the oral administration of hydrophilic macromolecular drugs. *Adv. Drug Deliv. Rev.* **2019**, *142*, 91–101. [CrossRef] [PubMed]
20. Meyer, J.D.; Manning, M.C. Hydrophobic ion pairing: Altering the solubility properties of biomolecules. *Pharm. Res.* **1998**, *15*, 188–193. [CrossRef]
21. Simberg, D.; Weisman, S.; Talmon, Y.; Barenholz, Y. DOTAP (and other cationic lipids): Chemistry, biophysics, and transfection. *Crit. Rev. Ther. Drug Carr. Syst.* **2004**, *21*, 257–317. [CrossRef]

22. Lobovkina, T.; Jacobson, G.B.; Gonzalez-Gonzalez, E.; Hickerson, R.P.; Leake, D.; Kaspar, R.L.; Contag, C.H.; Zare, R.N. In vivo sustained release of siRNA from solid lipid nanoparticles. *ACS Nano* **2011**, *5*, 9977–9983. [CrossRef]
23. Wong, F.M.P.; Reimer, D.L.; Bally, M.B. Cationic Lipid Binding to DNA: Characterization of Complex Formation. *Biochemistry* **1996**, *35*, 5756–5763. [CrossRef]
24. Marty, R.; N'soukpoé-Kossi, C.N.; Charbonneau, D.; Weinert, C.M.; Kreplak, L.; Tajmir-Riahi, H.A. Structural analysis of DNA complexation with cationic lipids. *Nucleic Acids Res.* **2009**, *37*, 849–857. [CrossRef] [PubMed]
25. Xu, Y.; Szoka, F.C. Mechanism of DNA release from cationic liposome/DNA complexes used in cell transfection. *Biochemistry* **1996**, *35*, 5616–5623. [CrossRef]
26. Liang, W.W.; Lam, J.K. Endosomal Escape Pathways for Non-Viral Nucleic Acid Delivery Systems. In *Molecular Regulation of Endocytosis*; InTech: London, UK, 2012; Volume 2, p. 64. ISBN 9789537619992.
27. Kiptoo, P.; Calcagno, A.M.; Siahann, T.J. Drug delivery: Principles and applications. In *Drug Delivery: Principles and Applications*; John Wiley & Sons, Ltd.: Hoboken, NJ, USA, 2016; pp. 19–34. ISBN 1118833236.
28. Maher, S.; Brayden, D.J.; Casettari, L.; Illum, L. Application of permeation enhancers in oral delivery of macromolecules: An update. *Pharmaceutics* **2019**, *11*, 1–23. [CrossRef]
29. Hayashi, M.; Sakai, T.; Hasegawa, Y.; Nishikawahara, T.; Tomioka, H.; Iida, A.; Shimizu, N.; Tomita, M.; Awazu, S. Physiological mechanism for enhancement of paracellular drug transport. *J. Control. Release* **1999**, *62*, 141–148. [CrossRef]
30. Sha, X.; Yan, G.; Wu, Y.; Li, J.; Fang, X. Effect of self-microemulsifying drug delivery systems containing Labrasol on tight junctions in Caco-2 cells. *Eur. J. Pharm. Sci.* **2005**, *24*, 477–486. [CrossRef] [PubMed]
31. Hauptstein, S.; Prüfert, F.; Bernkop-Schnürch, A. Self-nanoemulsifying drug delivery systems as novel approach for pDNA drug delivery. *Int. J. Pharm.* **2015**, *487*, 25–31. [CrossRef] [PubMed]
32. Mahmood, A.; Prüfert, F.; Efiana, N.A.; Ashraf, M.I.; Hermann, M.; Hussain, S.; Bernkop-Schnürch, A. Cell-penetrating self-nanoemulsifying drug delivery systems (SNEDDS) for oral gene delivery. *Expert Opin. Drug Deliv.* **2016**, *13*, 1503–1512. [CrossRef] [PubMed]
33. Bligh, E.G.; Dyer, W.J. A rapid method of total lipid extraction and purification. *Can. J. Biochem. Physiol.* **1959**, *37*, 911–917. [CrossRef]
34. Gilmore, J.; Deguchi, K.; Takeyasu, K. Nanoimaging of RNA Molecules with Atomic Force Microscopy. *Microsc. Imaging Sci. Pract. Approaches Appl. Res. Educ.* **2017**, *54*, 300–306.
35. Lyubchenko, Y.L.; Shlyakhtenko, L.S.; Ando, T. Imaging of nucleic acids with atomic force microscopy. *Methods* **2011**, *54*, 274–283. [CrossRef]
36. Niu, Z.; Tedesco, E.; Benetti, F.; Mabondzo, A.; Montagner, I.M.; Marigo, I.; Gonzalez-Touceda, D.; Tovar, S.; Diéguez, C.; Santander-Ortega, M.J.; et al. Rational design of polyarginine nanocapsules intended to help peptides overcoming intestinal barriers. *J. Control. Release* **2017**, *263*, 4–17. [CrossRef]
37. Amara, S.; Patin, A.; Giuffrida, F.; Wooster, T.J.; Thakkar, S.K.; Bénarouche, A.; Poncin, I.; Robert, S.; Point, V.; Molinari, S.; et al. In vitro digestion of citric acid esters of mono- and diglycerides (CITREM) and CITREM-containing infant formula/emulsions. *Food Funct.* **2014**, *5*, 1409–1421. [CrossRef] [PubMed]
38. Zangenberg, N.H.; Müllertz, A.; Gjelstrup, K.H.; Hovgaard, L. A dynamic in vitro lipolysis model. II: Evaluation of the model. *Eur. J. Pharm. Sci.* **2001**, *14*, 237–244. [CrossRef]
39. Siqueira, J.S.D.; Al Sawaf, M.; Graeser, K.; Mu, H.; Müllertz, A.; Rades, T. The ability of two in vitro lipolysis models reflecting the human and rat gastro-intestinal conditions to predict the in vivo performance of SNEDDS dosing regimens. *Eur. J. Pharm. Biopharm.* **2018**, *124*, 116–124. [CrossRef]
40. Berthelsen, R.; Klitgaard, M.; Rades, T.; Müllertz, A. In vitro digestion models to evaluate lipid based drug delivery systems; present status and current trends. *Adv. Drug Deliv. Rev.* **2019**, *142*, 35–49. [CrossRef] [PubMed]
41. Michaelsen, M.H.; Siqueira, J.S.D.; Abdi, I.M.; Wasan, K.M.; Rades, T.; Müllertz, A. Fenofibrate oral absorption from SNEDDS and super-SNEDDS is not significantly affected by lipase inhibition in rats. *Eur. J. Pharm. Biopharm.* **2019**, *142*, 258–264. [CrossRef] [PubMed]
42. Fountain, K.J.; Gilar, M.; Budman, Y.; Gebler, J.C. Purification of dye-labeled oligonucleotides by ion-pair reversed-phase high-performance liquid chromatography. *J. Chromatogr. B Anal. Technol. Biomed. Life Sci.* **2003**, *783*, 61–72. [CrossRef]
43. Schön, P. Atomic force microscopy of RNA: State of the art and recent advancements. *Semin. Cell Dev. Biol.* **2018**, *73*, 209–219. [CrossRef] [PubMed]
44. Seeman, N.C. An Overview of Structural DNA Nanotechnology. *Mol. Biotechnol.* **2007**, *37*, 246–257. [CrossRef]
45. Berg, J.; Tymoczko, J.; Stryer, L. Fatty Acids Are Key Constituents of Lipids. In *Biochemistry*, 5th ed.; WH Freeman: New York, NY, USA, 2002.
46. Banyay, M.; Sarkar, M.; Gräslund, A. A library of IR bands of nucleic acids in solution. *Biophys. Chem.* **2003**, *104*, 477–488. [CrossRef]
47. Choosakoonkriang, S.; Wiethoff, C.M.; Anchordoquy, T.J.; Koe, G.S.; Smith, J.G.; Middaugh, C.R. Infrared Spectroscopic Characterization of the Interaction of Cationic Lipids with Plasmid DNA. *J. Biol. Chem.* **2001**, *276*, 8037–8043. [CrossRef]
48. Coates, J. Interpretation of Infrared Spectra, A Practical Approach. *Encycl. Anal. Chem.* **2004**, 1–23.
49. Taillandier, E.; Liquier, J. Vibrational Spectroscopy of Nucleic Acids. In *Handbook of Vibrational Spectroscopy*; John Wiley & Sons, Ltd.: Hoboken, NJ, USA, 2006; ISBN 9780470027325.

50. Wu, Y.; Manna, S.; Petrochenko, P.; Koo, B.; Chen, L.; Xu, X.; Choi, S.; Kozak, D.; Zheng, J. Coexistence of oil droplets and lipid vesicles in propofol drug products. *Int. J. Pharm.* **2020**, *577*, 118998. [CrossRef]
51. de Ilarduya, C.T.; Sun, Y.; Düzgüneş, N. Gene delivery by lipoplexes and polyplexes. *Eur. J. Pharm. Sci.* **2010**, *40*, 159–170. [CrossRef]
52. Bouxsein, N.F.; McAllister, C.S.; Ewert, K.K.; Samuel, C.E.; Safinya, C.R. Structure and gene silencing activities of monovalent and pentavalent cationic lipid vectors complexed with siRNA. *Biochemistry* **2007**, *46*, 4785–4792. [CrossRef] [PubMed]
53. Lv, H.; Zhang, S.; Wang, B.; Cui, S.; Yan, J. Toxicity of cationic lipids and cationic polymers in gene delivery. *J. Control. Release* **2006**, *114*, 100–109. [CrossRef]
54. Lobo, B.A.; Davis, A.; Koe, G.; Smith, J.G.; Middaugh, C.R. Isothermal Titration Calorimetric Analysis of the Interaction between Cationic Lipids and Plasmid DNA. *Arch. Biochem. Biophys.* **2001**, *386*, 95–105. [CrossRef]
55. Reimer, D.L.; Zhang, Y.P.; Kong, S.; Wheeler, J.J.; Graham, R.W.; Bally, M.B. Formation of Novel Hydrophobic Complexes between Cationic Lipids and Plasmid DNA. *Biochemistry* **1995**, *34*, 12877–12883. [CrossRef]
56. Belletti, D.; Tonelli, M.; Forni, F.; Tosi, G.; Vandelli, M.A.; Ruozi, B. AFM and TEM characterization of siRNAs lipoplexes: A combinatory tools to predict the efficacy of complexation. *Colloids Surfaces A Physicochem. Eng. Asp.* **2013**, *436*, 459–466. [CrossRef]
57. Scholz, C.; Wagner, E. Therapeutic plasmid DNA versus siRNA delivery: Common and different tasks for synthetic carriers. *J. Control. Release* **2012**, *161*, 554–565. [CrossRef]
58. Kubackova, J.; Zbytovska, J.; Holas, O. Nanomaterials for direct and indirect immunomodulation: A review of applications. *Eur. J. Pharm. Sci.* **2020**, *142*, 105–139. [CrossRef]
59. Tran, T.; Xi, X.; Rades, T.; Müllertz, A. Formulation and characterization of self-nanoemulsifying drug delivery systems containing monoacyl phosphatidylcholine. *Int. J. Pharm.* **2016**, *502*, 151–160. [CrossRef] [PubMed]
60. Fatouros, D.G.; Bergenstahl, B.; Mullertz, A. Morphological observations on a lipid-based drug delivery system during in vitro digestion. *Eur. J. Pharm. Sci.* **2007**, *31*, 85–94. [CrossRef] [PubMed]
61. Armand, M. Lipases and lipolysis in the human digestive tract: Where do we stand? *Curr. Opin. Clin. Nutr. Metab. Care* **2007**, *10*, 156–164. [CrossRef]
62. McCartney, F.; Jannin, V.; Chevrier, S.; Boulghobra, H.; Hristov, D.R.; Ritter, N.; Miolane, C.; Chavant, Y.; Demarne, F.; Brayden, D.J. Labrasol® is an efficacious intestinal permeation enhancer across rat intestine: Ex vivo and in vivo rat studies. *J. Control. Release* **2019**, *310*, 115–126. [CrossRef]
63. Liu, J.; Werner, U.; Funke, M.; Besenius, M.; Saaby, L.; Fanø, M.; Mu, H.; Müllertz, A. SEDDS for intestinal absorption of insulin: Application of Caco-2 and Caco-2/HT29 co-culture monolayers and intra-jejunal instillation in rats. *Int. J. Pharm.* **2019**, *560*, 377–384. [CrossRef]
64. Maher, S.; Geoghegan, C.; Brayden, D.J. Intestinal permeation enhancers to improve oral bioavailability of macromolecules: Reasons for low efficacy in humans. *Expert Opin. Drug Deliv.* **2020**, *18*, 273–300. [CrossRef]
65. Li, P.; Nielsen, H.M.; Müllertz, A. Impact of Lipid-Based Drug Delivery Systems on the Transport and Uptake of Insulin Across Caco-2 Cell Monolayers. *J. Pharm. Sci.* **2016**, *105*, 2743–2751. [CrossRef]
66. Swain, S.; Patra, C.N.; Rao, M.E.B. *Pharmaceutical Drug Delivery Systems and Vehicles*; Woodhead Publishing India: New Delhi, India, 2016; ISBN 987-93-85059-00-1.
67. van Hoogevest, P. Review–An update on the use of oral phospholipid excipients. *Eur. J. Pharm. Sci.* **2017**, *108*, 1–12. [CrossRef] [PubMed]
68. Fröhlich, E. The role of surface charge in cellular uptake and cytotoxicity of medical nanoparticles. *Int. J. Nanomed.* **2012**, *7*, 5577–5591. [CrossRef] [PubMed]

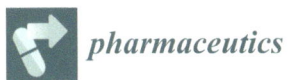

Article

Cyanocobalamin Ultraflexible Lipid Vesicles: Characterization and In Vitro Evaluation of Drug-Skin Depth Profiles

Antonio José Guillot, Enrique Jornet-Mollá, Natalia Landsberg, Carmen Milián-Guimerá, M. Carmen Montesinos, Teresa M. Garrigues and Ana Melero

1. Department of Pharmacy and Pharmaceutical Technology and Parasitology, Faculty of Pharmacy, University of Valencia, Avda. Vicent Andrés Estellés s/n, 46100 Burjassot, Spain; antonio.guillot@uv.es (A.J.G.); enjormo@alumni.uv.es (E.J.-M.); landsbergnat95@gmail.com (N.L.); carmenmilianguimera@gmail.com (C.M.-G.); ana.melero@uv.es (A.M.)
2. Department of Pharmacology, Faculty of Pharmacy, University of Valencia, Avda. Vicent Andrés Estellés s/n, 46100 Burjassot, Spain
3. Center of Molecular Recognition and Technological Development (IDM), Polytechnic University of Valencia and University of Valencia, Avda. Vicent Andrés Estellés s/n, 46100 Burjassot, Spain
* Correspondence: m.carmen.montesinos@uv.es (M.C.M.); teresa.garrigues@uv.es (T.M.G.)

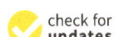

Citation: Guillot, A.J.; Jornet-Mollá, E.; Landsberg, N.; Milián-Guimerá, C.; Montesinos, M.C.; Garrigues, T.M.; Melero, A. Cyanocobalamin Ultraflexible Lipid Vesicles: Characterization and In Vitro Evaluation of Drug-Skin Depth Profiles. *Pharmaceutics* **2021**, *13*, 418. https://doi.org/10.3390/pharmaceutics13030418

Academic Editors: Maria Camilla Bergonzi and Ana Catarina Silva

Received: 4 February 2021
Accepted: 16 March 2021
Published: 20 March 2021

Publisher's Note: MDPI stays neutral with regard to jurisdictional claims in published maps and institutional affiliations.

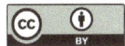

Copyright: © 2021 by the authors. Licensee MDPI, Basel, Switzerland. This article is an open access article distributed under the terms and conditions of the Creative Commons Attribution (CC BY) license (https://creativecommons.org/licenses/by/4.0/).

Abstract: Atopic dermatitis (AD) and psoriasis are the most common chronic inflammatory skin disorders, which importantly affect the quality of life of patients who suffer them. Among other causes, nitric oxide has been reported as part of the triggering factors in the pathogenesis of both conditions. Cyanocobalamin (vitamin B_{12}) has shown efficacy as a nitric oxide scavenger and some clinical trials have given positive outcomes in its use for treating skin pathologies. Passive skin diffusion is possible only for drugs with low molecular weights and intermediate lipophilicity. Unfortunately, the molecular weight and hydrophilicity of vitamin B_{12} do not predict its effective diffusion through the skin. The aim of this work was to design new lipid vesicles to encapsulate the vitamin B_{12} to enhance its skin penetration. Nine prototypes of vesicles were generated and characterized in terms of size, polydispersity, surface charge, drug encapsulation, flexibility, and stability with positive results. Additionally, their ability to release the drug content in a controlled manner was demonstrated. Finally, we found that these lipid vesicle formulations facilitated the penetration of cyanocobalamin to the deeper layers of the skin. The present work shows a promising system to effectively administer vitamin B_{12} topically, which could be of interest in the treatment of skin diseases such as AD and psoriasis.

Keywords: cyanocobalamin; vitamin B12; atopic dermatitis; psoriasis; liposomes; transferosomes; lipid vesicles; skin topical delivery

1. Introduction

Eczema or atopic dermatitis (AD) and psoriasis are the most common chronic inflammatory skin diseases. AD is characterized by pruritus, dry skin, eczematous injuries, and lichenification [1]. The onset of AD commonly occurs during childhood, and it is associated with a significant morbidity and reduced quality of life. The prevalence of AD has increased over the past 30 years, and its incidence has increased 2- to 3-fold in recent years. Approximately, 20% of children and 1–3% of adults are affected by this disorder [2]. Although the pathogenesis of AD is not completely understood, it has been associated with various factors: alteration of the skin barrier function, immune dysregulation, infections, and environmental processes. The alterations in the skin barrier function may be caused by deficient levels of ceramides and proteins involved in keratinocyte differentiation and prevention of transepidermal water loss [3,4]. Several genetic factors, such as mutations in filaggrin genes, could cause this situation [5]. The defective barrier function allows the penetration of allergens and irritant agents that trigger inflammation through Th2 responses (with increased interleukins: IL-4, IL-5, IL-13 cytokines) in the acute phase and Th1 responses (with increased Interferon (IFN)-gamma and IL-12) in chronic injuries [6]. In addition, the usual scratching stimulates keratinocytes to release other inflammatory cytokines like Tumoral Necrosis Factor (TNF)-alpha, IL-1, and IL-6, which perpetuate chronic inflammation. Ultimately, the modified state of the skin contributes to bacteria colonization, which further worsens the disorder [6].

Likewise, psoriasis is a chronic and inflammatory skin disease with a marked immune component. Its most typical skin manifestation consists in erythematous plaques, often spread over large areas of the body. The worldwide prevalence varies from 1% to 8%, depending on the geographical areas. Although it can begin at any age, its onset frequently occurs in adulthood, with one out of three cases during childhood [7]. A major characteristic in psoriasis pathogenesis is the inappropriate activation of the immune system, which leads to keratinocyte hyperplasia, altered T cell function and angiogenesis, among others [8–10]. Besides, oxidative stress and increased expression of insulin-like growth factor-1 (IGF-1) and epidermal growth factor (EGF) also participate in the pathogenesis [11].

The main goals of the treatment of these pathologies include restoring skin barrier, limiting itching, decreasing inflammation, and controlling immune alterations. To achieve them, a wide plethora of drugs may be used, with systemic immunosuppressive agents, topical corticosteroids, and topical calcineurin inhibitors (TCIs) being the first-line drugs in the pharmacological management of AD and psoriasis [12]. However, systemic treatments are not exempt of potential serious adverse side effects, such as kidney and liver dysfunction or myelosuppression, which complicate the management of severe cases [13–15]. Local side effects associated with long-term use of topical steroids and TCIs are relatively common, such as skin atrophy, ecchymosis, erosions, striae, delayed wound healing, purpura, easy bruising, and acne [16]. In addition, the Food and Drug Administration (FDA) has reported warnings for the use of some TCIs due to the potential risk of skin cancer and lymphomas [17].

The proinflammatory cytokines involved in AD and psoriasis stimulate the expression of inducible nitric oxide synthase (iNOS) in keratinocytes. In consequence, skin lesions of AD and psoriasis present higher levels of nitric oxide, which has been implicated in the pathogenesis of atopic eczema and psoriasis [18]. Oral and topical cyanocobalamin (B12) have been used as an alternative for preventing or ameliorating AD and psoriasis [19]. Although the first trials dated from the 1960s, not many studies have been carried out recently [20]. Januchowski et al. compared the effect of B12 cream (0.07%) with a moisturizer base for the treatment of childhood eczema in a double-blinded randomized trial using the SCORAD scale (Scoring of Atopic Dermatitis). Intraindividual comparisons showed significant differences in reduction of SCORAD values between B12 cream and placebo. Particularly, topical B12 significantly improved treated skin more than placebo at 2 and 4 weeks. Recently, mild-to-moderate plaque psoriasis has been treated with topical B12 ointments for 12 weeks in two clinical randomized trials [21]. Strücker et al. compared the effect of B12 with calcipotriol (vitamin D_3 analogue), obtaining similar decreases in the PASI score (Psoriasis Area Severity Index) after the studied period. Moreover, there was a marked diminution of the efficacy of calcipotriol after 4 weeks of therapy, whereas the efficacy of B12 remained largely constant over the whole observation period, making it more suitable for long-term use [22]. Similarly, a positive outcome was obtained when comparing B12 and emollient cream in the study done by Del Luca et al. The differences in PASI reduction were noticeable at week 2 and increased during the following 10 weeks. Two weeks after the end of the treatment, the psoriatic lesions evolved negatively (especially the ones treated with B12), proving the potential role of cyanocobalamin-based formulation in the treatment of epidermal disorders [23].

Despite these promising results, the molecular weight (1355 Da) and hydrophilicity of B12 limit its diffusion through intact human skin, given that one of the main functions of the skin is to prevent the penetration of exogenous substances to the body [24]. As the barrier function is recovered during treatment, B12 permeability might be gradually reduced.

Research on cutaneous permeability has shown that skin diffusion may be improved by using a suitable formulation, and it can even be used for systemic administration [25]. The strategies to overcome the limitations for drug permeation through the skin are addressed to disrupt the barrier function of the stratum corneum or to change the drug physicochemical properties. In this sense, although water-based vehicles have been reported to be suitable for B12 topical delivery, other studies suggest that the use of chemical enhancers, such as ethanolic solutions and oleic acid/propyleneglycol-based formulations, provide a better diffusion through the skin [26,27]. In addition, other active strategies, such as iontophoresis and microneedeling, showed higher penetration rates for B12 as well [27,28].

Nanosystems are another strategy to enhance drug delivery through the skin, consisting of the design of different types of nanocarriers, such as lipid nanoparticles, polymeric micelles, and poly (β-amino ester) [29–34]. Among those, liposomal-type systems have shown promising results in transdermal purposes [35,36]. Liposomes are microscopic vesicles with an aqueous core surrounded by one or more outer layers composed of non-toxic and biodegradable phospholipids, which are commonly used for their ability to encapsulate hydrophilic and lipophilic drugs [37]. Biomedical research has led to the development of modified lipid vesicles that include surfactants (transfersomes) or ethanol (ethosomes) in their composition, which provide greater flexibility, causing different carrier–skin interactions and thus enhancing skin drug delivery [38,39]. Cyanocobalamin liposomes have already been prepared by Arsalan et al. to improve its photostability and by Vitetta et al. to achieve systemic absorption after oral administration [40,41].

Based on these criteria, the aim of this study was to prepare and characterize stable lipid vesicles—liposomes, transfersomes, and ethosomes—to improve cyanocobalamin skin penetration.

2. Materials and Methods

2.1. Materials

Phospholipon 90G (soybean phosphatidylcholine) (P90G) was kindly donated by Lipoid (Steinhausen, Switzerland). Cholesterol and B12 (purity 95%) were purchased from Acofarma (Madrid, Spain). Tween 80, phosphate salts, and sodium chloride to prepare buffers were from Scharlab (Sentmenat, Spain). Regenerated cellulose dialysis membranes with a cut-off of 14kDa (Spectra/Por® molecular porous membrane tubing) for the in vitro release studies were acquired from Repligen (Waltham, MA, USA). HPLC-quality water obtained by Milli-Q purification (Millipore, Madrid, Spain) with resistance > 18 MΩ cm and TOC < 10 ppb was used for liposome reconstitution and HPLC analysis. Methanol for the HPLC mobile phase was purchased at VWR International (Radnor, PA, USA). For the tape-stripping studies, adhesive tape Tesafilm kristall-klar (33 mm × 19 mm, cut to 30 mm × 19 mm sections) was obtained from Tesa (Hamburg, Germany); Parafilm Sealing Film—50 mm (2″) Film Width × Roll Length 75 m (Parafilm, Madrid, Spain) was used; glass beads were obtained from MERCK (Madrid, Spain). Pig ears were procured from a local slaughterhouse (Mercavalencia, Valencia, Spain).

2.2. Cyanocobalamin Quantification. Development and Validation of a HPLC Method

B12 was quantified by HPLC using a PerkinElmer® Series 200 equipped with a UV detector settled at 360nm and a Kromasil® C18 HPLC column of 5 μm particle size, pore size 100 Å, L × I.D. 150 mm × 4.6 mm. The volume injection was 50 μL, and the mobile phase consisted of a isocratic mixture of methanol:water (30:70), delivered at a flow rate of 1 mL min^{-1}. The B12 retention time was 3.6 min, and the analysis duration was 5 min.

For the validation of the method, a stock standard solution of B12 (100 μg/mL) was prepared by dissolving 0.01 g of the drug in 100 mL of water. Ten working solutions (100, 10, 5, 2.5, 1.25, 0.625, 0.312, 0.156, 0.078, and 0.039 μg/mL) were prepared by diluting an adequate amount of stock standard solution with water. All analyses were performed in triplicate ($n = 3$).

2.3. Preparation of Liposomes, Transferosomes and Ethosomes

Several formulations of liposomes (L), transferosomes (T), and ethosomes (E) were prepared by the classic film-hydration method [42,43]. Their quantitative composition, reconstitution conditions, and the methods used to purify them are shown in Table 1. Three batches of each lipid vesicle type were prepared, empty and loaded with a variable amount of B12. Cyanocobalamin was added to the organic phase dispersion or included in the liposomal reconstitution solution (80% *w/v* of the solubility limit to achieve the maximum loading possible). Briefly, P90G, cholesterol (P90G:Chol molar ratio 17:1) or surfactants (15% *w/w* of lipid), and cyanocobalamin (except in the blank formulations and formulations reconstituted with B12 solution) were dissolved in methanol. The solvent was evaporated using a rotary evaporator (BUCHI R-210) under stirring (Heidolph RZR-2021) at 50 °C and 100 mbar. The resulting thin film was hydrated by addition of PBS 7.4 pH or B12 solution and then stirred for 1 h at 50 °C to obtain a multi-lamellar vesicle (MLV) dispersion. Transfersome batches were prepared by the same process with the exception that cholesterol was replaced by Tween 80. The ethosomal batches were prepared by the Touitou method [44], dissolving P90G and B12 in ethanol. Then, an appropriate amount of water was added at 12 ± 0.5 mL/h in a sealed beaker under stirring (710 ± 5 rpm), in a water bath tempered at 30 °C. Concurrently, the option of adding B12 dissolved in the water flow was also explored. The system was kept under stirring for 5 min after the addition of the water.

Table 1. Quantitative composition of the different lipid vesicle systems, reconstitution conditions, and purification method.

Components (% w/v)	Formulations								
	L1	L2	L3	T1c	T2c	T1d	T2d	E1	E2
Phospholipon 90G®	4.5	4.5	4.5	4.5	4.5	4.5	4.5	3	3
Cholesterol	0.135	0.135	0.135	-	-	-	-	-	-
Tween 80	-	-	-	0.675	0.675	0.675	0.675	-	-
B12 [1]	1 [1]	0.2 [2]	0.2 [1]	1 [1]	0.2 [2]	1 [1]	0.2 [2]	0.2 [2]	0.2 [3]
Reconstitution solvent (mL)	10 mL PBS	10 mL PBS	10 mL PBS	10 mL PBS	10 mL PBS	10 mL PBS	10 mL PBS	20 mL Water	20 mL Water
Purification method [4]	C	C	C	C	C	D	D	C	C

[1] B12 added in reconstitution solution. [2] B12 added in the organic-lipid phase. [3] B12 added dropwise in solution. [4] C: centrifugation; D: dialysis (24 h). PBS: Phosphate Buffer Saline.

Once MLV were obtained, their size was reduced by sonication and membrane extrusion. In the case of L and T, they were firstly sonicated at 50 °C for 2 h (Elmasonic S60H), then cooled down to 4 °C and extruded through a 200 μm membrane at 30 °C, using a LiposoFast-Basic Extruder, Avestin (20 times) [45]. Ethosomes were sonicated for 1 h at room temperature and reduced by the same extrusion process. After size reduction, the samples were purified by centrifugation (12,800× *g*, 30 min) or washed in 2 L PBS at 4 °C for 24 h to compare both methods [46,47]. The batches were then stored at 4 °C protected from the light.

2.4. Characterization of the Lipid Vesicles

2.4.1. Determination of Entrapment Efficiency

Entrapment efficiency (EE) was determined directly by calculating the amount of B12 encapsulated in lipid vesicle dispersions using the following equation (Equation (1)) [48]:

$$EE(\%) = (Q_e/Q_t) \cdot 100 \tag{1}$$

where Q_e is the amount of B12 encapsulated, and Q_t is the amount of B12 used for batch preparation.

For this, 0.5 mL of lipid vesicles dispersion was incubated for 1 h with a mixture of water:methanol:sodium doceyl sulfate 1% (45:45:10) to dissolve all the vesicle components [49–51]. The final mixture was filtered, and B12 content was analysed by HPLC.

2.4.2. Determination of Particle Size, Polidispersity Index (PDI) and Zeta-Potential

Vesicular size (average diameter), polydispersity index (PDI), and zeta potential were measured by means of a Malvern nanozetasizer (Malvern, UK). Dynamic light scattering (DLS) mode was used to measure the vesicular size and PDI, while laser doppler electrophoresis (LDE) was used to determine the zeta potential. The temperature was set at 25 °C in all cases, and each sample ($n = 3$) was analysed in triplicate [52].

2.4.3. Determination of Phospholipid Content of Lipid Vesicles

The method of Rouser et al. was used to determine the amount of phosphatidylcholine (PC) incorporated into the different vesicles ($n = 3$) [53]. Briefly, 100 μl of the liposomal aqueous samples was heated at 270 °C until complete liquid evaporation, followed by addition of 450 μL of $HClO_4$ (70% v/v). Next, the mixture was heated to 250 °C for 30 min. After cooling down, 3.5 mL of water, 500 μL of ammonium molybdate (2.5% w/v), and 500 μL of ascorbic acid (10% w/v) were added. The mixture was vortexed and incubated at 100 °C for 7 min. After the tubes were cooled down, the absorbance was measured at 820 nm (spectrophotometer HITACHI U-2900, Milan, Italy).

2.4.4. Evaluation of Lipid Vesicle Flexibility

The flexibility of the different lipid vesicles was estimated indirectly by extrusion through a 100 nm membrane in cold. For this, 500 μL of each formulation ($n = 3$) was extruded 9 times at room temperature. The final collected volume was also recorded and the relative decrease ratio in particle size was calculated [54].

2.4.5. Stability Studies

The physical stability of the vesicles was checked weekly during 60 days in terms of size and PDI by DLS. The stability of the vesicle suspensions was determined using Turbiscan™ LAB Stability Analyzer (Formulaction SA, L'Union, France) by checking the phenomena of coalescence, flocculation, creaming, sedimentation, and clarification during the 24 h after the suspension was formulated [55]. The chemical stability of the B12 was assessed by determination of drug content every week for 3 months.

2.5. Release Studies

In vitro release studies were carried out using static Franz-type diffusion cells with an effective diffusion area of 1.76 cm^2. A 500 μL of each formulation was added to the donor chamber, and the receptor chamber was filled with 12 mL of PBS (pH 7.4) ($n = 6$). Temperature was maintained at 32 °C throughout the experiment. A Spectra/Por® molecular porous membrane was used to separate donor and acceptor compartments. Both the donor compartment and the sampling port were covered with Parafilm® to avoid leakage and solvent evaporation. Samples of 400 μL were collected at 1, 2, 3, 4, 5, 6, 7, 8, 9, 10, 24, 48, and 72 h. At every sampling time, the volume was replaced with pre-warmed PBS to guarantee sink conditions [56].

The released B12 was quantified using the same HPLC analytical method described above, and the cumulative amounts of B12 versus time were calculated. The total drug amount released was calculated according to the previous determination of the drug content and plotted versus time. The release profiles were fitted to different mathematical kinetic models: Higuchi, Korsmeyer–Peppas, Kim, Peppas–Sahlin, zero order and first order. For each case, the Akaike information criterion (AIC) was calculated to determine the optimal models to explain the experimental data. The correlation coefficient (R^2) of the most accurate model was reported as an indicator of the proportion of variation of the results that could be explained by the model [57,58].

The Higuchi model assumes that the release process is carried out only by passive diffusion and is governed by the following equation (Equation (2)) [59]:

$$M_t/M_\infty = k \cdot \sqrt{t} \tag{2}$$

where M_t is the amount released at time t, M_∞ is the maximum amount of drug released, M_t/M_∞ is the fraction of the amount of drug released at time t, k is the constant that governs the process.

The Korsmeyer–Peppas model or power-law is described with the following equation (Equation (3)) [60,61]:

$$M_t/M_\infty = k \cdot t^n \tag{3}$$

where M_t is the amount released at time t, M_∞ is the maximum amount of drug released, M_t/M_∞ is the fraction of the amount of drug released at time t, k is the constant that governs the process and explains the characteristics of the system, and n is the diffusion release exponent. Values of n < 0.5 are indicative that the release process is carried out by passive diffusion; values of 0.85 < n < 1 show that the process is governed mainly by relaxation, and intermediate values 0.5 < n < 0.85 indicate the existence of both phenomena (anomalous transport).

As a variation of the Korsmeyer–Peppas equation, Kim et al. proposed a modification (Equation (4)) to assess the possible burst effect of the formulation [62]:

$$M_t/M_\infty = k \cdot t^n + n \tag{4}$$

where b is the parameter corresponding to the burst effect.

The Peppas–Sahlin model considers that release may occur through the processes of passive diffusion and relaxation, each represented by a constant (Equation (5)) [63]:

$$M_t/M_\infty = k_1 \cdot t^n + k_2 \cdot t^n \tag{5}$$

where k_1 and k_2 are, respectively, the constants associated with the processes of drug release by passive diffusion and relaxation, and n is the diffusion release exponent.

Representative theoretical models, zero order (Equation (6)) and first order (Equation (7)), are described by the following equations [64]:

$$M_t/M_\infty = k_d \cdot t \tag{6}$$

$$M_t/M_\infty = 1 - e^{-kd \cdot t} \tag{7}$$

where k_d is the constant of diffusion release that governs the process.

2.6. Tape-Stripping Studies. Drug Penetration through the Skin and Stratum Corneum Depth

The assay was performed using porcine skin samples. Skin was removed from the connective tissues and placed onto a glass slide, with the outside layer facing upwards. An aluminium mask was placed over it, leaving the application area uncovered. One hundred microliters of each formulation containing lipid vesicles was applied to the delimited application area of skin. The system was then incubated at 32 °C for 2, 4, and 6 h. Each test was performed in triplicate (*n* = 3). After incubation, 20 strips of adhesive tape were applied sequentially to the skin using a roller, according to the standardized procedure in our lab, and then removed with a forceps [65]. The amount of stratum corneum removed was determined by infrared densitometry (SquameScan™ 850A device, Wetzlar, Germany), and strips were grouped in different pools, following the sequence: 1, 2, 3–5, 6–10, 11–15, 16–20 [66]. The B12 amount present in each sample was extracted overnight from the strips using a methanol:water mixture (50:50 *v/v*) as extraction solvent, since it afforded an optimal B12 recovery ratio within the established range (100 ± 20%) [67]. Subsequently, B12 was quantified by HPLC with no interferences with the analytical method.

2.7. Data Analysis and Statistical Analysis

All data processing was performed in Microsoft Excel 2016 (Redmond, WA, USA) and SPSS version 22.0 (IBM Corp, Armonk, NY, USA). Data are expressed as the mean ± standard deviation (SD) unless otherwise stated. Statistical differences were determined using one-way ANOVA followed by Tukey's post hoc analysis for tests with two variables or two-way ANOVA followed by Bonferroni's post hoc analysis for tests with three variables, where p-values below 5% ($p < 0.05$) were considered significant.

3. Results and Discussion

3.1. Characterization of Lipid Vesicles

During the lipid vesicle design stage, different factors were considered that could potentially influence their properties, based on previous knowledge about this type of nanocarriers. In this sense, two essential factors are the composition and proportion of components, since they can affect important properties, such as the size, stability, or releasing ability of the drug. It is well known that by increasing the proportion of cholesterol located in the lipid bilayers, the particle size [68,69] and the vesicle rigidity also increase [69,70]. Considering that one of the main reasons why lipid vesicles improve drug absorption through the skin is their ability to deform and penetrate between the cells of the stratum corneum, we sought to produce flexible vesicles of the smallest possible size [71,72]. For this, a low ratio of cholesterol to phospholipid (molar ratio 1:17) was chosen for conventional liposomes, since it provides small and ultraflexible vesicles with enough stability. Besides, 85:15% w/w lipid:surfactant ratio was used since Ahad et al. demonstrated that it is the most suitable for transdermal delivery of eprosartan mesylate in transferosomes based on P90G:Tween 80 [43]. Additionally, different proportions of ethanol have been studied for preparing ethosomes (20–50% w/w). In this case, intermediate concentration (30% w/w) was used, considering that it is the most promising ratio for transdermal absorption purposes, according to the characterization results [73].

The initial results (day 0) of size, PDI, zeta potential, drug loading, and phospholipid content are reported in Table 2.

Table 2. Characterization of the B12 lipid vesicles in terms of size, polydispersity index (PDI), zeta-potential, drug loading, and phospholipid content (PC). All results are expressed as mean ± SD ($n = 3$).

	Formulations								
	L1	L2	L3	T1c	T2c	T1d	T2d	E1	E2
Size (nm)	283 ± 6	278 ± 13	275 ± 9	175 ± 5	169 ± 10	177 ± 4	171 ± 3	150 ± 5	141 ± 11
PDI	0.269 ± 0.07	0.205 ± 0.002	0.215 ± 0.009	0.239 ± 0.02	0.261 ± 0.03	0.223 ± 0.01	0.244 ± 0.03	0.200 ± 0.003	0.193 ± 0.01
Zeta potential (mV)	−11.2 ± 0.12	−10.1 ± 0.3	−9.55 ± 0.84	−4.77 ± 0.13	−5.01 ± 0.21	−5.51 ± 0.17	−5.17 ± 0.37	−4.63 ± 0.75	−5.35 ± 1.58
Drug loading (mg per mL)	1.9 ± 0.3	0.75 ± 0.07	0.17 ± 0.09	0.52 ± 0.02	0.14 ± 0.04	2.2 ± 0.2	0.60 ± 0.02	0.22 ± 0.03	0.23 ± 0.04
PC (%)	80 ± 4	84 ± 7	77 ± 2	33 ± 3	30 ± 0.9	86 ± 8	82 ± 5	66 ± 2	60 ± 5

In accordance with other works, size measurements were in the expected range for these types of lipid vesicles. Wu et al. obtained conventional liposomes in a range of 236–374 nm, depending on the percentage of cholesterol included in the formulation [74]. The transferosomal and ethosomal particle dimensions obtained were smaller than those of conventional liposomes, because the presence of the edge-activating substances in the lipid bilayer of the vesicles causes a reduction in the surface tension [75]. Transferosome sizes obtained were similar to the values previously reported by Carreras et al. [75], and ethosomal batches reproduced at exactly the size described by Touitou et al., the original research for this vesicle type (30% w/w ethanol content) [44].

PDI values as a measure of the variability in size of the particle populations were always below 0.3, which is the limit value to consider homogeneous populations for lipid-based carriers in drug delivery applications [76,77].

Zeta-potential values of all formulations were negative, as expected, due to the negative charge of the phospholipids. Liposomes showed the strongest charge, probably due to the bigger size and higher phospholipid amount. It has also been reported that the surface charge decreases when increasing the level of cholesterol in a phospholipid membrane [78]. Consequently, our prototypes presented lower values in comparison with other reports where lipid vesicles contained cholesterol in higher proportion [75]. Regarding the transferosomes and ethosomes, they presented a size reduction (probably because of an edge-activator), which implies a lower concentration in phospholipids, thus reducing the negative charge. These results are consistent with the ranges described by Ahad et al. and Touitou et al., who reported values from -5.91 to -14.0 and 4.6 to -4.3 mV for the same type of transferosomes and ethosomes, respectively [43,44].

Following the work of Jain et al., we used the vesicle size reduction rate and volume loss after cold extrusion as an indirect measurement of the vesicles deformability capacity [54]. Results are presented in Figure 1a,b. Significant differences were obtained between liposomes and ultraflexible vesicles, as expected [79,80]. Liposomes were retained in the 100 nm filters and forced to split into smaller particles to pass the pores. On the contrary, transferosomes and ethosomes—whose initial size was higher than 100 nm—maintained their size during the passage thanks to their flexibility. Likewise, the final volume collected after cold extrusion was inversely related to the vesicle flexibility. As such, no differences were observed in transferosomal or ethosomal batches, while all liposomal prototypes presented a significant reduction compared to their initial volumes. Thus, both techniques confirm the flexibility of transferosomes and ethosomes.

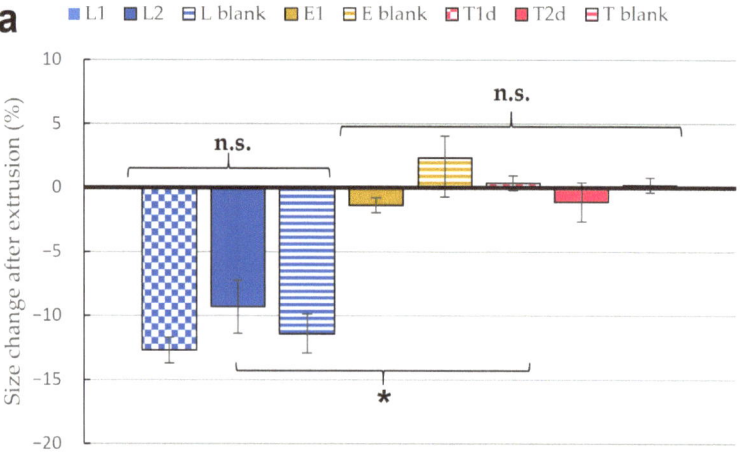

Figure 1. *Cont.*

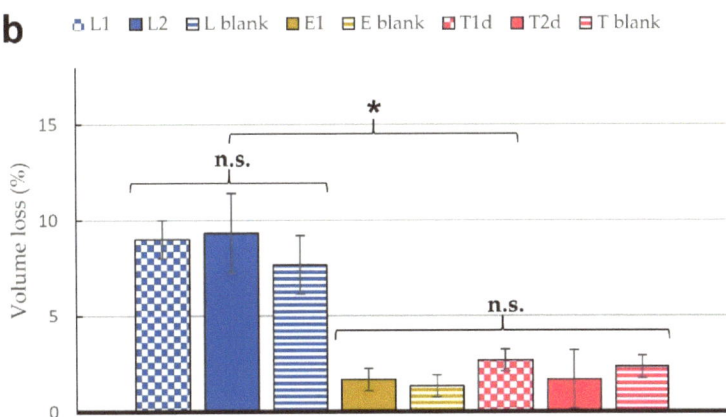

Figure 1. (a) Size change after extrusion through 100 nm membrane; (b) Volume loss after extrusion through 100 nm membrane (9 passages). All results are expressed as mean ± SD (n = 3). * means statistically significant differences ($p < 0.05$), n.s. means no statistically significant differences ($p > 0.05$) using one-way ANOVA followed by Tukey's multiple comparison test.

The entrapment efficiency percentage and total amount of encapsulated B12 are also graphically presented in Figure 2a,c. Hydrophilic compounds often show lower entrapment rates than lipophilic ones. This happens because the entrapment is more efficient if the compound is retained in the phospholipid bilayers, which depends on its primary affinity [48,81]. Arsalan et al. reported a maximum entrapment efficacy of 40% in B12 liposomes when maximizing the amount of lipid included during the vesicle formulation [40]. This result is clearly superior to our L1 data (Figure 2a). To overcome this issue and considering the ability of B12 to solve in aqueous and organic solvents such as methanol, we explored the option of formulating B12 in the organic phase to check any possible difference. In our case, the L2 formulation showed the maximum efficiency in the entrapment process compared to our other prototypes, being significantly different from the other formulations. The comparison between L2 and L1 analyzes the effect of including the B12 in every phase, and the result was higher when the addition was in the lipid one. We also tested the possible influence of differences in the initial dose by preparing L3 formulation. The poor entrapment efficiency in L3 formulation seems to indicate a destabilization of the vesicles with such strategy. T1d and T2d presented an entrapment value within the expected range. At this point, the differences between both transferosomes and L2 could be attributed either to the differences in size, which allowed the incorporation of a higher amount of B12 in the vesicle core, or to the purification method used to remove the non-entrapped drug. While liposomal formulations were centrifuged, T1d and T2d were dialyzed over 24 h [47]. This latter reason is also checked through the EE% and PC% results of T1c and T2c. Both values were lower than expected, probably because of the unsuitability of the centrifugation method for transferosomes. In fact, the supernatant obtained after centrifugation was not completely clear, as it was in the conventional liposomes, and contained still an important amount of liposomes, as demonstrated by a poor phospholipid recovery. The specific encapsulation efficiency parameter was calculated by dividing EE% by PC% [82] (Figure 2b). We could assume that the centrifugation method is adequate for liposomes, as this method is usually successfully used in our laboratories, and the expected amount of phospholipid was recovered after the process. Based on our results, we could conclude that centrifugation was only suitable for liposomal formulations. Ethosomes were not dialyzed because the dialysis process could extract the ethanol from the vesicles [75]. The recovered PC% in ethosomes was around 60% of the initial amount, and the EE% was reasonable for a hydrophilic molecule. In the other samples, phosphatidylcholine was not incorporated in a complete manner, presumably due to material loss during the manufacturing and extrusion processes (Table 2).

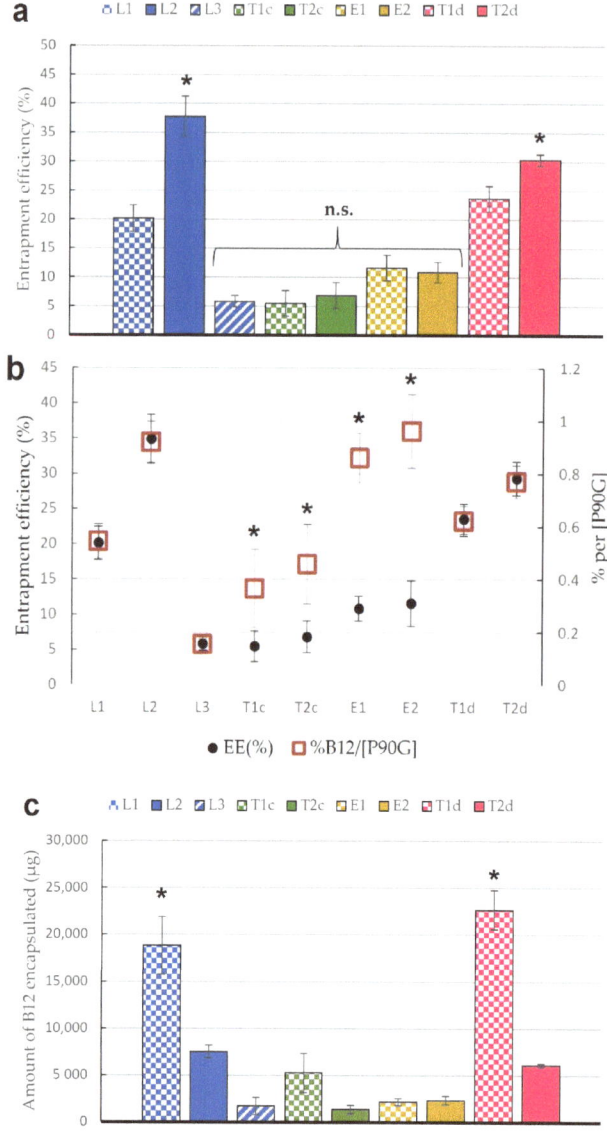

Figure 2. (**a**) Entrapment efficiency (EE) (expressed as a percentage) of the nine prototypes of liposomes, transferosomes, and ethosomes; (**b**) Specific entrapment efficiency rate of the nine prototypes of liposomes, transferosomes, and ethosomes; (**c**) Total amount of B12 encapsulated in 10 mL of liposomal suspension (µg). All results are expressed as mean ± SD ($n = 3$). * means statistically significant differences ($p < 0.05$), n.s. means no statistically significant differences ($p > 0.05$) using one-way ANOVA followed by Tukey's multiple comparison test.

However, it should be considered that the objective of this project was to obtain flexible lipid vesicles with the highest possible B12 dose, as saturated systems provide highest skin permeability rates [83]. Figure 2c represents the final amount of B12 per 10 mL of liposomal suspension. Here, we observed that, regardless the encapsulation efficiency values obtained, the highest B12 load was obtained when B12 was introduced in the aqueous phase in a saturated PBS solution (L1 and T1d) (Figure 2c). The higher water volume entrapped by the liposome core contains higher total amounts of B12 compared to the incorporation of the drug in the thin film layer.

The short-term stability behavior of the formulations was studied by the Turbiscan Stability Index (TSI), a parameter offered by Turbiscan^{TM} LAB Stability Analyzer device. TSI allows the comparison of samples that present different progression phenomena [84]. Transferosomes were found to be the most stable formulation since no changes in light transmission and backscattering lines were reported over 24 h (Figure 3c,d). A flocculation phenomenon was observed for the ethosomal samples through the backscattering graph (Figure 3f). Its evolution over the whole height of the sample proves a global increase of the particles size (Figure 3e,f). Flocculates could be easily redispersed by gentle shaking. Other aggregative processes, such as coalescence, were discarded, given that no significant long-term size changes were observed after periodically redispersing the samples. On the contrary, liposomal vesicles experienced first a sedimentation process, as the backscattering increases at the bottom of the sample, due to an increase of the concentration in the dispersed phase (sediment) and a decrease at the top of the sample, due to a reduction of the concentration (clarified layer) (Figure 3a,b). Additionally, the smallest particles that remained at the clarified phase showed a tiny flocculation at the end of the investigated times (yellow-red frame). Transmission and backscattering profiles in the work of Cristiano et al. were similar and showed comparable phenomena of flocculation for ethosomes and stability for transferosomes [85]. Therefore, the global destabilization kinetics (Figure 4) confirmed the stability indexes about B12 vesicles (liposome < ethosome < transferosome).

3.2. Stability Studies

Physical and chemical long-term stability was monitored by measuring the vesicle size, PDI, and EE% every week for 2 months and the drug content for 3 months. Figure 5a shows that no significant differences in size as a function of storage time at 4 °C, except for the liposomal formulations after 4 weeks of storage. This fact has been previously reported by other authors [86,87]. On the other hand, intra-type significant changes in PDI were not observed, pointing out a homogeneous evolution in size of vesicles populations (Figure 5b).

Significant changes in drug content related to the initial amount were detected in all prototypes between weeks 7 and 8 (Figure 6). Recent works have also reported a drug leakage and an effective content loss, especially for liposomes containing hydrophilic drugs, thus supporting our observations [87,88]. Considering these findings, B12 lipid vesicles seemed to exhibit short- and medium-term stability (at least 1 month for all the parameters checked), which makes them suitable for clinical applications. However, to increase the stability for longer-term use, liposome lyophilization could be investigated in the future for these B12 lipid vesicles, since it has been shown as an excellent method for ensuring liposome long-term stability [89,90].

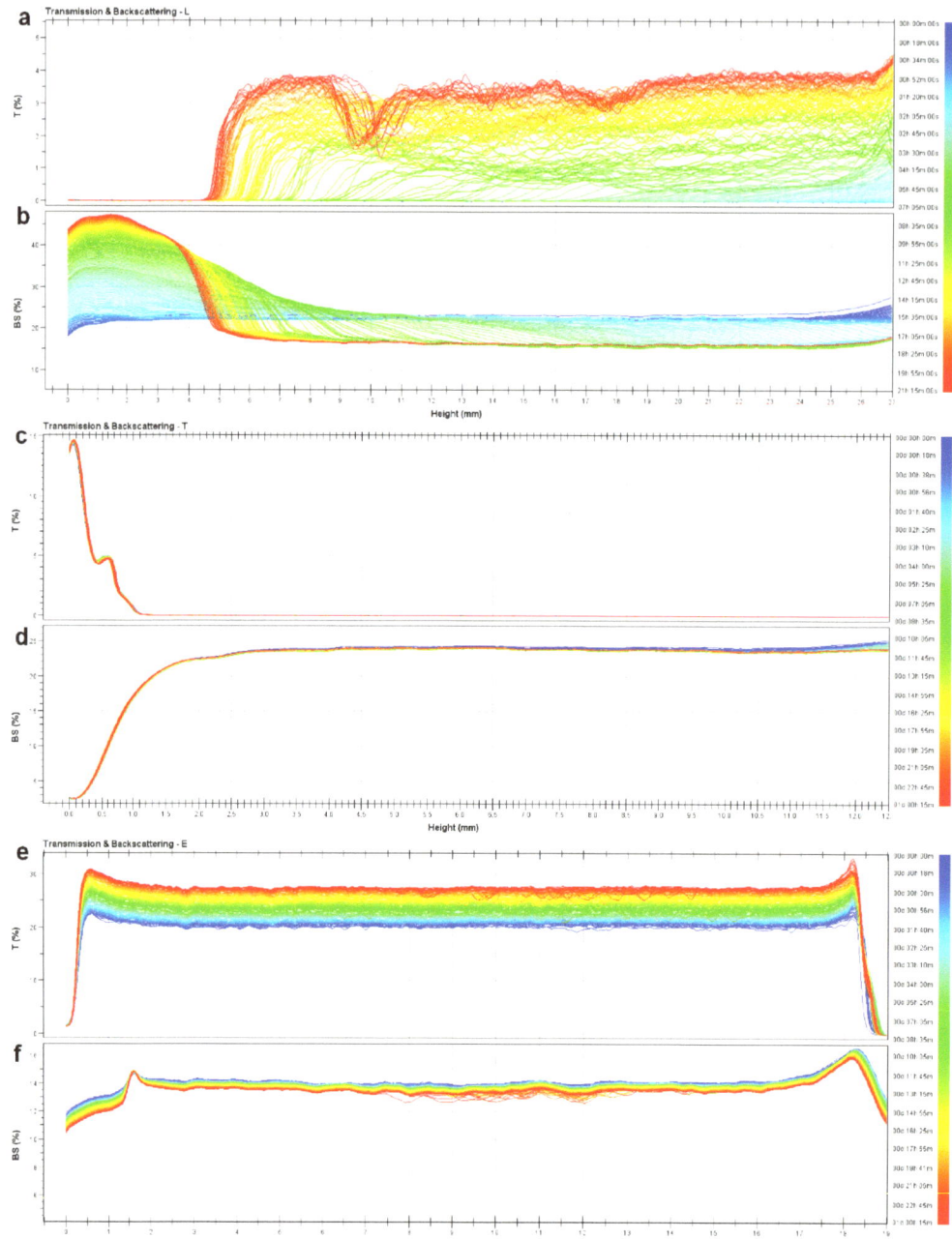

Figure 3. Short-term stability data: (**a**) L1 transmission data; (**b**) L1 backscattering data; (**c**) T1d transmission data; (**d**) T1d backscattering data; (**e**) E1 transmission data; (**f**) E1 backscattering data.

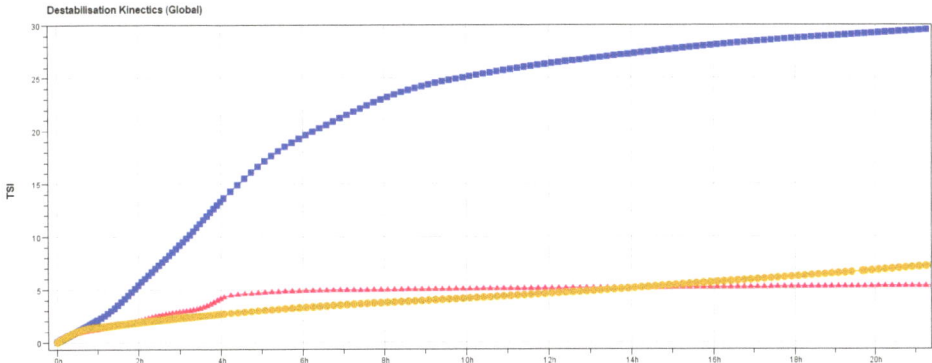

Figure 4. Short-term stability data; L1 TSI (blue), E1 TSI (yellow), and T1d TSI (red).

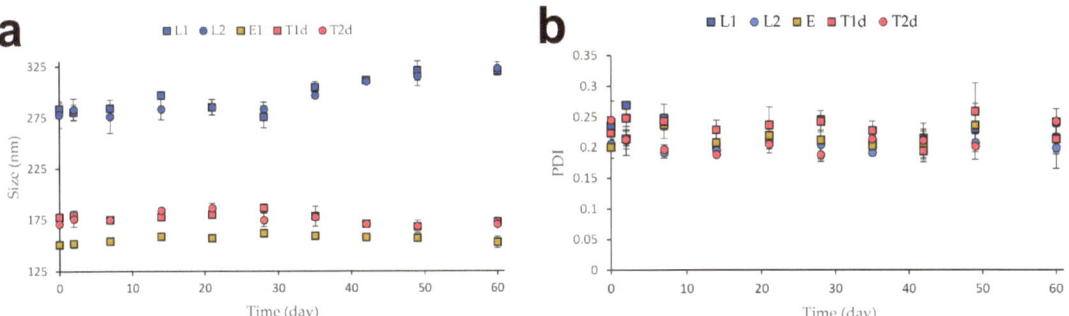

Figure 5. (**a**) Vesicle size over 2 months of storage (4 °C); (**b**) PDI over 2 months of storage (4 °C). All results are expressed as mean ± SD (n = 3). * means statistically significant differences when compared to the initial values ($p < 0.05$) using one-way ANOVA followed by Tukey's multiple comparison test.

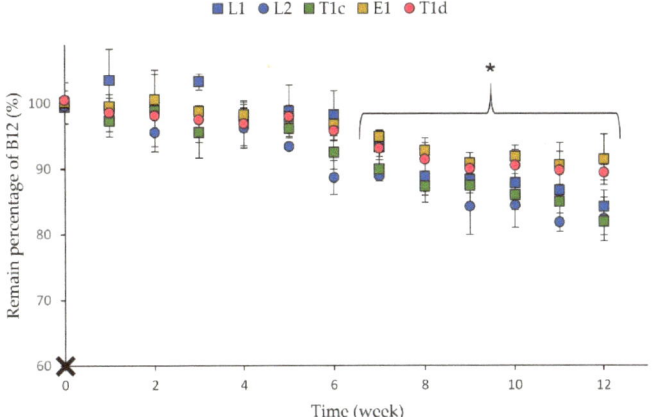

Figure 6. Remaining percentage of B12 amounts during 2 months of storage (4 °C). All results are expressed as mean ± SD (n = 3). * means statistically significant differences when compared to initial values ($p < 0.05$) using one-way ANOVA followed by Tukey's multiple comparison test.

3.3. In Vitro Drug Release Studies

In vitro drug release studies are regularly used in the optimization process of pharmaceutical forms [91]. In this work, the cumulative drug release profiles of the preselected optimized formulations were estimated by a dialysis method using the Franz diffusion cell set-up [92] and presented in Figure 7 and Tables S1 and S2 (Supplementary Materials section). Dialysis methods are appropriate and well accepted to study drug release profiles. Two processes are involved in drug transfer from the donor to the receiver chamber: drug release from the drug reservoir and molecule diffusion through the dialysis membrane, K' (diffusion rate) and K (release rate) being their respective experimental constants. Using the fitting models, in which K > K' for first orders transports and K ≈ K' for zero order transport, we observed that K was higher than K'. Therefore, the limiting step in all cases presented is the drug release from the drug carrier [74].

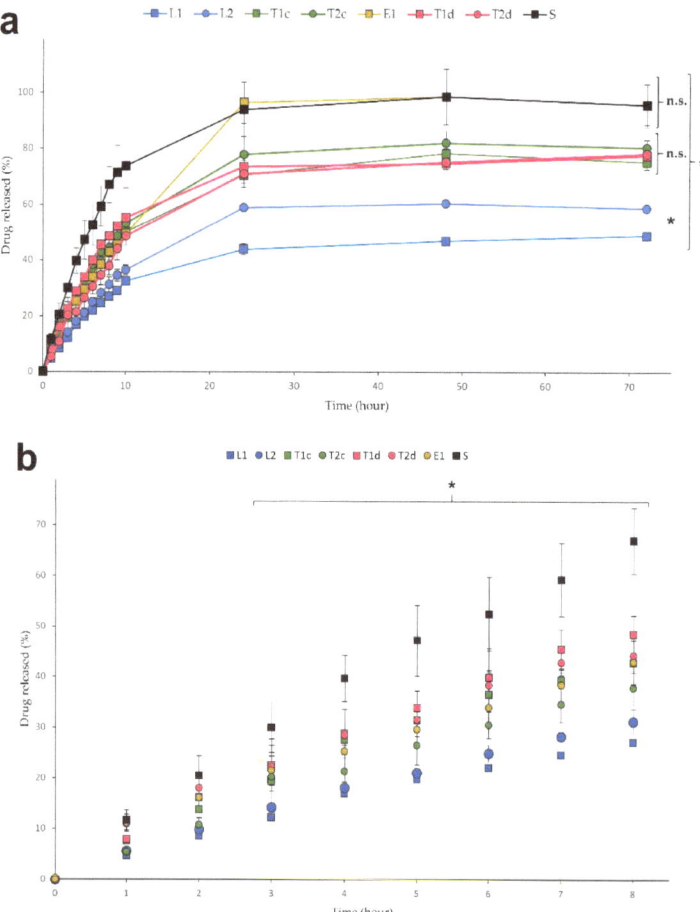

Figure 7. Release profiles from liposomes, transferosomes, ethosomes, and solution after 72 h (**a**) and 8 h (**b**). All results are expressed as mean ± SD (n = 6). * means statistically significant differences ($p < 0.05$), n.s. means no statistically significant differences ($p > 0.05$) using two-way ANOVA followed by Bonferroni's multiple comparison test.

The B12 solution (S) was used as a control as it represents the drug diffusion profile without limitations. The rest of the lipid vesicle formulations showed a controlled release of drug, as shown in Figure 7b. B12 was released faster during the initial hours from all the tested formulations due to the concentration gradient established between the donor and the receiver media [93]. After 3 h, the B12 amount detected in the receptor medium was significantly higher for the solution than the liposomes, transferosomes, and ethosomes, as expected [94]. Moreover, differences between the release from liposomal and ultraflexible vesicles were also observed, being lower from the liposomes, probably due to their different rigidity. It has been reported that vesicles with considerable bilayer rigidity exhibit higher resistance to drug transport through the liposomal bilayer [95]. The long-term percentage of drug released is probably also affected by this vesicle property. The lowest percentage of drug released corresponded to the liposomes and the highest to the ethosomes, which were able to release around 100% of the encapsulated B12. Nevertheless, the final percentages of released B12 between transferosomes and ethosomes were different (Figure 7a) even though no differences were found in vesicle flexibility during the characterization stage (Figure 1a,b). Possible reasons for this are: the difference of entrapped drug amounts (higher in transferosomes than in ethosomes) that led to different gradients and the vesicle structure and components. We found similar results in B12 release from L1 and L2 formulations profiles at the initial stage (<10 h) even though the B12 entrapped amount in L1 was higher than L2 formulation (Figure 2c). Differences are observed when reaching the plateau. However, the B12 cumulative amounts found in the last L1 samples (44, 46, and 48% at 24, 48, and 72 h, respectively) rose, suggesting that the plateau was not reached and differences may be reduced if the release were extended.

3.4. Model Fitting: Kinetic Drug Release Mechanisms

The experimental release data were fitted to different kinetic models to better understand the release profiles: Higuchi, Korsmeyer–Peppas, Kim, Peppas–Sahlin, zero order, and first order. This point is highly recommended since mathematical modeling could help to understand the further in vivo performance of the formulations [96]. Fitting parameters of all the models using the first 10 h data and 72 h data are listed in Table S1, Supplementary Materials section. The AIC was used as a comparative of the goodness of fit (also listed in Table S1, Supplementary Materials section). In general, the Korsmeyer–Peppas model presented the lowest AIC values, indicating an accurate fitting, for almost all formulations. However, in certain cases (T1d 10 h, T2c 72 h, E1 72 h and S), the first order was the best model. The Kim model is a modification of the Korsmeyer–Peppas one that considers a possible burst effect. This burst effect (represented by parameter "b") was neglected by the fitting, and the results of both models match. Burst release effect of drugs is frequently related to "dose dumping", an event to avoid in a controlled release system that was demonstrated not to happen in our prototypes [97,98].

The main difference between the first order model and the Korsmeyer–Peppas one is the mechanisms underlying the release process. First order only reflects a passive diffusion, while Korsmeyer–Peppas also considers other effects, such as relaxation or matrix erosion. Contrary to what was expected for ultraflexible vesicles, the Korsmeyer–Peppas model was more suitable for most of the cases, pointing out that they present a mixed release mechanism. It seems that relaxation has a stronger influence during the first steps and gets diluted during longer sampling times, in favor of passive diffusion. This behavior can be deduced from the values of the release exponent "n", which presents intermediate values (0.5–0.85) when the initial 10 h data are fitted and low values (<0.5) when 72 h data are included. Finally, the R^2 values from both models are also listed in Table S2 (Supplementary Materials section). We could observe from their analysis that the models used are suitable for explaining the release process (they account for >90% of the experimental data variation) [57,58].

3.5. Tape-Stripping Drug Penetration Studies

The stratum corneum layers depth in porcine skin was determined by infrared densitometry using a standardized procedure [66]. The total thickness obtained was around

20 µm, according with the standard values between 17–28 µm, previously reported by Jacobi et al. [99]. Tape-stripping studies were performed using the most promising formulations according to the afore-presented data: L1, L2, T1d, T2d, and E1. As incubation times, 2 h, 4 h, and 6 h were selected, covering the longest time a topical formulation would be maintained onto the skin. Besides, longer incubation times lead to overhydration of the skin and removal of the whole stratum corneum in a single strip [83]. The B12 solution 0.5% *w/v* (S) was used as a reference since it represents the free diffusion, and no enhancing absorption effects are expected from the vehicle.

Figure 8 shows the progressive B12 penetration in the different layers of the stratum corneum at different incubation periods. In general, the amounts of B12 detected in the deeper layers of the skin increased as a function of the incubation time, as expected. As shown, B12 solution presented the highest amount of B12 extracted in the first strip regardless of the incubation time. Two reasons can explain this fact: immediate availability of B12 on the skin leading to a quick distribution over the first stratum corneum layer, where it is retained; and a deficient cleaning of the skin surface. Concerning the latter, many authors discard this strip because the inaccuracy of the data is typically high and considered as an experimental artifact [100]. However, the rest of B12 from the solution did not penetrate the stratum corneum nor the deeper skin layers, and only low quantifiable concentrations were detected up to the third strip, which corresponds to 6 µm depth, after 6 h. These findings confirm the inability of B12 to diffuse through intact skin. The ethosome samples presented the lowest quantifiable amounts among all the vesicles tested, probably due to the low B12 load and the gradual release. Samples could have easily been under the detection/quantification limits.

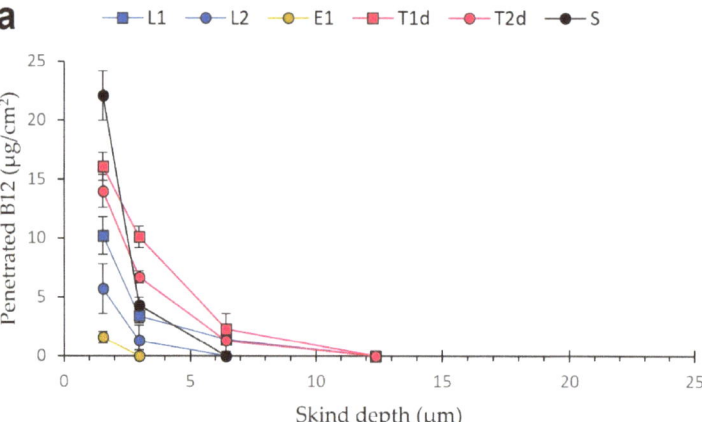

Figure 8. *Cont.*

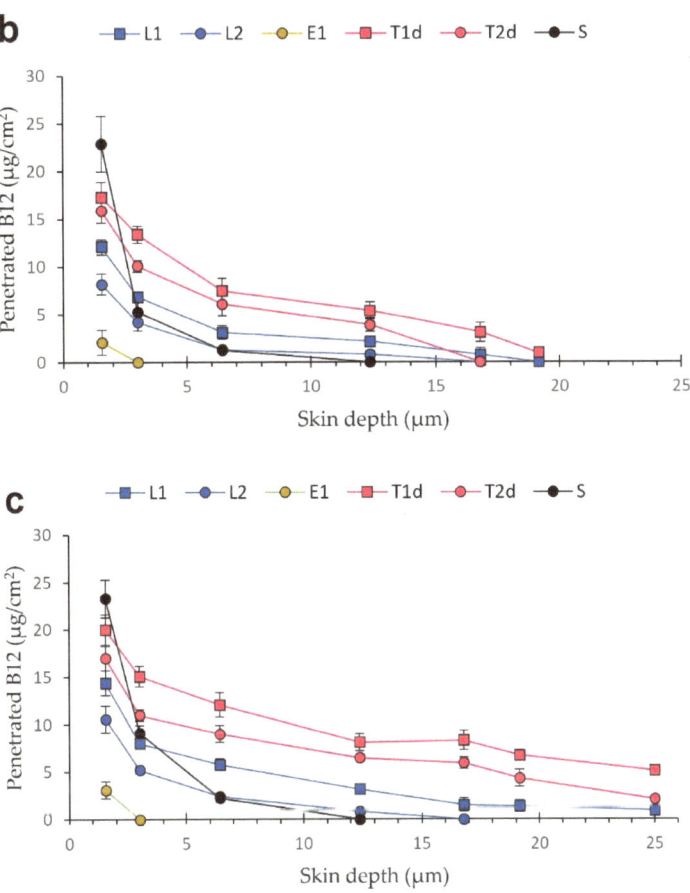

Figure 8. Penetration profiles of B12 delivered from liposomes, transferosomes, ethosomes, and solution after 2 h (**a**), 4 h (**b**), and 6 h (**c**). All results are expressed as mean ± SD (*n* = 3).

The best penetration results were obtained using liposomes and transferosomes. L2 carries less B12 amounts than the other prototypes, consequently showing a considerably lower B12 penetration amounts, only until approximately 15 µm depth (Figure 8c). Nevertheless, L1, T1d, and T2d vesicles allowed the B12 to reach the dermis (>25 µm). L1 and T2d contained similar B12 doses, but after 4 and 6 h of incubation, the transferosomes showed higher permeation rates up to the deepest layers (Figure 8b,c). This means that the stratum corneum is saturated in B12 at that time point, and a diffusion gradient to the deeper layers starts. T1d showed the highest permeation profiles. Our penetration results suggest that transferosome enhancing effect was much higher than the one of liposomes and are in agreement with Abd et al. [101], who compared the penetration of a hydrophilic drug (caffeine) delivered from liposomes, transferosomes, and solution.

B12 has been delivered through the skin using chemical and physical methods by other authors. Recently, Ramöller et al. achieved an effective delivery of B12 to plasma in a rat model. Rapidly dissolving microneedle allowed the permeation of 60% of dose after 2 h post-insertion, achieving 0.4 µg/mL plasma levels [28]. Yang et al. studied in vitro the effects of chemical enhancers and physical methods in topical administration of B12. Chemical enhancers (ethanol, oleic acid, and propylene glycol) allowed an effective permeability of B12 in comparison with passive diffusion. The permeability enhancement offered by iontophoresis was around 2-fold in comparison with a combination of all enhancers (50% ethanol, 10% oleic acid, and 40% propylene glycol) [27]. Although these methods have proven to effectively delivery B12, they present several inconveniences in B12 delivery for atopic dermatitis. For example, they were not able to localize their effects in the epidermis and dermis leading to an absorption of B12 to systemic circulation, which is unnecessary for psoriatic and atopic dermatitis patients. Additionally, local skin reactions and poor effectiveness in combination with hydrophilic molecules has been reported for chemical enhancers [102]. Moreover, ultraflexible lipid vesicles are technically easier to produce and a low cost in comparison to microneedles and iontophoresis devices [102].

From the results presented here, it can be concluded that the developed formulations are able to efficiently deliver B12 to the deeper skin layers after 6 h, as desired. We also demonstrate that B12 does not diffuse through the stratum corneum if formulated in water media. Further studies should be performed to formulate these vesicles in adequate dosage forms for an effective topical application of B12 that can be transferred to the clinic.

4. Conclusions

Enhanced penetration of B12 through the skin is possible using the lipid vesicle formulations (L1, T2d, and T1d) designed in this work, which opens the possibility to improve the clinical results obtained in previous studies and to investigate its utility for topical treatment of atopic dermatitis and psoriasis. Several particle properties such as size, stability, and purification method were revealed as key parameters to achieve a suitable and efficient production of lipid vesicles. Skin permeability studies should be further investigated to elucidate if these nanosystems are able not only to increase the penetration in the skin but also to allow the passage of B12 to the systemic circulation, thus broadening the possible applications of the systems for the treatment of other pathologies related with B12 deficiencies.

Supplementary Materials: The following are available online at https://www.mdpi.com/1999-4923/13/3/418/s1, Figure S1: Release parameters (10 and 72 h) for release kinetic models: Higuchi, Korsmeyer–Peppas, Kim, Peppas–Sahlin, zero order, and first order; Figure S2: R^2 values of Korsmeyer–Peppas and first order models for the B12 vesicles release data (10 and 72 h).

Author Contributions: Conceptualization, A.J.G., E.J.-M., T.M.G., and A.M.; methodology, A.J.G., T.M.G., and A.M.; software, A.J.G.; formal analysis, A.J.G., T.M.G., and A.M.; investigation and visualization, A.J.G., N.L., E.J.-M., and C.M.-G.; resources, M.C.M. and A.M.; writing—original draft preparation, A.J.G.; writing—review and editing, A.M., T.M.G., and M.C.M.; supervision, M.C.M., T.M.G., and A.M.; funding acquisition, M.C.M. and A.M. All authors have read and agreed to the published version of the manuscript.

Funding: A.J.G acknowledges the support of the "Atracció de Talent" fellowship of the University of Valencia (grant UV-INV-PREDOC-18F2-743816). A.J.G., T.M.G., and A.M. would also like to thank the University of Valencia and the Valencian Government (grants UV-19-INV-AE19 and GV2015-054). M.C.M., A.J.G., and A.M. acknowledge the Spanish Ministry of Science and Innovation-FEDER (SAF2017-85806-R). All authors acknowledge the support from AIMPLAS (project 3D-Future: IMDEEA/2019/90).

Institutional Review Board Statement: Not applicable.

Informed Consent Statement: Not applicable.

Data Availability Statement: Data is contained within the article.

Acknowledgments: All illustrations were created with Biorender.com.

Conflicts of Interest: The authors declare no conflict of interest.

References

1. Adler-Neal, A.L.; Cline, A.; Frantz, T.; Strowd, L.; Feldman, S.R.; Taylor, S. Complementary and Integrative Therapies for Childhood Atopic Dermatitis. *Children* **2019**, *6*, 121. [CrossRef]
2. Kapur, S.; Watson, W.; Carr, S. Atopic Dermatitis. *Allergy Asthma Clin. Immunol.* **2018**, *14* (Suppl. 2). [CrossRef]

3. Hirabayashi, T.; Anjo, T.; Kaneko, A.; Senoo, Y.; Shibata, A.; Takama, H.; Yokoyama, K.; Nishito, Y.; Ono, T.; Taya, C.; et al. PNPLA1 Has a Crucial Role in Skin Barrier Function by Directing Acylceramide Biosynthesis. *Nat. Commun.* **2017**, *8*, 14609. [CrossRef] [PubMed]
4. Agrawal, R.; Woodfolk, J.A. Skin Barrier Defects in Atopic Dermatitis. *Curr. Allergy Asthma Rep.* **2014**, *14*, 433. [CrossRef]
5. Zaniboni, M.C.; Samorano, L.P.; Orfali, R.L.; Aoki, V. Skin Barrier in Atopic Dermatitis: Beyond Filaggrin. *An. Bras. Dermatol.* **2016**, *91*, 472–478. [CrossRef]
6. Kolb, L.; Ferrer-Bruker, S.J. Atopic Dermatitis. In *StatPearls*; StatPearls Publishing: Treasure Island, FL, USA, 2020.
7. Parisi, R.; Symmons, D.P.M.; Griffiths, C.E.M.; Ashcroft, D.M.; Identification and Management of Psoriasis and Associated ComorbidiTy (IMPACT) Project Team. Global Epidemiology of Psoriasis: A Systematic Review of Incidence and Prevalence. *J. Investig. Dermatol.* **2013**, *133*, 377–385. [CrossRef]
8. Arima, K.; Ohta, S.; Takagi, A.; Shiraishi, H.; Masuoka, M.; Ontsuka, K.; Suto, H.; Suzuki, S.; Yamamoto, K.-I.; Ogawa, M.; et al. Periostin Contributes to Epidermal Hyperplasia in Psoriasis Common to Atopic Dermatitis. *Allergol. Int.* **2015**, *64*, 41–48. [CrossRef]
9. Heidenreich, R.; Röcken, M.; Ghoreschi, K. Angiogenesis Drives Psoriasis Pathogenesis. *Int. J. Exp. Pathol.* **2009**, *90*, 232–248. [CrossRef] [PubMed]
10. Nussbaum, L.; Chen, Y.L.; Ogg, G.S. Role of Regulatory T Cells in Psoriasis Pathogenesis and Treatment. *Br. J. Dermatol.* **2021**, *184*, 14–24. [CrossRef] [PubMed]
11. Badri, T.; Kumar, P.; Oakley, A.M. Plaque Psoriasis. In *StatPearls*; StatPearls Publishing: Treasure Island, FL, USA, 2020.
12. Thomsen, S.F. Atopic Dermatitis: Natural History, Diagnosis, and Treatment. *Int. Sch. Res. Not.* **2014**, *2014*, 354250. [CrossRef] [PubMed]
13. Fiore, M.; Leone, S.; Maraolo, A.E.; Berti, E.; Damiani, G. Liver Illness and Psoriatic Patients. *BioMed Res. Int.* **2018**, *2018*, 3140983. [CrossRef] [PubMed]
14. Grandinetti, V.; Baraldi, O.; Comai, G.; Corradetti, V.; Aiello, V.; Bini, C.; Minerva, V.; Barbuto, S.; Fabbrizio, B.; Donati, G.; et al. Renal Dysfunction in Psoriatic Patients. *G. Ital. Nefrol.* **2020**, *37*, 1–12.
15. Jindal, N.; Arora, K.; Jindal, P.; Jain, V.K.; Ghosh, S. Inflamed Psoriatic Plaques: Drug Toxicity or Disease Exacerbation? *Indian J. Pharmacol.* **2013**, *45*, 410–411. [CrossRef]
16. Oray, M.; Abu Samra, K.; Ebrahimiadib, N.; Meese, H.; Foster, C.S. Long-Term Side Effects of Glucocorticoids. *Expert Opin. Drug Saf.* **2016**, *15*, 457–465. [CrossRef]
17. Siegfried, E.C.; Jaworski, J.C.; Hebert, A.A. Topical Calcineurin Inhibitors and Lymphoma Risk: Evidence Update with Implications for Daily Practice. *Am. J. Clin. Dermatol.* **2013**, *14*, 163–178. [CrossRef]
18. Sirsjö, A.; Karlsson, M.; Gidlöf, A.; Rollman, O.; Törmä, H. Increased Expression of Inducible Nitric Oxide Synthase in Psoriatic Skin and Cytokine-Stimulated Cultured Keratinocytes. *Br. J. Dermatol.* **1996**, *134*, 643–648. [CrossRef] [PubMed]
19. Brescoll, J.; Daveluy, S. A Review of Vitamin B12 in Dermatology. *Am. J. Clin. Dermatol.* **2015**, *16*, 27–33. [CrossRef]
20. Baker, H.; Comaish, J.S. Is Vitamin B12 of Value in Psoriasis? *Br. Med. J.* **1962**, *2*, 1729–1730. [CrossRef]
21. Januchowski, R. Evaluation of Topical Vitamin B(12) for the Treatment of Childhood Eczema. *J. Altern Complement. Med.* **2009**, *15*, 387–389. [CrossRef]
22. Stücker, M.; Memmel, U.; Hoffmann, M.; Hartung, J.; Altmeyer, P. Vitamin B(12) Cream Containing Avocado Oil in the Therapy of Plaque Psoriasis. *Dermatology* **2001**, *203*, 141–147. [CrossRef] [PubMed]
23. Del Duca, E.; Farnetani, F.; De Carvalho, N.; Bottoni, U.; Pellacani, G.; Nisticò, S.P. Superiority of a Vitamin B12-Containing Emollient Compared to a Standard Emollient in the Maintenance Treatment of Mild-to-Moderate Plaque Psoriasis. *Int. J. Immunopathol. Pharmacol.* **2017**, *30*, 439–444. [CrossRef]
24. Moore, R.; Harry, R. *Harry's Cosmeticology*, 7th ed.; Chemical Publishing: New York, NY, USA, 1982; pp. 1–41.
25. Paudel, K.S.; Milewski, M.; Swadley, C.L.; Brogden, N.K.; Ghosh, P.; Stinchcomb, A.L. Challenges and Opportunities in Dermal/Transdermal Delivery. *Ther. Deliv.* **2010**, *1*, 109–131. [CrossRef]
26. Howe, E.E.; Dooley, C.L.; Geoffroy, R.F.; Rosenblum, C. Percutaneous Absorption of Vitamin B12 in the Rat and Guinea Pig. *J. Nutr.* **1967**, *92*, 261–266. [CrossRef] [PubMed]
27. Yang, Y.; Kalluri, H.; Banga, A.K. Effects of Chemical and Physical Enhancement Techniques on Transdermal Delivery of Cyanocobalamin (Vitamin B12) In Vitro. *Pharmaceutics* **2011**, *3*, 474–484. [CrossRef]
28. Ramöller, I.K.; Tekko, I.A.; McCarthy, H.O.; Donnelly, R.F. Rapidly Dissolving Bilayer Microneedle Arrays—A Minimally Invasive Transdermal Drug Delivery System for Vitamin B12. *Int. J. Pharm.* **2019**, *566*, 299–306. [CrossRef]
29. Kim, M.-H.; Jeon, Y.-E.; Kang, S.; Lee, J.-Y.; Lee, K.W.; Kim, K.-T.; Kim, D.-D. Lipid Nanoparticles for Enhancing the Physicochemical Stability and Topical Skin Delivery of Orobol. *Pharmaceutics* **2020**, *12*, 845. [CrossRef]
30. Yotsumoto, K.; Ishii, K.; Kokubo, M.; Yasuoka, S. Improvement of the Skin Penetration of Hydrophobic Drugs by Polymeric Micelles. *Int. J. Pharm.* **2018**, *553*, 132–140. [CrossRef]
31. Cutlar, L.; Zhou, D.; Hu, X.; Duarte, B.; Greiser, U.; Larcher, F.; Wang, W. A Non-Viral Gene Therapy for Treatment of Recessive Dystrophic Epidermolysis Bullosa. *Exp. Dermatol.* **2016**, *25*, 818–820. [CrossRef]
32. Zeng, M.; Alshehri, F.; Zhou, D.; Lara-Sáez, I.; Wang, X.; Li, X.; Xu, Q.; Zhang, J.; Wang, W. Efficient and Robust Highly Branched Poly(β-Amino Ester)/Minicircle COL7A1 Polymeric Nanoparticles for Gene Delivery to Recessive Dystrophic Epidermolysis Bullosa Keratinocytes. *ACS Appl. Mater. Interfaces* **2019**, *11*, 30661–30672. [CrossRef] [PubMed]
33. Zhou, D.; Gao, Y.; Aied, A.; Cutlar, L.; Igoucheva, O.; Newland, B.; Alexeeve, V.; Greiser, U.; Uitto, J.; Wang, W. Highly Branched Poly(β-Amino Ester)s for Skin Gene Therapy. *J. Control. Release* **2016**, *244*, 336–346. [CrossRef] [PubMed]

34. Zeng, M.; Zhou, D.; Alshehri, F.; Lara-Sáez, I.; Lyu, Y.; Creagh-Flynn, J.; Xu, Q.; Zhang, J.; Wang, W. Manipulation of Transgene Expression in Fibroblast Cells by a Multifunctional Linear-Branched Hybrid Poly(β-Amino Ester) Synthesized through an Oligomer Combination Approach. *Nano Lett.* **2018**, *19*, 381–391. [CrossRef]
35. Mostafa, M.; Alaaeldin, E.; Aly, U.F.; Sarhan, H.A. Optimization and Characterization of Thymoquinone-Loaded Liposomes with Enhanced Topical Anti-Inflammatory Activity. *AAPS PharmSciTech* **2018**, *19*, 3490–3500. [CrossRef] [PubMed]
36. Peralta, M.F.; Guzmán, M.L.; Pérez, A.P.; Apezteguia, G.A.; Fórmica, M.L.; Romero, E.L.; Olivera, M.E.; Carrer, D.C. Liposomes Can Both Enhance or Reduce Drugs Penetration through the Skin. *Sci. Rep.* **2018**, *8*, 13253. [CrossRef] [PubMed]
37. Bozzuto, G.; Molinari, A. Liposomes as Nanomedical Devices. *Int. J. Nanomed.* **2015**, *10*, 975–999. [CrossRef]
38. Cevc, G.; Blume, G. Lipid Vesicles Penetrate into Intact Skin Owing to the Transdermal Osmotic Gradients and Hydration Force. *Biochim. Biophys. Acta* **1992**, *1104*, 226–232. [CrossRef]
39. Touitou, E.; Godin, B. Ethosomes for Skin Delivery. *J. Drug Deliv. Sci. Technol.* **2007**, *17*, 303–308. [CrossRef]
40. Arsalan, A.; Ahmad, I.; Ali, S.A.; Qadeer, K.; Mahmud, S.; Humayun, F.; Beg, A.E. The Kinetics of Photostabilization of Cyanocobalamin in Liposomal Preparations. *Int. J. Chem. Kinet.* **2020**, *52*, 207–217. [CrossRef]
41. Vitetta, L.; Zhou, J.; Manuel, R.; Dal Forno, S.; Hall, S.; Rutolo, D. Route and Type of Formulation Administered Influences the Absorption and Disposition of Vitamin B12 Levels in Serum. *J. Funct. Biomater.* **2018**, *9*, 12. [CrossRef]
42. Castoldi, A.; Herr, C.; Niederstraßer, J.; Labouta, H.I.; Melero, A.; Gordon, S.; Schneider-Daum, N.; Bals, R.; Lehr, C.-M. Calcifediol-Loaded Liposomes for Local Treatment of Pulmonary Bacterial Infections. *Eur. J. Pharm. Biopharm.* **2017**, *118*, 62–67. [CrossRef] [PubMed]
43. Ahad, A.; Al-Saleh, A.A.; Al-Mohizea, A.M.; Al-Jenoobi, F.I.; Raish, M.; Yassin, A.E.B.; Alam, M.A. Formulation and Characterization of Novel Soft Nanovesicles for Enhanced Transdermal Delivery of Eprosartan Mesylate. *Saudi Pharm. J.* **2017**, *25*, 1040–1046. [CrossRef]
44. Touitou, E.; Dayan, N.; Bergelson, L.; Godin, B.; Eliaz, M. Ethosomes—Novel Vesicular Carriers for Enhanced Delivery: Characterization and Skin Penetration Properties. *J. Control. Release* **2000**, *65*, 403–418. [CrossRef]
45. El Maghraby, G.M.; Williams, A.C.; Barry, B.W. Oestradiol Skin Delivery from Ultradeformable Liposomes: Refinement of Surfactant Concentration. *Int. J. Pharm.* **2000**, *196*, 63–74. [CrossRef]
46. Ong, S.G.M.; Ming, L.C.; Lee, K.S.; Yuen, K.H. Influence of the Encapsulation Efficiency and Size of Liposome on the Oral Bioavailability of Griseofulvin-Loaded Liposomes. *Pharmaceutics* **2016**, *8*, 25. [CrossRef]
47. Lin, M.; Qi, X.-R. Purification Method of Drug-Loaded Liposome. In *Liposome-Based Drug Delivery Systems*; Lu, W.-L., Qi, X.-R., Eds.; Biomaterial Engineering; Springer: Berlin/Heidelberg, Germany, 2018. [CrossRef]
48. Panwar, P.; Pandey, B.; Lakhera, P.C.; Singh, K.P. Preparation, Characterization, and In Vitro Release Study of Albendazole-Encapsulated Nanosize Liposomes. *Int. J. Nanomed.* **2010**, *5*, 101–108. [CrossRef]
49. Keller, S.; Heerklotz, H.; Jahnke, N.; Blume, A. Thermodynamics of Lipid Membrane Solubilization by Sodium Dodecyl Sulfate. *Biophys. J.* **2006**, *90*, 4509–4521. [CrossRef]
50. Hernández-Borrell, J.; Pons, M.; Juarez, J.C.; Estelrich, J. The Action of Triton X-100 and Sodium Dodecyl Sulphate on Lipid Layers. Effect on Monolayers and Liposomes. *J. Microencapsul.* **1990**, *7*, 255–259. [CrossRef] [PubMed]
51. Igarashi, T.; Shoji, Y.; Katayama, K. Anomalous Solubilization Behavior of Dimyristoylphosphatidylcholine Liposomes Induced by Sodium Dodecyl Sulfate Micelles. *Anal. Sci.* **2012**, *28*, 345–350. [CrossRef]
52. Sabeti, B.; Noordin, M.I.; Mohd, S.; Hashim, R.; Dahlan, A.; Javar, H.A. Development and Characterization of Liposomal Doxorubicin Hydrochloride with Palm Oil. *Biomed Res. Int.* **2014**, *2014*, 765426. [CrossRef]
53. Rouser, G.; Fkeischer, S.; Yamamoto, A. Two Dimensional Then Layer Chromatographic Separation of Polar Lipids and Determination of Phospholipids by Phosphorus Analysis of Spots. *Lipids* **1970**, *5*, 494–496. [CrossRef]
54. Jain, S.; Jain, P.; Umamaheshwari, R.B.; Jain, N.K. Transfersomes–a Novel Vesicular Carrier for Enhanced Transdermal Delivery: Development, Characterization, and Performance Evaluation. *Drug Dev. Ind. Pharm.* **2003**, *29*, 1013–1026. [CrossRef]
55. Celia, C.; Trapasso, E.; Cosco, D.; Paolino, D.; Fresta, M. Turbiscan Lab Expert Analysis of the Stability of Ethosomes and Ultradeformable Liposomes Containing a Bilayer Fluidizing Agent. *Colloids Surf. B Biointerfaces* **2009**, *72*, 155–160. [CrossRef]
56. Nava, G.; Piñón, E.; Mendoza, L.; Mendoza, N.; Quintanar, D.; Ganem, A. Formulation and in Vitro, Ex Vivo and in Vivo Evaluation of Elastic Liposomes for Transdermal Delivery of Ketorolac Trometamine. *Pharmaceutics* **2011**, *3*, 954–970. [CrossRef]
57. Akaike, H. Information Theory and an Extension of the Maximum Likelihood Principle. In *Selected Papers of Hirotugu Akaike*; Parzen, E., Tanabe, K., Kitagawa, G., Eds.; Springer Series in Statistics; Springer: New York, NY, USA, 1998; pp. 199–213. [CrossRef]
58. Hamilton, D.F.; Ghert, M.; Simpson, A.H.R.W. Interpreting Regression Models in Clinical Outcome Studies. *Bone Joint Res.* **2015**, *4*, 152–153. [CrossRef]
59. Higuchi, T. Rate of Release of Medicaments from Ointment Bases Containing Drugs in Suspension. *J. Pharm. Sci.* **1961**, *50*, 874–875. [CrossRef]
60. Ritger, P.L.; Peppas, N.A. A Simple Equation for Description of Solute Release I. Fickian and Non-Fickian Release from Non-Swellable Devices in the Form of Slabs, Spheres, Cylinders or Discs. *J. Control. Release* **1987**, *5*, 23–36. [CrossRef]
61. Ritger, P.L.; Peppas, N.A. A Simple Equation for Description of Solute Release II. Fickian and Anomalous Release from Swellable Devices. *J. Control. Release* **1987**, *5*, 37–42. [CrossRef]
62. Kim, H.; Fassihi, R. Application of Binary Polymer System in Drug Release Rate Modulation. 2. Influence of Formulation Variables and Hydrodynamic Conditions on Release Kinetics. *J. Pharm. Sci.* **1997**, *86*, 323–328. [CrossRef]
63. Peppas, N.A.; Sahlin, J.J. A Simple Equation for the Description of Solute Release. III. Coupling of Diffusion and Relaxation. *Int. J. Pharm.* **1989**, *57*, 169–172. [CrossRef]

64. Jain, A.; Jain, S.K. In vitro release kinetics model fitting of liposomes: An insight. *Chem. Phys. Lipids* **2016**, *201*, 28–40. [CrossRef]
65. Carolina Oliveira dos Santos, L.; Spagnol, C.M.; Guillot, A.J.; Melero, A.; Corrêa, M.A. Caffeic Acid Skin Absorption: Delivery of Microparticles to Hair Follicles. *Saudi Pharm. J.* **2019**, *27*, 791–797. [CrossRef]
66. Melero, A.; Hahn, T.; Schaefer, U.F.; Schneider, M. In Vitro Human Skin Segmentation and Drug Concentration-Skin Depth Profiles. *Methods Mol. Biol.* **2011**, *763*, 33–50. [CrossRef]
67. Melero, A.; Ferreira Ourique, A.; Stanisçuaski Guterres, S.; Raffin Pohlmann, A.; Lehr, C.-M.; Ruver Beck, R.C.; Schaefer, U. Nanoencapsulation in Lipid-Core Nanocapsules Controls Mometasone Furoate Skin Permeability Rate and Its Penetration to the Deeper Skin Layers. *Skin Pharmacol. Physiol.* **2014**, *27*, 217. [CrossRef]
68. Shaker, S.; Gardouh, A.R.; Ghorab, M.M. Factors Affecting Liposomes Particle Size Prepared by Ethanol Injection Method. *Res. Pharm. Sci.* **2017**, *12*, 346–352. [CrossRef]
69. Lee, S.-C.; Lee, K.-E.; Kim, J.-J.; Lim, S.-H. The Effect of Cholesterol in the Liposome Bilayer on the Stabilization of Incorporated Retinol. *J. Liposome Res.* **2005**, *15*, 157–166. [CrossRef] [PubMed]
70. Coderch, L.; Fonollosa, J.; De Pera, M.; Estelrich, J.; De La Maza, A.; Parra, J.L. Influence of Cholesterol on Liposome Fluidity by EPR. Relationship with Percutaneous Absorption. *J. Control. Release* **2000**, *68*, 85–95. [CrossRef]
71. Opatha, S.A.T.; Titapiwatanakun, V.; Chutoprapat, R. Transfersomes: A Promising Nanoencapsulation Technique for Transdermal Drug Delivery. *Pharmaceutics* **2020**, *12*, 855. [CrossRef]
72. Fernández-García, R.; Lalatsa, A.; Statts, L.; Bolás-Fernández, F.; Ballesteros, M.P.; Serrano, D.R. Transferosomes as Nanocarriers for Drugs across the Skin: Quality by Design from Lab to Industrial Scale. *Int. J. Pharm.* **2020**, *573*, 118817. [CrossRef]
73. Ascenso, A.; Raposo, S.; Batista, C.; Cardoso, P.; Mendes, T.; Praça, F.G.; Bentley, M.V.L.B.; Simões, S. Development, Characterization, and Skin Delivery Studies of Related Ultradeformable Vesicles: Transfersomes, Ethosomes, and Transethosomes. *Int. J. Nanomed.* **2015**, *10*, 5837–5851. [CrossRef]
74. Wu, I.Y.; Bala, S.; Škalko-Basnet, N.; di Cagno, M.P. Interpreting Non-Linear Drug Diffusion Data: Utilizing Korsmeyer-Peppas Model to Study Drug Release from Liposomes. *Eur. J. Pharm. Sci.* **2019**, *138*, 105026. [CrossRef]
75. Carreras, J.J.; Tapia-Ramirez, W.E.; Sala, A.; Guillot, A.J.; Garrigues, T.M.; Melero, A. Ultraflexible Lipid Vesicles Allow Topical Absorption of Cyclosporin A. *Drug Deliv. Transl. Res.* **2020**, *10*, 486–497. [CrossRef] [PubMed]
76. Danaei, M.; Dehghankhold, M.; Ataei, S.; Hasanzadeh Davarani, F.; Javanmard, R.; Dokhani, A.; Khorasani, S.; Mozafari, M.R. Impact of Particle Size and Polydispersity Index on the Clinical Applications of Lipidic Nanocarrier Systems. *Pharmaceutics* **2018**, *10*, 57. [CrossRef] [PubMed]
77. Chen, C.; Han, D.; Cai, C.; Tang, X. An Overview of Liposome Lyophilization and Its Future Potential. *J. Control. Release* **2010**, *142*, 299–311. [CrossRef] [PubMed]
78. Magarkar, A.; Dhawan, V.; Kallinteri, P.; Viitala, T.; Elmowafy, M.; Róg, T.; Bunker, A. Cholesterol Level Affects Surface Charge of Lipid Membranes in Saline Solution. *Sci. Rep.* **2014**, *4*, 5005. [CrossRef]
79. Abdulbaqi, I.M.; Darwis, Y.; Khan, N.A.K.; Assi, R.A.; Khan, A.A. Ethosomal Nanocarriers: The Impact of Constituents and Formulation Techniques on Ethosomal Properties, in Vivo Studies, and Clinical Trials. *Int. J. Nanomed.* **2016**, *11*, 2279–2304. [CrossRef] [PubMed]
80. Iskandaryah, I.; Masrijal, C.; Harmita, H. Effects of sonication on size distribution and entrapment of lynestrenol transferosome. *Int. J. Appl. Pharm.* **2020**, 245–247. [CrossRef]
81. Xu, X.; Khan, M.A.; Burgess, D.J. Predicting Hydrophilic Drug Encapsulation inside Unilamellar Liposomes. *Int. J. Pharm.* **2012**, *423*, 410–418. [CrossRef] [PubMed]
82. Kirby, C.; Gregoriadis, G. Dehydration-Rehydration Vesicles: A Simple Method for High Yield Drug Entrapment in Liposomes. *Nat. Biotechnology* **1984**, *2*, 979–984. [CrossRef]
83. Melero, A.; Garrigues, T.M.; Almudever, P.; Villodre, A.M.; Lehr, C.M.; Schäfer, U. Nortriptyline Hydrochloride Skin Absorption: Development of a Transdermal Patch. *Eur. J. Pharm. Biopharm.* **2008**, *69*, 588–596. [CrossRef]
84. Wu, C.-S.; Guo, J.-H.; Lin, M.-J. Stability Evaluation of PH-Adjusted Goat Milk for Developing Ricotta Cheese with a Mixture of Cow Cheese Whey and Goat Milk. *Foods* **2020**, *9*, 366. [CrossRef] [PubMed]
85. Cristiano, M.C.; Froiio, F.; Spaccapelo, R.; Mancuso, A.; Nisticò, S.P.; Udongo, B.P.; Fresta, M.; Paolino, D. Sulforaphane-Loaded Ultradeformable Vesicles as A Potential Natural Nanomedicine for the Treatment of Skin Cancer Diseases. *Pharmaceutics* **2019**, *12*, 6. [CrossRef]
86. Elsana, H.; Olusanya, T.O.B.; Carr-Wilkinson, J.; Darby, S.; Faheem, A.; Elkordy, A.A. Evaluation of Novel Cationic Gene Based Liposomes with Cyclodextrin Prepared by Thin Film Hydration and Microfluidic Systems. *Sci. Rep.* **2019**, *9*, 15120. [CrossRef]
87. Liang, T.; Guan, R.; Quan, Z.; Tao, Q.; Liu, Z.; Hu, Q. Cyanidin-3-o-Glucoside Liposome: Preparation via a Green Method and Antioxidant Activity in GES-1 Cells. *Food Res. Int.* **2019**, *125*, 108648. [CrossRef] [PubMed]
88. Muppidi, K.; Pumerantz, A.S.; Wang, J.; Betageri, G. Development and Stability Studies of Novel Liposomal Vancomycin Formulations. *Int. Sch. Res. Not.* **2012**, *2012*, 636743. [CrossRef]
89. Franzé, S.; Selmin, F.; Samaritani, E.; Minghetti, P.; Cilurzo, F. Lyophilization of Liposomal Formulations: Still Necessary, Still Challenging. *Pharmaceutics* **2018**, *10*, 139. [CrossRef] [PubMed]
90. Chen, M.; Liu, X.; Fahr, A. Skin Penetration and Deposition of Carboxyfluorescein and Temoporfin from Different Lipid Vesicular Systems: In Vitro Study with Finite and Infinite Dosage Application. *Int. J. Pharm.* **2011**, *408*, 223–234. [CrossRef]

91. Cunha, S.; Costa, C.P.; Loureiro, J.A.; Alves, J.; Peixoto, A.F.; Forbes, B.; Sousa Lobo, J.M.; Silva, A.C. Double Optimization of Rivastigmine-Loaded Nanostructured Lipid Carriers (NLC) for Nose-to-Brain Delivery Using the Quality by Design (QbD) Approach: Formulation Variables and Instrumental Parameters. *Pharmaceutics* **2020**, *12*, 599. [CrossRef]
92. Spagnol, C.M.; Zaera, A.M.; Isaac, V.L.B.; Corrêa, M.A.; Salgado, H.R.N. Release and Permeation Profiles of Spray-Dried Chitosan Microparticles Containing Caffeic Acid. *Saudi Pharm. J.* **2018**, *26*, 410–415. [CrossRef] [PubMed]
93. Gulati, K.; Kant, K.; Findlay, D.; Losic, D. Periodically Tailored Titania Nanotubes for Enhanced Drug Loading and Releasing Performances. *J. Mater. Chem. B* **2015**, *3*, 2553–2559. [CrossRef] [PubMed]
94. Nounou, M.M.; El-Khordagui, L.K.; Khalafallah, N.A.; Khalil, S.A. In Vitro Release of Hydrophilic and Hydrophobic Drugs from Liposomal Dispersions and Gels. *Acta Pharm.* **2006**, *56*, 311–324.
95. Leite, N.B.; Martins, D.B.; Fazani, V.E.; Vieira, M.R.; Dos Santos Cabrera, M.P. Cholesterol Modulates Curcumin Partitioning and Membrane Effects. *Biochim. Biophys. Acta Biomembr.* **2018**, *1860*, 2320–2328. [CrossRef]
96. Lu, T.; ten Hagen, T.L.M. A Novel Kinetic Model to Describe the Ultra-Fast Triggered Release of Thermosensitive Liposomal Drug Delivery Systems. *J. Control. Release* **2020**, *324*, 669–678. [CrossRef]
97. Kaur, G.; Grewal, J.; Jyoti, K.; Jain, U.K.; Chandra, R.; Madan, J. Chapter 15—Oral Controlled and Sustained Drug Delivery Systems: Concepts, Advances, Preclinical, and Clinical Status. In *Drug Targeting and Stimuli Sensitive Drug Delivery Systems*; Grumezescu, A.M., Ed.; William Andrew Publishing: Norwich, NY, USA, 2018; pp. 567–626. [CrossRef]
98. Brazel, C.S.; Huang, X. The Cost of Optimal Drug Delivery: Reducing and Preventing the Burst Effect in Matrix Systems. In *Carrier-Based Drug Delivery*; ACS Symposium Series; American Chemical Society: Washington, DC, USA, 2004; Volume 879. [CrossRef]
99. Jacobi, U.; Kaiser, M.; Toll, R.; Mangelsdorf, S.; Audring, H.; Otberg, N.; Sterry, W.; Lademann, J. Porcine Ear Skin: An in Vitro Model for Human Skin. *Skin Res. Technol.* **2007**, *13*, 19–24. [CrossRef]
100. Surber, C.; Schwarb, F.P.; Smith, E.W. Tape-Stripping Technique. *J. Toxicol. Cutan. Ocul. Toxicol.* **2001**, *20*, 461–474. [CrossRef]
101. Abd, E.; Roberts, M.S.; Grice, J.E. A Comparison of the Penetration and Permeation of Caffeine into and through Human Epidermis after Application in Various Vesicle Formulations. *Skin Pharmacol. Physiol.* **2016**, *29*, 24–30. [CrossRef]
102. Guillot, A.J.; Cordeiro, A.S.; Donnelly, R.F.; Montesinos, M.C.; Garrigues, T.M.; Melero, A. Microneedle-Based Delivery: An Overview of Current Applications and Trends. *Pharmaceutics* **2020**, *12*, 569. [CrossRef]

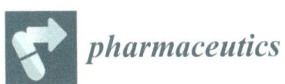

Article

The Impact of Lipid Handling and Phase Distribution on the Acoustic Behavior of Microbubbles

Simone A.G. Langeveld, Inés Beekers, Gonzalo Collado-Lara, Antonius F. W. van der Steen, Nico de Jong and Klazina Kooiman

1. Thorax Center, Biomedical Engineering, Erasmus University Medical Center, 3000 CA Rotterdam, The Netherlands; inesbeekers@gmail.com (I.B.); g.colladolara@erasmusmc.nl (G.C.-L.); a.vandersteen@erasmusmc.nl (A.F.W.v.d.S.); n.dejong@erasmusmc.nl (N.d.J.); k.kooiman@erasmusmc.nl (K.K.)
2. Acoustical Wavefield Imaging, Delft University of Technology, 2628 CJ Delft, The Netherlands
* Correspondence: s.a.g.langeveld@erasmusmc.nl

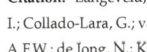

Citation: Langeveld, S.A.G.; Beekers, I.; Collado-Lara, G.; van der Steen, A.F.W.; de Jong, N.; Kooiman, K. The Impact of Lipid Handling and Phase Distribution on the Acoustic Behavior of Microbubbles. *Pharmaceutics* **2021**, *13*, 119. https://doi.org/10.3390/pharmaceutics13010119

Received: 18 December 2020
Accepted: 14 January 2021
Published: 19 January 2021

Publisher's Note: MDPI stays neutral with regard to jurisdictional claims in published maps and institutional affiliations.

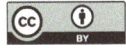

Copyright: © 2021 by the authors. Licensee MDPI, Basel, Switzerland. This article is an open access article distributed under the terms and conditions of the Creative Commons Attribution (CC BY) license (https://creativecommons.org/licenses/by/4.0/).

Abstract: Phospholipid-coated microbubbles are ultrasound contrast agents that can be employed for ultrasound molecular imaging and drug delivery. For safe and effective implementation, microbubbles must respond uniformly and predictably to ultrasound. Therefore, we investigated how lipid handling and phase distribution affected the variability in the acoustic behavior of microbubbles. Cholesterol was used to modify the lateral molecular packing of 1,2-distearoyl-*sn*-glycero-3-phosphocholine (DSPC)-based microbubbles. To assess the effect of lipid handling, microbubbles were produced by a direct method, i.e., lipids directly dispersed in an aqueous medium or indirect method, i.e., lipids first dissolved in an organic solvent. The lipid phase and ligand distribution in the microbubble coating were investigated using confocal microscopy, and the acoustic response was recorded with the Brandaris 128 ultra-high-speed camera. In microbubbles with 12 mol% cholesterol, the lipids were miscible and all in the same phase, which resulted in more buckle formation, lower shell elasticity and higher shell viscosity. Indirect DSPC microbubbles had a more uniform response to ultrasound than direct DSPC and indirect DSPC-cholesterol microbubbles. The difference in lipid handling between direct and indirect DSPC microbubbles significantly affected the acoustic behavior. Indirect DSPC microbubbles are the most promising candidate for ultrasound molecular imaging and drug delivery applications.

Keywords: ultrasound contrast agents; phospholipid coating; ligand distribution; cholesterol; acoustic response; microbubble; lipid phase

1. Introduction

Microbubbles are small gas bubbles (diameter 1–10 μm) that are clinically used as ultrasound contrast agents for non-invasive diagnostic imaging of blood perfusion [1]. Targeted microbubbles are employed for molecular imaging of inflammation, tumors, and cardiovascular disease [2]. Other types of microbubbles are being developed specifically for drug delivery [3]. All of these applications make use of the compression and expansion of the microbubble gas core upon ultrasound insonification. These microbubble vibrations produce a nonlinear response, including super- and subharmonic oscillations, which can be differentiated from the surrounding tissue to form a contrast-enhanced image [1]. Additionally, this acoustic response can induce bioeffects on nearby cells–resulting in enhanced uptake or extravasation of drug molecules [4]. Successful translation to the clinical use of microbubbles for molecular imaging and enhanced drug delivery is currently challenged, however, by the microbubbles' unpredictable acoustic behavior.

To stabilize the gas core, microbubbles are usually coated with a phospholipid monolayer, proteins, or polymers. For a schematic representation, the reader is referred to recent reviews on microbubbles [5,6]. The coating reduces surface tension and gas diffusion [7].

If phospholipids or polymers are used as microbubble coating, a ligand can be attached for molecular imaging [8], and they can be loaded with a drug for localized delivery [3]. The physicochemical properties of the microbubble coating, such as the shell elasticity and viscosity, are related to the acoustical properties, such as the resonance frequency and the damping coefficient [9,10]. Therefore, the composition of the microbubble coating can affect the acoustical properties. For instance, the use of a phospholipid molecule with a longer acyl chain length, 1,2-distearoyl-*sn*-glycero-3-phosphocholine (DSPC; C18), resulted in a higher shell elasticity and more acoustic stability than the use of a shorter acyl chain length phospholipid, 1,2-dipalmitoyl-*sn*-glycero-3-phosphocholine (DPPC; C16) [11]. Besides the shell elasticity, acyl chain length has also been shown to affect the half-life of microbubbles, with longer acyl chain length resulting in more stable size distribution and ultrasound signal over time [12].

Since microbubbles are generally coated with a mixture of phospholipids and a PEGylated emulsifier, the physicochemical properties are determined by the miscibility and lipid phase behavior. Molecules in the microbubble coating can be in the liquid expanded (LE) or liquid condensed (LC) phase, resulting in distinctive microstructures. These microstructures can be altered by using different types of phospholipids [13], changing the ratio between phospholipid and emulsifier, or heating and cooling of the microbubble coating [14]. Microstructures formed by lipid phase separation have been shown to affect the subharmonic response to ultrasound [15]. The effect of lipid phase separation on the subharmonic response to ultrasound has been characterized previously in three types of microbubbles with different levels of lipid phase separation: 20%, 50% or 80% of the microbubbles had LC phase domains. Each microbubble type had a peak subharmonic response at a different microbubble size, suggesting that microstructures in the coating affect the acoustical properties of a microbubble [15]. The microbubble coating can also be altered by the distribution of the phospholipid and PEGylated-emulsifier molecules over the microbubble coating, depending on the lipid handling prior to microbubble production by probe sonication. The use of organic solvent resulted in a more homogeneous ligand distribution than the use of aqueous solutions only [16]. The effect of lipid handling on the acoustic response of microbubbles, however, has not been investigated.

For both ultrasound molecular imaging and drug delivery, it is important that all microbubbles respond uniformly and predictably to ultrasound. Currently available microbubbles respond to ultrasound in a heterogeneous way [11,17], even when they are the same size [18]. While it is thought this variability in response could be due to the microstructures in the microbubble coating, this is challenging to confirm because it can only be investigated by looking at single microbubbles. Different approaches have been used to record a single microbubble's response to ultrasound, including an ultra-high-speed camera to image the microbubble during insonification [19], recording the acoustic response [15] or optical scattering [20], and photo-acoustic techniques [21]. Until recently, however, no techniques were available to image both the lipid phase distribution in 3D and the acoustic response of the same microbubble. In this regard, the challenge lies in the time scale (µs) and optical resolution (µm) needed to record the lipid phase distribution and response to ultrasound of a single microbubble.

The purpose of this study was to relate the effects of lipid handling and phase distribution before microbubble production to the acoustic behavior of phospholipid-coated microbubbles. Cholesterol can modify the lateral molecular packing of phospholipids in a monolayer, resulting in a single liquid phase [22–24]. While microbubbles with cholesterol in their coating have been produced before [25,26], the effect of cholesterol on the lipid phase separation in microbubbles has not been studied. To determine this effect in the microbubble coating, we made microbubbles by probe sonication with DSPC as the main lipid and varying concentrations of cholesterol. The lipid phase distribution and ligand distribution in the microbubble coating were imaged using high-axial-resolution 4Pi confocal microscopy. To assess the acoustic response and variability in the acoustic behavior, we used a unique system combining a confocal microscope with the Brandaris

128 ultra-high-speed camera. With this system, the lipid phase separation (in nanometer resolution) and acoustic response to ultrasound (in nanosecond resolution) were captured at a single microbubble level.

2. Materials and Methods

2.1. Materials

DSPC was provided by Lipoid GmbH (Ludwigshafen, Germany). PEG40-stearate and cholesterol were purchased from Sigma-Aldrich (Zwijndrecht, The Netherlands), 1,2-distearoyl-*sn*-glycero-3-phosphoethanolamine-*N*-carboxy-(polyethylene glycol) (DSPE-PEG2000) was purchased from Iris Biotech GmbH (Marktredwitz, Germany), and 1,2-distearoyl-*sn*-glycero-3-phosphoethanolamine-*N*-biotinyl(polyethylene glycol) (DSPE-PEG2000-biotin) was purchased from Avanti Polar Lipids (Alabaster, AL, USA). Perfluoro butane (C_4F_{10}) was purchased from F2 Chemicals (Preston, UK), and argon gas was purchased from Linde Gas Benelux (Schiedam, the Netherlands). Streptavidin Oregon Green 488 was purchased from BioSynthesis (Louisville, TX, USA), and Lissamine rhodamine B 1,2-dihexadecanoyl-*sn*-glycero-3-phosphoethanolamine, triethylammonium salt (rhodamine-DHPE) was purchased from Thermo Fisher (Waltham, MA, USA).

2.2. Microbubble Production

Biotinylated lipid-coated microbubbles with a C_4F_{10} gas core were made as described previously [27], by probe sonication at 20 kHz with a Sonicator ultrasonic processor XL2020 at a power setting 10 (HeatSystems, Farmingdale, NY, USA) for 10 s. Three types of microbubbles were made by altering the production method or adding cholesterol to the microbubble coating. For microbubbles without cholesterol, the coating components (84.8 mol% DSPC; 8.2 mol% PEG40-stearate; 5.9 mol% DSPE-PEG2000; 1.1 mol% DSPE-PEG2000-biotin) were prepared with either an indirect or a direct method as described previously [16]. In short, for the indirect method, the components were dissolved in chloroform/methanol (9:1 vol/vol), the solvent was evaporated using argon gas, and the obtained lipid film was dried overnight under vacuum. The lipid film was then dispersed in saline solution (0.9% NaCl, saturated with C_4F_{10}) with a final concentration of 2.5 mg/mL DSPC, 0.625 mg/mL PEG40-stearate, 0.625 mg/mL DSPE-PEG2000 and 0.125 mg/mL DSPE-PEG2000-biotin. The fluorescent dye rhodamine-DHPE (0.01 mol%) was added to image the lipid phase separation in the microbubble coating. The solution was placed in a sonicator bath for 10 min, and the probe sonicator was used at power setting 3 for 5 min. For the direct method, the coating components (84.8 mol% DSPC; 8.2 mol% PEG40-stearate; 5.9 mol% DSPE-PEG2000; 1.1 mol% DSPE-PEG2000-biotin) were dispersed directly in C_4F_{10}-saturated saline solution with a final concentration of 2.5 mg/mL DSPC, 0.625 mg/mL PEG40-stearate, 0.625 mg/mL DSPE-PEG2000 and 0.125 mg/mL DSPE-PEG2000-biotin. Fluorescent dye rhodamine-DHPE (0.01 mol%) was added before sonication.

Microbubbles with cholesterol, referred to as DSPC-cholesterol microbubbles, were produced with the indirect method only since cholesterol is insoluble in an aqueous medium, and the organic solvent was required to mix all microbubble coating components [28]. Cholesterol was added (7, 10, 12, 14, or 32 mol%) to the ternary mixture of coating components: DSPC, PEG40-stearate, DSPE-PEG2000, and DSPE-PEG2000-biotin (molar ratio 84.8/8.2/5.9/1.1) in chloroform/methanol (9:1 vol/vol). The lipids were then dried to form a lipid film and dispersed in saline solution, as described above, with 0.02 mol% rhodamine-DHPE added for fluorescent labeling of the microbubbles. All types of microbubbles were produced by sonicating under a constant flow of C_4F_{10}.

2.3. Physicochemical Characterization

To image the ligand distribution, fluorescent ligand streptavidin Oregon Green 488 was conjugated to the biotinylated microbubbles as described previously [29]. Briefly, microbubbles were first washed by flotation: 0.9 mL microbubble suspension was placed in a 3 mL syringe and topped with 2.1 mL saline solution saturated with C_4F_{10}. After 45 min, the subnatant was drained, and the microbubbles were resuspended in 0.3 mL saline solution saturated with C_4F_{10}. Then, 22.5 µL of streptavidin-Oregon Green 488 (2 mg/mL) was allowed to incubate with $0.7–1.0 \times 10^8$ microbubbles for 30 min on ice. The excess of streptavidin was washed away by flotation as described above, with resuspension of the microbubbles in 0.2 mL saline solution.

To measure the microbubble size distribution and concentration, a Coulter Counter Multisizer 3 (Beckman Coulter, Mijdrecht, The Netherlands) was used. To quantify particles between 1 and 30 µm, a 50 µm aperture tube was used. To evaluate the polydispersity of the samples, the span value was calculated, defined as $(d90 - d10\%)/d50\%$, where $d90$, $d10$ and $d50\%$ are the microbubble diameters below which 90, 10 and 50% of the cumulative number of microbubbles was found. Samples were measured after the first flotation wash and again after conjugation with streptavidin Oregon Green 488.

The streptavidin-conjugated microbubbles were imaged by microscopy as described by Langeveld et al. [16]. In short, the microbubbles were placed between quartz glass in 87% glycerol (v/v in phosphate-buffered saline) to reduce Brownian motion and imaged with a Leica TCS 4Pi confocal laser-scanning microscope [30]. An axial resolution up to 90 nm was achieved with a matched pair of aligned opposing 100× glycerol HCX PL APO objective lenses (numerical aperture 1.35). For excitation of Oregon Green 488, a 488 nm laser was used, and for excitation of rhodamine-DHPE, a 561 nm laser was used. Images were recorded in 3D as y-stacked xz-scans in a green (500–550 nm) and red (580–640 nm) spectral channel. The "voltex" function was used to volume-render the image stacks with AMIRA (Version 2020.2, FEI, Mérignac Cedex, France).

Quantitative analysis was performed on the 4Pi microscopy data using custom-developed image analysis software in MATLAB (Mathworks, Natick, MA, USA), based on the method described by Langeveld et al. [16]. The microbubble coating was subdivided into 32 parts, of which the mean fluorescence pixel intensity (I_{part} for the green channel and $I_{part\text{-}rhod}$ for the red channel) was calculated. The median intensity of all parts (I_{median} for the green channel and $I_{median\text{-}rhod}$ for the red channel) was calculated per microbubble. To evaluate the ligand distribution, parts were classified as inhomogeneous when the absolute difference between I_{part} and I_{median} was more than two-thirds times the value of I_{median} (i.e., $|I_{part} - I_{median}| > 2/3 \times I_{median}$), and the percentage of inhomogeneous parts was calculated per microbubble. To evaluate the lipid phase distribution, parts were classified as LC phase when the value of $I_{part\text{-}rhod}$ was less than one-third of $I_{median\text{-}rhod}$ (i.e., $I_{part\text{-}rhod} < 1/3 \times I_{median\text{-}rhod}$). The LC phase surface area was first calculated in µm², and then a percentage of the total analyzed surface area per microbubble. Before evaluating the ligand distribution or the lipid phase distribution, an additional normalization step was included in the image analysis. This step corrected for a difference in fluorescence intensity between the center and the top or bottom of the microbubbles, likely caused by attenuation of the laser light leading to a lower fluorescence signal at the center of the sample. The normalization factor was calculated based on the median I_{part} (for the green channel) or the median $I_{part\text{-}rhod}$ (for the red channel) per angular part from all microbubbles (Supplemental Figure S1). To determine the number of microbubbles with buckles, the microbubble coating was manually scored for fluorescent signal outside and attached to the microbubble coating, based on the red channel (rhodamine-DHPE signal). Only bright spots with 1 µm diameter or larger were classified as a buckle.

2.4. Acoustical Characterization

To study both the acoustical behavior and the lipid phase separation of single microbubbles simultaneously, the combined confocal microscopy and Brandaris 128 ultra-high-speed camera system was used [31]. Microbubble spectroscopy was employed to characterize the acoustic behavior of single microbubbles as described previously [11,32]. Microbubbles were washed by flotation once and counted using the Coulter Counter Multisizer 3, as described above. An acoustically compatible [32] CLINIcell (MABIO, Tourcoing,

France) with 50 µm membranes (25 µm²) was first blocked with 12 mL of 2% (w/v) bovine serum albumin (BSA) in phosphate-buffered saline (PBS) for 1 h, to avoid unspecific microbubble binding to the membranes. The CLINIcell was washed three times with PBS before inserting 12 mL of 10^5 microbubbles/mL in PBS. Next, the CLINIcell was placed underwater in the experimental setup and kept at room temperature for up to 2 h. To study the lipid phase separation, the custom-built confocal microscope (Nikon Instruments, Amsterdam, The Netherlands) was used with a 561 nm laser to excite rhodamine-DHPE and emitted light was detected in a 595/50 nm channel. Z-stacks with 0.4 µm steps were acquired with a CFI Plan 100 × W objective of single microbubbles directly before and after insonification. To perform microbubble spectroscopy, each individual microbubble was insonified over a range of transmitting frequencies (f_T) from 1 to 4 MHz in steps of 200 kHz. The microbubbles were insonified with 8-cycle Gaussian tapered sine wave bursts either at 50 kPa or first at 20 kPa and then at 150 kPa external peak negative pressure (PNP), generated by a Tabor 8026 arbitrary waveform generator (AWG, Tabor Electronics, Tel Hanan, Israel). The signal was first attenuated by a 20-dB attenuator (Mini-Circuits, Brooklyn, New York, NY, USA), then amplified by a broadband amplifier (ENI A-500, Electronics and Innovation, Rochester, New York, NY, USA), and finally transmitted to the microbubble sample at a 45° incidence angle with a single-element transducer (1–9 MHz bandwidth, 25 mm focal distance, −6 dB beamwidth at 1 MHz of 1.3 mm, PA275, Precision Acoustics, Dorchester, UK), which was calibrated using a 1-mm needle hydrophone (Precision Acoustics, Dorchester, UK) in water. The Brandaris 128 ultra-high-speed camera [33], coupled with the confocal microscope [31], was used to record the microbubble oscillation behavior at approximately 17 million frames/s. First, a recording was made without ultrasound to establish the initial microbubble size. Next, 16 recordings at 50 kPa PNP, or 16 recordings at 20 kPa PNP and then 16 recordings at 150 kPa PNP were made of a single microbubble upon ultrasound insonification at the different transmit frequencies with 80 ms in between recordings. To avoid any effects from nearby microbubbles on the oscillation behavior, only microbubbles which were at least 0.7 mm from other microbubbles were investigated.

To quantify microbubble oscillation, custom-developed image analysis software in MATLAB was used to determine the change in microbubble radius as a function of time (R–t curve) [19]. As previously described, the resonance frequency and shell parameters can be obtained from the spectroscopy dataset [11,19]. Briefly, the relative oscillation amplitude (x_0) of each microbubble was defined as the maximum of the filtered R-t curve (a third-order Butterworth bandpass filter centered at f_T with a 300 kHz bandwidth) and divided by the resting size of the microbubble (R_0; mean size of the first five frames). Next, for each f_T, the x_0 obtained at 50 kPa were fitted to the harmonic oscillator model:

$$x_0 = \frac{|P|/(4\pi^2 \rho R_0^2)}{\sqrt{(f_0^2 - f_T^2)^2 + (\delta f_T f_0)^2}} \quad (1)$$

with P being the acoustic pressure and $\rho = 10^3$ kg/m³ being the density of water. The eigenfrequency (f_0) of the microbubble is defined as:

$$f_0 = \frac{1}{2\pi}\sqrt{\frac{1}{\rho R_0^2}\left[3\gamma P_0 + \frac{2(3\gamma - 1)\sigma_w}{R_0} + \frac{4\chi}{R_0}\right]} \quad (2)$$

with $\gamma = 1.07$, the ratio of specific heats for C_4F_{10}, $P_0 = 10^5$ Pa the ambient pressure, $\sigma_w = 0.072$ N/m the surface tension in water, and χ the microbubble shell elasticity. The damping coefficient (δ) is given by:

$$\delta = \frac{\omega_0 R_0}{c} + 2\frac{4\mu}{R_0^2 \rho \omega_0} + \frac{4\kappa_s}{R_0^3 \rho \omega_0} \quad (3)$$

with $\omega_0 = 2\pi f_0$, $c = 1500$ m/s the speed of sound in water, $\mu = 10^{-3}$ Pa·s the viscosity of water and κ_s the microbubble shell viscosity. The resonance frequency is defined by $f_{res} = f_0\sqrt{1 - \delta^2/2}$.

The variability in the acoustical response of each microbubble type was quantified by determining the interquartile range (IQR) of the relative oscillation amplitude (x_0) at each f_T and in diameter bins of 0.5 µm ($N > 3$ per bin). Since the microbubbles deflated after insonification, the acoustic stability was evaluated by quantifying the relative diameter decrease upon insonification as $(D_0 - D_{end})/D_0$, with D_0 the mean microbubble diameter of all 128 frames of the first recording without ultrasound and D_{end} the mean microbubble diameter of the last ten frames of the last recording.

The nonlinear behavior of microbubbles was assessed by calculating the fast fourier transforms (FFTs) of the R-t curves. The noise level of each microbubble was determined by the FFT of the first recording before the ultrasound. A microbubble was categorized as exhibiting nonlinear behavior when in at least two recordings it showed a detectable peak in the FFT (using the *islocalmax* function in MATLAB) around $\frac{1}{2} \cdot f_T$ for the subharmonic or around $2 \cdot f_T$ for the second harmonic and the peak's amplitude was at least 6 dB above the noise level. If so, then the amplitude of the nonlinear component was defined as the maximum FFT amplitude in a 300 kHz bandwidth around $\frac{1}{2} \cdot f_T$ for the subharmonic component and around $2 \cdot f_T$ for the second harmonic component and normalized to the fundamental at f_T.

Finally, the confocal microscopy recordings were scored manually for the presence of buckles (none, single, multiple, or extensive) before and after the ultrasound and for change in the microbubble coating before and after ultrasound (unchanged, buckles formed, coating material shed). Only bright spots with 1 µm diameter or larger were classified as the buckle (Supplemental Figure S2). Microbubbles between 4.5 and 6.0 µm in diameter were manually scored for the LC domain size as well (mostly large, large and small, undefined). The relationship between these classifications and the acoustical data were evaluated to determine the effect of the lipid phase distribution and buckling in the microbubble coating on the resulting acoustic response. To rule out size-dependent differences in oscillation amplitude, only microbubbles with an initial diameter in the range of 4.5–6.0 µm were included in this analysis.

2.5. Statistics

Statistical analysis was performed using IBM SPSS Statistics 25 for all 4Pi microscopy image analysis. Statistical analysis for the acoustical characterization was performed using MATLAB. A Shapiro–Wilk test was used to assess the distribution of the data. For data that were normally distributed, a regular *t*-test was used to analyze the differences between groups. For all other data, the Mann–Whitney *U* test was used to test the difference between groups. Differences between groups were only tested for $N > 2$. Pearson's correlation tests were performed to assess the correlation between parameters.

3. Results
3.1. Physicochemical Characterization

Figure 1A presents the number weighted size distributions of indirect DSPC-based microbubbles with and without cholesterol. For microbubbles without cholesterol (0 mol%; $N = 5$) and microbubbles with 12 mol% cholesterol ($N = 6$), the size distributions of batches for 4Pi microscopy and for acoustic experiments are both included, and the mean number (%) per diameter is shown with the standard error of the mean (SEM). For microbubbles with 7, 10, and 14 mol% cholesterol a representative curve is shown from 2 batches, as these types of microbubbles were produced for 4Pi microscopy only. The concentration of microbubbles ranged from 2.78×10^8 to 1.17×10^9 microbubbles per mL (Supplemental Table S1). The indirect DSPC-based microbubbles without cholesterol had more particles with diameter >3 µm than all types of microbubbles with cholesterol in the coating. Indirect DSPC-based microbubbles with 32 mol% cholesterol in the coating were highly unstable, with a concentration too low for measurement of the size distribution. Therefore, indirect DSPC-based microbubbles with 32 mol% cholesterol were not investigated further.

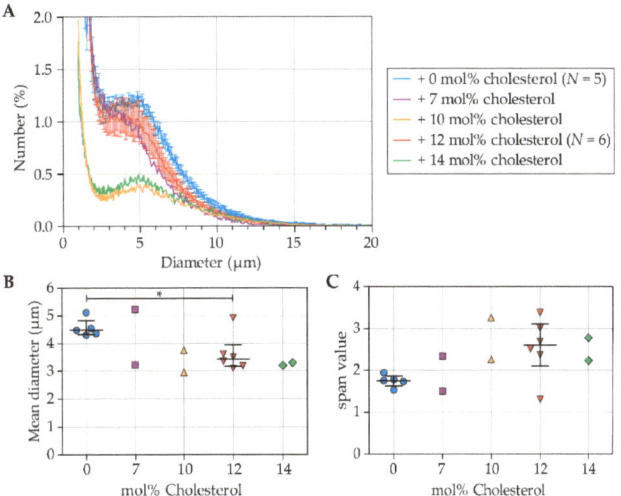

Figure 1. (**A**) Number weighted size distribution, (**B**) number weighted mean diameter (μm), and (**C**) span value of indirect DSPC-based microbubbles with cholesterol in a range from 0 to 14 mol%. In B and C, each symbol represents one batch of microbubbles; jittering was applied to avoid overlapping. The overlaid black lines represent the median and interquartile range. Statistical significance is indicated with * $p < 0.05$.

Figure 1B shows the mean diameter (μm) of indirect DSPC-based microbubbles without cholesterol and with 7, 10, 12, or 14 mol% cholesterol. Microbubbles with 12 mol% cholesterol had a smaller mean diameter than those without cholesterol ($p = 0.045$). Figure 1C shows the width of the size distributions represented as the span value. The size distributions of microbubbles with 12 mol% cholesterol were more polydisperse than those of microbubbles without cholesterol ($p = 0.068$).

The ligand and lipid phase distribution in the microbubble coating were imaged in indirect DSPC-based microbubbles without cholesterol ($N = 58$), with 7 mol% cholesterol ($N = 34$), with 10 mol% cholesterol ($N = 40$), with 12 mol% cholesterol ($N = 61$), and with 14 mol% cholesterol ($N = 45$). Images were recorded of at least two batches of microbubbles for all formulations, with microbubble diameters ranging from 2.2 μm to 8.7 μm. Typical examples of all formulations are presented in Figure 2. The ligand distribution is shown in the top row, the LE phase in the middle row, and a composite of both channels in the bottom row. Figure 3 shows a quantitative analysis of the 4Pi confocal microscopy images, with the calculated ligand distribution inhomogeneity in Figure 3A and the LC phase relative to the total surface area analyzed per microbubble in Figure 3B. Indirect DSPC-based microbubbles without cholesterol had a homogeneous ligand distribution (Figure 2A, Figure 3A). The inhomogeneity of the ligand distribution can be observed in Figure 2B,C,E, where the ligand is enriched in some areas of the microbubble surface. All indirect DSPC-cholesterol microbubbles had a significantly more heterogeneous ligand distribution compared to those without cholesterol (Figure 2B–E, Figure 3A). Microbubbles with 12 mol% cholesterol had a more homogeneous ligand distribution than those with 7 mol% cholesterol ($p = 0.070$), 10 mol% cholesterol ($p = 0.040$), and 14 mol% cholesterol ($p < 0.001$).

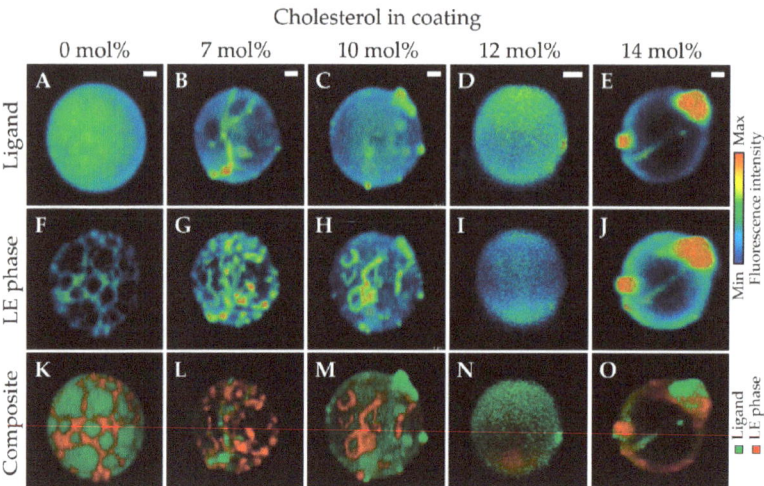

Figure 2. Selected views of 4Pi confocal microscopy y-stacks of indirect 1,2-distearoyl-sn-glycero-3-phosphocholine (DSPC)-based microbubbles without cholesterol (**A,F,K**, diameter (d) = 6.4 μm, liquid condensed (LC) phase area 35%), with 7 mol% cholesterol (**B,G,L**, d = 5.6 μm, LC phase area 22%), with 10 mol% cholesterol (**C,H,M**, d = 6.1 μm, LC phase area 22%), with 12 mol% cholesterol (**D,I,N**, d = 3.6 μm, LC phase area 7%), and with 14 mol% cholesterol (**E,J,O**, d = 5.8 μm, LC phase area 22%) in the phospholipid coating. Images show the ligand distribution (**A–E**; Oregon Green 488), liquid expanded (LE) phase (**F–J**; rhodamine-DHPE), and composite view (**K–O**). Scale bars are 1 μm.

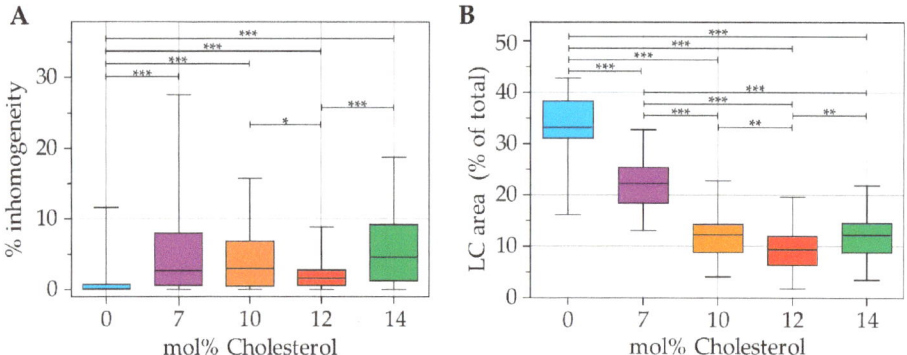

Figure 3. (**A**) Parts classified as inhomogeneity (%) in the ligand distribution, and (**B**) size of the LC area (% of total surface area) of indirect DSPC microbubbles without cholesterol (N = 58), with 7 mol% (N = 34), 10 mol% (N = 40), 12 mol% (N = 61), and with 14 mol% (N = 45) cholesterol in the coating. Boxplots show the median and interquartile range with whiskers from minimum to maximum. Statistical significance is indicated with * $p < 0.05$, ** $p < 0.01$, or *** $p < 0.001$.

The lipids were phase-separated in indirect DSPC-based microbubbles without cholesterol, as shown in Figure 2F and quantified in Figure 3B. The fluorescent dye rhodamine-DHPE was enriched in bright interdomain regions (i.e., LE phase) and absent in LC domains. In indirect DSPC-cholesterol microbubbles, the LC domains were less pronounced compared to those without cholesterol (Figure 2G–J). With increasing concentrations of cholesterol up to 12 mol%, the lipid phase distribution was increasingly affected, as reflected by quantification of the LC phase area (Figure 3B). Microbubbles without cholesterol had a significantly larger surface area in the LC phase than those with cholesterol in their coating. Microbubbles with 7 mol% cholesterol displayed LE phase areas with an enriched fluorescent dye (Figure 2G) and had a significantly larger surface area in the LC phase than those with more cholesterol in their coating. Microbubbles with 10 mol% cholesterol displayed LE phase areas as well (Figure 2H). Microbubbles with 12 mol% cholesterol had a homogeneous distribution of the fluorescent dye rhodamine-DHPE (Figure 2I), with the smallest LC phase area per microbubble of all formulations (Figure 3B). In microbubbles with 14 mol% cholesterol, rhodamine-DHPE was not only distributed homogeneously in the coating but also present in buckles on the outside of the coating (Figure 2J). The LC phase area in microbubbles with 14 mol% cholesterol was comparable to the LC phase area in microbubbles with 10 mol% cholesterol (Figure 3B).

Figure 4 shows the percentage of indirect DSPC-based microbubbles with buckles per batch. An example of a microbubble with buckles is shown in Figure 2J,O. Microbubbles without cholesterol in the coating had the lowest incidence of buckles. Microbubbles with 12 mol% cholesterol in the coating had a higher incidence of buckles ($p = 0.050$) than those without cholesterol. Furthermore, the variability between batches increased with higher concentrations of cholesterol.

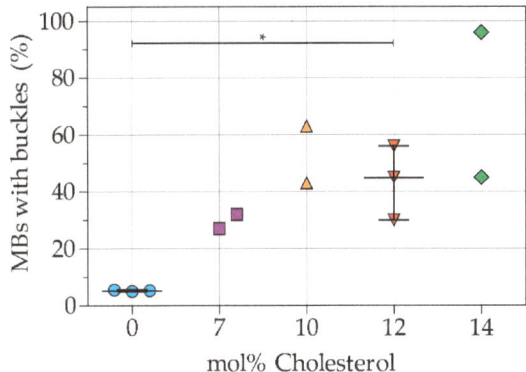

Figure 4. Percentage of microbubbles (MBs) with buckles per batch of indirect DSPC-based microbubbles without cholesterol and with 7, 10, 12, or 14 mol% cholesterol. Each symbol represents one batch of microbubbles. Overlaid black lines represent the median and interquartile range. Statistical significance is indicated with * $p < 0.05$.

3.2. Acoustical Characterization

Based on the physicochemical characterization described above, indirect DSPC-based microbubbles with 12 mol% cholesterol were chosen for acoustical characterization because they had the most homogeneous ligand and lipid phase distribution. They were compared to the direct and indirect DSPC-based microbubbles without cholesterol, and for each type of microbubble, data were acquired from at least two separate batches. Figure 5 shows a typical example of a 3D confocal acquisition before and after ultrasound with the corresponding R-t curve obtained from the ultra-high-speed recording at 50 kPa PNP for a direct DSPC (top row), indirect DSPC (middle row), and indirect DSPC-cholesterol (bottom row) microbubble. The coating of direct and indirect DSPC microbubbles was phase-separated into dark LC domains with a bright interdomain region, while the coating of indirect DSPC-cholesterol microbubbles was in one homogeneous lipid phase. This was in line with the results obtained by 4Pi confocal microscopy. The direct DSPC microbubble shown in Figure 5 had one bright spot present in the coating before and after the ultrasound, which was classified as a buckle. The coating of the indirect DSPC microbubble in Figure 5 had one large and several smaller LC phase domains. For the indirect DSPC-cholesterol microbubble in Figure 5, the maximum intensity projection of the confocal z-stacks resulted in more brightness near the edge of the microbubble than in the center. However, when looking at the separate z-slices, the fluorescent signal was homogeneous over the microbubble coating (Supplemental Figure S3).

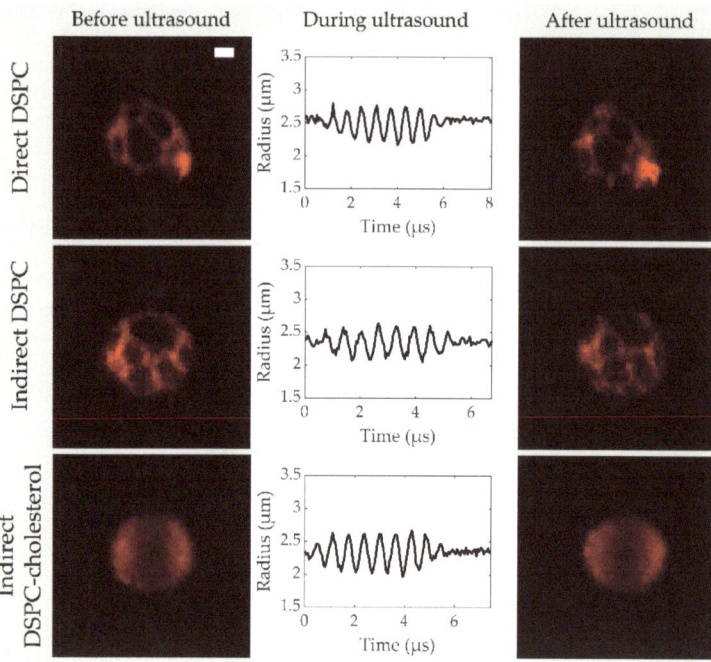

Figure 5. Maximum intensity projections of confocal z-stack from direct DSPC, indirect DSPC, and indirect DSPC-cholesterol (12 mol%) microbubbles with the LE phase in red, before and after ultrasound, with the microbubble radius as a function of time obtained from the Brandaris 128 ultra-high-speed recordings during ultrasound (50 kPa peak negative pressure (PNP), 1.6 MHz). Scale bar is 1 µm and applies to all images.

Oscillation amplitudes at frequencies between 1 and 4 MHz and acoustic pressure of 50 kPa were obtained per microbubble from the R-t curves and fitted to the harmonic oscillator model at each f_T (examples at 1.2, 1.6. and 2.0 MHz shown in Supplemental Figure S4). Resonance frequencies resulting from the fit to the harmonic oscillator model are presented in Figure 6, with the obtained shell elasticity and viscosity parameters listed in Table 1. The shell elasticity of direct DSPC microbubbles was the highest, while the shell elasticity of indirect DSPC-cholesterol microbubbles was close to that of an uncoated microbubble. The shell viscosity parameter is related to the damping of the oscillation and was lowest for the direct DSPC microbubbles, which had the highest oscillation amplitudes.

Table 1. Microbubble (MB) spectroscopy results at 50 kPa.

MB Type	N	Shell Elasticity [1] (N/m)	Shell Viscosity [1] ($\times 10^{-8}$ kg/s)	Max IQR of Oscillation Amplitude (%)	Median IQR of Oscillation Amplitude (%)
Direct DSPC	44	0.14 (0.12–0.15)	0.43 (0.38–0.61)	8.0	1.5
Indirect DSPC	49	0.03 (0.01–0.06)	0.99 (0.89–1.40)	4.5	0.6
DSPC-cholesterol [2]	50	0.01 (0.01–0.02)	1.39 (0.97–1.55)	10.2	0.7

[1] presented as median (IQR); [2] indirect DSPC-cholesterol microbubbles with 12 mol% cholesterol.

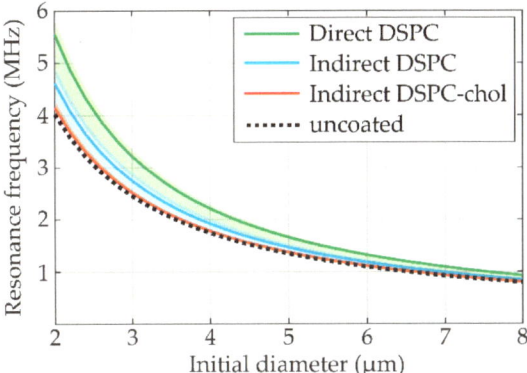

Figure 6. Resonance frequency (MHz) per initial diameter (μm) at 50 kPa of direct DSPC (green), indirect DSPC (blue), and indirect DSPC-cholesterol (red, 12 mol%) microbubbles. The dotted line represents the resonance frequency of uncoated microbubbles. The shaded areas indicate the range of individual microbubble resonance frequencies obtained by fitting at each f_T.

Figure 7 illustrates the variability in acoustical response within the three types of microbubbles. The variability was quantified as the interquartile range (IQR) of the oscillation amplitude from different microbubbles of the same size at the same transmit frequency ($N > 3$ per bin). The maximum and median IQR values for each type of microbubble are listed in Table 1. Indirect DSPC-cholesterol microbubbles had the highest maximum IQR, while direct DSPC microbubbles had the highest median IQR. Overall, indirect DSPC microbubbles exhibited the lowest variability in acoustical response.

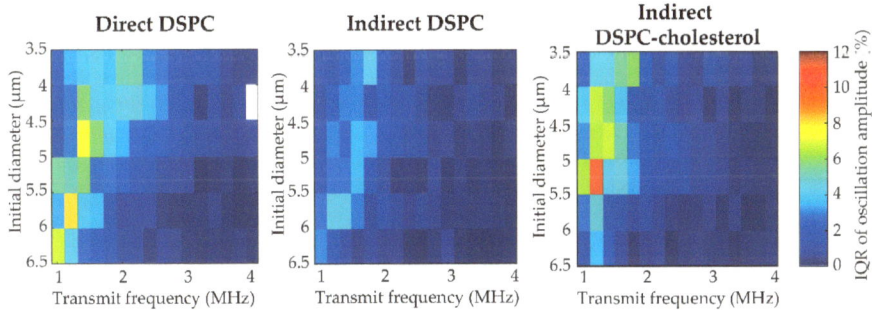

Figure 7. Variability in acoustic response represented as the IQR of the oscillation amplitude at 50 kPa of direct DSPC, indirect DSPC, and indirect DSPC-cholesterol (12 mol%) microbubbles of different sizes (3.5–6.5 μm) at different transmit frequencies (1–4 MHz). All bins are based on $N > 3$; bins with $N < 3$ are blank.

Figure 8 shows the deflation of the microbubble, quantified as the diameter decrease relative to the initial diameter, for direct DSPC, indirect DSPC, and indirect DSPC-cholesterol microbubbles. At 50 kPa, direct DSPC microbubbles deflated significantly more than the indirect DSPC and DSPC-cholesterol microbubbles, while no statistically significant difference in deflation was found between the indirect DSPC and DSPC-cholesterol microbubbles. However, at 50 kPa, the direct DSPC microbubbles had higher oscillation amplitudes than the other two groups. When comparing the deflation of microbubbles with similar oscillation amplitudes, marked as a gray area in Figure 8B, no statistically significant differences were found. Therefore, the statistical differences found at 50 kPa can be explained by a difference in oscillation amplitude, not acoustical stability. At 150 kPa, all types of microbubbles deflated significantly more than at 50 kPa. Furthermore, the indirect DSPC microbubbles deflated significantly less than both other groups, also when comparing only microbubbles with similar oscillation amplitudes (Figure 8C). No statistically significant difference in deflation was found between direct DSPC and indirect DSPC-cholesterol microbubbles.

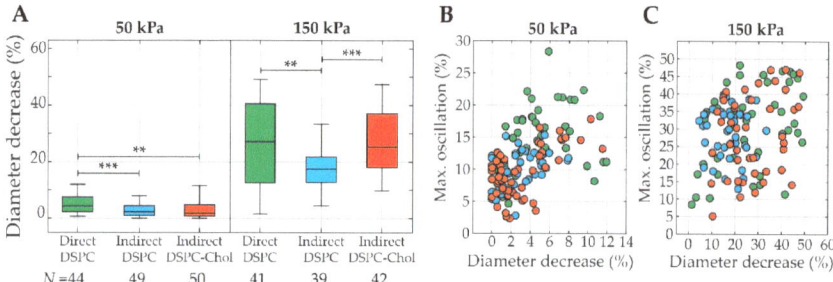

Figure 8. (**A**) Diameter decrease (%) for direct DSPC (green), indirect DSPC (blue), and indirect DSPC-cholesterol (red, 12 mol% cholesterol) microbubbles at 50 kPa (left panel) and 150 kPa (right panel). Boxplots represent the median and IQR. ** $p < 0.01$. *** $p < 0.001$. (**B**,**C**) Maximum oscillation (%) as a function of diameter decrease (%) for direct DSPC (green), indirect DSPC (blue), and DSPC-cholesterol (red, 12 mol% cholesterol) microbubbles at 50 kPa (**B**) and 150 kPa (**C**). Gray areas indicate the range of maximum oscillation values reached by all three types of microbubbles.

The nonlinear behavior was studied by looking at the acoustic response at the subharmonic and second harmonic frequencies at 50 and 150 kPa. At subharmonic frequencies, all types of microbubbles had a low response rate, and no statistical differences were found between the groups (Supplemental Figure S5). The percentages of microbubbles with a response at the second harmonic frequency are presented in Figure 9A. At 50 kPa, the direct DSPC microbubbles exhibited the highest number of second harmonic responses (68%), while this number was considerably lower for the indirect DSPC (26%) and the indirect DSPC-cholesterol (38%) microbubbles. At 150 kPa, all three types had similar percentages of microbubbles with a second harmonic response, and all occurrences were higher than those at 50 kPa. The second harmonic amplitudes were similar for all microbubble types at 50 kPa (Figure 9B). At 150 kPa, however, the direct DSPC microbubbles had significantly higher second harmonic amplitudes than both other microbubble types. Additionally, the indirect DSPC-cholesterol microbubbles had a significantly higher second harmonic amplitude than the indirect DSPC microbubbles.

Confocal z-stacks of each microbubble were manually scored for the presence of buckles (none, single, multiple, or extensive with examples provided in Supplemental Figure S2) before and after ultrasound insonification (Figure 10). Indirect DSPC microbubbles ($N = 49$ at 50 kPa; $N = 39$ at 150 kPa) had the lowest occurrence of buckles both before and after ultrasound insonification, which was comparable to that of the direct DSPC microbubbles ($N = 44$ at 50 kPa; $N = 41$ at 150 kPa). Indirect DSPC-cholesterol microbubbles ($N = 50$ at 50 kPa; $N = 42$ at 150 kPa) had a notably higher occurrence of buckles than both other groups at both 50 and 150 kPa. Further analysis did not reveal a direct correlation between the oscillation amplitude and the presence of buckles in the shell before ultrasound insonification (Supplemental Figure S6). The maximum oscillation amplitude was compared between microbubbles without buckles, with a single buckle, with multiple buckles, or with extensive buckles in the coating before ultrasound insonification. For all types of microbubbles, at 50 and 150 kPa, no statistically significant differences in oscillation amplitude were found between the groups. Next, the correlation between the change in microbubble coating upon ultrasound insonification and the maximum oscillation amplitude was evaluated, as shown in Figure 11. The median excursion amplitude of microbubbles that experienced a change, either by forming a buckle or by shedding lipids from the coating, was significantly larger ($p < 0.001$) than the excursion amplitude of unchanged microbubbles for all microbubble types. For direct DSPC microbubbles, the difference between changed and unchanged coatings was the most explicit, with a threshold amplitude of approximately 20% above which most microbubbles were changed after ultrasound insonification. For indirect DSPC microbubbles, the threshold amplitude was similar, albeit less pronounced. The indirect DSPC-cholesterol microbubbles also exhibited the formation of buckles and shedding of lipid material in microbubbles oscillating with amplitudes <20%.

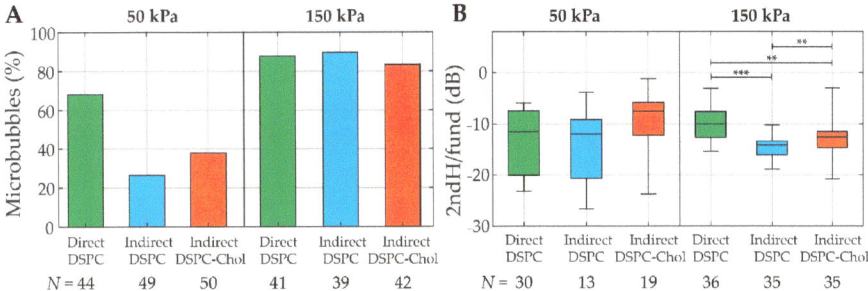

Figure 9. (A) Percentage of direct DSPC (green), indirect DSPC (blue), and indirect DSPC-cholesterol (red, 12 mol% cholesterol) microbubbles with a second harmonic response at 50 kPa (left panel) and 150 kPa (right panel). (B) Second harmonic amplitude normalized to the fundamental (dB) of direct DSPC (green), indirect DSPC (blue), and indirect DSPC-cholesterol (red, 12 mol% cholesterol) microbubbles at 50 kPa (left panel) and 150 kPa (right panel). Boxplots represent the median and interquartile range (IQR), with whiskers ranging from maximum to minimum. ** $p < 0.01$. *** $p < 0.001$.

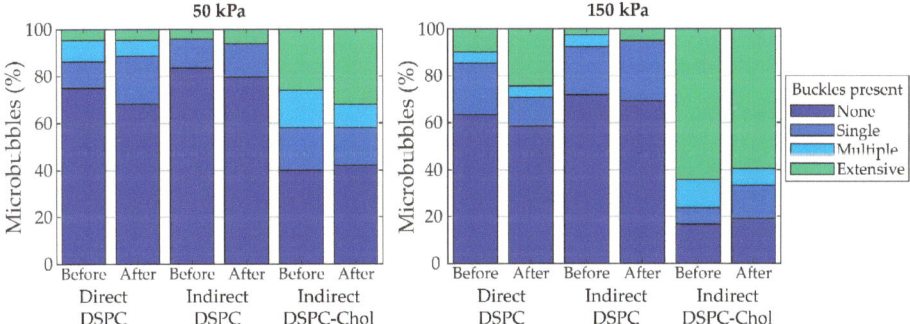

Figure 10. Percentage of microbubbles with buckles (none, single, multiple, or extensive) before and after insonification at 50 kPa (left panel) and 150 kPa (right panel). Indirect DSPC-cholesterol microbubbles contained 12 mol% cholesterol.

Finally, the correlation between LC domain size and oscillation amplitude was investigated for a limited size range of microbubbles, ruling out size-dependent differences in oscillation (Figure 12). Since the indirect DSPC-cholesterol microbubbles were lacking LC domains, they could not be scored for their LC domain size. Unscored microbubbles are shown as black dots in Figure 12. For the direct and indirect DSPC microbubbles of 4.5–6.0 μm (initial diameter), the lipid phase distribution was scored as "only large LC domains", "large and small LC domains", or "undefined" (Supplemental Figure S7). Both the direct ($N = 11$) and indirect ($N = 14$) DSPC microbubbles with large and small LC domains had a significantly higher oscillation amplitude than those with only large LC domains (direct: $N = 4$, indirect: $N = 15$).

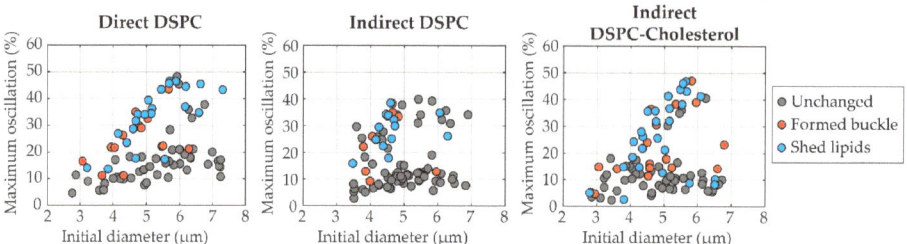

Figure 11. Maximum oscillation amplitude (%) of single direct DSPC (**left**, $N = 85$), indirect DSPC (**middle**, $N = 88$), and indirect DSPC-cholesterol (**right**, 12 mol% cholesterol, $N = 92$) microbubbles as a function of the initial microbubble diameter (μm). Microbubbles imaged by confocal microscopy directly before and after insonification (1–4 MHz, 50 or 150 kPa) were compared and scored as unchanged (gray), formed a buckle (red) or shed lipid material (blue).

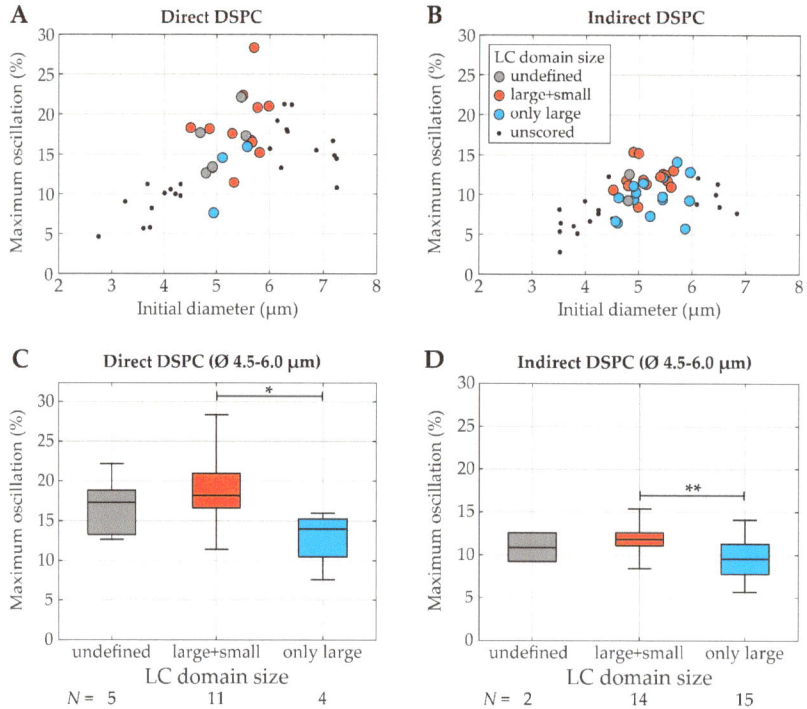

Figure 12. Maximum oscillation amplitude (%) at 50 kPa (over 1–4 MHz) as a function of initial diameter (μm) (**A,B**) for single direct DSPC (left) and indirect DSPC (right) microbubbles of 4.5–6.0 μm in diameter with LC domain size score as undefined (gray), large and small (red) or only large LC domains (blue), and as boxplot (**C,D**) representing the median and IQR with whiskers ranging from maximum to minimum. In A and B, the unscored microbubbles outside the 4.5–6.0 μm range are shown as black dots. * $p < 0.05$. ** $p < 0.01$.

4. Discussion

The results of this study showed that cholesterol significantly affected the ligand and lipid phase distribution in DSPC-based phospholipid-coated microbubbles made by the indirect method. The lipid handling prior to microbubble production also affected the ligand distribution, as shown previously [16]. Both the addition of cholesterol and the lipid handling prior to microbubble production were shown to influence the acoustic behavior of the microbubbles, as reflected in the apparent elasticity and viscosity values and resonance frequencies. Finally, the variability in acoustic response was enhanced for the microbubbles without lipid phase separation in the coating, namely the indirect DSPC-based microbubbles with 12 mol% cholesterol.

4.1. Physicochemical Characterization

The first part of this study revolved around the production and physicochemical characterization of DSPC-based microbubbles with cholesterol. Results indicated that the mean size of the microbubbles decreased with increasing concentrations of cholesterol. In contrast, Kaur et al. found that microbubbles with DSPC and cholesterol (1:1 molar ratio) were not significantly different in size from microbubbles with DSPC only [25]. However, those microbubbles were air-filled and did not contain any emulsifier such as PEG40-stearate or DSPE-PEG2000 like the microbubbles investigated in the present study. In our study, the span value increased with increasing concentrations of cholesterol, indicating that microbubbles with cholesterol were more polydisperse than those without cholesterol. Furthermore, the variability in polydispersity was larger between batches of microbubbles with cholesterol than those without cholesterol.

The addition of cholesterol to the indirect DSPC-based microbubble coating affected both the ligand and the lipid phase distribution. Indirect DSPC microbubbles without cholesterol had a mostly homogeneous ligand distribution as shown by fluorescence microscopy imaging, which is in agreement with results from Langeveld et al. [16]. However, all types of microbubbles with cholesterol had significantly more heterogeneous and variable ligand distribution than those without cholesterol. While the ligand distribution of microbubbles with 12 mol% cholesterol was the most homogeneous and comparable to that of the indirect DSPC microbubbles without cholesterol, indirect DSPC microbubbles with 14 mol% cholesterol had a more heterogeneous ligand distribution. The increased number of buckles in the coating is likely the reason for this increase in heterogeneity.

The indirect DSPC microbubbles without cholesterol had a lipid phase distribution similar to previous reports, with dark LC domains and a bright interdomain LE region [14,16]. All types of microbubbles with cholesterol had a significantly smaller LC phase area than those without cholesterol, indicating that cholesterol molecules modified the lateral molecular packing of the microbubble coating. The impact of cholesterol on the lipid phase distribution was most evident in microbubbles with 12 mol% cholesterol, where all components appeared to be miscible and in a single homogeneous phase. With a higher concentration of cholesterol, specifically 14 mol%, the quantified LC phase area was larger than in microbubbles with 12 mol% cholesterol. A previously reported analysis of the lipid phase behavior in binary monolayers of DPPC or DSPC with cholesterol suggested a three-state phase model [23], where cholesterol either reduced or increased the lateral molecular packing. According to that study, the lateral molecular packing of a lipid monolayer is expected to decrease with low concentrations of cholesterol and increase with higher concentrations of cholesterol. This is in agreement with our results of the lateral molecular packing, quantified here as LC phase area, decreasing up to 12 mol% and then increasing at 14 mol% cholesterol. Other work focused on lipid phase behavior in monolayers includes atomic force microscopy images of monolayers with DPPC and 33 mol% cholesterol, showing a homogeneous phase distribution [22]. While we found microbubbles with 32 mol% cholesterol to be highly unstable, those with 12 mol% had a homogeneous phase distribution. This suggests that the phase behavior of phospholipids in a monolayer cannot be directly translated to the phase behavior of phospholipids in a microbubble coating, which is supported by a direct comparison of lipid phase behavior in monolayers and microbubble coatings with the same ternary mixture of DPPC or DSPC with DSPE-PEG2000 and PEG40-stearate [16].

Interestingly, cholesterol (10–50 mol%) has been used for many years to stabilize liposomes with DPPC or DSPC by increasing the lateral molecular packing [34], emphasizing the difference in lamellar structures, i.e., bilayers, of a liposome compared to the phospholipid monolayer coating of a microbubble. DSPC forms lamellar structures when suspended in water at room temperature [35]. However, during microbubble production by probe sonication, the lamellar structures are disrupted, and the molecules self-assemble as a monolayer of phospholipids at the gas–liquid interface [36]. In a model membrane system with monolayer-bilayer junctions, cholesterol was shown to be involved in lipid-driven budding of the membrane, with higher concentrations of cholesterol resulting in increased budding [37]. These findings are in agreement with the increased budding and formation of buckles we found in microbubbles with higher concentrations of cholesterol in the coating. In this context, budding refers to the formation of lipid bilayer-coated vesicles, while buckle formation refers to bilayers that are still attached to the lipid monolayer coating of the microbubble.

The present study includes a normalization factor in the analysis of the 4Pi microscopy data to compensate for a difference in fluorescence intensity between the middle and the top or bottom of the microbubbles. The normalization factor did not affect the proper quantification of the LC phase area in microbubbles without cholesterol. Since the difference in fluorescence signal between LC and LE phase in those microbubbles was much larger than the difference in signal between the middle and top or bottom of the microbubble, the LC phase area could easily be quantified in microbubbles with clear separation of the lipids into LC and LE phase. The imaging artifact only became evident during the analysis of microbubbles with a homogeneous lipid phase distribution, i.e., containing cholesterol. All experiments in this study were performed at a room temperature of 19–21 °C. Since the 4Pi confocal microscope operates at a limited range of temperature, this practice facilitated comparison of the data obtained from the 4Pi confocal microscopy and the acoustic characterization with the combined confocal and Brandaris 128 system and was in accordance with previous microscopy studies on lipid and ligand distribution in microbubble coatings [14,16]. Slight fluctuations in the temperature of the sample due to, for instance, the light or ultrasound are not expected to affect the lipid phase distribution, since the transition temperature for DSPC is 55 °C [38]. Furthermore, it was previously reported that in lipid bilayers of DPPC and cholesterol (10 or 20 mol%), the lipid phase distribution was only affected by temperatures above 40 °C [39]. Processing of lipid films in the sonicator bath and with the probe sonicator at power 3 did not affect the temperature of the samples.

4.2. Acoustical Characterization

Microbubble spectroscopy was performed on direct DSPC, indirect DSPC, and indirect DSPC-cholesterol (12 mol%) microbubbles to characterize their acoustic behavior. The shell parameters found here can be directly compared to a previous study by van Rooij et al. [11], which used a similar method and included the same direct DSPC microbubbles as the current study. The shell elasticity found in the present study (0.14 (0.12–0.15) N/m) (median (IQR)) was slightly lower and the shell viscosity (0.43 (0.38–0.61) $\times 10^{-8}$ kg/s) slightly higher than previously published (0.26 $\pm$ 0.13 N/m, mean $\pm$ SD; 1.0 (0.7) $\times 10^{-8}$ kg/s, median (IQR)), however, still within the error margins. The indirect DSPC microbubbles had a shell elasticity approaching that of an uncoated microbubble, similar to the DPPC-based microbubbles studied by van Rooij et al. [11]. As the shell elasticity was lower, the resonance frequency was also lower (Equation (2)). Both the indirect DSPC and the indirect DSPC-cholesterol microbubbles had a higher shell viscosity than the direct DSPC microbubbles. This was reflected in the oscillation amplitudes at 50 kPa, which were higher for the direct DSPC microbubbles than for the other groups, indicating lower damping and, therefore, lower viscosity (Equation (1)).

The influence of lipid phase distribution and lipid handling on the variability in acoustic response was assessed by comparing microbubbles with lipid phase separation, i.e., indirect DSPC, to those without lipid phase separation, i.e., indirect DSPC-cholesterol (12 mol%), and to those made with a different way of lipid handling prior to microbubble production, i.e., direct DSPC. While indirect DSPC-cholesterol microbubbles had the highest maximum variability in response, the median variability was highest for the direct DSPC microbubbles. These results suggest that lipid handling prior to microbubble production can reduce the variability in response and that although the maximum variability was highest in the indirect DSPC-cholesterol microbubbles, the difference in lipid phase separation did not affect the variability in acoustic response overall. Due to their more uniform response, the indirect DSPC microbubbles would be the most suitable candidate for drug delivery applications. Two maxima can be observed in the variability in the response of direct and indirect DSPC microbubbles to ultrasound insonification. While this may be explained as a size-dependent effect, it is not a distinct trend and perhaps more likely due to the limited sample size. Apart from differences between the microbubble types, all microbubbles exhibited the highest variability in response at the resonance frequency. Thus, to insonify microbubbles at a frequency other than their resonance frequency could be a new strategy to achieve a more uniform response to ultrasound, although monodisperse microbubbles are needed for this strategy to yield a uniform and predictive response of a bulk of microbubbles.

Acoustical stability was studied using the decrease in diameter after ultrasound, i.e., deflation. For this analysis, the mean microbubble diameter of 128 frames without ultrasound was regarded as the initial diameter. Since the final diameter was determined based on the last recording of each microbubble, i.e., the recording of ultrasound insonification at 4 MHz, only the last 10 frames were used to calculate the mean microbubble diameter. The microbubble size in these last frames was stable, and the difference in sample size is therefore not expected to influence the results. At 50 kPa, statistical differences in deflation could be explained by differences in the oscillation amplitude. At 150 kPa, however, the indirect DSPC microbubbles were significantly more stable than the direct DSPC and indirect DSPC-cholesterol microbubbles. Since no statistical differences were found between the direct DSPC and indirect DSPC-cholesterol microbubbles, the difference in acoustical stability was not caused by a difference in coating microstructure, which is in accordance with previous studies [40]. As the composition of direct and indirect DSPC microbubbles was exactly the same, the difference in acoustical stability must have been caused by the difference in lipid handling prior to microbubble production, which is known to alter the ligand distribution, synonymous to the distribution of DSPE-PEG2000 [16].

The nonlinear behavior of microbubbles is imperative for successful contrast-enhanced ultrasound imaging and ultrasound molecular imaging. At 50 kPa, the direct DSPC microbubbles had a more frequent second harmonic response than the other types of microbubbles. At 150 kPa, the majority of all types of microbubbles had a second harmonic response. The differences in variability in the acoustic response between the types of microbubbles, as presented in Figure 7, are also reflected in the range of the second harmonic response at 150 kPa, presented in Figure 9B. Indirect DSPC microbubbles had the lowest variability in second harmonic amplitude at 150 kPa, while the response at 50 kPa was comparable to the other types. This could be due to the low amplitudes of the second harmonic response at 50 kPa, which translates to a larger experimental error. The percentage of direct DSPC microbubbles with a nonlinear response, subharmonic or second harmonic, at 50 kPa was lower than published before [11]. This may be explained by the different pulse lengths (8 cycle- instead of 10-cycle pulse) or the fact that as a lower amount of light reaches the Brandaris 128 camera in the current imaging system, the noise level is slightly higher. More experiments focused on nonlinear behavior are needed for a comprehensive assessment of indirect DSPC microbubbles for ultrasound molecular imaging. However, this lies outside the scope of the present study.

4.3. Lipid Phase Distribution and Acoustical Behavior

The homogeneous lipid phase distribution in indirect DSPC-cholesterol microbubbles found by 4Pi confocal microscopy was confirmed with confocal microscopy of the microbubbles also analyzed acoustically. Besides the homogeneous lipid phase distribution, indirect DSPC-cholesterol microbubbles had buckles in their coating before insonification more frequently and more extensively than microbubbles without cholesterol, demonstrated by 4Pi confocal microscopy as well. The DSPC-cholesterol microbubbles insonified at 150 kPa had more buckles than those insonified at 50 kPa, underlining the heterogeneity between different indirect DSPC-cholesterol microbubbles from the same batch. The variable buckle incidence may be explained by the low stability of the DSPC-cholesterol coating. Due to the low amount of LC phase area in their coating, indirect DSPC-cholesterol microbubbles are expected to dissolve at a faster rate than those without cholesterol [41]. Different collapse and shedding mechanisms, such as budding, folding, and buckling, have been proposed to explain how the phospholipid monolayer around the gas core responds to the spontaneous dissolution of the microbubble [42].

Next, the correlation between maximum oscillation amplitude and change in the microbubble coating was investigated. After combining the data from microbubbles insonified at 50 and 150 kPa, the oscillation amplitude of microbubbles that experienced change due to ultrasound insonification was found to be significantly higher than that of unchanged microbubbles for all microbubble types, with a threshold amplitude of approximately 20%. Other studies investigating the lipid coating behavior in microbubbles during ultrasound insonification found comparable results, namely a threshold oscillation amplitude of 30% [43,44]. The difference in threshold amplitude may be explained by the microbubble formulation as microbubbles in other studies were coated with DPPC [43] or DSPC [44] and DSPE-PEG2000, without PEG40-stearate. Another explanation could be a difference in the production method, as the microbubbles for the present study were all made by probe sonication, in contrast to the vial shaker method used for previous studies.

This study is the first to record both the lipid phase distribution and acoustic response in single microbubbles with the combined confocal microscope and Brandaris 128 camera system. Whereas no correlation could be confirmed between the oscillation amplitude and the amount of buckles present before insonification, the LC domain size did correlate with the oscillation amplitude. Microbubbles with small-sized LC domains had higher oscillation amplitudes, which is in accordance with previous reports on phospholipid-coated microbubbles with different sized LC domains, where those with smaller LC domains had a lower resistance to deformation [45]. By contrast, another study found no significant differences in the behavior or stability of microbubbles during ultrasound insonification when they related the lateral molecular packing to the acoustic behavior of microbubbles in different formulations, even though the method of production did affect the lipid packing significantly [46]. The reason for this could be the quantification of the lateral molecular packing, as this was done by calculating the generalized polarization value for single microbubbles, which does not account for lipid phase separation or microstructures in the coating. Before the DSPC-based microbubbles with and without cholesterol studied here can be used for in vivo applications, several differences between the in vitro setting and the in vivo situation need to be considered. Besides the temperature, these differences also include the blood flow, blood viscosity, and soft boundaries affecting the microbubbles' acoustic behavior. Furthermore, the targeting strategy must be adapted to avoid an immune response to streptavidin, a foreign protein [47].

4.4. Implications of the Study

The addition of cholesterol to the indirect DSPC-based microbubble coating increased the variability in ligand distribution, acoustic response, polydispersity, and buckle formation. These effects can be explained by the altered lipid phase distribution as described above and imply that the indirect DSPC-cholesterol microbubbles are less stable than those without cholesterol. Because the indirect DSPC-cholesterol microbubbles had heterogeneities in the form of buckles, they could not be regarded as microbubbles with a uniform lipid distribution when comparing their acoustic behavior to that of the microbubbles with heterogeneous lipid phase distribution, i.e., the direct and indirect DSPC microbubbles. Thus, reduced stability of the microbubble coating is expected when the components are all miscible and in the same LE phase, which will increase the heterogeneity of the microbubble population and thereby increase the variability of the acoustical response. Therefore, a different approach will be required to achieve a more uniform microbubble response to ultrasound, possibly by tailoring the LC phase domains, as our results suggest that differences in LC domain size can predict the relative oscillation amplitude.

5. Conclusions

We produced indirect DSPC-based microbubbles with 7, 10, 12, and 14 mol% cholesterol in the coating. Cholesterol reduced lipid phase separation in the microbubble coating, resulting in a single phase at 12 mol% where all components were miscible. Buckle formation was increased with the reduction of the LC phase area, suggesting increased spontaneous dissolution of the microbubbles. As the acoustic behavior of DSPC-based microbubbles made by the direct and indirect method was compared to that of indirect DSPC-based microbubbles with 12 mol% cholesterol, indirect DSPC microbubbles had the most uniform response to the ultrasound and were the most stable acoustically. They had a lower shell elasticity and higher shell viscosity than the direct DSPC microbubbles. The modified lateral molecular packing of indirect DSPC-cholesterol microbubbles resulted in the lowest shell elasticity and highest shell viscosity of all microbubble types. Direct DSPC microbubbles displayed more nonlinear acoustic behavior than the indirect DSPC and indirect DSPC-cholesterol microbubbles. Based on these results, we can conclude that both the lipid phase separation and lipid handling prior to microbubble production significantly affected the acoustic behavior of microbubbles. The indirect DSPC microbubbles had the most promising results with regard to stability and uniform ultrasound response. These are important traits for an ultrasound molecular imaging agent and for drug delivery applications, as the acoustic behavior of the microbubble must be predictable and controllable.

Supplementary Materials: The following are available online at https://www.mdpi.com/1999-4923/13/1/119/s1, Figure S1: Normalization factors for quantitative analysis of 4Pi confocal microscopy data, Figure S2: Examples of buckle score based on confocal microscopy, Figure S3: Confocal slices from z-stack acquisition of indirect DSPC-cholesterol (12 mol%) microbubble, Figure S4: Relative oscillation amplitude of single microbubbles as a function of the initial diameter, Figure S5: Percentage of microbubbles with subharmonic responses and amplitudes of subharmonic response, Figure S6: Shell buckles versus oscillation amplitude, Figure S7: examples of LC domain size score based on confocal microscopy. Table S1. Concentration of indirect DSPC microbubbles (MBs).

Author Contributions: Conceptualization, S.A.G.L., I.B., N.d.J. and K.K.; methodology, S.A.G.L., I.B. and G.C.-L.; software, I.B.; validation, S.A.G.L., I.B. and G.C.-L.; formal analysis, S.A.G.L. and I.B.; investigation, S.A.G.L. and I.B.; resources, A.F.W.v.d.S. and K.K.; data curation, S.A.G.L.; writing—original draft preparation, S.A.G.L.; writing—review and editing, S.A.G.L., I.B., G.C.-L., A.F.W.v.d.S., N.d.J. and K.K.; visualization, S.A.G.L.; supervision, N.d.J. and K.K.; project administration, S.A.G.L.; funding acquisition, A.F.W.v.d.S. and K.K. All authors have read and agreed to the published version of the manuscript.

Funding: This research was funded in part by the Phospholipid Research Center in Heidelberg, grant number KKO-2017-057/1-1, and in part by the Thorax Center of Erasmus University Medical Center in Rotterdam.

Institutional Review Board Statement: Not applicable.

Informed Consent Statement: Not applicable.

Data Availability Statement: The data presented in this study are available on request from the corresponding author. The data are not publicly available due to the complex nature and tailored analysis for the unique experimental set-ups used in this study.

Acknowledgments: The authors thank F. Mastik and R. Beurskens from the Department of Biomedical Engineering, Erasmus University Medical Center, Rotterdam, the Netherlands, for their technical assistance during the experiments. The authors thank the Erasmus Optical Imaging Centre of Erasmus MC for the use of their facilities and Gert van Cappellen and Alex Nigg for their help. Finally, the authors thank Lipoid GmbH for providing a free sample of DSPC phospholipid.

Conflicts of Interest: The authors declare no conflict of interest.

References

1. Chong, W.K.; Papadopoulou, V.; Dayton, P.A. Imaging with ultrasound contrast agents: Current status and future. *Abdom. Radiol.* **2018**, *43*, 762–772. [CrossRef] [PubMed]
2. Kosareva, A.; Abou-Elkacem, L.; Chowdhury, S.; Lindner, J.R.; Kaufmann, B.A. Seeing the Invisible—Ultrasound Molecular Imaging. *Ultrasound Med. Biol.* **2020**, *46*, 479–497. [CrossRef]
3. Kooiman, K.; Roovers, S.; Langeveld, S.A.G.; Kleven, R.T.; Dewitte, H.; O'Reilly, M.A.; Escoffre, J.M.; Bouakaz, A.; Verweij, M.D.; Hynynen, K.; et al. Ultrasound-Responsive Cavitation Nuclei for Therapy and Drug Delivery. *Ultrasound Med. Biol.* **2020**, *46*, 1296–1325. [CrossRef] [PubMed]
4. Kooiman, K.; Vos, H.J.; Versluis, M.; de Jong, N. Acoustic behavior of microbubbles and implications for drug delivery. *Adv. Drug Deliv. Rev.* **2014**, *72*, 28–48. [CrossRef] [PubMed]
5. Stride, E.; Segers, T.; Lajoinie, G.; Cherkaoui, S.; Bettinger, T.; Versluis, M.; Borden, M. Microbubble Agents: New Directions. *Ultrasound Med. Biol.* **2020**, *46*, 1326–1343. [CrossRef]
6. Versluis, M.; Stride, E.; Lajoinie, G.; Dollet, B.; Segers, T. Ultrasound Contrast Agent Modeling: A Review. *Ultrasound Med. Biol.* **2020**, *46*, 2117–2144. [CrossRef]
7. Klibanov, A.L. Ultrasound Contrast Agents: Development of the Field and Current Status. In *Contrast Agents II: Optical, Ultrasound, X-ray and Radiopharmaceutical Imaging*; Krause, W., Ed.; Springer Berlin Heidelberg: Berlin/Heidelberg, Germany, 2002; pp. 73–106.
8. Van Rooij, T.; Daeichin, V.; Skachkov, I.; de Jong, N.; Kooiman, K. Targeted ultrasound contrast agents for ultrasound molecular imaging and therapy. *Int. J. Hyperth.* **2015**, *31*, 90–106. [CrossRef] [PubMed]
9. Overvelde, M.; Garbin, V.; Sijl, J.; Dollet, B.; de Jong, N.; Lohse, D.; Versluism, M. Nonlinear shell behavior of phospholipid-coated microbubbles. *Ultrasound Med. Biol.* **2010**, *36*, 2080–2092. [CrossRef] [PubMed]
10. Marmottant, P.; Meer, S.; Emmer, M.; Versluis, M.; Jong, N.; Hilgenfeldt, S.; Lohse, D. A model for large amplitude oscillations of coated bubbles accounting for buckling and rupture. *J. Acoust. Soc. Am.* **2005**, *118*, 3499–3505. [CrossRef]
11. van Rooij, T.; Luan, Y.; Renaud, G.; van der Steen, A.F.; Versluis, M.; de Jong, N.; Kooiman, K. Non-linear response and viscoelastic properties of lipid-coated microbubbles: DSPC versus DPPC. *Ultrasound Med. Biol.* **2015**, *41*, 1432–1445. [CrossRef]
12. Garg, S.; Thomas, A.A.; Borden, M.A. The effect of lipid monolayer in-plane rigidity on in vivo microbubble circulation persistence. *Biomaterials* **2013**, *34*, 6862–6870. [CrossRef] [PubMed]
13. Borden, M.A.; Pu, G.; Runner, G.J.; Longo, M.L. Surface phase behavior and microstructure of lipid/PEG-emulsifier monolayer-coated microbubbles. *Colloids Surf. B Biointerfaces* **2004**, *35*, 209–223. [CrossRef] [PubMed]
14. Borden, M.A.; Martinez, G.V.; Ricker, J.; Tsvetkova, N.; Longo, M.; Gillies, R.J.; Dayton, P.A.; Ferrara, K.W. Lateral phase separation in lipid-coated microbubbles. *Langmuir* **2006**, *22*, 4291–4297. [CrossRef] [PubMed]
15. Helfield, B.L.; Cherin, E.; Foster, F.S.; Goertz, D.E. Investigating the subharmonic response of individual phospholipid encapsulated microbubbles at high frequencies: A comparative study of five agents. *Ultrasound Med. Biol.* **2012**, *38*, 846–863. [CrossRef]
16. Langeveld, S.A.G.; Schwieger, C.; Beekers, I.; Blaffert, J.; van Rooij, T.; Blume, A.; Kooiman, K. Ligand Distribution and Lipid Phase Behavior in Phospholipid-Coated Microbubbles and Monolayers. *Langmuir* **2020**, *36*, 3221–3233. [CrossRef]
17. van Rooij, T.; Beekers, I.; Lattwein, K.R.; van der Steen, A.F.W.; de Jong, N.; Kooiman, K. Vibrational Responses of Bound and Nonbound Targeted Lipid-Coated Single Microbubbles. *IEEE Trans. Ultrason. Ferroelectr. Freq. Control* **2017**, *64*, 785–797. [CrossRef] [PubMed]
18. Emmer, M.; Vos, H.J.; Versluis, M.; de Jong, N. Radial modulation of single microbubbles. *IEEE Trans. Ultrason. Ferroelectr. Freq. Control* **2009**, *56*, 2370–2379. [CrossRef]
19. Van der Meer, S.M.; Dollet, B.; Voormolen, M.M.; Chin, C.T.; Bouakaz, A.; de Jong, N.; Versluism, M.; Lohse, D. Microbubble spectroscopy of ultrasound contrast agents. *J. Acoust. Soc. Am.* **2007**, *121*, 648–656. [CrossRef]
20. Lum, J.S.; Dove, J.D.; Murray, T.W.; Borden, M.A. Single Microbubble Measurements of Lipid Monolayer Viscoelastic Properties for Small-Amplitude Oscillations. *Langmuir* **2016**, *32*, 9410–9417. [CrossRef] [PubMed]
21. Lum, J.S.; Stobbe, D.M.; Borden, M.A.; Murray, T.W. Photoacoustic technique to measure temperature effects on microbubble viscoelastic properties. *Appl. Phys. Lett.* **2018**, *112*, 111905. [CrossRef] [PubMed]
22. Yuan, C.; Johnston, L.J. Phase evolution in cholesterol/DPPC monolayers: Atomic force microscopy and near field scanning optical microscopy studies. *J. Microsc.* **2002**, *205*, 136–146. [CrossRef] [PubMed]
23. Miyoshi, T.; Kato, S. Detailed Analysis of the Surface Area and Elasticity in the Saturated 1,2-Diacylphosphatidylcholine/Cholesterol Binary Monolayer System. *Langmuir* **2015**, *31*, 9086–9096. [CrossRef] [PubMed]
24. Veatch, S.L.; Keller, S.L. Separation of liquid phases in giant vesicles of ternary mixtures of phospholipids and cholesterol. *Biophys. J.* **2003**, *85*, 3074–3083. [CrossRef]
25. Kaur, R.; Morris, R.; Bencsik, M.; Vangala, A.; Rades, T.; Perrie, Y. Development of a Novel Magnetic Resonance Imaging Contrast Agent for Pressure Measurements Using Lipid-Coated Microbubbles. *J. Biomed. Nanotechnol.* **2009**, *5*, 707–715. [CrossRef] [PubMed]

26. Lee, H.J.; Yoon, T.J.; Yoon, Y.I. Synthesis of ultrasound contrast agents: Characteristics and size distribution analysis (secondary publication). *Ultrasonography* **2017**, *36*, 378–384. [CrossRef] [PubMed]
27. Klibanov, A.L.; Rasche, P.T.; Hughes, M.S.; Wojdyla, J.K.; Galen, K.P.; Wible, J.H.; Brandenburger, G.H. Detection of Individual Microbubbles of Ultrasound Contrast Agents. *Investig. Radiol.* **2004**, *39*, 187–195. [CrossRef]
28. Chapman, D. Handbook of Lipid Research, Volume 4: The Physical Chemistry of Lipids. *Biochem. Soc. Trans.* **1987**, *15*, 184–185. [CrossRef]
29. Kooiman, K.; Kokhuis, T.J.A.; van Rooij, T.; Skachkov, I.; Nigg, A.; Bosch, J.G.; van der Steen, A.F.W.; van Cappellen, W.A.; de Jong, N. DSPC or DPPC as main shell component influences ligand distribution and binding area of lipid-coated targeted microbubbles. *Eur. J. Lipid Sci. Tech.* **2014**, *116*, 1217–1227. [CrossRef]
30. Hell, S.; Stelzer, E.H.K. Fundamental improvement of resolution with a 4Pi-confocal fluorescence microscope using two-photon excitation. *Opt. Commun.* **1992**, *93*, 277–282. [CrossRef]
31. Beekers, I.; Lattwein, K.R.; Kouijzer, J.J.P.; Langeveld, S.A.G.; Vegter, M.; Beurskens, R.; Mastik, F.; Verduyn Lunel, R.; Verver, E.; van der Steen, A.F.W. Combined Confocal Microscope and Brandaris 128 Ultra-High-Speed Camera. *Ultrasound Med. Biol.* **2019**, *45*, 2575–2582. [CrossRef]
32. Beekers, I.; van Rooij, T.; van der Steen, A.; Jong, N.; Verweij, M.; Kooiman, K. Acoustic Characterization of the CLINIcell for Ultrasound Contrast Agent Studies. *IEEE Trans. Ultrason. Ferroelectr. Freq. Control* **2018**, *66*, 244–246. [CrossRef] [PubMed]
33. Chin, C.T.; Lancée, C.; Borsboom, J.; Mastik, F.; Frijlink, M.E.; de Jong, N.; Versluis, M.; Lohse, D. Brandaris 128: A digital 25 million frames per second camera with 128 highly sensitive frames. *Rev. Sci. Instrum.* **2003**, *74*, 5026–5034. [CrossRef]
34. Demel, R.A.; De Kruyff, B. The function of sterols in membranes. *Biochim. Biophys. Acta* **1976**, *457*, 109–132. [CrossRef]
35. Ferrara, K.W.; Borden, M.A.; Zhang, H. Lipid-shelled vehicles: Engineering for ultrasound molecular imaging and drug delivery. *Acc. Chem. Res.* **2009**, *42*, 881–892. [CrossRef] [PubMed]
36. Sirsi, S.; Borden, M. Microbubble Compositions, Properties and Biomedical Applications. *Bubble Sci. Eng. Technol.* **2009**, *1*, 3–17. [CrossRef] [PubMed]
37. Lee, Y.K.; Yu, E.-S.; Ahn, D.J.; Ryu, Y.-S. Elasticity-Driven Membrane Budding through Cholesterol Concentration on Supported Lipid Monolayer–Bilayer Junction. *Adv. Mater. Interfaces* **2020**, *7*, 2000937. [CrossRef]
38. Silvius, J.R. Thermotropic Phase Transitions of Pure Lipids in Model Membranes and Their Modifications by Membrane Proteins. In *Lipid-Protein Interactions*; John Wiley & Sons, Inc.: New York, NY, USA, 1982.
39. Redondo-Morata, L.; Giannotti, M.I.; Sanz, F. Influence of Cholesterol on the Phase Transition of Lipid Bilayers: A Temperature-Controlled Force Spectroscopy Study. *Langmuir* **2012**, *28*, 12851–12860. [CrossRef]
40. Borden, M.A.; Kruse, D.E.; Caskey, C.F.; Shukui, Z.; Dayton, P.A.; Ferrara, K.W. Influence of lipid shell physicochemical properties on ultrasound-induced microbubble destruction. *IEEE Trans. Ultrason. Ferroelectr. Freq. Control* **2005**, *52*, 1992–2002. [CrossRef]
41. Pu, G.; Longo, M.L.; Borden, M.A. Effect of Microstructure on Molecular Oxygen Permeation through Condensed Phospholipid Monolayers. *J. Am. Chem. Soc.* **2005**, *127*, 6524–6525. [CrossRef]
42. Pu, G.; Borden, M.A.; Longo, M.L. Collapse and Shedding Transitions in Binary Lipid Monolayers Coating Microbubbles. *Langmuir* **2006**, *22*, 2993–2999. [CrossRef]
43. Luan, Y.; Lajoinie, G.; Gelderblom, E.; Skachkov, I.; van der Steen, A.F.; Vos, H.J.; Versluis, M.; de Jong, N. Lipid shedding from single oscillating microbubbles. *Ultrasound Med. Biol.* **2014**, *40*, 1834–1846. [CrossRef] [PubMed]
44. Kooiman, K.; van Rooij, T.; Qin, B.; Mastik, F.; Vos, H.J.; Versluis, M.; Klibanov, A.L.; de Jong, N.; Villanueva, F.S.; Chen, X. Focal areas of increased lipid concentration on the coating of microbubbles during short tone-burst ultrasound insonification. *PLoS ONE* **2017**, *12*, e0180747. [CrossRef] [PubMed]
45. Kim, D.H.; Costello, M.J.; Duncan, P.B.; Needham, D. Mechanical Properties and Microstructure of Polycrystalline Phospholipid Monolayer Shells: Novel Solid Microparticles. *Langmuir* **2003**, *19*, 8455–8466. [CrossRef]
46. Browning, R.J.; Aron, M.; Booth, A.; Rademeyer, P.; Wing, S.; Brans, V.; Shrivastava, S.; Carugo, D.; Stride, E. Spectral Imaging for Microbubble Characterization. *Langmuir* **2020**, *36*, 609–617. [CrossRef] [PubMed]
47. Paganelli, G.; Belloni, C.; Magnani, P.; Zito, F.; Pasini, A.; Sassi, I.; Meroni, M.; Mariani, M.; Vignali, M.; Siccardi, A.G.; et al. Two-step tumour targetting in ovarian cancer patients using biotinylated monoclonal antibodies and radioactive streptavidin. *Eur. J. Nucl. Med.* **1992**, *19*, 322–329. [CrossRef]

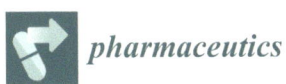

Article

Solid Lipid Particles for Lung Metastasis Treatment

Lourdes Valdivia, Lorena García-Hevia, Manuel Bañobre-López, Juan Gallo, Rafael Valiente and Mónica López Fanarraga

1 Nanomedicine Group, University of Cantabria—IDIVAL, Herrera Oria s/n, 39011 Santander, Spain; lourdes.valdivia@unican.es (L.V.); lgarcia@idival.org (L.G.-H.); rafael.valiente@unican.es (R.V.)
2 Advanced (Magnetic) Theranostic Nanostructures Laboratory, Nanomedicine Unit, International Iberian Nanotechnology Laboratory (INL), Av. Mestre José Veiga s/n, 4715-330 Braga, Portugal; manuel.banobre@inl.int (M.B.-L.); juan.gallo@inl.int (J.G.)
3 Applied Physics Department, Faculty of Sciences, Avda. de Los Castros 48, 39005 Santander, Spain
* Correspondence: fanarrag@unican.es; Tel.: +34-94-220-2067
† These authors contributed equally to this work.

Abstract: Solid lipid particles (SLPs) can sustainably encapsulate and release therapeutic agents over long periods, modifying their biodistribution, toxicity, and side effects. To date, no studies have been reported using SLPs loaded with doxorubicin chemotherapy for the treatment of metastatic cancer. This study characterizes the effect of doxorubicin-loaded carnauba wax particles in the treatment of lung metastatic malignant melanoma in vivo. Compared with the free drug, intravenously administered doxorubicin-loaded SLPs significantly reduce the number of pulmonary metastatic foci in mice. In vitro kinetic studies show two distinctive drug release profiles. A first chemotherapy burst-release wave occurs during the first 5 h, which accounts for approximately 30% of the entrapped drug rapidly providing therapeutic concentrations. The second wave occurs after the arrival of the particles to the final destination in the lung. This release is sustained for long periods (>40 days), providing constant levels of chemotherapy in situ that trigger the inhibition of metastatic growth. Our findings suggest that the use of chemotherapy with loaded SLPs could substantially improve the effectiveness of the drug locally, reducing side effects while improving overall survival.

Keywords: nanomedicine; cancer; doxorubicin; melanoma; drug delivery

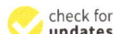

1. Introduction

In cancer, surgery is the treatment of choice. However, it is often not an option because many cancer cells have already escaped from the primary tumor and colonized distant tissues. Most patients with advanced metastatic disease confront a terminal illness. In fact, metastasis is the greatest challenge to a cancer patient's survival. There are currently no effective treatments to stop or prevent this process, so there is an urgent need to find new diagnostic and therapeutic approaches. To inhibit metastasis, local treatment is generally complemented by radiation therapy and high doses of chemotherapy that cause numerous side effects [1,2], limiting the success of metastasis treatment [3]. However, systemically applied cytotoxic drugs are not effective in preventing the spread of metastatic cells that cause 90% of cancer deaths [4].

Melanoma is an example of a fatal malignancy with rapid systemic dissemination. The 5-year survival rate for metastatic melanoma is less than 15%, and the median survival after developing pulmonary metastasis is on average 7.3 months [5]. The high recurrence of the tumor (one-third of all patients) and the low survival rate are due to the failure of chemotherapy as a systemic treatment for metastasis [6]. Recently, hormone therapy and immunotherapy have produced effective results boosting cell-mediated innate and adaptive antitumor immunity [7,8]. Thus, while understanding the molecular mechanisms behind cancer cell invasion of distal vital organs [1,9], new treatments must be developed to prevent/reduce the rate of metastasis.

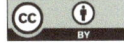

One possible solution to this issue could be the use of encapsulated drugs in nanosystems to reduce the systemic toxicity and improve the local effect and drug stability through a sustained and controlled drug release. In this sense, nanotechnology can greatly contribute by the development of delivery nanosystems which can inhibit primary tumors and, at the same time, prevent metastases before they sprout. Nanomedicine offers interesting opportunities to design different drug delivery systems, such as liposomes [3], carbon nanotubes [10], or gold nanoparticles [11], among others. These nanosystems can help in (i) reducing the toxicity of the treatment, (ii) preventing the premature elimination or degradation of the therapeutic compound, and (iii) significantly modifying the biodistribution of the encapsulated drug [12–15]. In this way, drugs with extraordinary pharmacological interest, but discarded due to their poor pharmacological properties or high systemic toxicity, can be reformulated into new nanocomposites showing multifunctional properties and improved therapeutic outputs [16]. Here, we have encapsulated doxorubicin (DOX) in lipidic particles. This drug has already been encapsulated in liposomes in previous studies that have been approved by the U. S. Food and Drug Administration (FDA) (Doxil® [16], Myocet® [17], and LipoDox® [18]). The advantages of these formulations are mainly to do with toxicity. They have less severe side effects than the free drug.

Numerous types of nanocarriers that allow the encapsulation of drugs to be systemically administered have been described. Among these, the most employed are liposomes [3,6], dendrimers [12–14], polymeric micelles [5–8], and silica-based materials [19–21]. Most of these nanomaterials have similar drug release patterns. In most examples, encapsulated therapeutic compounds are released at once, upon detachment, degradation, or permeabilization of the nanocarrier and/or its seal [22,23]. This "burst-release effect" triggers a fast peak of drug activity at the local or systemic level that closely mimics the effect caused by the free drug. Unfortunately, the effect of the drug is not sustained over time, selecting surviving cells and so generating resistant clones able to travel and colonize distant tissues. Thus, the development of drug carriers providing an initial delivery together with a sustained and controlled therapeutic release for long periods to obtain a level of drug higher than the minimum effective concentration is highly desirable. This suggests that the design of two-stage-release drug delivery systems could improve the prevention of metastasis.

Here, we used solid lipid particles (SLPs), which are aqueous colloidal dispersions with a matrix composed of solid biodegradable lipids. These nanoformulations present several advantages compared with other nanovehicles. Among the advantages, they show great biocompatibility, high drug-loading capacity, improved pharmaceutic stability, and excellent reproducibility [24]. Furthermore, the natural carnauba wax chosen in this study represents one of the best options to obtain excellent drug encapsulation efficiencies while maintaining the plasma drug concentration within the therapeutic window during a prolonged period [25].

In this study, we have investigated the antimetastatic effect of carnauba wax DOX-loaded SLPs. This drug is the first-line treatment for a wide range of cancers including lymphomas, leukemias, and solid tumors in the bladder, breast, stomach, lung, and ovaries, among others [26]. However, DOX use is currently decreasing due to its side effects, which include cardiotoxicity and nephrotoxicity [27,28]. This encapsulation system has already proved its efficacy in vitro in malignant melanoma cell cultures (2D and 3D melanoma models) [29] compared to the free DOX. Herein, we have studied the in vivo efficacy of the encapsulated DOX in a melanoma metastatic model.

2. Materials and Methods

2.1. Synthesis and Characterization of SLPs

The synthesis of SLPs was made by a modified melt emulsification method (Figure S1) as previously described [29]. Briefly, 100 mg of carnauba wax (T1 E00018; Koster Keunen, Watertown, CT, USA) was mixed with (i) a total of 30 mg of iron oxide (Fe_3O_4) nanoparticles, prepared following the coprecipitation method [30], with 13.02 ± 0.24 nm of diameter in a chloroform solution (99.5%, C2432; Sigma, St. Louis, MO, USA); (ii) 250 µL of 3,3′-dioctadecyloxacarbocyanine perchlorate (DiO) (D275; Invitrogen, Waltham, MA, USA) at 1 mg/mL in chloroform; and (iii) DOX (A14403; Adooq Bioscience, Irvine, CA, USA) (20 mg/mL). This mixture was heated until complete wax melting and chloroform (C2432; Sigma, Darmstadt, Germany) evaporation was achieved. Then, 2.25 mL of Milli-Q water and 250 µL of a 50 mg/mL water solution of Tween80 (P4780; Sigma, Darmstadt, Germany) were added to the vial. The sample was ultrasonicated (Branson 250; Emerson, St. Louis, MO, USA) at 25% power for 2 min at 20 s working intervals. The vial was cooled by a digital sonifier by immersion in ice to solidify the lipid particles. Finally, the formulation was centrifuged (Hettich Zentrifugen Universal 320, Tuttlingen, Germany) (3000 rpm, 10 min) and the supernatant was freeze-dried in the presence of sucrose (0.9% w/w) as a cryoprotectant.

Hydrodynamic diameters, ζ potential values and the polydispersity index of the SLPs were measured using dynamic light scattering (DLS) (Horiba Scientific SZ-100 instrument; Kyoto, Japan), and morphology was observed through transmission electron microscopy (TEM) images using a JEOL JEM-2100 (Tokyo, Japan) microscope at an accelerating voltage of 200 kV (Figure S2). The amount of DOX loaded from the SLPs was determined by high-performance liquid chromatography (UHPLC; Agilent 1290 Infinity II LC System; Santa Clara, CA, USA) using a gradient of water:acetonitrile (from 100% to 25:75%) and an Aeris 1.7 µm peptide XB-C18 column (Phenomenex; Torrance, CA, USA). Graphics were designed by BioRender.com.

2.2. Murine Malignant Melanoma Cells

Murine malignant melanoma B16-F10 cells (ATCC CRL-6475) were grown in Iscove's Modified Dulbecco's Medium (IMDM; P04-20350; Panbiotech; Aidenbach, Germany) supplemented with 10% fetal bovine serum (FBS; 26140079; Fisher Scientific; Waltham, MA, USA) and antibiotics. Cells were incubated under 37 °C with an atmosphere of 5% CO_2. B16-F10 cells were treated at a final concentration of 2 µg/mL of DOX-loaded SLPs (SLPs-DOX) for 2, 16, or 48 h. For confocal fluorescence imaging purposes, cells were fixed with 4% paraformaldehyde (43368; Alfa Aesar; Haverhill, MA, USA) and were immunolabeled with the anti-α-tubulin (B512; Sigma; Germany) antibody to recognize the microtubules. A secondary goat anti-mouse 647 (A21236; Invitrogen; USA) was used. Fluorescent images were obtained with a Nikon A1R confocal microscope (Tokyo, Japan). All images were pseudocolored.

2.3. In Vitro Drug Release

DOX release profile was studied in triplicate using dialysis (14 kDa cut-off cellulose membranes; Sigma; Germany) in phosphate-buffered saline media (PBS, pH 7.4). A total of 0.3 mL of DOX-loaded SLPs (SLPs-DOX) dispersion at a concentration of 20 mg/mL of DOX were added into the membrane bags that were submerged in PBS and stirred at 300 rpm at ca. 37 °C. The dialysis membrane allowed drug diffusion into the PBS while retaining the SLPs. Samples of 1 mL were taken at different times and measured using fluorescence spectroscopy in an Edinburgh Inst. FLSP920 spectrofluorometer (Livingston, UK). Values were compared to those of the calibration curve prepared for DOX (Figure S3). Finally, DOX release data in PBS pH 7.4 were fitted to a Korsmeyer–Peppas kinetic model.

2.4. Animal Studies, In Vivo Model

In vivo experiments were designed and performed to minimize the use of animals. C57BL/6 mice (12–16 weeks old) were housed with a 12 h light/dark cycle with free provision of food and water at the Experimentation Service (SEEA) of the University of Cantabria. Animals were maintained, handled, and sacrificed following the directive 2010/63/UE. The B16-F10 lung metastasis model in the C57BL/6 strain of mice is well established in the literature [31–34]. This cell line was derived from a spontaneous melanoma developed in C57BL/6 mice [31]. Metastatic foci were produced upon intravenous B16-F10 malignant melanoma cell transplantation. For this purpose, ca. 100,000 B16-F10 melanoma cells (50 µL/mouse) were injected in the retro-orbital venous sinus using a 0.3 mL microsyringe (BD Micro-Fine™; USA). Ten days after intravenous cancer cell injection, mice were randomly divided into four groups: untreated controls, mice injected with free DOX, mice injected with control SLPs, and finally, mice injected with SLPs-DOX. Animals were treated 3 times every 2 days at a concentration of 2.5 mg/kg DOX (each doses). Mice were euthanized 20 days after the transplant and had their tissues collected and fixed in formalin for histology. Lung metastatic colonies were easily recognized as black spots on the lung surface [35]. Histopathological evaluation was performed on hematoxylin (1.09249.0500; Merck; Kenilworth, NJ, USA) and eosin (256879; Panreac; Barcelona, Spain) stained paraffin-embedded lung tissue sections. Graphics were designed by BioRender.com.

2.5. Quantification of Metastasis and Statistical Analysis

The metastasis affection in the lungs was quantified using ImageJ software. Upon lung extraction, the lungs were photographed, and lesions were quantified automatically using the ImageJ software. Values were compared using a Student's two-tailed t test statistical analysis. The significance was established for (*) $p = 0.001$. The total number of events and the confidence levels obtained in the experiment (n) are all indicated in the figure captions. Results are expressed as mean values with their corresponding standard errors.

2.6. In Vivo SLP Distribution

The Fe_3O_4 nanoparticles in the nanocarrier allowed the determination of the SLP distribution in the different tissues using inductively coupled plasma optical emission spectrometry (ICP-OES) (ICPE-9000 SHIMADZU; Kyoto, Japan). For this purpose, tissues of 4 mice per treatment were collected at 20 days postinjection, fixed in formalin, weighed, and calcined at 450 °C for 12 h to remove all the organic matter. The obtained ashes were dispersed in concentrated chlorhydric acid (HCl 37%) overnight. Finally, samples were diluted to 10 mL with Milli-Q water and analyzed via ICP-OES.

Confocal microscopy imaging was used to visualize particles in lungs 3 and 8 h after intravenous administration. They were embedded in tissue-Tek® O.C.T (optimum cutting temperature) solution (Sakura, Japan), frozen, and cut into 15 µm sections with cryostat. Sections were then fixed in paraformaldehyde (4%) and stained with Hoechst (33258; Sigma; Germany).

3. Results

3.1. Preparation and Characterization of the Control and DOX-Loaded SLPs

The SLPs were synthesized using the melt emulsification method described in the Materials and Methods section (Figure S1). The hydrophobic organic matrix of the SLPs consisted of carnauba wax containing iron oxide nanoparticles. The wax matrix chosen is a natural complex wax obtained from a Brazilian palm tree widely used in food [36], pharmaceutical applications [8], and other technologies [37]. The SLPs were labeled with a fluorescent dye (3,3′-dioctadecyloxacarbocyanine perchlorate (DiO)), which was used for detection and imaging purposes. DiO has been widely used due to its biocompatibility and great stability in living and fixed tissues [38]. This dye allows particle localization using fluorescence technologies in processed cells and tissues [39]. The encapsulation of iron nanoparticles inside the wax matrix allowed us to know the biodistribution of SLPs in in vivo studies. Concentrations of iron were measured in different tissues of mice by the ICP technique. In this study, particles were loaded with 20% (w/w) of DOX to study if a drug delivery system can decrease the toxicity and improve the antineoplastic and antimetastatic effects of traditional chemotherapy (Figure 1a).

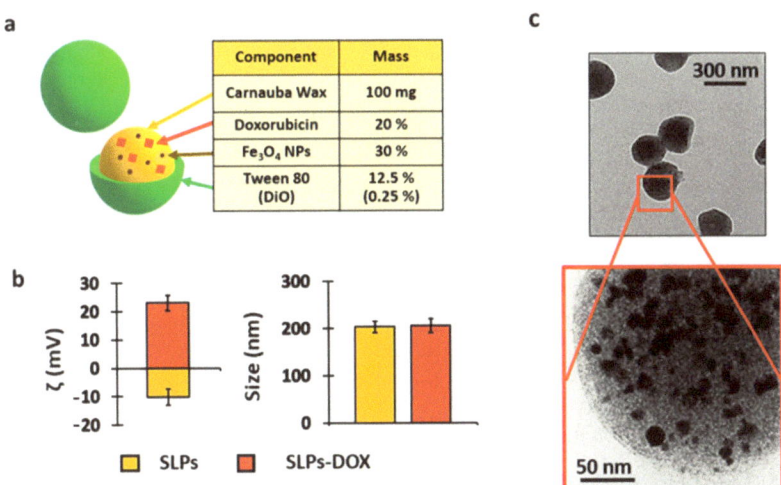

Figure 1. Solid lipid particle (SLP) characterization. (**a**) Composition of the SLPs. (**b**) Hydrodynamic particle size (right) and ζ potential (left) of the control SLPs (yellow) and SLPs loaded with doxorubicin (DOX) (red). (**c**) Representative TEM micrographs of SLPs. The Fe_3O_4 nanoparticles are visible as dark structures inside the composite (inset).

Upon SLPs-DOX synthesis, particle characterization revealed a DOX and Fe_3O_4 nanoparticle encapsulation efficiency of 86.5% ± 1.4 and 99%, respectively. The SLPs presented a hydrodynamic diameter of ca. 200 nm and an estimated ζ potential value of −10 and +23 mV for the control SLPs and SLPs-DOX, respectively. This charge change can be attributed to the positive charge of DOX at physiological pH (Figure 1b). The values of the polydispersity index were 0.36 ± 0.04 for the control SLPs and 0.16 ± 0.1 for the SLPs-DOX (Figure S2). Electron microscopy images show the rounded shape of particles. This technique also allowed the identification of the iron oxide nanoparticles inside the wax matrix (Figure 1c, dark hypointense spots).

3.2. Lung Targeting of SLPs

It is described that SLPs present several advantages in the treatment of pulmonary pathologies, stemming from their adequate size, the potential for deep lung deposition, low toxicity, and prolonged drug release [40].

To study the biodistribution of SLPs after intravenous injection (Figure S3), we administered in lung tissues fluorescent control SLPs particles and analyzed the presence of DiO fluorescence in lung tissue cryosections using fluorescence confocal microscopy. Figure S3a shows confocal Z-projection images of lung slides from SLP-treated mice. The particles are identified as small green spots in the vicinities of the nuclei of the cells. Particles were identified in the lung tissue at both 3 and 8 h after intravenous injection. To confirm this lung distribution after a long period (20 days after injection), we performed an additional biodistribution test quantifying the iron content by ICP-OES. This analysis revealed a broad distribution in the analyzed organs but also lung accumulation of the particles 20 days after injection (Figure S3b). Together, these results confirm that SLPs targeted the lung tissues.

3.3. A Two-Stage Drug Release Effect of SLPs

A few nanocarriers have been proposed capable of transporting and releasing an encapsulated drug upon activation by different stimuli. Two approaches can be adopted in designing stimuli-responsive drug nanosystems. In one approach, endogenous stimuli can be exploited for enhancing drug release. These include pH or enzymatic degradation [41]. This effect requires the selection of appropriate materials for designing the nanocarriers, which should respond to a specific endogenous stimulus releasing all of the encapsulated drug simultaneously (the so-called "burst release"). In the second approach, physical stimuli are applied externally to targeted tissue after administration of drug-loaded specific nanocarriers. These exogenous stimuli include temperature, light, magnetic field, electric field, and ultrasound [42]. The application of these exogenous stimuli is responsible for the alteration of the structure of specifically designed nanocarriers, which leads to drug release at targeted tissues [43,44]. In some nanosystems such as liposomes [45], the drug is released in two steps. The first is upon contact with blood, releasing the drug adsorbed on their surfaces producing a "burst-release effect" that triggers a peak of drug activity at the local or systemic level that is somewhat similar to the effect seen when the free drug is administered. During the second phase, the intraparticle cargo is released.

To investigate the effect of these DOX-loaded SLPs in vitro, we used malignant melanoma cells. Fluorescence confocal microscopy imaging of the cultures revealed that the specific DOX fluorescence progressively accumulated in the cell nucleus during the first 48 h (Figure 2a, red channel), showing an efficient release of drug from the SLPs in the cells.

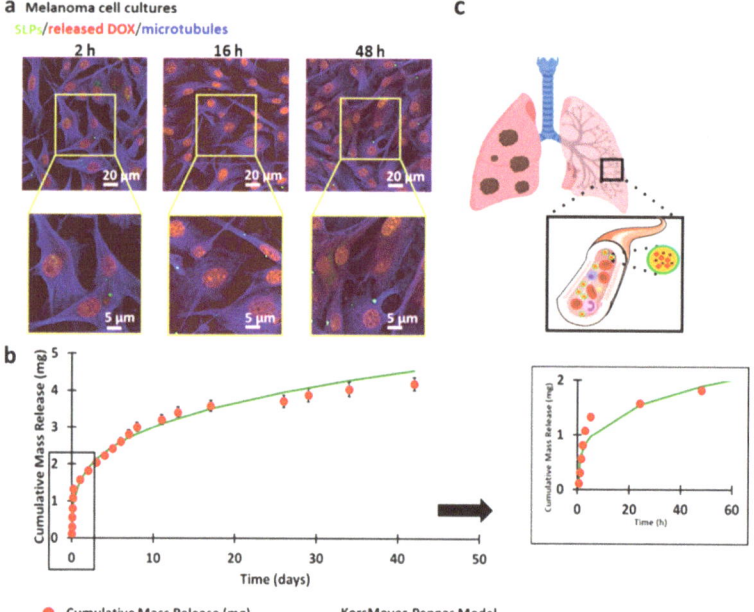

Figure 2. DOX release from DOX-loaded SLPs (SLPs-DOX) in cultured cells and in vitro. (**a**) Fluorescence confocal microscopy projection images of malignant melanoma cells treated with SLPs-DOX for 2, 16, and 48 h. The SLPs appear in the green channel, and microtubules are shown in the blue channel. The red nuclear fluorescence is indicative of the presence of released DOX. (**b**) In vitro drug release profile of the SLPs-DOX particles in physiological conditions (PBS at 37 °C). The results are mean ± SEM of three experimental replicas. (**c**) Scheme of treatment with SLPs-DOX against metastasis in the lungs.

Drug release from SLPs-DOX was also quantified in vitro (Figure S4). To that purpose, 0.3 mL of SLPs-DOX was resuspended in PBS at a concentration of 20 mg DOX/mL and incubated in rotation at 37 °C inside dialysis membranes. Figure 2b shows how DOX-loaded SLPs present an initial burst-release phase, where ca. one-third of the encapsulated drug is released in the media during the first 5 h. After this initial step, a pattern of prolonged and sustained drug release was observed that lasted for more than 40 days. Drug release data were fitted to a Korsmeyer–Peppas model [46]. The release profile of

DOX can be explained by this model, with a release exponent value of 0.28 and R^2 value of 0.96. The mechanism of drug release confirmed that the SLP drug release mechanism was diffusion (Fickian model) with a slope of <0.5. These release results are consistent with other systems based on lipid matrix particles described elsewhere [47–49].

3.4. Inhibition of Metastasis Growth or Antimetastatic Efficacy In Vivo by SLPs-DOX

To investigate the ability of SLPs-DOX to inhibit melanoma metastasis in the lungs, we used a well-established mouse metastatic model using B16-F10 melanoma cells as described in Section 2.4. For the study, metastasis-bearing animals were treated intravenously with 3 doses of 2.5 mg/kg of free DOX, or the equivalent amount of encapsulated drug in SLPs-DOX, at 10, 12, and 14 days after metastasis induction (Figure 3). Animals were sacrificed 20 days after the initial cell transplant. Lungs were collected, photographed, and preserved by fixation in formalin. After 20 days of intravenous injection of the cells, black colonies of metastatic cells were clearly observable on the surface of the lungs of all injected mice (Figure 4, negative control).

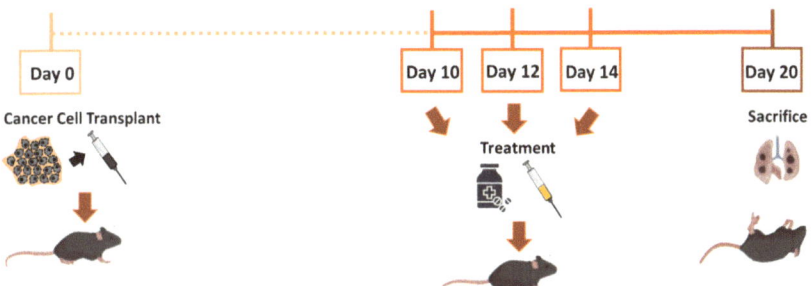

Figure 3. Schematic representation of the metastasis growth inhibition experiment.

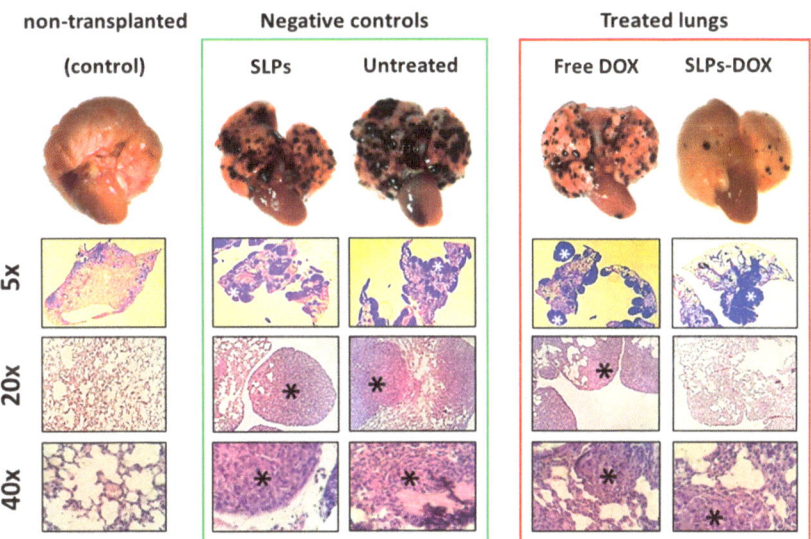

Figure 4. Representative images of metastatic lungs for each experimental group. In the first row, metastatic foci are recognized as black spots on the fresh lung surface. Hematoxylin–eosin-stained histological sections of the lung tissues are shown. Metastatic tissues are indicated by asterisks.

Figure 4 shows a representative example of the lungs after the different treatments. DOX-treated lungs (whether free or SLPs-DOX) present less metastatic spots than negative controls. In fact, SLPs-DOX-treated lungs present the lowest amount of metastasis. Histological analysis corroborates the results from fresh lung images.

ImageJ software was used to quantify the affected area in the lungs to evaluate the effect of treatment on metastasis. The ratio of affected area/total lung area was calculated in 120 animals. Figure 4 shows representative images of the lungs of mice treated with SLPs-DOX, where approximately a 60% reduction of the affected area was observed compared with mice treated with free DOX. These data, together with the differences between the SLPs-DOX-treated mice and the untreated mice, are statistically significant (Figure 5). It is also important to note that no significant differences were found in the survival rates (Figure S5) or body weight (Figure S6) between mice from the different treatment groups, indicating no detectable SLPs-DOX in vivo toxicity during the timeframe of these tests.

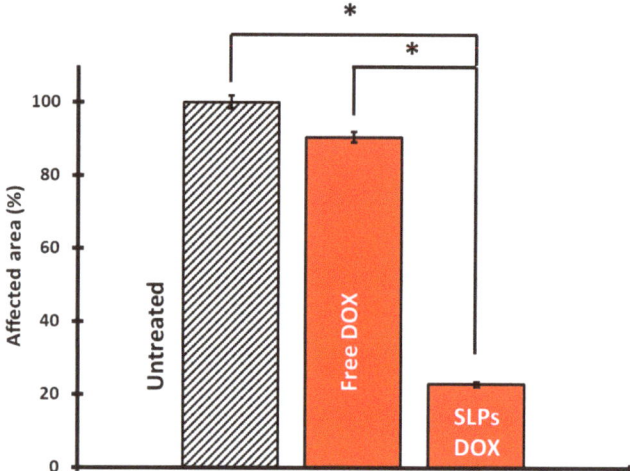

Figure 5. SLPs significantly reduce metastasis in the lungs. Representation of lung metastasis is expressed as the affected area with respect to the total area of the lung. Reduction in metastasis can be observed when the lungs are treated with the SLPs-DOX compared with the lungs treated with the free drug ($t = 5.94$; $n = 170$; * $t_{0.001}$). These differences are also significant between the lungs treated with SLPs-DOX with respect to untreated lungs.

4. Discussion

Considerable therapeutic effort in oncology has been focused on stopping cancer growth. Currently, patients with advanced metastasis have a low probability of recovery because there are no treatments to stop or prevent this process. Conventional drug systems and conventional drug carrier production methods have several limitations, such as frequent dosing, poor bioavailability, or poor patient compliance [50]. These formulations are designed in such a way that the therapeutic concentration of the drug must always be within the therapeutic window while trying to avoid the toxic effects that are produced by an overdose [51].

For this purpose, it is essential to study the drug concentration level in blood. On one hand, a high single dose of the drug could cause toxic side effects. On the other hand, lower administrated doses at different times can maintain the drug concentration in plasma, but without an efficient response from the clinical point of view. Therefore, targeted and maintained frequent drug administration with low doses could be a possible solution. In this scenario, smart delivery systems can make a significant contribution. The benefits of such delivery systems are (i) lower dosing frequency dictated by the matrix that releases the drug at a predetermined rate, (ii) higher bioavailability, (iii) improved drug stability,

(iv) reduced toxic effect of the drug due to chronic and repetitive use, and (v) reduced drug loss due to continuous elimination [52]. In this context, there are numerous types of drug delivery nanocarriers but there are also many issues associated with them: toxicity, low encapsulation efficacy, lack of drug stability, inability to encapsulate more than one drug, or rapid and ineffective release.

The SLPs chosen in this work are stable, inert, and safe, and most importantly, they provide long-term retention of drugs [53], with the ability to encapsulate drugs with limited solubility. The results presented here show that the drug encapsulation efficacy was 86% with a sustained release for more than 40 days at a predetermined rate (Figure 2). This is an important advantage of these systems compared with other nanocarriers such as liposomes that, in general, cannot achieve such high encapsulation efficiency values (recently developed high-pressure processes [54] can achieve drug encapsulation above 90% but are still not common practice). Furthermore, as shown in Figure S2a, these SLPs are retained in the lungs, allowing sustained release of the drug directly in tissues with a high risk of metastasis.

In this study, we encapsulated DOX for different reasons. It is a well-known drug that is commonly used in a variety of cancers; also, its encapsulation contains its undesirable effects such as low specificity to tumor cells, toxic effect in healthy tissues, and an initial burst release followed by a strong decrease in drug concentration when administered on its own [47]. In fact, its clinical use is limited due to its cardiotoxicity and nephrotoxicity [55,56]. We demonstrate that the encapsulation of the drug in SLPs improves the antimetastatic effect of the free drug (Figure 5), improving the biocompatibility in the mice (Figures S5 and S6).

As mentioned above, stable and controlled long-term sustained drug release provides superior therapeutic outcomes than periodically supplied individual higher doses [6,7]. Intravenous administration of conventional drugs usually leads to initial high concentrations followed by a rapid concentration drop below therapeutic limits as a result of drug metabolization or elimination [22]. Thus, our system hypothesizes that the drug release occurs in two well-differentiated steps. The initial one, attributed to the first 5 h of release observed in vitro, occurs while the nanocarrier is circulating in the bloodstream. This allows the elimination of most of the circulating cancer cells. The second, a sustained-release step, takes place upon nanocarrier arrival at the target destination. This surely inhibits tissue colonization by metastatic cells. This drug release pattern would significantly reduce the initial drug dosages and decrease the adverse effects of chemotherapy. Since in the preparation of these solid lipid particles the drug is both integrated within the matrix and adsorbed on the surface of the particles, as concluded by the significant change in the ζ potential from -10 to $+23$ mV, our system is able to provide this unique two-step drug release effect.

It is well known that mouse models are an important tool to understand the complex mechanism involved in the metastatic process and to identify new targets or improve therapeutic approaches [57]. Previous studies have already established the antitumor efficacy of this kind of formulation in melanoma models [26,27]. Here, we have focused on the effect of SLPs-DOX on metastasis inhibition. To evaluate this antimetastatic effect in vivo, a melanoma lung metastasis model was generated according to Figure 4. This model presents the advantage of producing naked-eye-visible black spots on the lung tissue corresponding to metastatic tumor metastatic colonies.

In previous studies, SLPs have been demonstrated to be effective against metastasis using chemotherapeutic drugs such as paclitaxel [58], etoposide [59], and gallic acid ester derivatives [60], among others. Our results indicate that these particles exhibit a higher antimetastatic effect than unformulated DOX without any detectable toxicity. This antimetastatic effect may be due to the stable drug release over time from these SLPs. This rate of drug release is particularly interesting because it maintains the drug level in blood within the therapeutic window, which is crucial for primary tumor inhibition. This drug release rate in combination with local accumulation in the lungs exerts an improved antimetastatic therapeutic output compared with that of the conventional drug; specifically, SLPs-DOX show 60% more antimetastatic effect than free DOX.

Liposomal doxorubicin formulations (Doxil®, Caelyx®, and Myocet®) are an encapsulated form of doxorubicin, with an improved pharmacokinetic profile and the ability to selectively accumulate in tumor tissue [61]. As a result, the tolerated dose of the drug can be increased, followed by a lower incidence of neutropenia and cardiotoxicity compared with treatment with free doxorubicin. However, the common adverse effect that limits the treatment dose regimen is palmoplantar erythrodysesthesia syndrome [62]. This side effect is a distinctive and relatively common toxic reaction associated with some chemotherapeutic agents. Doxorubicin, cytarabine, docetaxel, and fluorouracil are the agents most frequently implicated. This syndrome appears to be dose dependent, and its occurrence is determined by both the maximum drug concentration and the total cumulative dose. Withdrawal or reduction of the dose of the involved drug usually leads to an improvement in symptoms [63].

In summary, we have demonstrated here the ability to encapsulate DOX in SLPs and evaluated the potential of these particles to release the drug in metastatic tumors in mice. We have shown how the lipid fraction of the particles can significantly improve drug loading and thus generate formulations with improved drug loading and superior stability. We showed how these SLPs allow high retention of the drug in the matrix triggering sustained DOX release upon target tissue arrival [62]. We also demonstrated a significant reduction of the potential adverse effects of the encapsulated DOX, as is the case for the FDA-approved liposomal formulations. However, more interestingly, we demonstrated how the sustained release of the drug upon particle arrival to the target tissue results in an improved antimetastatic effect. This sustained in situ release effect allows improved local efficacy and reduced toxicity compared with that reported for liposomal formulations, where the release is faster and with a higher drug concentration, causing possible adverse effects such as palmoplantar erythrodysesthesia syndrome.

Finally, SLPs can also be prepared with encapsulated iron nanoparticles inside, which in future works will serve not only to trigger on-demand drug release but also for use in imaging techniques or hyperthermia therapy, enhancing the effect of DOX in the tumor [42].

5. Conclusions

The goal of this study was to evaluate the metastasis inhibition activity of DOX-loaded SLPs. The results show that these particles synthesized with natural compounds efficiently target lung tissue after only 2 h of intravenous administration. Furthermore, these particles stably release the drug during a long period of over 40 days. This translates into an important reduction in the number of metastases in the lungs compared with unformulated DOX, triggering no detectable toxic effect. The observed antitumor activity in melanoma models [29], together with the metastatic reduction upon treatment with SLPs-DOX, suggest that these particles are an excellent alternative as adjuvant or coadjuvant treatments for numerous systemic cancers.

Supplementary Materials: The following are available online at https://www.mdpi.com/1999-4923/13/1/93/s1, Figure S1. Scheme of the synthesis procedure followed to obtain magnetic DOX-loaded SLPs. Figure S2. Characterization of SLPs. (a) Size distribution of SLP control (left) and SLPs-DOX (right). (b) Transmission electron microscopy image of SLPs. Figure S3. SLPs reach lung tissue. (a) Fluorescent confocal microscopy images in cryostat lungs sections after 3 and 8 h of intravenous administration. The SLPs (green channel) appear close to cell nuclei (stained with Hoechst, blue channel). (b). Inductively coupled plasma spectroscopy (ICP) quantification of Fe in tissues indicative of the biodistribution of the two types of SLPs after 20 days postinjection ($n = 56$). The plot shows the amount of Fe ($\mu g/g$) in the liver (L), heart (H), kidneys (K), intestines (I), spleen (S), lungs (Lu), and brain (B). The results were normalized with respect to control tissues (saline serum). Figure S4. Calibration curve of DOX at 597 nm using fluorimetry. Figure S5. Plot of survival rate of mice after 20 days of the experiment; $n = 167$. The results show that SLPs with DOX did not have toxicity at the time of the experiment with respect to untreated mice. Figure S6. Loss of weight mice after 20 days of the experiment; $n = 13$.

Author Contributions: Conceptualization, J.G. and M.L.F.; methodology, L.V., L.G.-H. and M.L.F.; software, L.V.; validation, L.V. and L.G.-H.; formal analysis, L.V. and L.G.-H.; investigation, L.V., J.G. and L.G.-H.; resources, M.B.-L. and M.L.F.; data curation, L.V. and L.G.-H.; writing/original draft preparation, L.V., L.G.-H. and M.L.F.; writing/review and editing, J.G., M.B.-L. and R.V.; visualization, L.V. and L.G.-H.; supervision, M.L.F.; project administration, M.L.F.; funding acquisition, M.B.-L. and M.L.F. All authors have read and agreed to the published version of the manuscript.

Funding: This research was funded by the European Regional Development Fund (ERDF) and the Spanish MINECO Refs. PI16/00496 (AES 2016), PI19/00349 (AES 2019), and DTS19/00033; IDIVAL Refs. INNVAL17/11 and INNVAL19/12. J.G. and M.B.-L. also acknowledge financial support from the Fundação para a Ciência e a Tecnologia and the ERDF through NORTE2020 (2014–2020 North Portugal Regional Operational Program) through the projects UTAP-EXPL/NTec/0038/2017 (NANOTHER) and NORTE-01-0145-FEDER-031142 (MAGTARGETON). Nano2clinics COST Action CA17140.

Institutional Review Board Statement: The study was carried out in accordance with the guidelines of the Declaration of Helsinki and was approved by the Ethics Committee of the University of Cantabria (protocol code 2013-21 and acceptance date 24 January 2013).

Informed Consent Statement: Not applicable.

Data Availability Statement: Not applicable.

Acknowledgments: We thank Débora Muñoz Guerra and Begoña Ubilla for their technical assistance. We also want to thank Koster Keunen Holland BV (Raambrug 3, 5531 AG Bladel, The Netherlands) for providing us with T1 pharmaceutical grade *Carnauba wax*. Schematic representations were generated in BioRender software.

Conflicts of Interest: The authors declare no conflict of interest.

Abbreviations

SLPs	Solid lipid particles
DOX	Doxorubicin
FDA	Food and drug administration
DiO	3,3′-dioctadecyloxacarbocyanine perchlorate
DLS	Dynamic light scattering
TEM	Transmission electron microscopy
HPLC	High-performance liquid chromatography
IMDM	Iscove's modified Dulbecco's medium
FBS	Fetal bovine serum
PBS	Phosphate-buffered saline
SEEA	Animal establishment and experimentation service
ICP-OES	Inductively coupled plasma optical emission spectrometry
OCT	Optimum cutting temperature

References

1. Gupta, G.P.; Massagué, J. Cancer Metastasis: Building a Framework. *Cell* **2006**, *127*, 679–695. [CrossRef] [PubMed]
2. Wehner, R.; Bitterlich, A.; Meyer, N.; Kloß, A.; Schäkel, K.; Bachmann, M.; Schmitz, M. Impact of chemotherapeutic agents on the immunostimulatory properties of human 6-sulfo LacNAc+ (slan) dendritic cells. *Int. J. Cancer* **2013**, *132*, 1351–1359. [CrossRef]
3. Seyfried, T.N.; Huysentruyt, L.C. On the origin of cancer metastasis. *Crit. Rev. Oncog.* **2013**, *18*, 43–73. [CrossRef] [PubMed]
4. Zou, L.; Wang, H.; He, B.; Zeng, L.; Tan, T.; Cao, H.; He, X.; Zhang, Z.; Guo, S.; Li, Y. Current approaches of photothermal therapy in treating cancer metastasis with nanotherapeutics. *Theranostics* **2016**, *6*, 762–772. [CrossRef] [PubMed]
5. Sandru, A.; Voinea, S.; Panaitescu, E.; Blidaru, A. Survival rates of patients with metastatic malignant melanoma. *J. Med. Life* **2014**, *7*, 572–576. [PubMed]
6. Tas, F. Metastatic behavior in melanoma: Timing, pattern, survival, and influencing factors. *J. Oncol.* **2012**, 647684. [CrossRef] [PubMed]
7. Weber, G.F. Why does cancer therapy lack effective anti-metastasis drugs? *Cancer Lett.* **2013**, *328*, 207–211. [CrossRef]

8. Morrison, V.A. Immunosuppression associated with novel chemotherapy agents and monoclonal antibodies. *Clin. Infect. Dis.* **2014**, *59*, S360–S364. [CrossRef]
9. Fidler, I.J. The pathogenesis of cancer metastasis: The "seed and soil" hypothesis revisited. *Nat. Rev. Cancer* **2003**, *3*, 453–458. [CrossRef]
10. Beg, S.; Rahman, M.; Jain, A.; Saini, S.; Hasnain, M.S.; Swain, S.; Imam, S.; Kazmi, I.; Akhter, S. Emergence in the functionalized carbon nanotubes as smart nanocarriers for drug delivery applications. In *Fullerens, Graphenes and Nanotubes*; William Andrew Publishing: Norwich, UK, 2018; pp. 105–133.
11. Parvathy, R.; Chandran, R.; Thankam, T. Gold Nanoparticles in Cancer Drug Delivery. In *Nanotechnology Applications for Tissue Engineering*; William Andrew Publishing: Norwich, UK, 2015; pp. 221–237.
12. Wells, A.; Grahovac, J.; Wheeler, S.; Ma, B.; Lauffenburger, D. Targeting tumor cell motility as a strategy against invasion and metastasis. *Trends Pharmacol. Sci.* **2013**, *34*, 283–289. [CrossRef]
13. Remião, M.H.; Segatto, N.V.; Pohlmann, A.; Guterres, S.S.; Seixas, F.K.; Collares, T. The potential of nanotechnology in medically assisted reproduction. *Front. Pharmacol.* **2018**, *8*, 994. [CrossRef]
14. Tran, S.; DeGiovanni, P.J.; Piel, B.; Rai, P. Cancer nanomedicine: A review of recent success in drug delivery. *Clin. Transl. Med.* **2017**, *5*, 44. [CrossRef] [PubMed]
15. Wang, R.; Billone, P.S.; Mullett, W.M. Nanomedicine in Action: An Overview of Cancer Nanomedicine on the Market and in Clinical Trials. *J. Nanomater.* **2012**, *2013*, 12. [CrossRef]
16. Barenholz, Y. Doxil—The first fda-approved nano-drug: Lessons learned. *J. Control. Release* **2012**, *160*, 117–134. [CrossRef] [PubMed]
17. Lammers, T.; Hennink, W.E.; Storm, G. Tumour-targeted nanomedicines: Principles and practice. *British J. Cancer* **2008**, *99*, 392–397. [CrossRef]
18. Chang, H.I.; Yeh, M.K. Clinical development of liposome-based drugs: Formulation, characterization and therapeutic efficacy. *Int. J. Nanomed.* **2012**, *7*, 49–60.
19. Iturrioz-Rodríguez, N.; Correa-Duarte, M.A.; Fanarraga, M.L. Controlled drug delivery systems for cancer based on mesoporous silica particles. *Int. J. Nanomed.* **2019**, *14*, 3389–3401. [CrossRef]
20. Zhou, J.; Zhang, W.; Hong, C.; Pan, C. Silica Nanotubes Decorated by pH-Responsive Diblock Copolymers for Controlled Drug Release. *ACS Appl. Mater. Interfaces* **2015**, *7*, 3618–3625. [CrossRef] [PubMed]
21. Vallet-Regí, M.; Colilla, M.; Izquierdo-Barba, I.; Manzano, M. Mesoporous Silica Nanoparticles for Drug Delivery: Current Insights. *Molecules* **2018**, *23*, 47. [CrossRef] [PubMed]
22. Lee, J.H.; Yeo, Y. Controlled drug release from pharmaceutical nanocarriers. *Chem. Eng. Sci.* **2015**, *125*, 75–84. [CrossRef]
23. Hasan, A.S.; Socha, M.; Lamprecht, A.; El Ghazouani, F.; Sapin, A.; Hoffman, M.; Maincent, P.; Ubrich, N. Effect of the microencapsulation of nanoparticles on the reduction of burst release. *Int. J. Pharm.* **2007**, *344*, 53–61. [CrossRef] [PubMed]
24. Yadav, N.; Khatak, S.; Singh Sara, U.V. Solid lipid nanoparticles—A review. *Int. J. Appl. Pharm.* **2013**, *3*, 5–12.
25. Kheradmandnia, S.; Vasheghani-Farahani, E.; Nosrati, M.; Atyabi, F. Preparation and characterization of ketoprofen-loaded solid lipid nanoparticles made from beeswax and carnauba wax. *Nanomedicine* **2010**, *6*, 753–759. [CrossRef] [PubMed]
26. Blum, R.H.; Carter, S.K. Adriamycin. A new anticancer drug with significant clinical activity. *Ann. Intern. Med.* **1974**, *80*, 249–259. [CrossRef] [PubMed]
27. Weiss, R.B. The anthracyclines: Will we ever find a better doxorubicin? *Semin. Oncol.* **1992**, *19*, 670–686.
28. Carvalho, C.; Santos, R.; Cardoso, S.; Correia, S.; Oliveira, P.; Santos, M.; Moreira, P. Doxorubicin: The Good, the Bad and the Ugly Effect. *Curr. Med. Chem.* **2009**, *16*, 3267–3285. [CrossRef]
29. Jiménez-López, J.; García-Hevia, L.; Melguizo, C.; Prados, J.; Bañobre-López, M.G.J. Extensive in vitro validation of novel magnetic wax nanocomposite vehicles as cancer combinatorial therapy agents. Evaluation of novel doxorubicin-loaded magnetic wax nanocomposite vehicles as cancer combinatorial therapy agents. *Pharmaceutics* **2020**, *12*, 637.
30. Jadhav, N.V.; Prasad, A.I.; Kumar, A.; Mishra, R.; Dhara, S.; Babu, K.R.; Prajapat, C.L.; Misra, N.L.; Ningthoujam, R.S.; Pandey, B.N.; et al. Synthesis of oleic acid functionalized Fe3O4 magnetic nanoparticles and studying their interaction with tumor cells for potential hyperthermia applications. *Colloids Surf. B Biointerfaces* **2013**, *108*, 158–168. [CrossRef] [PubMed]
31. Fidler, I.J. Selection of successive tumour lines for metastasis. *Nat. New Biol.* **1973**, *242*, 148–149. [CrossRef] [PubMed]
32. Poste, G.; Doll, J.; Hart, I.R.; Fidler, I.J. In vitro selection of murine B16 melanoma variants with enhanced tissue-invasive properties. *Cancer Res.* **1980**, *40*, 1636–1644. [PubMed]
33. Overwijk, W.W.; Restifo, N.P. B16 as a Mouse Model for Human Melanoma. *Curr. Protoc. Immunol.* **2000**, *39*, 20–21. [CrossRef]
34. Gautam, A.; Waldrep, J.; Densmore, C.; Koshkina, N.; Melton, S.; Roberts, L.; Gilbert, B.; Knight, V. Growth inhibition of established B16-F10 lung metastases by sequential aerosol delivery of p53 gene and 9-nitrocamptothecin. *Gene Ther.* **2002**, *9*, 353–357. [CrossRef] [PubMed]
35. Bibby, M.C. Orthotopic models of cancer for preclinical drug evaluation: Advantages and disadvantages. *Eur. J. Cancer* **2004**, *40*, 852–857. [CrossRef]
36. Mo, R.; Jiang, T.; Gu, Z. Enhanced Anticancer Efficacy by ATP-Mediated Liposomal Drug Delivery. *Angew. Int. Ed. Engl.* **2014**, *5*, 5815–5820. [CrossRef] [PubMed]

37. Dicheva, B.M.; ten Hagen, T.L.M.; Seynhaeve, A.L.B.; Amin, M.; Eggermont, A.M.M.; Koning, G.A. Enhanced Specificity and Drug Delivery in Tumors by cRGD—Anchoring Thermosensitive Liposomes. *Pharm. Res.* **2015**, *32*, 3862–3876. [CrossRef] [PubMed]
38. Honig, M.G.; Hume, R.I. Dil and DiO: Versatile fluorescent dyes for neuronal labelling and pathway tracing. *Trends Neurosci.* **1989**, *12*, 333–335. [CrossRef]
39. Von Bartheld, C.S.; Cunningham, D.E.; Rubel, E.W. Neuronal tracing with DiI: Decalcification, cryosectioning, and photoconversion for light and electron microscopic analysis. *J. Histochem. Cytochem.* **1990**, *38*, 725–733. [CrossRef] [PubMed]
40. Weber, S.; Zimmer, A.; Pardeike, J. Solid Lipid Nanoparticles (SLN) and Nanostructured Lipid Carriers (NLC) for pulmonary application: A review of the state of the art. *Eur. J. Pharm. Biopharm.* **2014**, *86*, 7–22. [CrossRef]
41. Swainson, S.M.E.; Taresco, V.; Pearce, A.K.; Clapp, L.H.; Ager, B.; McAllister, M.; Bosquillon, C.; Garnett, M.C. Exploring the enzymatic degradation of poly(glycerol adipate). *Eur. J. Pharm. Biopharm.* **2019**, *142*, 377–386. [CrossRef] [PubMed]
42. Iglesias, G.R.; Reyes-Ortega, F.; Checa Fernández, B.L.; Delgado, A.V. Hyperthermia-triggered gemcitabine release from polymer-coated magnetite nanoparticles. *Polymers* **2018**, *10*, 269. [CrossRef] [PubMed]
43. Hu, X.; Tian, J.; Liu, T.; Zhang, G.; Liu, S. Photo-triggered release of caged camptothecin prodrugs from dually responsive shell cross-linked micelles. *Macromolecules* **2013**, *46*, 6243–6256. [CrossRef]
44. Kundu, J.K.; Surh, Y.J. Nrf2-Keap1 signaling as a potential target for chemoprevention of inflammation-associated carcinogenesis. *Pharm. Res.* **2010**, *27*, 999–1013. [CrossRef] [PubMed]
45. Kaddha, S.; Khreich, N.; Kaddah, F.; Charcosset, C.; Greige-Gerges, H. Chloresterol modulates the liposome membrane fluidity and permeability for a hydrophilic molecule. *Food Chem. Toxicol.* **2018**, *113*, 40–48. [CrossRef] [PubMed]
46. Korsmeyer, R.W.; Gurny, R.; Doelker, E.; Buri, P.; Peppas, N.A. Mechanisms of solute release from porous hydrophilic polymers. *Int. J. Pharm.* **1983**, *15*, 25–35. [CrossRef]
47. Kashanian, S.; Azandaryani, A.H.; Derakhshandeh, K. New surface-modified solid lipid nanoparticles using N-glutaryl phosphatidylethanolamine as the outer shell. *Int. J. Nanomed.* **2011**, *6*, 2393–2401.
48. De Almeida, R.R.; Gallo, J.; Da Silva, A.C.C.; Da Silva, A.K.O.; Pessoa, O.D.L.; Araújo, T.G.; Leal, L.K.A.M.; Fechine, P.B.A.; Bañobre-López, M.; Ricardo, N.M.P.S. Preliminary Evaluation of Novel Triglyceride-Based Nanocomposites for Biomedical Applications. *J. Braz. Chem. Soc.* **2017**, *28*, 1–10. [CrossRef]
49. Wen, H.; Jung, H.; Li, X. Drug Delivery Approaches in Addressing Clinical Pharmacology-Related Issues: Opportunities and Challenges. *AAPS J.* **2015**, *17*, 1327–1340. [CrossRef] [PubMed]
50. Weisser, J.R.; Saltzman, W.M. Controlled release for local delivery of drugs: Barriers and models. *J. Control. Release* **2014**, *190*, 664–673. [CrossRef]
51. Mitragotri, S.; Burke, P.A.; Larger, R. Overcoming the challenges in administering biopharmaceuticals: Formulation and delivery strategies. *Nat. Rev. Drug Discov.* **2014**, *13*, 655–672. [CrossRef] [PubMed]
52. Mellema, M.; Van Benthum, W.A.J.; Boer, B.; Von Harras, J.; Visser, A. Wax encapsulation of water-soluble compounds for application in foods. *J. Microencapsul.* **2006**, *23*, 729–740. [CrossRef] [PubMed]
53. De M. Barbosa, R.; Ribeiro, L.N.M.; Casadei, B.R.; Da Silva, C.M.G.; Queiróz, V.A.; Duran, N.; de Araújo, D.R.; Severino, P.; De Paula, E. Solid Lipid Nanoparticles for Dibucaine Sustained Release. *Pharmaceutics* **2018**, *10*, 231.
54. Trucillo, P.; Campardelli, R.; Reverchon, E. Liposomes: From bangham to supercritical fluids. *Processes* **2020**, *8*, 1022. [CrossRef]
55. Bae, Y.; Diezi, T.A.; Zhao, A.; Kwon, G.S. Mixed polymeric micelles for combination cancer chemotherapy through the concurrent delivery of multiple chemotherapeutic agents. *J. Control. Release* **2007**, *122*, 324–330. [CrossRef] [PubMed]
56. Kakinoki, A.; Kaneo, Y.; Ikeda, Y.; Tanaka, T.; Fujita, K. Synthesis of poly(vinyl alcohol)-doxorubicin conjugates containing cis-aconityl acid-cleavable bond and its isomer dependent doxorubicin release. *Biol. Pharm. Bull.* **2008**, *31*, 103–110. [CrossRef] [PubMed]
57. Gomez-Cuadrado, L.; Tracey, N.; Ma, R.; Qian, B.; Brunton, V.G. Mouse models of metastasis: Progress and prospects. *DMM Dis. Model. Mech.* **2017**, *10*, 1061–1074. [CrossRef]
58. Ma, P.; Benhabbour, S.R.; Feng, L.; Mumper, R.J. 2′-Behenoyl-paclitaxel conjugate containing lipid nanoparticles for the treatment of metastatic breast cancer. *Cancer Lett.* **2013**, *334*, 253–262. [CrossRef] [PubMed]
59. Athawale, R.B.; Jain, D.S.; Singh, K.K.; Gude, R.P. Etoposide loaded solid lipid nanoparticles for curtailing B16F10 melanoma colonization in lung. *Biomed. Pharmacother.* **2014**, *68*, 231–240. [CrossRef] [PubMed]
60. Cordova, C.A.S.; Locatelli, C.; Winter, E.; Silva, A.H.; Zanetti-Ramos, B.G.; Jasper, R.; Mascarello, A.; Yunes, R.A.; Nunes, R.J.; Creczynski-Pasa, T.B. Solid lipid nanoparticles improve octyl gallate antimetastatic activity and ameliorate its renal and hepatic toxic effects. *Anticancer Drugs* **2017**, *27*, 977–988. [CrossRef] [PubMed]
61. Waterhouse, D.N.; Tardi, P.G.; Mayer, L.D.; Bally, M.B. A comparison of liposomal formulations of doxorubicin with drug administered in free form: Changing toxicity profiles. *Drug Saf.* **2001**, *24*, 903–920. [CrossRef]
62. Stella, B.; Peira, E.; Dianzani, C.; Gallarate, M.; Battaglia, L.; Gigliotti, C.L.; Boggio, E.; Dianzani, U.; Dosio, F. Development and Characterization of Solid Lipid Nanoparticles Loaded with a Highly Active Doxorubicin Derivative. *Nanomaterials* **2018**, *8*, 110. [CrossRef]
63. Lorusso, D.; Di Stefano, A.; Carone, V.; Fagotti, F.; Pisconti, F.; Scambia, G. Pegylated liposomal doxorubicin-related palmar-plantar erythrodysesthesia ('hand-foot' syndrome). *Ann. Oncol.* **2007**, *18*, 1159–1164. [CrossRef] [PubMed]

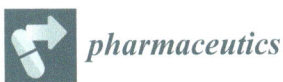

Article

Oral Gel Loaded by Fluconazole–Sesame Oil Nanotransfersomes: Development, Optimization, and Assessment of Antifungal Activity

Hala M. Alkhalidi, Khaled M. Hosny and Waleed Y. Rizg

1 Department of Clinical Pharmacy, Faculty of Pharmacy, King Abdulaziz University, Jeddah 21589, Saudi Arabia; halkhaldi@kau.edu.sa
2 Department of Pharmaceutics, Faculty of Pharmacy, King Abdulaziz University, Jeddah 21589, Saudi Arabia; wrizq@kau.edu.sa
3 Center of Excellence for Drug Research and Pharmaceutical Industries, King Abdulaziz University, Jeddah 21589, Saudi Arabia
* Correspondence: kmhomar@kau.edu.sa; Tel.: +966-592722634

Abstract: Candidiasis is one of the frequently encountered opportunistic infections in the oral cavity and can be found in acute and chronic presentations. The study aimed to develop fluconazole-loaded sesame oil containing nanotransfersomes (FS-NTF) by the thin-layer evaporation technique to improve the local treatment of oral candidiasis. Optimization of the formulation was performed using the Box-Behnken statistical design to determine the variable parameters that influence the vesicle size, entrapment efficiency, zone of inhibition, and ulcer index. Finally, the formulated FS-NTF was embedded within the hyaluronic acid-based hydrogel (HA-FS-NTF). The rheological behavior of the optimized HA-FS-NTF was assessed and the thixotropic behavior with the pseudoplastic flow was recorded; this is desirable for an oral application. An in vitro release study revealed the rapid release of fluconazole from the HA-FS-NTF. This was significantly higher when compared with the fluconazole suspension and hyaluronic acid hydrogel containing fluconazole. Correspondingly, the ex vivo permeation was also found to be higher in HA-FS-NTF in sheep buccal mucosa (400 μg/cm^2) when compared with the fluconazole suspension (122 μg/cm^2) and hyaluronic acid hydrogel (294 μg/cm^2). The optimized formulation had an inhibition zone of 14.33 ± 0.76 mm and enhanced antifungal efficacy for the ulcer index (0.67 ± 0.29) in immunocompromised animals with *Candida* infection; these findings were superior to those of other tested formulations. Hence, it can be summarized that fluconazole can effectively be delivered for the treatment of oral candidiasis when it is entrapped in a nanotransfersome carrier and embedded into cross-linked hyaluronic acid hydrogel.

Keywords: fluconazole; Box-Behnken design; nanotransfersome; ulcer index; zone of inhibition; rheological behavior; ex vivo permeation

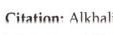

Citation: Alkhalidi, H.M.; Hosny, K.M.; Rizg, W.Y. Oral Gel Loaded by Fluconazole-Sesame Oil Nanotransfersomes: Development, Optimization, and Assessment of Antifungal Activity. *Pharmaceutics* 2020, 13, 27. https://doi.org/10.3390/pharmaceutics13010027

Received: 2 December 2020
Accepted: 22 December 2020
Published: 25 December 2020

Publisher's Note: MDPI stays neutral with regard to jurisdictional claims in published maps and institutional affiliations.

Copyright: © 2020 by the authors. Licensee MDPI, Basel, Switzerland. This article is an open access article distributed under the terms and conditions of the Creative Commons Attribution (CC BY) license (https://creativecommons.org/licenses/by/4.0/).

1. Introduction

Oral candidiasis is a frequently encountered infection of the oral mucosa. It can be caused by the overgrowth of 150 species of *Candida*; however, 95% cases are caused by *Candida* albicans [1,2]. This is sometimes mild in nature, but may be resistant to therapies and is frequently vulnerable to relapse.

The drug of choice for the treatment of oral candidiasis is fluconazole, a fluorinated bis-triazole derivative. This agent has been found to be effective against several species of *Candida* in both immunocompromised and immunocompetent patients [3]. The mechanism of inhibiting *Candida* spp. infection involves the inhibitory effect of 14-α-demethylase, which is required for ergosterol biosynthesis and thereby interrupts the cell wall synthesis of the fungi. The common route of administration of conventional fluconazole is oral; however, this route is known to produce gastrointestinal disturbances, such as abdominal discomfort, bloating, vomiting, and severe hepatotoxicity [4]. Localized delivery of the medication for the treatment of oral candidiasis could reduce the development of drug resistance and also reduce the associated side effects [3]. Conventional local forms of delivery of fluconazole (e.g., sprays, lotions, gels, and creams) are associated with major limitations in dosing accuracy and length of time at the site of application, as well as variations in performance. Lozenges, troches, rinses, and mouth paints are the alternate treatment options for oral candidiasis; however, maintenance of the salivary concentration of the medication is difficult because salivary secretions can wash away these substances and shorten the contact time of the formulation, leading to poor efficacy and poor patient compliance [4,5]. Therefore, novel formulations with properties that are retained at the site of application and release the entrapped drug for a desired period would be a possible alternative to conventional deliveries. Researchers have used various approaches to deliver fluconazole effectively and with improved efficacy. They used mucoadhesive platforms, such as fluconazole-loaded oral strips [3], mucoadhesive nanoparticles [4], hydrogels [6], and natural rubber latex biomembranes [7], among others.

In view of the advantages of longer retainment at the site of application for the mucoadhesive components and the superior release characteristics of the nanotechnology-based products, the present study aimed to formulate fluconazole-loaded sesame oil containing nanotransfersomes (FS-NTF) embedded in a cross-linked hyaluronic acid hydrogel. A new field of research on topical delivery was opened with the use of liposomes for dermal delivery, and since then, a wide range of novel lipid-based vesicles, such as deformable liposomes in nanosizes, which are currently known as nanotransfersomes, have been developed. The addition of nonionic surfactants to the liposomal bilayer structure of liposomes provides the flexibility necessary for liposomes, and this new structure is called the nanotransfersome [8]. In the proliferation phase, in which granulation tissue is formed, hyaluronic acid is synthesized mainly by fibroblasts, and this allows, within the framework of a temporary extracellular matrix, the diffusion of nutrients and the elimination of waste products. Hyaluronic acid facilitates the migration and proliferation of fibroblasts and keratinocytes and is a reservoir of growth factors. This is due to the ability of hyaluronic acid to absorb water, maintain wound moisture, and limit cellular adhesion to extracellular matrix molecules [9]. Hyaluronic acid has also been shown to possess antifungal efficacy, especially fungistatic efficacy [10]. Therefore, it was expected that superior efficacy would be achieved by the FS-NTF embedded in hyaluronic acid (HA-FS-NTF). It was expected that the formulation would remain at the site of application because of the swelling properties of hyaluronic acid [11]. Additionally, incorporation of sesame oil in the formulation would be advantageous for its established antifungal efficacy [12]. To reach this goal, the optimization of the FS-NTF was performed by the Box-Behnken statistical design to determine the various parameters that influence the vesicle size, entrapment efficiency, zone of inhibition, and ulcer index. Finally, the HA-FS-NTF was formulated and evaluated for its rheological behavior, in vitro release pattern, ex vivo permeability, inhibitory zone of *Candida* growth, and ulcer index in an immunocompromised animal model.

2. Materials and Methods

2.1. Materials

Fluconazole was purchased from Sigma-Aldrich Co. (St Louis, MO, USA). Tween 20® was acquired as a generous gift from Saudi Drugs and Medical Instruments Company (SPIMACO), in Qassim, Saudi Arabia. Sesame oil and Lecithin were procured from Avanti Polar Liquids (Alabaster, AL, USA). High-performance liquid chromatography (HPLC)-grade solvents were collected form Merck (Darmstadt, Germany). All other reagents and chemicals used were of analytical grade.

2.2. Methods

2.2.1. Optimization of Fluconazole-Sesame Oil Nanotransfersomes Using the Box–Behnken Statistical Design

A response surface Box–Behnken statistical design was adopted for our current investigation using Design-Expert® software version 12.0.6.0 (2019, Stat-Ease, Inc., Minneapolis, MN, USA). Three factors at three levels were incorporated to optimize the fluconazole nanotransfersome formulations. Based on data in the literature, higher and lower levels of the independent variables, such as the lecithin concentration and amounts of fluconazole and sesame oil, were selected for the identification of the optimized FS-NTF formulation [10,13]. The software generated 19 batches with various combinations of the three independent variables at their low (−1), medium (0), and high (+1) levels. The batches were developed and analyzed for the four dependent variables, which were the globule size of the prepared FS-NTF (Y1), entrapment efficiency (EE%) of fluconazole within the prepared FS-NTF (Y2), zone of inhibition against *C. albicans* (Y3), and ulcer index score (Y4) (Table 1). Experimental data for the four dependent variables were included in the software. The interactions of the independent variables at their different levels with the dependent variables were analyzed to gain insight into the composition of the optimized formulation. The significance of the data was statistically analyzed using the analysis of variance (ANOVA). The effect of the three independent variables at their different levels was assessed by the generated perturbation plot, contour plots, and three-dimensional surface plot [14,15]. The best fitting model was used based on data on the adequate precision ratio and the predicted and adjusted determination coefficients for the dependent variables.

The software generated a polynomial equation consisting of three factors, and the responses are depicted in the following Equation (1):

$$Y = b_0 + b_1A + b_2B + b_3C + b_{12}AB + b_{13}AC + b_{23}BC + b_{11}A^2 + b_{22}B^2 + b_{33}C^2 \quad (1)$$

where Y was the measured response associated with each factor level combination, b_0 was the intercept, b_1 to b_3 were the regression coefficients [16], and A, B, and C were the coded levels of the independent variables.

Table 1. Experimental runs in Box–Behnken statistical design: The independent variables and experimental dependent variables.

Run	Values of Independent Variables			Dependent Variable (Y)							
	A: Lecithin	B: Fluconazole	C: Sesame Oil	Globule Size (nm) (Actual)	Globule Size (nm) (Predicted)	EE (%) (Actual)	EE (%) (Predicted)	Inhibition Zone (mm) (Actual)	Inhibition Zone (mm) (Predicted)	Ulcer Index Score (Point) (Actual)	Ulcer Index Score (Point) (Predicted)
1	75	50	25	146.00	144.45	68.00	68.54	10.50	10.36	4.00	4.03
2	150	25	25	186.00	187.24	60.00	59.93	3.50	3.53	5.00	4.68
3	150	50	50	218.00	219.67	75.00	75.19	11.00	10.83	2.50	2.55
4	150	75	25	266.00	263.03	54.00	54.01	15.00	15.01	3.00	3.34
5	75	25	50	110.00	112.84	57.00	56.96	4.50	4.31	3.00	3.24
6	225	50	25	240.00	244.65	77.00	76.72	10.00	9.82	4.00	4.00
7	225	25	50	200.00	193.54	64.00	64.64	3.50	3.53	3.00	3.21
8	225	50	75	232.00	235.11	79.00	78.70	12.00	12.16	1.00	1.07
9	225	75	50	293.00	291.53	58.00	58.17	15.50	15.69	2.00	1.87
10	150	25	75	173.00	175.00	63.00	62.96	5.50	5.44	2.00	1.76
11	150	75	75	252.00	250.99	56.00	56.49	18.50	18.35	0.50	0.4190
12	75	50	75	134.00	129.72	72.00	72.08	13.00	13.26	1.00	1.11
13	150	50	50	221.00	219.67	76.00	75.19	10.50	10.83	2.50	2.55
14	75	50	50	160.00	166.64	52.00	51.05	16.50	16.55	2.00	1.90
15	75	25	25	120.00	118.63	55.00	54.79	3.50	3.78	5.00	4.70
16	75	50	50	141.00	138.72	70.00	70.58	11.50	11.24	2.50	2.57
17	150	25	50	181.00	182.75	62.00	61.71	4.00	3.91	3.00	3.22
18	150	75	50	260.00	258.64	55.00	55.52	16.00	16.11	2.00	1.88
19	225	75	75	285.00	285.18	59.00	58.76	18	17.79	0.5	0.4024

Dependent variables: Y1 = globule size of the prepared fluconazole-loaded sesame oil containing nanotransfersomes (FS-NTF); Y2 = Entrapment Efficiency Percentage (EE%) of fluconazole within the prepared FS-NTF; Y3 = zone of inhibition against *Candida albicans*; Y4 = ulcer index score.

2.2.2. Preparation of Fluconazole-Sesame Oil Nanotransfersomes (FS-NTF)

Development of the drug-loaded NTF was approached by the thin-layer evaporation technique using the optimized ratios of the components suggested by the statistical design [17]. In brief, accurately measured quantities of Tween 20®, as an edge activator, were incorporated with the phospholipid to form the vesicular structure of the nanotransfersome. The Tween® and phospholipid were placed in a round-bottom flask, along with the sesame oil and fluconazole, using the solvent mixture of chloroform:methanol at a ratio of 1:1 (v/v). The organic solvents in the round-bottom flask were evaporated at reduced pressure using the rotary vacuum evaporator (BUCHI Rotavapor R-205, Marshall Scientific, Hampton, NH, USA) at 45 °C, and the rotation of the flask was maintained at 80 rpm. Later, following the removal of traces of organic solvents in the mixture, a thin film of the components was formed within the inner wall of the round-bottom flask. Lastly, phosphate buffered saline (pH 7.4) was used to hydrate the thin layer in order to form the lipid vesicles at room temperature. The multilamellar vesicles were formed upon hydration, and they were further sonicated using a probe sonicator (Branson, Danbury, CT, USA) for 15 min to form our desired drug-loaded unilamellar vesicles (FS-NTF). Finally, the formulation was collected after it had passed through polycarbonate membranes of the desired size and stored at 4 °C for further characterization and experiments. Figure 1

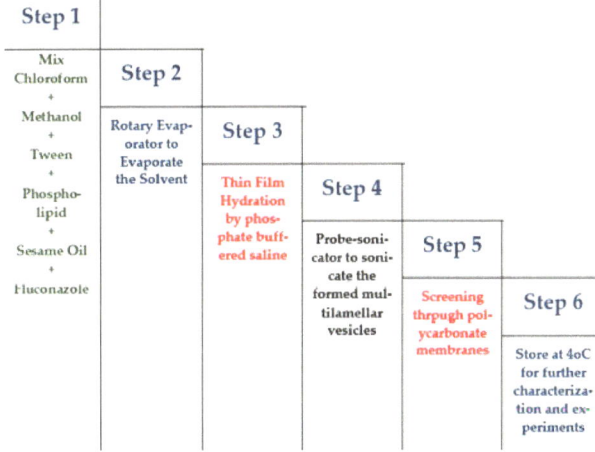

Figure 1. Schematic representation of steps of preparation of fluconazole-sesame oil nanotransfersomes (FS-NTF).

2.2.3. Characterization of the Fluconazole-Loaded Nanotransfersomes

Globule Size Measurements

The vesicle size of the developed FS-NTF was measured by appropriately diluting the mixture with purified water (10 times), and the mixture was agitated vigorously before measurement. The size of the formulated vesicles was finally determined by the dynamic light-scattering technique, in which 100 µL of the diluted sample was placed in the Microtrac® particle size analyzer (Microtrac, Inc., Montgomeryville, PA, USA) at 25 ± 1 °C. The average readings were recorded to correlate with our findings.

Entrapment Efficiency Percentage (EE%)

The EE% of the developed and optimized FS-NTF was determined using the indirect method [18], where the EE% was stated as the percentage of the total amount of drugs incorporated within the final formulation. To perform this experiment, the FS-NTF was freeze dried (Martin Christ Gefriertrocknungsanlagen GmbH, Osterode am Harz, Germany) first to remove the traces of the aqueous phase in the formulation. Later, it was dispersed with methanol and mixed cautiously. The mixture was centrifuged (Centurion, West Sussex, UK), and the supernatant was collected. The residue was washed again with the same solvent to recover the traces of the free fluconazole present in the developed formulation. The supernatant containing the drug was measured to determine the concentration of free fluconazole in the formulation using a UV-visible spectrophotometer (6705 UV/Vis spectrophotometer; JENWAY, Cole-Parmer, Stone, Staffordshire, UK) at 261.6 nm. The correlation coefficient was 0.9997, and the molar absorptivity equaled 0.735×10^3 L/mol/cm [19].

Finally, the EE% of the formulation was determined using Equation (2).

$$EE\% = \frac{C_{total} - C_{free}}{C_{total}} \times 100 \qquad (2)$$

where C_{total} and C_{free} are the total quantity of drug added in each formulation according to the experimental design mentioned in Table 1 (25, 50, or 75 mg) and the free drug available outside the formed nanotransfersome vesicles, respectively.

Development of Hyaluronic Acid Hydrogel of FS-NTF (HA-FS-NTF)

The formulated FS-NTF was embedded into the hyaluronic acid hydrogel by sprinkling it on the pH-induced hyaluronic acid hydrogel. This polymeric hydrogel was prepared with 2% hyaluronic acid using 0.5% Gantrez® S-97 (Mw = 1.2×10^6 Da) as a cross-linker in a phosphate buffer saline (PBS) media (pH 4.5) maintained at 37 ± 1 °C according to preliminary tests which were performed to determine the optimum levels for hyaluronic acid and cross linker. The polymeric mixture was left overnight to hydrate with continuous stirring at 110 rpm. Finally, the HA-FS-NTF was developed by mixing 10 mL of the formulated FS-NTF containing 600 mg of the drug into the prepared hydrogel (100 mL) to obtain the final 0.5% drug containing the transfersomal hydrogel preparation. The FS-NTF was dispersed in water, and this aqueous dispersion was sprinkled over the plain hydrogel base. Because hyaluronic acid has a higher affinity to absorb water molecules and swell, the state of the water in swollen hydrogels is an important factor that influences the absorption and diffusion of solutes through the hydrogel. Generally, water consists of bound water and free water in water-swollen systems. When a hydrogel network begins to swell, the hydrophilic and hydrophobic groups of polymer chains interact with the water molecules, leading to "bound water." Then the network will absorb additional water, due to the osmotic pressure, leading to "free water" that fills the space between the network chains. This HA-FS-NTF was refrigerated at 4 °C to 8 °C and tested for content uniformity by dividing a certain amount of the formed gel into pieces of equal weight and analyzing these pieces for fluconazole content. After ensuring the content uniformity, further evaluation was done.

2.2.4. Rheological Evaluation of the HA-FS-NTF Hydrogel

The rheological property, viscosity, of the HA-FS-NTF and the plain hyaluronic acid gel was measured using a Brookfield Viscometer fitted with a spindle 52. A quantity equivalent to 1 g of the swollen tested hydrogel sample was used to determine the desired parameters, and the run of the spindle was performed at 25 ± 5 °C [20]. The findings were recorded over a range of shear rates (2, 10, 20, 30, 40, 50, and 60 s^{-1}) to identify the flow pattern of the formulated gels. Thus, the shear rate (s^{-1}), shear stress (dyne/cm^2), and viscosity (cP) were recorded and plotted. The viscosity and degree of pseudoplasticity (Farrow's constant) were determined at a minimum rate of shear (ηmin) and a maximum rate of shear (ηmax) by Farrow's equation (Equation (3)) [21].

$$\text{Log} G = N \text{ Log} F - \text{Log } \eta \qquad (3)$$

where the shear rate, viscosity, and shear stress are expressed as G, η, and F, respectively, and Farrow's constant is expressed as N.

2.2.5. In Vitro Release of the FS-NTF-Loaded Hydrogel

In vitro release of the entrapped drug from the developed HA-FS-NTF containing the 0.5% marketed formulation of fluconazole and the suspension containing 0.5% fluconazole was studied using a Type I USP dissolution apparatus (basket type) (DT 700 LH device, ERWEKA GmbH DT 700, Heusenstamm, Germany). The samples were loaded into the respective cylindrical tubes (10 cm in length and 2.7 cm in diameter) and were attached to the apparatus instead of the basket, with the lower end of the tube closed tightly by a semipermeable membrane with a pore size of 100 µm. Before use, the dialysis membrane was activated by placing the dialysis membrane in boiling water containing 1 M $NaHCO_3$ for 1 h. Thereafter, it was washed thoroughly using tap water and stored in phosphate buffer (pH 7.4) for 1 h. The dialysis membranes were kept in the refrigerator in the phosphate buffer (pH 7.4) media overnight prior to performing the release study.

One gram of each sample was loaded in the cylindrical glass tube assembly as described above. The release study was performed in 250 mL phosphate buffered saline (pH 6.8), which was maintained at a physiological temperature (37 ± 0.5 °C) with the rotation of the stirring shaft fixed at 50 rpm. The release study was performed for 3 h, during which time 5-mL aliquots were withdrawn at intervals of 0.0, 0.25, 0.5, 1.0, 1.5, 2.0, 2.5, and 3.0 h. Fresh media were replaced during each withdrawal and maintained at room temperature. The collected samples were filtered using a 0.45-m membrane filter, and the rate of drug release was determined using a UV-visible spectrophotometer at 261.6 nm, with phosphate buffered saline as the blank.

2.2.6. Ex Vivo Skin Permeation Studies

An ex vivo permeability study was performed using sheep buccal mucous membrane by the Franz diffusion cell method (MicroettePlus®, Teledyne Hanson, Chatsworth, CA, USA). The freshly excised buccal mucous membrane was obtained from the slaughterhouse and kept in phosphate buffered saline. A prepared buccal mucous membrane of 2 × 2 cm was carefully arranged between the acceptor and donor compartments of the diffusion cell area (1.75 cm^2). The permeation characteristics were evaluated for the developed HA FS NTF containing the 0.5% marketed formulation of fluconazole and the suspension containing the 0.5% fluconazole. Eight milliliters of phosphate buffered saline (pH 6.8) prepared from disodium hydrogen phosphate (Na_2HPO_4 anhydrous) = 14.4 g sodium dihydrogen phosphate (KH_2PO_4 anhydrous) = 2.4 g sodium chloride (NaCl) = 80.0 g, and potassium chloride (KCl) = 2.0 g, was kept in the receptor chamber, which was maintained at 32 ± 2 °C with the help of a warm water jacket and stirred at 410 to 430 rpm using the magnetic bead. The samples were autosampled at predetermined time intervals and quantified in parallel using high-performance liquid chromatography (HPLC) [22]. Diffusion of the fluconazole from the donor compartment to the receptor compartment through the mounted mucous membrane was determined by plotting the cumulative release pattern of the drug per unit of time and area. We calculated the diffusion coefficient (D), enhancement factor (EF), permeability coefficient (Pc), and steady-state flux (Jss) to determine whether the developed formulation was superior. Finally, the percentage of fluconazole permeated and the total amount of fluconazole diffused across the receptor chamber was calculated using Equation (4):

$$Percent\ permeated = \frac{F_P}{F_T} \times 100 \quad (4)$$

where F_P and F_T are the permeated amount of fluconazole in the receptor chamber and the loaded amount of fluconazole in the donor chamber, respectively.

2.2.7. Determination of Zone of Inhibition against *Candida Albicans*

The antifungal efficacy of the formulated formulation was determined by the disk diffusion method. We used the Sabouraud dextrose agar medium to grow *C. albicans* strains for inoculum preparation and the conduction of in vitro antifungal evaluation using the fungal strains.

Preparation of Inoculum

Four to five colonies of standard *C. albicans* strains were selected and suspended in normal saline (2 mL) and mixed vigorously. The turbidity of the fungal suspension was maintained homogeneously by the use of the 0.6-meq McFarland standards. Thereafter, streaks were made on the Sabouraud dextrose agar plate by dipping a sterile swab into the prepared fungal suspension to get the lawn culture.

Disk Diffusion Method

Sterile filter paper discs of 5 mm in diameter were soaked with 100 μL of the FS-NTF and ethanol (99.9%) as test and positive control samples, respectively. The soaked paper disks were placed on inoculated Sabouraud dextrose agar plates. The inoculated plates were incubated at $24 \pm 2\,°C$ for 48 h and then examined for their respective zones of inhibition.

2.2.8. Determination of Ulcer Index

Animals

Male albino rats weighing between 160 and 240 g were selected for the in vivo determination of the ulcer index. The experimental animals were procured from the animal house facility of the Clinical Laboratory Center, Beni Suef, Egypt. The animals were housed in standard laboratory conditions (temperature, $25 \pm 2\,°C$; relative humidity, $55 \pm 5\%$) with free access to water and food for 7 days [16]. Thereafter, the animals were used for the current experiment following approval of the protocol by the Institutional Review Board for Animal Research/Studies Animals (Approval No.15-08-2020).

Preparation of Organisms for Inoculation in Animal Model

Four to five colonies of standard *C. albicans* strains were selected and suspended in normal saline (2 mL) and mixed vigorously. The suspended cells were collected by centrifugation at $2500 \times g$ for 10 min. Thereafter, the pelleted cells were washed with phosphate buffered saline thrice and finally suspended in the buffer to obtain the final cell concentration of 3×10^8 colony-forming units (CFU)/mL.

Formation of Oral Candidiasis in the Rat Model and Evaluation of the Developed Formulation

Preparation of Immunocompromised Model

The efficacy of the developed HA-FS-NTZ for the oral candidiasis model was evaluated in immunocompromised animal models following the protocol of Martinez and team [23]. The acclimatized animals were immunocompromised first by the consumption of dexamethasone with tetracycline. The initial dose of dexamethasone (0.5 mg/L) and tetracycline (1 g/L) was supplied to the animals via drinking water for 7 days, followed by an increase in the concentration of dexamethasone (1 mg/L) and a reduction in the concentration of tetracycline (0.1 g/L) 1 day before infecting the animals. The same dose of dexamethasone with tetracycline was continued until the end of the study.

Inoculation of *C. albicans* Strains to the Immunocompromised Animals

The oral cavities of the experimental animals were checked for infection with *C. albicans*. Following the confirmed absence of *C. albicans* infections, the animals were orally infected by rolling a cotton swab containing 0.1 mL of the prepared fungal suspension thrice over the entire oral cavity on days 3, 5, and 7. Confirmation of infection in the experimental animals and quantification of the number of CFUs in the oral cavity were performed by an oral swab test after 72 h from the last inoculation.

Treatment of the Infected Animals

The animals were divided into six groups. The control group was treated with normal saline, and the animals in the other five groups were treated with formulated HA-FS-NTF, hyaluronic acid hydrogel loaded with F-NTF (without sesame oil), hyaluronic acid hydrogel loaded with fluconazole, fluconazole aqueous suspension, and blank hyaluronic acid hydrogel. The treatments were continued for 3 consecutive days, and the ulcer indexes were determined on third day [24,25]. Scoring of the oral ulcer index in the experimental animals was measured as shown in Table 2.

Table 2. Scoring table of the oral ulcers created post-infection of *Candida albicans*.

Condition	Score
Normal-colored epithelial lining	0.5
Red coloration	1
Spot ulceration less than 1 mm	2
Ulcers between 1 and 2 mm without hemorrhagic streaks	2.5
Ulcers between 1 and 2 mm with hemorrhagic streaks	3
Ulcers > 2 mm but < 3 mm	4
Ulcers > 3 mm	5

The scores of the respective animals in each groups were recorded and analyzed.

2.2.9. Statistical Analysis

All of the presented results were expressed as the mean ± the standard deviation. The comparisons of results between the different groups were performed statistically using the paired *t*-test, where $p < 0.05$ was considered a significant difference between the compared groups.

3. Results and Discussion

3.1. Formulation of Fluconazole-Loaded Nanotransfersome

The edge activators in the nanotransfersome formulations played a definitive role. They make the formed vesicles ultraflexible so that they are capable of noninvasively penetrating the skin by virtue of their high level of self-optimizing deformability. An elastic nanotransfersomal carrier is described as a lipid droplet of such deformability that it permits easy penetration through pores much smaller than the droplet size, and, also, it is a highly adaptable and stress-responsive complex aggregate. The vesicles are elastic and very deformable; they consist of lecithin in combination with an edge-active surfactant such as Tween. An edge activator is usually a single-chain surfactant that causes the destabilization of the lipid bilayer of the vesicle and increases the vesicle elasticity or fluidity by lowering its interfacial tension. Amongst the various edge activators used widely by different researchers, Spans, Tweens, potassium glycyrrhizinate, sodium deoxycholate, and sodium cholate are widely incorporated for the development of stable and effective formulations [17]. The current approach of formulating fluconazole-loaded nanotransfersomes was achieved by incorporating Tween 20. Tween 20 is a nonionic polyoxyethylene sorbitol ester widely used in pharmaceutical preparations due to its biocompatible characteristics. The development of the nanotransfersomes progressed using this nonionic surfactant [26].

We also incorporated sesame oil in the nanotransfersome formulation. Sesame oil is traditionally used as a pulling agent for dentures; it prevents malodor, bleeding from the gums, tooth decay, and dryness of the lips and throat [27]. Further studies revealed a concentration-dependent antifungal role of sesame oil, specifically against *C. albicans* [10]. Therefore, a total of 19 formulations were prepared according to the Design of Experiment model to formulate an optimized formulation for the next stage of experiment.

3.2. Optimization of the Fluconazole-Sesame Oil Nanotransfersome: Box–Behnken Statistical Design

3.2.1. Optimization of the Globule Size of the Fluconazole-Sesame Oil Nanotransfersome Formulations

The globule size of a nanotransfersome formulation is one important parameter in formulation optimization because it can affect the solubility and drug permeation through the skin [28]. Therefore, we analyzed the interactions of the three independent variables in our formulation to determine the globule size of the FS-NTF. During the optimization process, the quadratic model was found to be the best fit. Table 3 shows the statistical outcome of the interactions between the amount of lecithin, fluconazole, and sesame oil in the formulation and the globule size of the FS-NTF. The statistical significance of the different model terms is represented by the p-value (<0.05). The model's F-value of 321.4 represents the significance of the model. A lack-of-fit F-value of 4.88 and a respective p-value (>0.05) indicated that the lack of fit was not significant relative to the pure error, and this was desirable because we wanted the model to be fit. Close agreement was observed between the actual and predicted globule sizes of the formulations, as shown in Table 1, and also in the predicted and adjusted R^2 values, with a difference of less than 0.2 for the dependent variable of globule size.

Table 3. Statistical outcome (ANOVA) of the interaction of three independent variables on globule size of FS-NTF.

Source	Mean Square	F-Ratio	p-Value
Model	6429.44	321.44	<0.0001
A-Lecithin	26,799.61	1339.85	<0.0001
B-Fluconazole	16,346.65	817.25	<0.0001
C-Sesame oil	346.17	17.31	0.0024
AB	581.84	29.09	0.0004
AC	8.04	0.4020	0.5418
BC	0.0114	0.0006	0.9815
A^2	3565.26	178.25	<0.0001
B^2	4.02	0.2010	0.6645
C^2	11.54	0.5770	0.4669
Residual	20.00		
Lack of Fit	21.94	4.88	0.3373
Pure Error	4.50		
Correlation Total			

The model terms A, B, C, AB, and A2 were significant; they represent the significant effects of the amounts of lecithin, fluconazole, and sesame oil on the globule size of the formulations. A desirable signal-to-noise ratio is higher than 4, and the suggested model has a value of 55.071, indicating an adequate signal. Therefore, this model could be used to navigate the design space.

The generated quadratic equation on the interactions of the three independent variables with the globule size of the formulations is shown in Equation (5).

$$Y1 = +219.67 + 51.40*A + 37.95*B - 6.07*C - 29.56*A^2 + 11.05*A*B + 1.30*A*C + 1.02*B^2 + 0.0489*B*C - 1.63*C^2 \quad (5)$$

Model terms A and B have positive coefficient values of +51.40 and +37.95, respectively, whereas model term C has a negative coefficient value (-6.07) (Equation (5)). The p-value for all the model terms was less than 0.05 (Table 3); this indicates a significant increase in the particle size with increasing amounts of lecithin and fluconazole and a decreasing amount of sesame oil in the formulation. The higher value of coefficient of model term A indicates a higher effect on the particle size with changes in the amount of lecithin, followed by the amounts of fluconazole and sesame oil in the formulations. Lecithin is a phospholipid that is responsible for the formation of the concentric lipid bilayers of the formed vesicles. This lipid bilayer is the medium in which the lipophilic drug is located.

For this reason, the increase in the lecithin concentration within the formulated liposomes leads to an increased number of bilayers of this multilamellar vesicle, and this leads to an increase in the size of the formed vesicles. A similar effect is reflected in the perturbation plot, where positive slopes are evident with model terms A and B and there is a flattened negative curve with model term C. The curve with model term A is stiffer than the curve with model term B, and this is per the respective coefficient value in Equation (2). Similar effects on the interaction of the amounts of lecithin and fluconazole are reflected by color changes in the contour plot (see Figure 2a) and by changes in the color and slope of the three-dimensional surface plot (see Figure 2b).

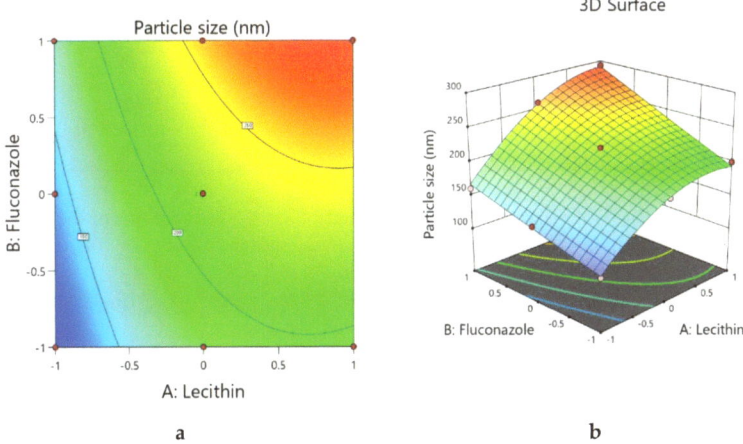

Figure 2. (**a**) Contour plot showing the interactions of lecithin and fluconazole with the globule size of the FS-NTF. (**b**) 3D surface plot showing the interactions of lecithin and fluconazole with the globule size of the FS-NTF.

3.2.2. Box–Behnken Statistical Designs: Optimization of the Entrapment Efficiency of the Fluconazole-Sesame Oil Nanotransfersome Formulations

The EE% of the nanoformulation is one of the hurdles in developing novel deliveries, where nanoformulations with a higher EE% are desirable [29]. Therefore, we analyzed the interactions of the three independent variables in our formulation to achieve a higher percentage of fluconazole to be successfully entrapped in the FS-NTF. During the optimization process, the quadratic model was found to be the best fit for a response such as the EE%. The statistical outcome of the interactions of the amounts of lecithin, fluconazole, and sesame oil in the formulation on the EE% of the FS-NTF is shown in Table 4. The model F-value of 386.29 represents the significance of the model. An F-value of 0.76 for the lack of fit and the respective p-value (>0.05) indicated that the lack of fit was not significant relative to the pure error; this was desirable as it indicated the model was fit. Close agreement was observed between the predicted and actual EE% of the formulations, as shown in Table 1, and the difference between the predicted and actual R^2 values was found to be less than 0.2.

In Table 4, the p-value indicates a significant effect of the amounts of lecithin, fluconazole, and sesame oil on the EE% of the formulations. When the coefficient value of model terms A, B, and C in the quadratic equation (Equation (6)) indicated that a desirable signal-to-noise ratio was more than 4, we found that the suggested model had a value of 60.699, indicating an adequate signal. Therefore, this model could be used to navigate the design space.

Table 4. Statistical outcome (ANOVA) of the interactions of three independent variables on the EE% of the FS-NTF.

Source	Mean Square	F-Value	p-Value
Model	152.40	386.29	<0.0001
A-Lecithin	138.98	352.26	<0.0001
B-Fluconazole	108.87	275.96	<0.0001
C-Sesame oil	17.88	45.32	<0.0001
AB	0.0908	0.2302	0.6428
AC	0.7177	1.82	0.2104
BC	0.0908	0.2302	0.6428
A^2	3.37	8.55	0.0169
B^2	1057.67	2680.86	<0.0001
C^2	0.3050	0.7730	0.4021
Residual	0.3945		
Lack of Fit	0.3813	0.7627	0.7147
Pure Error	0.5000		
Correlation Total			

The generated quadratic equation on the interactions of the three independent variables on the EE% of the formulations is shown in Equation (6).

$$Y2 = +75.19 + 3.70*A - 3.10*B + 1.38*C - 0.9091*A^2 - 0.1381*A*B - 0.3881*A*C - 16.57*B^2 - 0.1381*B*C - 0.2650*C^2 \quad (6)$$

From the equation, it can be seen that the model terms A and C have a positive coefficient value of +3.70 and +1.38, respectively, whereas model term B has a negative coefficient value (−3.10). The p-value for all the model terms was less than 0.05 (Table 4). This indicates a significant increase in the EE% with an increasing amount of lecithin and sesame oil and a decreasing amount of fluconazole in the formulation. A similar effect is reflected in the perturbation plot, where positive slopes are evident with model terms A and C and a positive slope is observed for model term C up to a certain extent and the curve of the model term goes down with an increasing amount of fluconazole. The curve with model term A is stiffer than the curve with model term C; this is per the respective coefficient value in Equation (3), so it can be inferred that the effect of the amount of lecithin is higher than for the amount of sesame oil in the EE% of the formulation. The effect of the interactions between the amounts of lecithin and fluconazole is reflected by the color changes in the contour plot (Figure 3a) and by the changes in color and slope in the three-dimensional surface plot (see Figure 3b). It is interesting to note that for the contour plot and three-dimensional surface plot (see Figure 3), an increasing amount of drug in the nanotransfersome formulation leads to an increase in the EE% up to a certain point; however, a further increase in drug concentration leads to a decrease in the EE% of the formulation. This phenomenon might be explained by the inefficiency of entrapping a higher amount of drug in the nanotransfersome formulation. At each level for the lecithin amount, the increase of fluconazole will increase the EE% until a certain level is reached, but then a further increase in the level of fluconazole will lead to a decrease in the EE%. This occurs as the space available for the incorporation of the added fluconazole becomes insufficient for the excess amount added, consequently leading to a decrease in the EE% at a higher level of fluconazole.

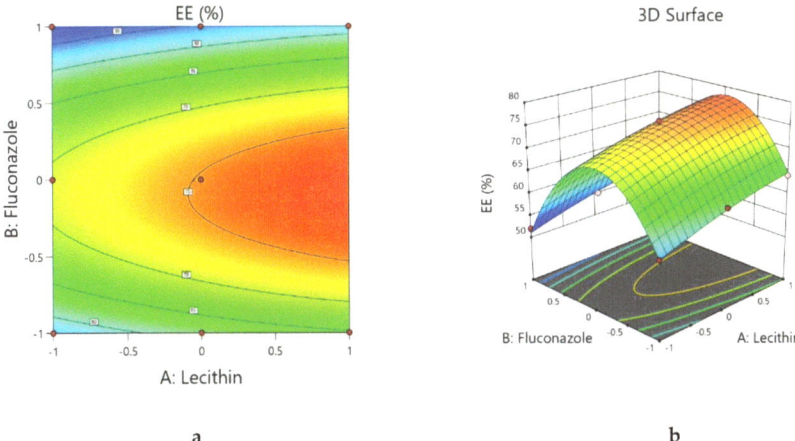

Figure 3. (**a**) Contour plot showing the interactions of lecithin and fluconazole with the EE% of the FS-NTF. (**b**) Three-dimensional surface plot showing the interactions of lecithin and fluconazole with the EE% of the FS-NTF.

3.2.3. Box–Behnken Statistical Designs: Optimization of Zone of Inhibition of Fluconazole-Sesame Oil Nanotransfersome Formulations

To assess the antifungal activity, we analyzed the interactions of the three independent variables of the zone of inhibition of the FS-NTF. During the optimization process, it was observed that the quadratic model was the best fit for the zone of inhibition of the formulation. The statistical outcome of the interactions of the amounts of lecithin, fluconazole, and sesame oil in the formulation's zone of inhibition of the FS-NTF is shown in Table 5. The model's F-value is 818.62, and the respective p-value of less than 0.05 represents the significance of the model. An F-value of 0.4747 for the lack of fit and respective p-value (>0.05) indicated the desirable lack of fit. The predicted R^2 value (0.9941) and adjusted R^2 value were in close agreement (0.9976). Close agreement was also observed for the predicted and actual zone of inhibition data in Table 1.

Table 5. Statistical outcome (ANOVA) of the interactions of three independent variables on the zone of inhibition of the FS-NTF.

Source	Mean Square	F-Value	p-Value
Model	54.55	818.62	<0.0001
A-Lecithin	1.69	25.35	0.0007
B-Fluconazole	422.36	6338.58	<0.0001
C-Sesame oil	16.17	242.74	0.0817
AB	0.0015	0.0223	0.8845
AC	0.0970	1.46	0.2583
BC	0.6086	9.13	0.0144
A^2	0.0002	0.0036	0.9536
B^2	2.55	38.23	0.0002
C^2	1.40	21.02	0.3413
Residual	0.0666		
Lack of Fit	0.0593	0.4747	0.8153
Pure Error	0.1250		

All three model terms had a significant effect on the zone of inhibition as per the p-value in Table 5. Further, when the coefficient value of model terms A, B, and C in the quadratic equation (Equation (4)) indicated that a desirable signal-to-noise ratio was higher than 4, the suggested model had a value of 79.149, indicating the adequate signal. Therefore, this model could be used to navigate the design space.

The generated quadratic equation on the interactions of the three independent variables on the zone of inhibition of the formulations is shown in Equation (7).

$$Y3 = +10.83 - 0.4081*A + 6.10*B + 1.31*C + 0.0076*A^2 - 0.0177*A*B - 0.1427*A*C - 0.8133*B^2 + 0.3573*B*C + 0.5681*C^2 \quad (7)$$

Model term B had the highest coefficient (+6.10) as was expected because as the fluconazole concentration increased the zone of inhibition also increased. Although model terms A and C exhibited a significant effect as per the *p*-value in Table 5, model term B had the maximum effect on the zone of inhibition. For the coefficient values, model term A exhibited an inverse effect whereas model term C exhibited a proportional relationship on the zone of inhibition. Similar findings on the effects of models A, B, and C are evident in the contour plot and three-dimensional surface plot (Figure 4a,b). In the contour plot and three-dimensional surface plot, no color changes were observed through the sesame oil axis.

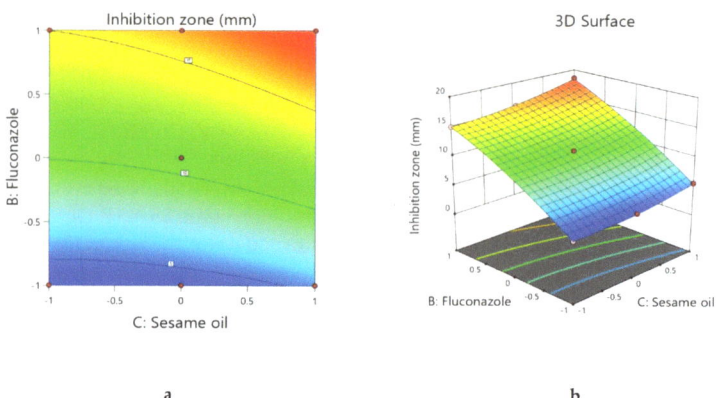

Figure 4. (**a**) Contour plot showing the interactions of sesame oil and fluconazole on the zone of inhibition of the FS-NTF. (**b**) Three-dimensional surface plot showing the interactions of sesame oil and fluconazole on the zone of inhibition of the FS-NTF.

3.2.4. Box–Behnken Statistical Designs: Optimization of the Ulcer Index of the Fluconazole–Sesame Oil Nanotransfersome Formulations

During optimization of the interactions of the three independent variables on the ulcer index of the FS-NTF, the linear model was found to be the best fit. The statistical outcome of the suggested linear model for the ulcer index is seen in Table 6. The model was found to be significant. Close agreement was observed in the predicted and actual ulcer indexes in Table 1 and in the adjusted R^2 value (0.9771) and predicted R^2 value (0.9671).

Table 6. Statistical outcome (ANOVA) for the linear model showing the interactions between the three independent variables and the ulcer index of the FS-NTF.

Source	Mean Square	*F*-Value	*p*-Value
Model	10.28	257.20	<0.0001
A-Lecithin	0.0028	0.0712	0.7932
B-Fluconazole	5.10	127.57	<0.0001
C-Sesame oil	20.12	503.27	<0.0001
Residual	0.0400		
Lack of Fit	0.0428		
Pure Error	0.0000		

It could be said that model terms B and C had a significant effect, whereas the effect of model term A was insignificant, as per the *p*-value in Table 6. The generated linear equation for the interactions of the three independent variables with the ulcer index of the formulations is shown in Equation (8).

$$Y4 = +2.55 - 0.0166*A - 0.6701*B - 1.46*C \tag{8}$$

The negative coefficient of significance for model terms B and C in Equation (8) represent a decrease in the ulcer index with an increasing amount of fluconazole and sesame oil, and this is in accordance with reported data [2,10]. Further, the maximum coefficient value of model term C represents a maximum effect of the sesame oil rather than the fluconazole, as per the contour plot and three-dimensional surface plot (Figure 5a,b), where the maximum effect of the sesame oil is reflected, followed by the amount of fluconazole.

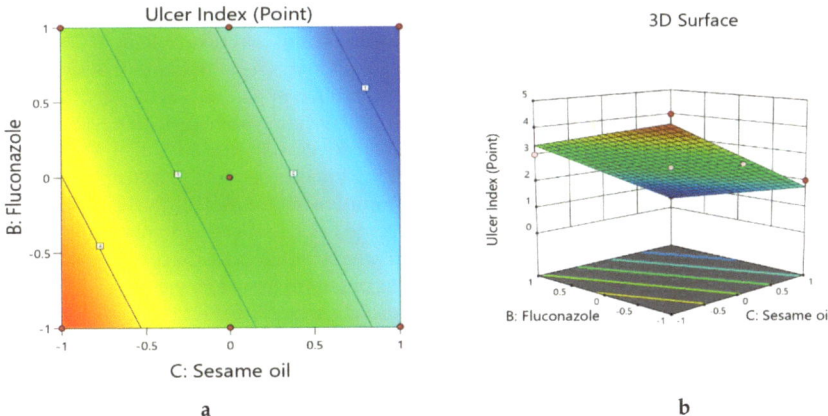

Figure 5. (**a**) Contour plot showing the interactions of the sesame oil and fluconazole on the ulcer index of the FS-NTF. (**b**) Three-dimensional surface plot showing the interactions of the sesame oil and fluconazole on the ulcer index of the FS-NTF.

3.3. Formulation of Optimized FS-NTF and FS-NTF-Loaded Hyaluronic Acid Hydrogel

Finally, the optimized nanotransfersome formulation was developed with the use of lecithin (level: $-0.99 \approx -1$) 75 mg, fluconazole (level: $0.32 \approx 0.3$) 60 mg, and sesame oil (level: $+0.99 \approx 1$) 75 mg. The predicted and observed values for the responses of the optimized formula are summarized in Table 7 as suggested by the software based on an analysis of the actual and predicted data. Values of the expected and adjusted R^2 of the studied responses were in close agreement, proving the significance and predictive capacity of the design. Moreover, the experimental and predicted ratios with a percentage error of less than 10% and acceptable residuals were found between the real and predicted responses, showing a lack of curvature in the responses and the validity of the model (Table 5).

Hyaluronic acid, a natural biomolecule, has shown its antimicrobial effectiveness against bacteria and fungi in a dose-dependent manner [30]. Another contemporary study revealed a fungistatic role of hyaluronic acid through its inhibitory effect on the fungal lysozyme and peroxidase system [11]. Further, hydrogel containing hyaluronic acid has an effective and safe coating, facilitating the proliferation of basal keratinocytes and promoting reepithelialization. This role of hyaluronic acid controls the hydration of ulcer tissues and also the inflammatory process [31]. Therefore, the hyaluronic acid hydrogel was formulated in the present study of the formulated FS-NTF and was incorporated to facilitate the application of the developed formulation at the oral mucosa.

Table 7. Composition of the actual and predicted responses of the optimal FS-NTF formulation.

Factor	Optimal Value	Response Variable	Actual Value	Predicted Value
A: Lecithin (mg)	75	Globule size of the prepared FS-NTF	140	138.6
B: Fluconazole (mg)	60	EE% of fluconazole within the prepared FS-NTF	70	69.2
C: Sesame oil (mg)	75	Zone of inhibition against *Candida albicans*	14.5	15.3
		Ulcer index score	1	0.88

3.4. Rheological Evaluation of the HA-FS-NTF Hydrogel

The naturally available polysaccharide hyaluronic acid has been explored for incorporation in several pharmaceutical preparations because of its unique viscoelastic properties and effective augmentation of soft tissues. However, the degree of cross-linking and preparation method, along with the molecular weight of the natural polymer, have been shown to have a direct relationship on the rheological properties of the final product [32]. Therefore, the impact of our method of preparation and the cross-linking with Gantrez® S-97 on the rheological property of the formulated hydrogel of hyaluronic acid was evaluated in the present study through an analysis of different parameters by the Brookfield viscometer.

It is clear from Figure 6a that there was an obvious increase in the rate of shear with the increase in the shear stress of the hyaluronic acid hydrogel. Further, incorporation of the FS-NTF within the formulated hydrogel was found to be associated with an increase in the shear rate of the developed formulation (Figure 6b). The ηmin for the FS-NTF-loaded hyaluronic acid hydrogel was recorded as 132,318 cp, a number much higher than that for the ηmin for the blank hyaluronic acid hydrogel (110,016 cp). Therefore, application of this formulation within the oral cavity might promote in increasing shear rate during talking, eating, or smiling [33]. This increasing shear rate might promote longer retention of the formulation at the site of application for the effective healing of the ulcers.

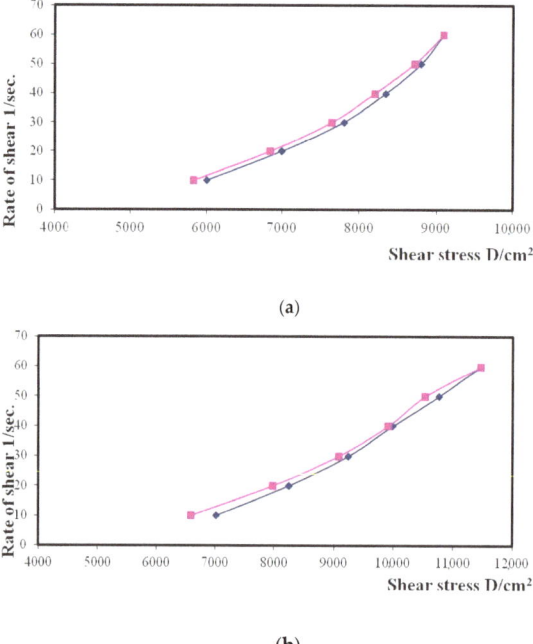

Figure 6. Rheogram of the (a) blank hyaluronic acid hydrogel and (b) HA-FS-NTF.

Values calculated by the Farrow's constant (N) indicate a deviation in the fluid of the Newtonian flow behavior, where an increased value indicates a change in the flow behavior toward a more non-Newtonian flow [34]. Calculations for the values of the Farrow's constant (N) were performed by plotting the logarithm of the shear rate (G) versus the logarithm of the shear stress (F), where the slope indicates the value of N (Figure 7). A value of less than 1 indicates dilatancy, and a value greater than 1 indicates pseudoplastic flow [34]. The flow behavior of the formulated hydrogels is presented in Table 8. All the hydrogel formulations had thixotropic behavior with pseudoplastic flow, and that is a desirable property for pharmaceutical gels for oral use. This special flow characteristic of hyaluronic acid hydrogel could be due to the breakdown of the structural configuration through the interruption of the existing intermolecular interactions between polymeric chains upon application of shear. There is further reoccurrence of polymerization between the molecules due to the force of the van der Waals interaction between the molecules upon removal of such shear [35,36]. The present study outcomes indicate that the optimal formulation of the HA-FS-NTF could facilitate the mean residence time within the oral cavity. This attribute is mostly due to the greater affinity of hyaluronic acid for the oral membrane due to its viscosity.

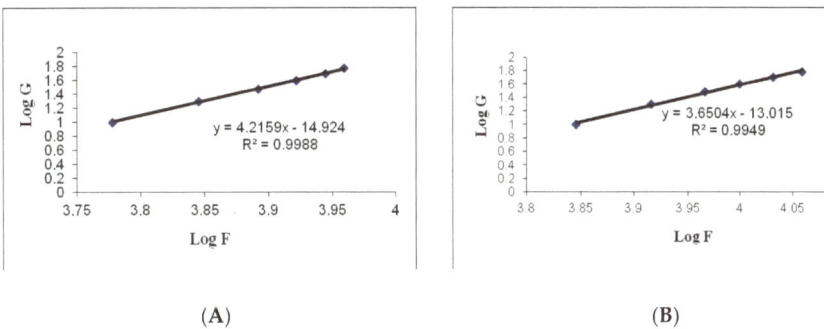

Figure 7. Representative plots of the logarithm of the rate of shear (G) versus the logarithm of the shearing stress (F) for (**A**) blank hyaluronic acid hydrogel and (**B**) HA-FS-NTF.

Table 8. Rheological parameters of blank hyaluronic acid hydrogel and HA-FS-NTF.

Formulations	Viscosity * (Minimum) (cP)	Viscosity * (Maximum) (cP)	Farrow's Constant (N)	Flow Behavior
Blank hyaluronic acid hydrogel	110,016 ± 7812	1535 ± 206	3.0111	Pseudoplastic
HA-FS-NTF	132,318 ± 9513	1907 ± 275	3.0024	Pseudoplastic

* Data are expressed as mean ± SD (n = 3).

The results in Table 8 show that the viscosity of the developed formulations had different values at a minimum rate of shear (ηmin) and maximum rate of shear (ηmax); the values of the ηmax were less than those for the ηmin for both the formulations. Therefore, it could be assumed from our previous result that there might be structural breakdown of the polymeric chains during shear. Figure 8 shows the relation between the viscosity and shear rate of different gel bases at various concentrations.

We previously discussed the non-Newtonian behavior of the hyaluronic acid hydrogel. Figure 8 demonstrates that there is an inverse relationship between the viscosity of hydrogel and the applied shear rate. Therefore, the pseudoplastic flow of the formulated hydrogel is confirmed from the obtained results. Our results are in agreement with the available information in the literature on the relationship between shear rate and viscosity [36].

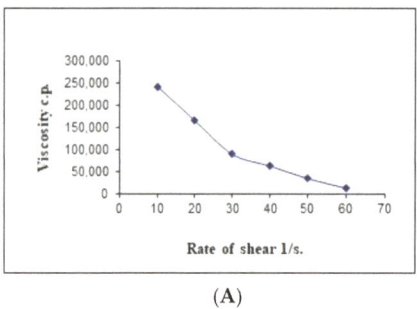
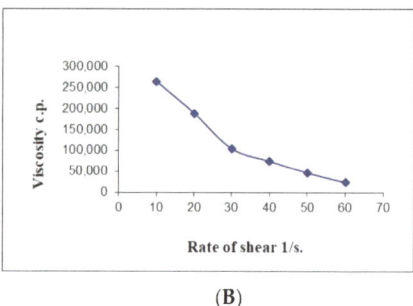

(A) (B)

Figure 8. Representative plots of the rate of shear (G) versus the viscosity (η) for the (**A**) blank hyaluronic acid hydrogel and (**B**) HA-FS-NTF.

3.5. In Vitro Release Profile of the HA-FS-NTF

The results of the in vitro release study of the formulated HA-FS-NTF containing the 0.5% marketed formulation of fluconazole and the HA suspension containing the 0.5% fluconazole using the Type I USP dissolution apparatus are presented in Figure 9. From the results, it could be clearly seen that the release of fluconazole from the HA-FS-NTF was faster and completed within the time frame of 3 h, when compared with the other two formulations. The release of drug from the marketed gel and aqueous suspension was slow, at approximately 43% and 12%, respectively. There was a significantly higher rate of release (<0.05) for our formulated FS-NTF-loaded hydrogel (~85%). From Figure 9, it can be demonstrated that the initial release rate of the drug from the HA-FS-NTF was retarded due to incomplete gel formation, but the release of fluconazole was gradual following complete hydration of the gel and remained at a steady state thereafter owing to pseudoplastic flow. Swelling of the polymer due to hydration led to a change in the physical and chemical parameters of the hydrogel configuration, to tune the porous structure uniformly [37]. The decreased release of fluconazole from the suspension and even from the gel might be due to a larger particle size or a less porous configuration, whereas the development of the nanotransfersome delivery facilitated the release of the drug from the semipermeable membrane owing to the smaller vesicle size and enhanced solubility. Our results are in agreement with those of the existing literature, where the release of an entrapped hydrophobic agent (resveratrol) was found to be improved when delivered via this nanotransfersome method [26].

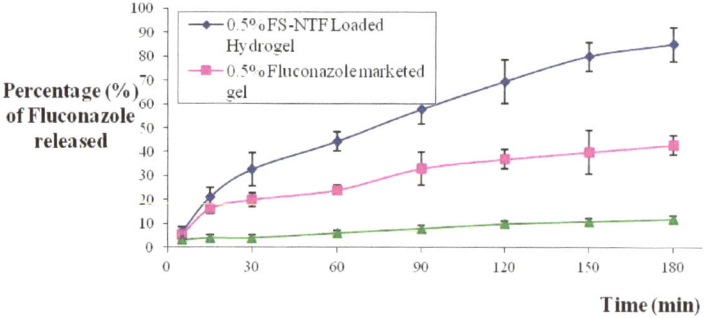

Figure 9. In vitro release profile of fluconazole from aqueous suspension, marketed gel, and HA-FS-NTF formulation. Data are expressed as mean ± SD (n = 3).

3.6. Permeation Parameters of Fluconazole from Optimized HA-FS-NTF by Ex Vivo Permeation Studies

The cumulative permeation of fluconazole through the sheep buccal mucosa was found to be 400 ± 57, 294 ± 34, and 122 ± 18 μg/cm^2 (Table 9) after 3 h of an experimental period from the 0.5% HA-FS-NTF optimized hydrogel, marketed 0.5% fluconazole gel, and aqueous 0.5% fluconazole suspension, respectively. With respect to the examined formulations, the optimized HA-FS-NTF hydrogel had maximum fluconazole permeation across the oral mucosa, and this is statistically significant ($p < 0.05$) when compared with the other two formulations. Our ex vivo permeation results of the tested formulations could be correlated with the in vitro release profile of the respective formulations, where the highest in vitro release from the HA-FS-NTF is reflected by the highest ex vivo permeability from the same formulation (400 μg/cm^2). The D, EF, Pc, and Jss of the optimized HA-FS-NTF were found to be superior when compared with those of the marketed gel and aqueous suspension (Table 9).

Table 9. Parameters of permeation for fluconazole across the buccal mucosa for different formulations.

Parameters of Permeation	Optimized HA-FS-NTF Formulation	Fluconazole 0.5% Marketed Gel	Fluconazole Aqueous Suspension (0.5%)
Cumulative amount permeated (μg/cm^2)	400 ± 57	294 ± 34	122 ± 18
Steady state flux, Jss, (μg/cm^2.min)	2.223	1.633	0.677
Permeability coefficient, Pc, (cm/min)	4.1×10^{-5}	3.2×10^{-5}	1.3×10^{-5}
Diffusion coefficient, D, (cm^2/min)	13.12×10^{-5}	8.11×10^{-5}	1.53×10^{-5}
Relative permeation rate (RPR)	1.36	-	0.414
Enhancement factor (EF)	3.278	2.409	-

The maximum permeation of fluconazole through the buccal mucosa could be explained by the fact that the presence of nanosized vesicles containing the drug provided a platform for rapid skin permeation, which could be through transcellular and paracellular pathways [28,38]. Additionally, the presence of an edge activator in the HA-FS-NTF formulation (i.e., a surfactant, Tween 20®) might also act as a penetration enhancer that might aid in drug transport across the skin [39]. The presence of the edge activator in the HA-FS-NTF interchange with keratin-based filaments with a disruption is advantageous for drug transport. Oral thrush is not just a superficial manifestation, but the fungal growth also affects deeper skin layers. Therefore, permeation of fluconazole into deeper layers is of the utmost importance.

3.7. Zone of Inhibition against Candida Albicans

The antifungal efficacy using the disk diffusion technique was established to monitor the susceptibility of fluconazole in different laboratory settings in a cost-saving manner [40,41]. The accuracy and precision of the method could be comparable to broth microdilution minimum inhibitory concentration MIC testing [41].

The inhibitory zone diameters of the respective samples were measured at transitional points where the growth of C. albicans abruptly decreased. The areas were distinguished by a marked decrease in colony sizes. The diameters of the zone were measured after 48 h, and the readings are presented in Figure 10. The figure clearly shows that the inhibitory zone was highest for the HA-FS-NTF, and that the lack of sesame oil (HA-F-NTF) in the formulation was associated with a significant decrease in the zone of inhibition. This could be explained by the lack of antifungal properties of sesame oil in the formulation [10]. Alternatively, the zone of inhibition of the fluconazole suspension (F-Suspension) and hyaluronic acid containing fluconazole (HA-F) showed similar results; however, a comparatively greater diameter was observed with the latter one. This might be due to the additional effect of hyaluronic acid on the growth of C. albicans [11,30], which was also evident in the results of the blank hydrogel (HA) of hyaluronic acid (1.33 ± 0.58 mm).

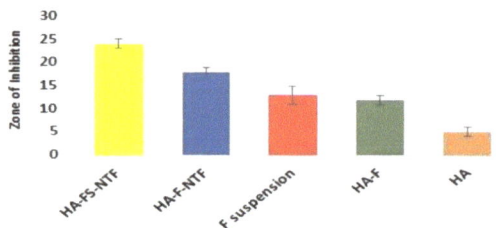

Figure 10. Representation of inhibitory zone diameters (mm) following 48 h of incubation of the agar plates containing *C. albicans*. Data are expressed as mean ± SD (n = 3).

Inhibitory Effect of Oral Candidiasis

Healthy rats were immunocompromised and tested for negative results of *Candida* in the oral cavity. Thereafter, confirmation of *Candida* infection was confirmed in the oral cavity of the immunocompromised animals. Daily treatment with five different formulations in the groups of animals with a sterile cotton swab revealed the improvement of oral infection as measured by the decrease in the ulcer index (Table 10). The results demonstrated that the HA-FS-NTF would be effective in controlling oral ulcers in the animals when compared with the other treatment options. The findings are quite similar to the in vitro inhibitory efficacy against *C. albicans*. Lack of sesame oil in the hyaluronic acid hydrogel loaded with F-NTF showed a marked difference in the ulcer index; however, the difference is statistically insignificant. Such a difference in efficacy in the HA-FS-NTF could be explained by the additional antifungal effect of sesame oil. Additionally, lack of hyaluronic acid in the fluconazole suspension was found be associated with a significant decrease in efficacy when compared with the hyaluronic acid hydrogel loaded with fluconazole; this could be illuminated by the additional role of hyaluronic acid in the control of *C. albicans* growth.

Table 10. In vivo ulcer index of the *Candida* albicans-infected immunocompromised animals after 3 days of treatment.

Tested Formula	Ulcer Index
HA-FS-NTF	0.67 ± 0.29
Hyaluronic acid hydrogel loaded with F-NTF (without sesame oil)	1.33 ± 0.28
Hyaluronic acid hydrogel loaded with fluconazole	2.17 ± 0.29
Fluconazole aqueous dispersion	2.83 ± 0.29
Blank hyaluronic acid hydrogel	4.67 ± 0.38

Data are expressed as mean ± SD (n = 3).

4. Conclusions

In summary, an optimal FS-NTF formulation was successfully developed by using the Design Experiment model, where the developed nanotransfersome was embedded into the hyaluronic acid hydrogel matrix. The in vitro drug release pattern and ex vivo permeation study through the sheep buccal mucosa of HA-FS-NTF showed a rapid release of the entrapped drug with significantly increased permeation parameters. These findings are positive indicators for local application in the oral cavity. The rheological properties of the HA-FS-NTF also support the localized application of the developed formulation. An in vitro antifungal assay and in vivo assessment of the ulcer index suggest a beneficial role for the developed formulation against oral candidiasis. The improved antifungal efficacy in our HA-FS-NTF might be due to the synergistic effect of hyaluronic acid, sesame oil, and fluconazole. Therefore, it can be summarized that fluconazole can effectively be delivered for the treatment of oral candidiasis when it is entrapped in a nanotransfersome carrier and embedded into cross-linked hyaluronic acid hydrogel.

Author Contributions: Conceptualization and methodology, H.M.A.; software and validation, K.M.H.; formal analysis, investigation, resources, and data curation, K.M.H.; writing—original draft preparation, W.Y.R.; writing—review and editing, K.M.H.; visualization, W.Y.R.; supervision and project administration, K.M.H. All authors have read and agreed to the published version of the manuscript.

Funding: This research work was funded by Institutional Fund Projects under grant no. (IFPHI-063-166-2020).

Institutional Review Board Statement: The study was conducted according to the guidelines of the Declaration of Helsinki, and approved by the Animal Ethics Committee of the Beni-Suef Clinical Laboratory (Approval No.15-08-2020, at August 2020).

Informed Consent Statement: Not applicable.

Data Availability Statement: Not applicable.

Acknowledgments: This research work was funded by Institutional Fund Projects under grant no. (IFPHI-063-166-2020). Therefore, authors gratefully acknowledge technical and financial support from the Ministry of Education and King Abdulaziz University, DSR, Jeddah, Saudi Arabia.

Conflicts of Interest: The authors declare no conflict of interest.

References

1. Chamorro-Petronacci, C.; García-García, A.; Lorenzo-Pouso, A.I.; Gómez-García, F.J.; Padín-Iruegas, M.E.; Gándara-Vila, P.; Blanco-Carrión, A.; Pérez-Sayáns, M. Management options for low-dose methotrexate-induced oral ulcers: A systematic review. *Med. Oral Patol. Oral Cir. Bucal* **2019**, *24*, e172–e180. [CrossRef] [PubMed]
2. Miranda-Cadena, K.; Marcos-Arias, C.; Mateo, E.; Aguirre, J.M.; Quindós, G.; Eraso, E. Prevalence and antifungal susceptibility profiles of *Candida* glabrata, *Candida* parapsilosis and their close-related species in oral candidiasis. *Arch. Oral Biol.* **2018**, *95*, 100–107. [CrossRef] [PubMed]
3. Rençber, S.; Karavana, S.Y.; Yilmaz, F.F.; Eraç, B.; Nenni, M.; Gurer-Orhan, H.; Limoncu, M.H.; Güneri, P.; Ertan, G. Formulation and evaluation of fluconazole loaded oral strips for local treatment of oral candidiasis. *J. Drug Deliv. Sci. Technol.* **2019**, *49*, 615–621. [CrossRef]
4. Rençber, S.; Karavana, S.Y.; Yılmaz, F.F.; Eraç, B.; Nenni, M.; Özbal, S.; Pekçetin, Ç.; Gurer-Orhan, H.; Hoşgör-Limoncu, M.; Güneri, P.; et al. Development, characterization, and in vivo assessment of mucoadhesive nanoparticles containing fluconazole for the local treatment of oral candidiasis. *Int. J. Nanomed.* **2016**, *11*, 2641–2653. [CrossRef] [PubMed]
5. Mohamed, S.P.; Muzzammil, S.; Pramod, K.T.M. Preparation of fluconazole buccal tablet and influence of formulation expedients on its properties. *Acta Pharm. Sin.* **2011**, *46*, 460–465.
6. Khan, S.; Gowda, B.H.H.; Deveswaran, R.; Mishra, S.; Sharma, A. Comparison of fluconazole and tea tree oil hydrogels designed for oral candidiasis: An in vitro study. *AIP Conf. Proc.* **2020**, *2274*, 050004.
7. Yonashiro Marcelino, M.; Azevedo Borges, F.; Martins Costa, A.F.; De Lacorte Singulani, J.; Ribeiro, N.V.; Barcelos Costa-Orlandi, C.; Garms, B.C.; Soares Mendes-Giannini, M.J.; Herculano, R.D.; Fusco-Almeida, A.M. Antifungal activity of fluconazole-loaded natural rubber latex against *Candida* albicans. *Future Microbiol.* **2018**, *13*, 359–367. [CrossRef]
8. Al Shuwaili, A.H.; Rasool, B.K.; Abdulrasool, A.A. Optimization of elastic transfersome formulations for transdermal delivery of pentoxifylline. *Eur. J. Pharm. Biopharm.* **2016**, *102*, 101–114. [CrossRef]
9. Price, R.D.; Myers, S.; Leigh, I.M.; Navsaria, H.A. The role of hyaluronic acid in wound healing: Assessment of clinical evidence. *Am. J. Clin. Dermatol.* **2005**, *6*, 393–402. [CrossRef]
10. Sakai, A.; Akifusa, S.; Itano, N.; Kimata, K.; Kawamura, T.; Koseki, T.; Takehara, T.; Nishihara, T. Potential role of high molecular weight hyaluronan in the anti-*Candida* activity of human oral epithelial cells. *Med. Mycol.* **2007**, *45*, 73–79. [CrossRef]
11. Griesser, J.; Hetényi, G.; Bernkop-Schnürch, A. Thiolated hyaluronic acid as versatile mucoadhesive polymer: From the chemistry behind to product developments-What are the capabilities? *Polymers* **2018**, *10*, 243. [CrossRef] [PubMed]
12. Ogawa, T.; Nishio, J.; Okada, S. Effect of edible sesame oil on growth of clinical isolates of *Candida* albicans. *Biol. Res. Nurs.* **2014**, *16*, 335–343. [CrossRef] [PubMed]
13. Kateh Shamshiri, M.; Momtazi-Borojeni, A.A.; Khodabandeh Shahraky, M.; Rahimi, F. Lecithin soybean phospholipid nano-transfersomes as potential carriers for transdermal delivery of the human growth hormone. *J. Cell. Biochem.* **2019**, *120*, 9023–9033. [CrossRef] [PubMed]
14. Alhakamy, N.A.; Badr-Eldin, S.M.; Fahmy, U.A.; Alruwaili, N.K.; Awan, Z.A.; Caruso, G.; Alfaleh, M.A.; Alaofi, A.L.; Arif, F.O.; Ahmed, O.A.A.; et al. Thymoquinone-Loaded soy-phospholipid-based phytosomes exhibit anticancer potential against human lung cancer cells. *Pharmaceutics* **2020**, *12*, 761. [CrossRef] [PubMed]

15. Akrawi, S.H.; Gorain, B.; Nair, A.B.; Choudhury, H.; Pandey, M.; Shah, J.N.; Venugopala, K.N. Development and optimization of naringenin-loaded chitosan-coated nanoemulsion for topical therapy in wound healing. *Pharmaceutics* **2020**, *12*, 893. [CrossRef]
16. Kumbhar, S.A.; Kokare, C.R.; Shrivastava, B.; Gorain, B.; Choudhury, H. Preparation, characterization, and optimization of asenapine maleate mucoadhesive nanoemulsion using Box-Behnken design: In vitro and in vivo studies for brain targeting. *Int. J. Pharm.* **2020**, *586*, 119499. [CrossRef]
17. Ahad, A.; Al-Saleh, A.A.; Al-Mohizea, A.M.; Al-Jenoobi, F.I.; Raish, M.; Yassin, A.E.B.; Alam, M.A. Formulation and characterization of novel soft nanovesicles for enhanced transdermal delivery of eprosartan mesylate. *Saudi Pharm. J.* **2017**, *25*, 1040–1046. [CrossRef]
18. Opatha, S.A.T.; Titapiwatanakun, V.; Chutoprapat, R. Transfersomes: A promising nanoencapsulation technique for transdermal drug delivery. *Pharmaceutics* **2020**, *12*, 855. [CrossRef]
19. Göğer, N.G.; Aboul-Enein, H.Y. Quantitative determination of fluconazole in capsules and IV solutions by UV spectrophotometric methods. *Anal. Lett.* **2001**, *34*, 2089–2098. [CrossRef]
20. Gorain, B.; Choudhury, H.; Kundu, A.; Sarkar, L.; Karmakar, S.; Jaisankar, P.; Pal, T.K. Nanoemulsion strategy for olmesartan medoxomil improves oral absorption and extended antihypertensive activity in hypertensive rats. *Colloids Surf. B Biointerfaces* **2014**, *115*, 286–294. [CrossRef]
21. Ibrahim, H.K. A novel liquid effervescent floating delivery system for sustained drug delivery. *Drug Discov. Ther.* **2009**, *3*, 168–175. [PubMed]
22. Jebaliya, H.; Patel, M.; Jadeja, Y.; Dabhi, B.; Shah, A. A Comparative Validation Study of Fluconazole by HPLC and UPLC with Forced Degradation Study. *Chromatogr. Res. Int.* **2013**, *2013*, 673150. [CrossRef]
23. Martinez, A.; Regadera, J.; Jimenez, E.; Santos, I.; Gargallo-Viola, D. Antifungal efficacy of GM237354, a sordarin derivative, in experimental oral candidiasis in immunosuppressed rats. *Antimicrob. Agents Chemother.* **2001**, *45*, 1008–1013. [CrossRef] [PubMed]
24. Al-Yahya, A.; Asad, M. Antiulcer activity of gum arabic and its interaction with antiulcer effect of ranitidine in rats. *Biomed. Res.* **2016**, *27*, 1102–1106.
25. Mostofa, R.; Ahmed, S.; Begum, M.M.; Rahman, M.S.; Begum, T.; Ahmed, S.U.; Tuhin, R.H.; Das, M.; Hossain, A.; Sharma, M.; et al. Evaluation of anti-inflammatory and gastric anti-ulcer activity of *Phyllanthus niruri* L. (*Euphorbiaceae*) leaves in experimental rats. *BMC Complement. Altern. Med.* **2017**, *17*, 267. [CrossRef]
26. Wu, P.S.; Li, Y.S.; Kuo, Y.C.; Tsai, S.J.J.; Lin, C.C. Preparation and evaluation of novel transfersomes combined with the natural antioxidant resveratrol. *Molecules* **2019**, *24*, 600. [CrossRef]
27. Asokan, S.; Rathan, J.; Muthu, M.; Rathna, P.; Emmadi, P.; Raghuraman; Chamundeswari. Effect of oil pulling on *Streptococcus mutans* count in plaque and saliva using Dentocult SM Strip mutans test: A randomized, controlled, triple-blind study. *J. Indian Soc. Pedod. Prev. Dent.* **2008**, *26*, 12–17. [CrossRef]
28. Marwah, H.; Garg, T.; Rath, G.; Goyal, A.K. Development of transferosomal gel for trans-dermal delivery of insulin using iodine complex. *Drug Deliv.* **2016**, *23*, 1636–1644. [CrossRef]
29. Panahi, Y.; Farshbaf, M.; Mohammadhosseini, M.; Mirahadi, M.; Khalilov, R.; Saghfi, S.; Akbarzadeh, A. Recent advances on liposomal nanoparticles: Synthesis, characterization and biomedical applications. *Artif. Cells Nanomed. Biotechnol.* **2017**, *45*, 788–799. [CrossRef]
30. Ardizzoni, A.; Neglia, R.G.; Baschieri, M.C.; Cermelli, C.; Caratozzolo, M.; Righi, E.; Palmieri, B.; Blasi, E. Influence of hyaluronic acid on bacterial and fungal species, including clinically relevant opportunistic pathogens. *J. Mater. Sci. Mater. Med.* **2011**, *22*, 2329–2338. [CrossRef]
31. Lee, J.; Jung, J.; Bang, D. The efficacy of topical 0.2% hyaluronic acid gel on recurrent oral ulcers: Comparison between recurrent aphthous ulcers and the oral ulcers of Behçet's disease. *J. Eur. Acad. Dermatol. Venereol.* **2008**, *22*, 590–595. [CrossRef] [PubMed]
32. Chernos, M.; Grecov, D.; Kwok, E.; Bebe, S.; Babsola, O.; Anastassiades, T. Rheological study of hyaluronic acid derivatives. *Biomed. Eng. Lett.* **2017**, *7*, 17–24. [CrossRef] [PubMed]
33. Gavard Molliard, S.; Bon Bétemps, J.; Hadjab, B.; Topchian, D.; Micheels, P.; Salomon, D. Key rheological properties of hyaluronic acid fillers: From tissue integration to product degradation. *Plast. Aesthetic Res.* **2018**, *5*, 17. [CrossRef]
34. El-Leithy, E.S.; Shaker, D.S.; Ghorab, M.K.; Abdel-Rashid, R.S. Evaluation of mucoadhesive hydrogels loaded with diclofenac sodium-chitosan microspheres for rectal administration. *AAPS PharmSciTech* **2010**, *11*, 1695–1702. [CrossRef]
35. Pisárčik, M.; Bakoš, D.; Čeppan, M. Non-Newtonian properties of hyaluronic acid aqueous solution. *Colloids Surf. A Physicochem. Eng. Asp.* **1995**, *97*, 197–202. [CrossRef]
36. Snetkov, P.; Zakharova, K.; Morozkina, S.; Olekhnovich, R.; Uspenskaya, M. Hyaluronic acid: The influence of molecular weight on structural, physical, physico-chemical, and degradable properties of biopolymer. *Polymers* **2020**, *12*, 1800. [CrossRef]
37. Bayer, I.S. Hyaluronic acid and controlled release: A review. *Molecules* **2020**, *25*, 2649. [CrossRef]
38. Choudhury, H.; Pandey, M.; Yin, T.H.; Kaur, T.; Jia, G.W.; Tan, S.Q.L.; Weijie, H.; Yang, E.K.S.; Keat, C.G.; Bhattamishra, S.K.; et al. Rising horizon in circumventing multidrug resistance in chemotherapy with nanotechnology. *Mater. Sci. Eng. C* **2019**, *101*, 596–613. [CrossRef]
39. Som, I.; Bhatia, K.; Yasir, M. Status of surfactants as penetration enhancers in transdermal drug delivery. *J. Pharm. Bioallied Sci.* **2012**, *4*, 2–9.

40. Kirkpatrick, W.R.; Turner, T.M.; Fothergill, A.W.; McCarthy, D.I.; Redding, S.W.; Rinaldi, M.G.; Patterson, T.F. Fluconazole disk diffusion susceptibility testing of *Candida* species. *J. Clin. Microbiol.* **1998**, *36*, 3429–3432. [CrossRef]
41. Pfaller, M.A.; Hazen, K.C.; Messer, S.A.; Boyken, L.; Tendolkar, S.; Hollis, R.J.; Diekema, D.J. Comparison of results of fluconazole disk diffusion testing for *Candida* species with results from a central reference laboratory in the ARTEMIS global antifungal surveillance program. *J. Clin. Microbiol.* **2004**, *42*, 3607–3612. [CrossRef] [PubMed]

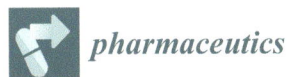

Article

Nanostructured Lipid Carriers Made of Ω-3 Polyunsaturated Fatty Acids: In Vitro Evaluation of Emerging Nanocarriers to Treat Neurodegenerative Diseases

Sara Hernando, Enara Herran, Rosa Maria Hernandez and Manoli Igartua

1. NanoBioCel Research Group, Laboratory of Pharmaceutics, School of Pharmacy University of the Basque Country (UPV/EHU), 01006 Vitoria-Gasteiz, Spain; sara.hernando@ehu.eus
2. Biomedical Research Networking Centre in Bioengineering, Biomaterials and Nanomedicine (CIBER-BBN), Institute of Health Carlos III, 28029 Madrid, Spain
3. Bioaraba, NanoBioCel Research Group, 01006 Vitoria-Gasteiz, Spain
4. Biokeralty Research Institute, C/Albert Einstein 25 bajo, Edificio E-3 Miñano, 01510 Álava, Spain; enara.herran@keralty.com
* Correspondence: rosa.hernandez@ehu.es (R.M.H.); manoli.igartua@ehu.es (M.I.); Tel.: +34-94501-3095 (R.M.H.); +34-94501-3007 (M.I.)

Received: 15 July 2020; Accepted: 26 September 2020; Published: 29 September 2020

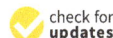

Abstract: Neurodegenerative diseases (ND) are one of the main problems of public health systems in the 21st century. The rise of nanotechnology-based drug delivery systems (DDS) has become in an emerging approach to target and treat these disorders related to the central nervous system (CNS). Among others, the use of nanostructured lipid carriers (NLCs) has increased in the last few years. Up to today, most of the developed NLCs have been made of a mixture of solid and liquid lipids without any active role in preventing or treating diseases. In this study, we successfully developed NLCs made of a functional lipid, such as the hydroxylated derivate of docohexaenoic acid (DHAH), named DHAH-NLCs. The newly developed nanocarriers were around 100 nm in size, with a polydispersity index (PDI) value of <0.3, and they exhibited positive zeta potential due to the successful chitosan (CS) and TAT coating. DHAH-NLCs were shown to be safe in both dopaminergic and microglia primary cell cultures. Moreover, they exhibited neuroprotective effects in dopaminergic neuron cell cultures after exposition to 6-hydroxydopamine hydrochloride (6-OHDA) neurotoxin and decreased the proinflammatory cytokine levels in microglia primary cell cultures after lipopolysaccharide (LPS) stimuli. The levels of the three tested cytokines, IL-6, IL-1β and TNF-α were decreased almost to control levels after the treatment with DHAH-NLCs. Taken together, these data suggest the suitability of DHAH-NLCs to attaining enhanced and synergistic effects for the treatment of NDs.

Keywords: nanostructured lipid carriers; nanocarrier; docohexaenoic acid; neuroprotection; neuroinflammation

1. Introduction

Neurodegenerative diseases (ND) cause progressive loss of brain functions and overlapping clinical syndromes. Among the many risk factors associated with neurodegeneration, the aging process itself has by far the most impact. However, other environmental and genetic aspects are associated with the risk of suffering these diseases. Indeed, the NDs are the result of a combination of different environmental risk factors, such as vascular risk, tobacco consumption, alcohol and aging, together with different genes involved in the development of these central nervous system (CNS) disorders.

For example, in Alzheimer's disease (AD), APOE4 (apolipoprotein E) is the major genetic risk factor. Moreover, mutations in APP, (amyloid precursor protein) PSEN1 (presenilin proteins) and PSEN2 probably accelerate the toxic accumulation of proteins that leads to the undergoing neurodegenerative process present in AD. Another example is mutation in GBA (glucocerebrosidase), which encodes β-glucocerebrosidase. Alterations in this gene lead to lysosomal enzyme deficiency and an increase in the prevalence of Parkinson diseases (PD). Other mutations in genes, such as LRRK2 (leucine-rich repeat kinase 2), parkin and SNCA, (alpha synuclein) which encodes the protein α-synuclein, are the most common causes of dominantly and recessively inherited PD. These NDs are age-dependent disorders that are becoming increasingly prevalent as life expectancy rises worldwide. This prevalence will increase, becoming a serious economic burden and public health problem. Despite AD and PD being the most common NDs, Huntington's disease (HD), amyotrophic lateral sclerosis (ALS), frontotemporal dementia and the spinocerebellar ataxias are also examples of NDs, with aging as the main risk factor for all of them [1–3]. Although they have different clinical manifestations and symptoms, they share common features and mechanisms of neurodegeneration, highlighting protein deposits, mitochondrial homeostasis, stress granules and synaptic toxicity, together with a maladaptive innate immune response that converges in the form of chronic inflammation characterized by reactive gliosis and an increase in proinflammatory cytokines [4,5].

Despite the significant public health issues NDs have, to date, the treatments for these diseases remain symptomatic without halting the progression of the disease. Moreover, the lack of an overall positive effect on the clinical manifestation of the disease, together with the presence of systemic side effects, has prompted the patients to abandon their therapies [6,7]. Due to the lack of an effective treatment for NDs, in the last few years, promising new molecules, such as neurotrophic factors (NTFs), antioxidant molecules and polyunsaturated fatty acids (PUFAs), have been raised as a feasible therapeutic options to target the undergoing oxidative stress and inflammatory status or to enhance neurogenesis [8–10].

Nevertheless, no matter the treatment, one of the most challenging obstacles for an effective therapy for NDs is the low penetration efficiency of drugs to the CNS due to the presence of the blood brain barrier (BBB). In the last few years, different strategies have been developed in order to achieve brain targeting. These strategies include direct and indirect methods. The direct or invasive techniques include surgical methods to administer drugs directly into the brain and the disruption of the BBB to open it. Meanwhile, the indirect or noninvasive techniques include nonaggressive approaches to access the brain without affecting this barrier integrity [11,12]. These noninvasive techniques include alternative systemic administration routes like intranasal administration [13,14]. Gartziandia et al. conducted a study that successfully showed the brain delivery of therapeutics after intranasal administration with lipid nanoparticles coated with chitosan (CS) [15]. Moreover, the combination of the formulation with cell-penetrating peptides (CPP) has been disclosed as a useful strategy to enter the brain [16,17]. Anyway, one of the most studied approaches to attain this goal are nanotechnology-based drug delivery systems [18,19]. Among them, nanoparticles (NPs) have been widely used as a promising approach for ND treatment. NPs are highly stable 3D encapsulation systems that can be loaded with drugs and functionalized with targeting ligands or antibodies, and they can be used as nanocarriers to deliver drugs to the CNS [20]. Among other materials, natural or synthetic polymers and lipids have been employed in NP development [11].

Indeed, numerous research papers have combined NPs with well-known treatments or therapeutic approaches that have recently appeared, such as growth factors (GFs), antioxidant molecules and PUFAs entrapped in the nanoformulation [21–24]. All these research papers support the use of nanoparticles, offering many advantages over traditional formulations, such as protecting the molecule from degradation, increasing the half-life of the therapeutic molecules and, therefore, limiting multiple dosing and decreasing side effects. Among others, the nanostructured lipid carriers (NLCs) are an unstructured solid lipid matrix made of a mixture of blended solid and liquid lipids and an aqueous phase with a mixture of surfactants [25]. In addition, they have gained the attention of researchers since they exhibit a lack of toxicity, high drug loading capacity of both hydrophobic and hydrophilic compounds and a natural tendency to pass across the BBB [26]. Moreover, the NLCs can be functionalized with different substances to increase their tendency to pass through the BBB [27]. Examples of these molecules are chitosan (CS) and the cationic cell-penetrating peptide TAT; both molecules have increased brain targeting of therapeutic molecules for NDs treatment, as we pointed out in previous publications [15,24].

Up to today, most of the lipids used for NLC formulation are inert excipients, without any active role in preventing or treating diseases [28]. Indeed, only a few research groups have described the use of functional lipids that could play a therapeutic role in forming the lipid matrix, i.e., Ω-9 oleic acid incorporated into a NLC formulation for dermal applications [29]. Other kinds of functional lipids are PUFAs, Ω-3 and Ω-6 polyunsaturated fatty acids. As previously pointed out, PUFAs have been raised as a promising new approach to target neurodegenerative diseases. Although the biochemical mechanism undergoing the beneficial effect in NDs is not clear at all, they have exhibited the positive effect of decreasing the neuroinflammation process undergoing NDs, improving memory in animal models of AD, sensory motor tests in PD animal models and inhibiting amyloid-β fibrils both in vitro and in vivo [30–32]. Such functional lipids, which are also called nutraceutical, have proved to be a useful tool to manage NDs [33]; although they cannot totally restore brain functions, they may be beneficial to manage some symptoms of the disease or just as a coadjutant treatment. Actually, in the last few years, numerous observational studies showed an association between a diet rich in PUFAs and a lower risk of PD. Moreover, dietary treatments with PUFAs have shown to decrease the inflammatory status of these NDs and decrease depressive symptoms, among others [34–36].

Therefore, taking into account the promising results obtained with PUFAs in ND treatment, along with the beneficial effects of NLCs modified with CS and TAT for brain targeting, the objective of this research article is to combine both strategies for ND treatment. More concretely, the goal of the present work is to develop NLC with a functional lipid, such as DHA (docohexaenoic acid) and its hydroxylated derivate (DHAH), so the nanoparticles themselves could exhibit neuroprotective and antiinflammatory effects. In summary, we aim to demonstrate the beneficial effect of PUFAs incorporated to the NLC matrix, generating a new functional nanocarrier for entrapping different therapeutic molecules in the future and acting as a synergetic therapy.

2. Materials and Methods

2.1. Materials

Precirol ATO 5® (glycerol disterate) (pharma grade) and Mygliol® (caprylic/capric triglyceride) (pharma grade) were a kind gift from Gattefosé (Lyon, France) and IOI Oleo GmbH, respectively. DHA (80% purity) and DHAH (85.4% purity) fatty acids in ethyl ester and triglyceride form were purchased from Medalchemy (Alicante, Spain). They were aliquoted in topaz vials in N_2 inert atmosphere conditions ready for one unique use in order to avoid oxidation during storage over the course of the experiment. Tween 80, Tween 20 and 3.7% paraformaldehyde were purchased from Panreac (Barcelona, Spain). Lutrol® F-68 (Poloxamer 188) (FDA-approved excipient) was acquired from VWR Avantor (Barcelona, Spain). Chitosan (CS) was obtained from NovaMatrix (Sandvika, Norway). Trehalose dehydrate, Triton X-110, bovine serum albumin (BSA), poly-l-lysine hydrobromide (PLL), deoxyribonuclease I from a bovine pancreas (DNase I), 6-hydroxydopamine hydrochloride (6-OHDA), Cell Counting Kit-8 (CCK-8), 2,2′-Azino-bis(3-ethylbenzthiazoline-6-sulfonic acid) (ABTS) and Fluoromount™ Aqueous Mounting Medium were acquired from Millipore Sigma Life Sciences (Madrid, Spain). Additionally, 4′,6-diamidino-2-phenylindole (DAPI), donkey anti-mouse IgG (H+L) cross-adsorbed secondary antibody, Alexa Fluor 555, goat anti-rabbit IgG (H+L) cross-adsorbed secondary antibody and Alexa Fluor 488 were purchased from Thermo Fisher Scientific (Madrid, Spain). Neurobasal™ medium, B-27™ supplement, glutamine 100X, penicillin-streptomycin (P/S), fetal bovine serum (FBS), DMEM GlutaMAX™, trypsin-EDTA 0.25% and Hank's Balanced Salt Solution (HBSS) were obtained from Gibco© by Life Technologies (Madrid, Spain). Anti-tyrosine-hydroxilase (TH) primary antibody and anti-glial fibrillary acidic protein (GFAP) primary antibodies were obtained from Abcam (Cambridge, UK). Anti-Iba1 (ionizing calcium-binding adaptor molecule 1) primary antibody was purchased from Synaptic Systems (Göttingen, Germany). Lipopolysaccharide (LPS) suitable for cell culture was bought from InvivoGen (Toulouse, France). Rat IL-6 Standard, Rat IL-1β Standard and Rat TNF-α Standard ABTS ELISA Development Kits were obtained from Peprotech (London, UK). Finally, TAT (>95% purity) was obtained from ChinaPeptides (Suzhou, China). All reagents used were of analytical grade.

2.2. NLC Preparation and Optimization

NLC were prepared based on a previously described melt-emulsification technique [16,24]. Four different formulations were developed, combining solid and liquid lipids. The solid lipid Precirol ATO 5® (melting point: 56 °C) was used in all formulations; however, different liquid lipids in a different solid:lipid ratio were used, as shown Table 1. All nanoformulations shown in Table 1 were performed in triplicate.

Table 1. The composition of the different nanoparticles, using Precirol® ATO 5 and different Ω-3 fatty acids or Mygliol® as a liquid lipid with different solid:liquid lipid ratios.

Liquid Lipid	Formulation	% Precirol ATO 5® (w/v)	% Liquid Lipid (w/v)	% T80 (w/v)	% Poloxamer 188 (w/v)
Mygliol®	A1	2.5	0.25	3	2
	A2	2	0.75	3	2
	A3	1.75	1	3	2
	A4	1.5	1.25	3	2
DHA	B1	2.5	0.25	3	2
	B2	2	0.75	3	2
	B3	1.75	1	3	2
	B4	1.5	1.25	3	2
DHAH-EE	C1	2.5	0.25	3	2
	C2	2	0.75	3	2
	C3	1.75	1	3	2
	C4	1.5	1.25	3	2
DHAH-TG	D1	2.5	0.25	3	2
	D2	2	0.75	3	2
	D3	1.75	1	3	2
	D4	1.5	1.25	3	2

DHA, its hydroxylated derivate in ethyl ester form (DHAH-EE) and Mygliol® (caprylic/capric glyceride) were liquid at room temperature; however, the hydroxylated derivate of DHA in triglyceride form (DHAH-TG) was slightly more viscous. We used two different variants of DHAH, its hydroxylated derivate in ethyl ester form (DHAH-EE) and triglyceride form (DHAH-TG) in order to select the most suitable one to develop our new nanocarrier.

The lipid phase, containing both the solid and the liquid lipid, was heated 5 °C above its melting point until a clear and homogeneous phase was obtained. The lipid phase was formed with a different solid:liquid lipid ratio, as described in Table 1. The aqueous solution was composed of Tween 80 (3% w/v) and poloxamer 188 (2% w/v) for a final volume of 4 ml. The aqueous phase was warmed and added to the melted oily phase and sonicated for 60 s at 50 W (Branson® Sonifier 250, Fisher Scientific, Madrid, Spain). The obtained nanoemulsion was maintained under magnetic stirring for 15 min at room temperature and stored at 4 °C overnight to allow the recrystallisation of the lipid for NLC formation. On the following day, the nanoparticle dispersion was centrifuged in an Amicon filter (Amicon, "Ultracel-100k", Millipore Sigma Life Sciences, Madrid, Spain) at 2500 rpm (MIXTASEL,

JP Selecta, Barcelona, Spain) for 15 min and the nanoparticles were washed three times with milli Q water. Finally, 15% *w/w* trehalose was added as cryoprotectant, and the NLCs were lyophilized for 42 h (LyoBeta 15, Telstar, Spain).

Prior to the NLC coating process, TAT was covalently linked to CS by a surface activation method previously described by our research group [16] The CS: TAT employed ratio was 1:0.01 (*w/w*). TAT conjugation with CS was prepared through a carbodiimide-mediated coupling reaction [37]. The reaction was made though the EDC/NHS technique, in which the reactive sulfo-NHS ester reacted with the amine functionality of proteins and peptides via the formation of an amide bond [38,39]. Briefly, 250 µL EDC (1-ethyl-3-(3-dimethylaminopropyl) carbodiimide hydrochloride) in solution (1 mg/mL) and 250 µL of sulfo-NHS (*N*-hydroxysulfosuccinimide) in 0.02 M phosphate buffered saline (PBS) were added dropwise to a 4 mL CS solution (0.5% *w/v* in PBS 0.02 M) under magnetic stirring (2 h at room temperature). For the coupling of TAT, a 250 µL TAT solution (1 mg/mL) in PBS (0.02 M; pH 7.4) was added dropwise to the activated CS under gentle agitation. The TAT-CS solution was maintained under agitation for another 4 h at room temperature and then incubated at 4 °C overnight. The next day, the NLC were coated with TAT-CS; for that purpose, an NLC dispersion previously prepared was added dropwise to the TAT-CS solution under continuous agitation for 20 min at room temperature. After the coating process, CS-NLC-TAT nanoformulation was centrifuged in Amicon filters (Amicon, "Ultracel-100k", Millipore, Millipore Sigma Life Sciences, Madrid, Spain) at 2500 rpm (MIXTASEL, JP Selecta, Barcelona, Spain) for 15 min and washed three times with Milli Q water. Finally, the nanoformulation was freeze-dried with the cryoprotectant trehalose at a final concentration of 15% (*w/w*) of the weighed lipid, and then it was lyophilized for 42 h (LyoBeta 15, Telstar, Terrassa, Spain). This final step, regarding the coating with CS and TAT, was only performed after the election of the lipid type and the solid:lipid ratio, resulting in the formulations named (CS-TAT) DHAH-NLC, or just DHAH-NLC, and (CS-TAT) Mygliol-NLC, or just Mygliol-NLC, used in the following described studies in primary cell cultures.

2.3. NLC Characterization

The mean particle size (Z-average diameter) and the polydispersity index (PDI) were measured by dynamic light scattering (DLS), and the zeta potential was determined through laser Doppler micro-electrophoresis (Malvern® Zetasizer Nano ZS, Model Zen 3600; Malvern Instruments Ltd., Malvern, UK). Three independent measurements were performed for each formulation. The data are represented as the mean ± SD. Nanoparticle surface characteristics and morphology were examined by transmission electron microscopy (JEOL JEM 1400 Plus, Izasa Scientific, Madrid, Spain). The thermal behavior of the nanoparticles and the excipients and components themselves were studied using differential scanning calorimetry (DSC) (DSC-50, Shimadzu, Kioto, Japan). Each sample was sealed in an aluminum pan and heated from 25 °C to 350 °C at a heating rate of 10 °C per minute. The sample size was 1–2 mg for each measurement. Finally, Fourier transform infrared (FTIR) spectra of Mygliol-NLC and DHAH-NLC with and without CS and TAT coating were carried out on a Nicolet Nexus FTIR spectrometer using ATR Golden Gate (Thermo Scientific, Madrid, Spain) with a crystal ZnSe. The sample was placed directly onto the ATR crystal and the spectrum was obtained in transmittance mode. Each spectrum was the result of an average of 32 scans at 4 cm^{-1} resolution. Measurements were recorded in the wavelength range of 4000–750 cm^{-1}.

2.4. Cell Cultures

2.4.1. Primary Dopaminergic Cell Culture

Dopaminergic neuronal cultures were prepared from Wistar rat embryos at 15, 16 or 17 days of gestation (E15–E17). Animal procedures were reviewed and approved (3 April 2017) by the Local Ethical Committee for Animal Research of the University of the Basque Country (UPV/EHU, CEEA, ref. M20/2017/019). All of the experiments were performed in accordance with the European Community

Council Directive on "The Protection of Animals Used for Scientific Purposes" (2010/63/EU) and with Spanish Law (RD 53/2013) for the care and use of laboratory animals.

To obtain primary dopaminergic cell cultures, the following protocols were followed with slight modifications [40,41] (Figure 1A). Pregnant rats were euthanized and, under no aseptic conditions, the whole brain was removed from the rat embryos and kept on ice in a Petri dish (10 cm ∅) with HBSS for removing the blood vessels and meninges. Petri dishes containing embryos' brains were put under the magnifying glass to select the brain areas of interest following Gaven et al. protocol [42]. The ventral portion of the mesencephalic flexure, a region of the developing brain rich in dopaminergic neurons, was used for cell preparations. After collecting the brain areas of interest, tissue was incubated with tryspin at 37 °C for 15 min under aseptic conditions. Then, it was also incubated with DNase for 30 s and, after that time, the trypsin was inactivated and the tissue was washed twice with DMEM GlutMAX^{TM} FBS 10%, P/S. Then, the tissue was mechanically dissociated by several passages through a 5 and 2 mL pipette. Finally, the cell suspension was passed through a 100 μm nylon strainer and centrifuged for obtaining a cell pellet. The cell pellet was resuspended in neurobasal medium supplemented with 0.5 mM glutamine, 1% antibiotic and 3% B27. Cells were seeded in 96-well culture plates (for the cell viability assay, neuroprotective activity assay and 6-OHDA toxin-induced assay) and in 24-well culture plates with glass coverslips (for the immunofluorescence assay), both previously coated with poly-l-lysine to promote cell adhesion, at a density of 40×10^3 cells/well and 150×10^3 cells/well, respectively.

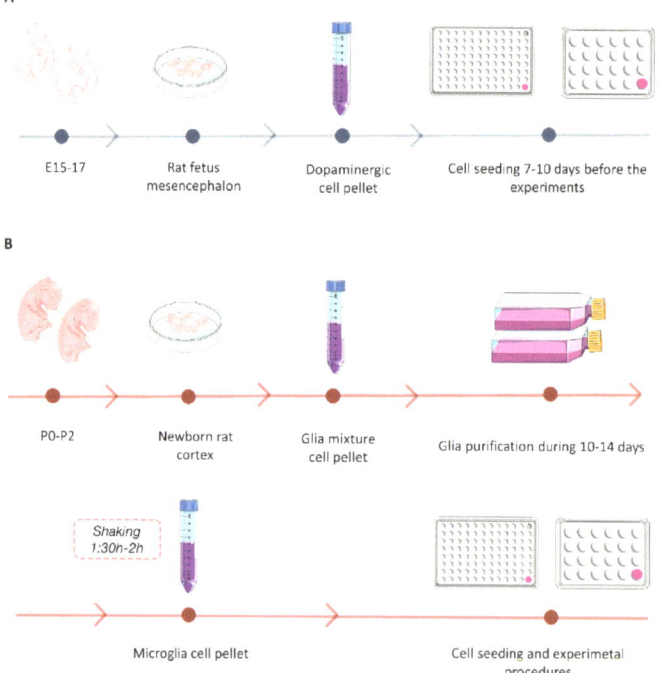

Figure 1. Schematic representation of primary cell culture protocols. (**A**) Primary dopaminergic neuron culture isolation and seeding. (**B**) Primary microglia cell culture isolation and seeding. This figure was created using Servier Medical Art templates, which are licensed under a Creative Commons Attribution 3.0 Unported License (https://smart.servier.com).

2.4.2. Primary Microglia Cell Culture

Microglia neuronal cultures were prepared from Wistar rat puppets at day 0 to 2 (P0–P2). Animal procedures were reviewed and approved by the Local Ethical Committee for Animal Research of the University of the Basque Country (UPV/EHU, CEEA, ref. M20/2017/035). All the experiments were performed in accordance with the European Community Council Directive on "The Protection of Animals Used for Scientific Purposes" (2010/63/EU) (22 September 2010) and with Spanish Law (RD 53/2013) (8 February 2013) for the care and use of laboratory animals.

Primary microglia cell cultures were obtained following Chen et al. protocol with slight modifications [43] (Figure 1B). Puppets' brains were removed and kept on ice in a Petri dish (10 cm ⌀) with HBSS under magnifying glasses for removing the meninges and selecting the brain area of interest. Then, the cortex of the brain was collected and incubated with trypsin for 15 min at 37 °C. The tissue was incubated with DNase for 30 s and, afterwards, the trypsin was inactivated and the tissue was washed twice with DMEM GlutMAX™ FBS 10%, P/S. Finally, the tissue was mechanically dissociated by several passages through a 5 and 2 mL pipette and, then, passed through a 70 µm nylon strainer and centrifuged for obtaining a cell pellet. The obtained pellet was resuspended in DMEM GlutMAX™ FBS 15%, P/S and incubated in a poly-l-lysine-coated flask at 37 °C in a humidified 5% CO_2 atmosphere. After 3 days, full media were changed to DMEM GlutMAX™ FBS 10%, P/S. After this, half media changes were done every 2–3 days for maintaining this glia mixture culture for 10–14 days. After that period, the flask media were removed and replaced with DMEM GlutMAX™ FBS 15% P/S 24 h before microglia cell isolation started. Microglia cells were detached from the astroglia layer by shaking the flasks at 250 rpm for 1.5–2 h. Then, primary microglia cells were removed from the flask, resuspended in complete DMEM with FBS 15% and seeded in poly-l-lysine-precoated 96-well culture plates (for cell viability and cytokine release assays) and in 24-well culture plates with glass coverslips (for the immunofluorescence assay) at a density of 50×10^3 cells/well and 150×10^3 cells/well, respectively.

2.5. Immunofluorescence

Primary cells were seeded at a density of 150×10^3 cells/well in 24-well culture plates with glass coverslips precoated with poly-l-lysine. At the time of interest, cells were fixed with 3.7% paraformaldehyde (PFA) for 10 min and, then, washed three times in PBS. Then, they were blocked and permeabilized with 1% (w/v) of BSA solution and 0.1% (v/v) Triton X-100 in PBS for 1 h at room temperature. After rinsing, they were incubated in rabbit polyclonal antibody Iba-1 (1:1000), mouse monoclonal anti-GFAP (1:2000) or rabbit polyclonal antibody TH (1:1000), respectively, with 1% (w/v) BSA and 0.1% Triton X-100 in PBS with agitation on at 4 °C. The following day, cells were incubated with the secondary antibody: anti-rabbit Alexa Fluor IgG 488 (1:1000) or anti-goat Alexa Fluor IgG 555 (1:1000), respectively, in PBS with 1% BSA and 0.1% Triton X-100 for 2 h at room temperature. After three rinsing steps, the fixed cells were incubated in DAPI (1:10,000) in PBS for 10 min. Then, they were washed twice with PBS and mounted with Fluoromount™.

2.6. Cell Viability Assay

As previously pointed out, for cell viability study, the cells were seed in 40×10^3 cells/well in poly-d-lysine-precoated 96-well culture plates. Dopaminergic cells were maintained for 7–10 days before performing the experiments and the medium was changed every 3 days, if necessary. At a determined time point, the media from the cells were removed and new fresh media were added with the different nanoparticle concentrations, DHAH-NLCs or Mygliol-NLCs, (100, 75, 50, 25, 12.5 and 5 µM) for 24 or 48 h. The concentration (µM) refers to the quantity of DHAH present in the NLC formulation. For dosing Mygliol NPs, an equal amount of NLCs was used as an internal control to observe the difference between using a functional lipid, such as DHAH, versus an inert lipid, such as Mygliol®.

Afterwards, the viability was assessed using the CCK-8 kit. Briefly, 10 µL of the CCK-8 reagent was added to the cells. After 4 h of incubation, the absorbance of the mixture was read at 450 nm, using 650 nm as the reference wavelength (Plate Reader Infinite M200, Tecan, Männedorf, Switzerland). The absorbance was directly proportional to the number of living cells in the culture. Cell viability for each condition is represented in a percentage related to the control positive (C^+), where no treatment was added to the cell media.

In the case of microglia, slight modifications were done in the cell viability assay protocol. After obtaining a pure microglial cell culture, as previously pointed out, the microglia cells were seeded in 50×10^3 cells/well density. Some 24 h after cell attachment, the media were removed and the cells were incubated for 24 or 48 h with the different concentrations of NLCs, as previously pointed out. Then, the viability CCK-8 test was performed as earlier described.

2.7. 6-OHDA Toxicity Assay

After 7–10 days of maintaining dopaminergic culture, the media were removed and different concentrations of 6-OHDA toxin were added (500, 100, 50, 25, 10 and 5 µM) for 24 h to correlate neurotoxin concentration to cell viability; for C^+, we just changed the media and, for control negative (C^-), DMSO 10% was added. To assess cell viability, after 24 h of incubation with 6-OHDA neurotoxin, the media were removed and the cells were fixed with 3.7% paraformaldehyde (PFA) for 10 min and, then, washed three times in PBS. DAPI staining (1:10,000) in PBS for 15 min was used to determine viable cells. For cell viability quantification, fluorescence microscopy images were obtained by means of an inverted microscope (Nikon TMS, Hampton, NH). Two images per well and three wells were used for each group; in total, six images were taken per group. Dopaminergic cells were scored as positive if they exhibited defined nuclear counterstaining. The data are expressed as the percentage of the C^+ group with no treatment, which was set as 100%.

2.8. Neuroprotective Assay

After 7–10 days of maintaining a dopaminergic culture, a neuroprotective assay was carried out with the developed nanocarriers (Figure 2A). The media were removed and different concentrations of DHAH-NLCs and Mygliol NLCs were added to the cells (50, 25 and 12.5 µM) 24 h before the 6-OHDA neurotoxin was added to the culture. 24 h after, the media were removed and fresh media were added, with a final concentration of 25 µM 6-OHDA neurotoxin and the previously tested concentrations for NLCs (50, 25 and 12.5 µM). To assess the neuroprotective effect of DHAH-NLCs against 6-OHDA neurotoxin, the media were removed 24 h later and cells were fixed with 3.7% paraformaldehyde (PFA) for 10 min and, then, washed three times in PBS. DAPI staining (1:10,000) in PBS for 15 min was used to determine viable cells. For cell viability quantification, fluorescence microscopy images were obtained by means of an inverted microscope (Nikon TMS, Hampton, NH). Two images per well and three wells were used for each group; in total, six images were taken per group. Dopaminergic cells were scored as positive if they exhibited defined nuclear counterstaining. The data are expressed as the percentage of the C^+ group with no treatment but just media change, which was set as 100%.

2.9. Proinflammatory Cytokine Release Quantification: TNF-α, IL-1β and IL-6

DHAH-NLCs antiinflammatory effect against LPS (lipopolysaccharide) was carried out in microglia primary cells (Figure 3A). To perform the assay, cells were pretreated for 24 h with DHAH-NLCs and Mygliol-NLCs at different concentrations selected from studies previously carried out in Section 2.6 (50 µM, 25 µM and 12.5 µM) or just media change. After that treatment, media were removed and cells were incubated for another 24 h with LPS 50 ng/mL and the different concentration of the nanoparticles. After that 24 h, the cell media supernatant was collected and stored at −80 °C. The levels of TNF-α, IL-1β and IL-6 were analyzed with ELISA assay (Peprotech, London, UK). The total amount of cytokine release was normalized according to cell viability measured with CCK-8 assay at the same time point.

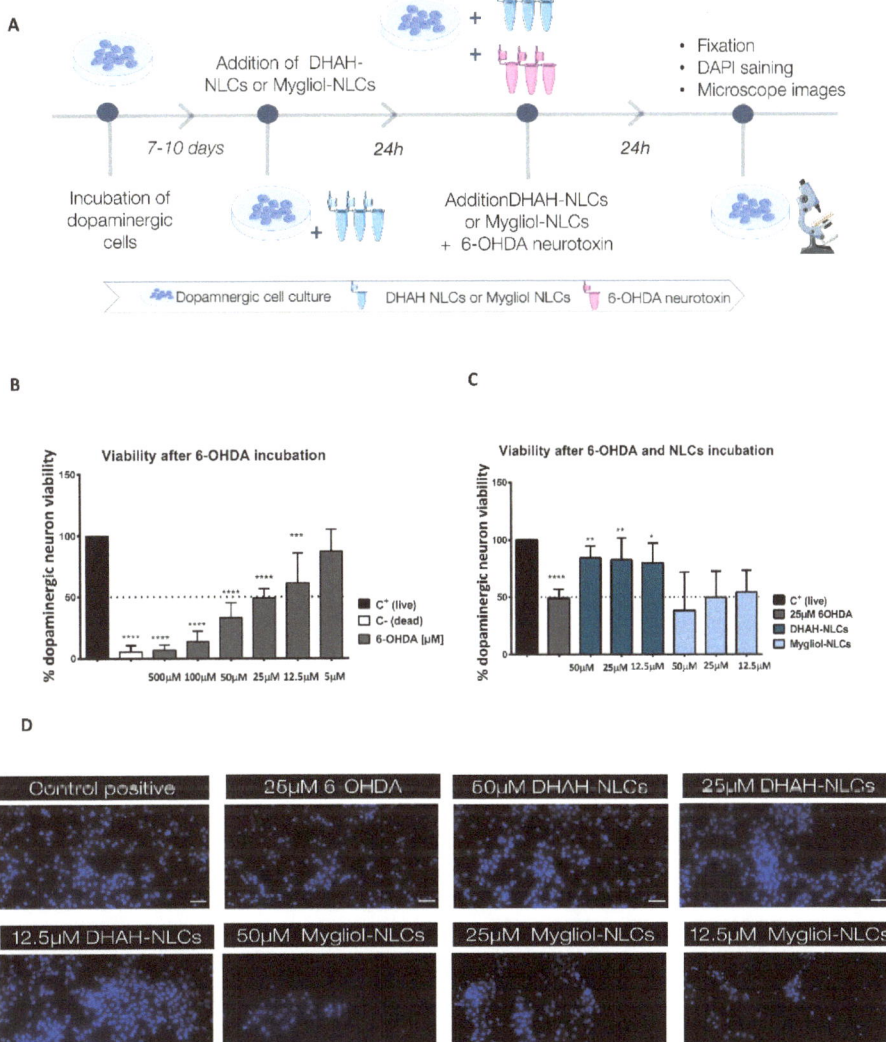

Figure 2. (**A**) Schematic representation of dopaminergic cell-based assays to evaluate the neuroprotective effects of DHAH-NLCs and Mygliol-NLCs. This figure was created using Servier Medical Art templates, which are licensed under a Creative Commons Attribution 3.0 Unported License (https://smart.servier.com). (**B**) Graphic representation of dopaminergic neuron viability after 24 h of incubation with different doses of 6-OHDA (**** $p < 0.0001$ C^+ vs C^-, 500 µM, 100 µM and 25 µM *** $p < 0.001$ C^+ vs 10 µM); one-way ANOVA. (**C**) Graphic representation of the neuroprotective effect of DHAH-NLCs (** $p < 0.01$ 25 µM 6-OHDA vs 50 µM DHAH-NLCs and 25 µM DHAH-NLCs, * $p < 0.05$ 25 µM 6-OHDA vs 12.5 µM DHAH-NLCs); one-way ANOVA. (**D**) Representative fluorescence images of the neuroprotective assay with DAPI staining. The scale bar indicates 50 µM.

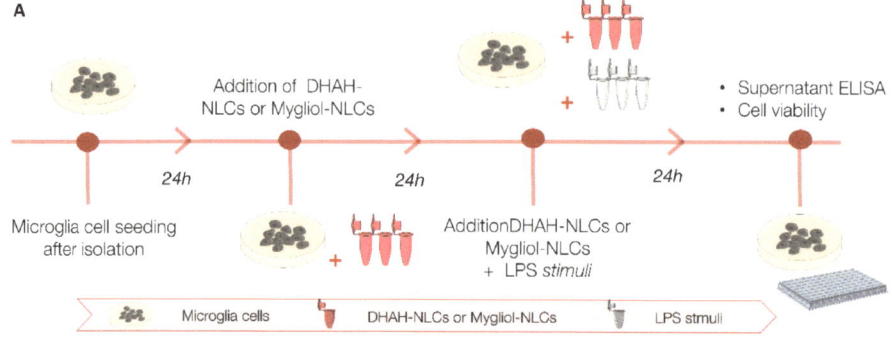
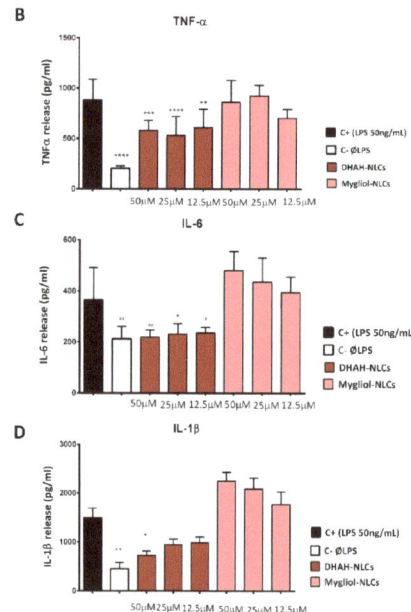

Figure 3. (**A**) Schematic representation of the antiinflammatory assay with DHAH-NLCs and Mygliol-NLCs. This figure was created using Servier Medical Art templates, which are licensed under a Creative Commons Attribution 3.0 Unported License (https://smart.servier.com). (**B**) Graphic representation of TNF-α values (pg/mL) for all the different tested concentrations and formulations (**** $p < 0.0001$ C$^+$ vs. C$^-$ and 25 μM DHAH-NLCs, *** $p < 0.001$ C$^+$ vs. 50 μM DHAH-NLCs, ** $p < 0.01$ C$^+$ vs. 12.5 μM DHAH-NLCs); one-way ANOVA. (**C**) Graphic representation of IL-6 values (pg/mL) for all the different tested concentrations and formulations (** $p < 0.01$ C$^+$ vs. C$^-$ and 50 μM DHAH-NLCs, * $p < 0.05$ C$^+$ vs. 25μM DHAH-NLCs and 12.5μM DHAH-NLCs); one-way ANOVA. (**D**) Graphic representation of IL-1β values (pg/mL) for all the different tested concentrations and formulations (** $p < 0.01$ C$^+$ vs. C$^-$ and * $p < 0.05$ C$^+$ vs. 5 μM DHAH-NLCs); one-way ANOVA.

2.10. Statistical Analysis

All results are expressed as mean ± SD. The results obtained from the cell culture have been performed in $n = 3$ biological replicates for all the experiments described in this article. Experimental data were analyzed using the computer program GraphPad Prism (v. 6.01, GraphPad Software,

San Diego, CA, USA). One-way ANOVA was used for analyzing all the data represented in this research article. *p* values <0.05 were considered significant.

3. Results

3.1. Nanoparticle Characterization

The aim of the present work was to develop a new nanocarrier enriched in functional lipids, such as Ω-3 fatty acids, to form the lipid matrix of NLCs. For that purpose, we tried to substitute the lipids of the nanoformulation with different kinds of Ω-3 fatty acids. Precirol ATO 5® was maintained as solid lipid. All modifications in the optimization process of the nanoformulation were performed in the liquid lipid, DHA, DHA-TG and DHA-EE, modifying the liquid lipid type and also the ratio of solid:lipid to formulate NLCs, since the main goal of this research was to increase the percentage of these functional lipids up to the maximum to form this new nanocarrier. In order to achieve this aim, we increased the percentage of lipid liquid from the 0.25% that we used in previous studies with Mygliol® [44–46] to 1.25%, as described in Table 1. We used DHA and two different types of DHAH to select the most suitable one to prepare the NLCs, and we worked with Mygliol®, the liquid lipid previously used in our research group for different clinical applications [15,47], as our control.

Between DHAH-EE and DHAH-TG, the ethyl ester form (DHAH-EE) was liquid at room temperature, and the obtained lyophilized NLCs were easy to handle. However, the NLCs prepared with DHAH-TG became a soggy and sticky powder at room temperature, and this was more difficult to handle after the lyophilization process. That is why the nanoformulations developed with DHAH-TG (C1–C4, Figure 4) were discarded to continue working.

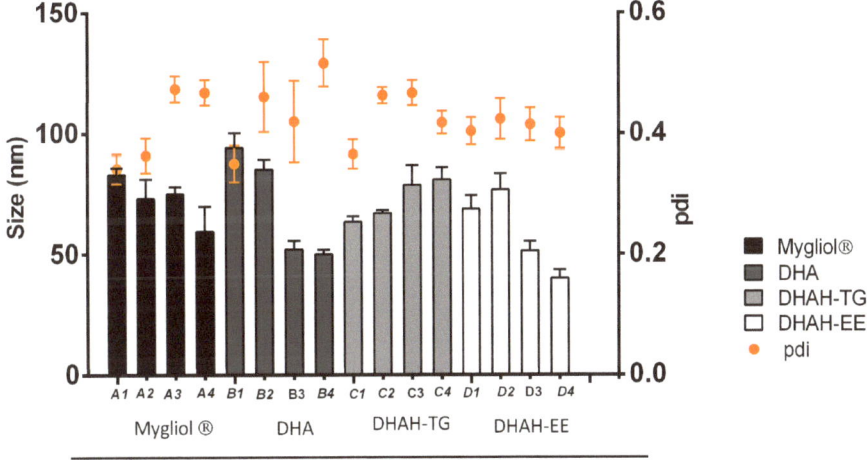

Figure 4. Characterization of the developed nanostructured lipids (NLCs) (*n* = 3 for all the nanoformulations).

NLCs formed with DHA and DHAH-EE showed similar pharmaceutical characteristics; however, as we probed in a previous in vivo study, DHA and DHAH functional lipids showed different biological activity [31]. Therefore, taking into account the remarkably beneficial effects of DHAH, we chose DHAH-EE nanoformulations to continue working. Among the different nanoformulations developed with DHAH-EE (D1–D4, Figure 4), we selected D3 (51.40nm ± 11.65 and 0.415 ± 0.082 for PDI values) since it was the formulation with the highest percentage of Ω-3 fatty acid incorporated into the lipid matrix of NLCs with the best resuspension characteristics, qualitatively determined. In order to confirm the therapeutic effect of DHAH-EE in the newly developed NLCs, we also chose Mygliol-based NLCs in the same proportion of solid:liquid lipid (A3, Figure 4), with a particle size of 75.02 ± 6.97 nm and 0.474 ± 0.023 PDI value, as the control formulation.

All the data regarding size, PDI and Z potential of all the developed nanoformulations have been summarized in Table 2. As seen, the size of NLC decreased when the percentage of liquid lipid was higher. Moreover, the Z potential of all nanoformulations was negative, which was reverted after CS and TAT coating (Table 3).

Table 2. Characterization of the developed NLCs ($n = 3$ for all the nanoformulations). The data are presented in media ± SD.

Formulation	Size after Lyoph (nm)	PDI	Z Potential (mV)
Formulation A1	83.07 ± 36.54	0.342 ± 0.061	−15.6 ± 1.7
Formulation A2	73.11 ± 19.51	0.364 ± 0.071	−16.0 ± 2.8
Formulation A3	75.02 ± 6.97	0.474 ± 0.023	−14.2 ± 19.2
Formulation A4	59.38 ± 25.39	0.468 ± 0.052	−14.4 ± 4.8
Formulation B1	94.19 ± 18.01	0.350 ± 0.092	−19.4 ± 1.8
Formulation B2	85.20 ± 12.20	0.461 ± 0.174	−19.9 ± 3.1
Formulation B3	51.98 ± 10.70	0.420 ± 0.202	−22.7 ± 3.5
Formulation B4	49.93 ± 5.36	0.587 ± 0.118	−22.8 ± 4.1
Formulation C1	63.34 ± 6.95	0.366 ± 0.073	−21.0 ± 5.8
Formulation C2	67.02 ± 4.10	0.463 ± 0.031	−16.5 ± 2.3
Formulation C3	78.63 ± 24.66	0.467 ± 0.062	−20.1 ± 3.4
Formulation C4	80.87 ± 15.15	0.418 ± 0.056	−20.4 ± 1.5
Formulation D1	68.62 ± 16.70	0.404 ± 0.068	−22.7 ± 2.6
Formulation D2	76.68 ± 20.12	0.425 ± 0.101	−24.2 ± 2.9
Formulation D3	51.40 ± 11.65	0.415 ± 0.082	−24.1 ± 2.9
Formulation D4	39.98 ± 10.39	0.401 ± 0.076	−24.9 ± 2.8

Table 3. Characterization of the final nanoformulations used for cell culture tests. ($n = 2$ independent experiments).

Formulation	Size after Lyoph (nm)	PDI	Z Potential (mV)
DHAH-NLC	97.80 ± 2.00	0.274 ± 1.26	12.63 ± 1.26
Mygliol-NLC	94.31 ± 0.43	0.454 ± 0.007	14.13 ± 0.21

In the next step, the CS and TAT coating process was performed. In Table 2, we can see the results from CS-TAT-NLC-DHAH-EE nanoformulation, called DHAH-NLCs, and from Mygliol-based nanoparticles with CS and TAT, called Mygliol-NLCs.

Both formulations were around 100 nm in size, with a PDI value below 0.5, and exhibited positive zeta values, indicating that the CS and TAT coating process has been successfully performed. In the external morphological study made by TEM (transmission electron microscopy), the nanoparticles showed a uniform size without irregularities (Figure 5). The DSC thermograms of the different excipients and formulations have been summarized in Appendix A Figure A1.

On the other hand, as seen in Figure A2, FTIR results exhibited a number of characteristic protein transmission bands (cm^{-1}). Mygliol-NLC and DHAH-NLC without CS and TAT coating showed typical peaks of lipid components, such as O–H stretching (3315), aliphatic C–H (2915, CH3 and CH2) asymmetrical stretching, aliphatic C–H (2852, CH3 and CH2) symmetrical stretching and C=O (1736, carboxylic group) stretching in addition to the vibrations associated with C–O and C–C (1150 and from 992 to 843) bonds. Moreover, CH2 and CH3 stretching (1466) and bending (1342) bands can be seen. Regarding nanoformulations with TAT and CS coating (CS-TAT-Mygliol-NLC and CS-TAT-DHAH-NLC), a new peak can be seen, concretely, in amide I (N–H stretching) (1645). This new peak is due to a chemical interaction. Indeed, it is related to the presence of the amide bond formed after TAT peptide conjugation through a cross linking reaction.

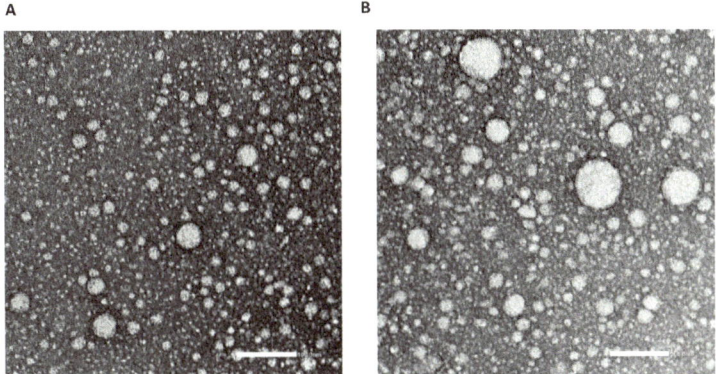

Figure 5. TEM (transmission electron microscopy) photographs of NLC (scale bar 100 nm). (**A**) hydroxylated derivate of docohexaenoic acid nanostructured lipids (DHAH-NLCs) (**B**) Mygliol-NLCs.

3.2. Cell Cultures

In order to assess the purity of our primary cultures, an immunofluoresce technique was performed in both dopaminergic and microglia cell cultures. The experiments were performed in triplicate and repeated at least three times independently ($n = 3$ biological replicates). Dopaminergic cell cultures were positive for TH dopaminergic marker, as shown in Figure 6A. In the case of the microglia cell culture, we tested both the microglia marker Iba1 and the astroglia maker GFAP. The culture was shown to be specific in a high percentage to microglia marker (Figure 6B. iv). However, it must be noted that, after this isolation method, the culture is not 100% specific for microglia cells, and also some astrocytes can be seen in a non-noteworthy way.

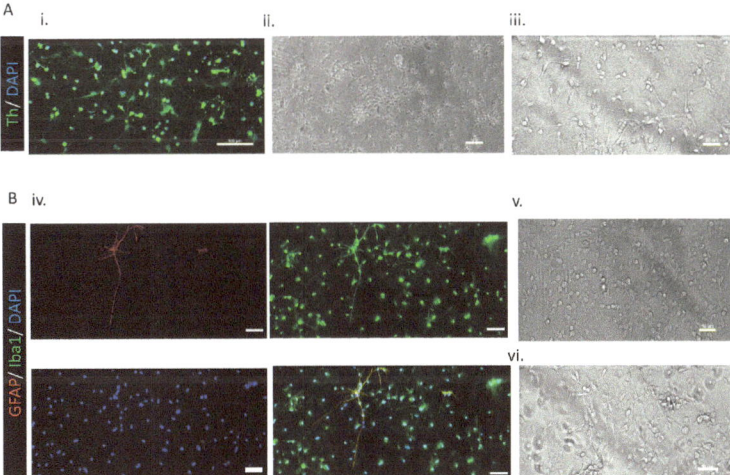

Figure 6. (**A**) Images of the primary dopaminergic cell culture. i: Immunofluorescence staining: positive for TH dopaminergic marker. (Scale bar 100 μM) ii: (scale bar 100 μM) and iii: (scale bar 50 μM) Bright field images of primary dopaminergic cell cultures. (**B**) Images of the primary microglia cell culture. Iv: Immunofluorescence staining. (Scale bar 50 μM) v: Bright field images of glia mix culture. (Scale bar 50 μM). vi: Bright field images of the primary microglia cell culture after isolation. (Scale bar 50 μM).

3.3. In Vitro Cell Viability Study

In order to assess the cytocompatibility of the nanoparticles, they were incubated with the dopaminergic and microglia cell cultures. After 24 and 48 h, cell viability was measured through the CCK-8 assay. Figure 7A,B illustrates the results obtained in the CCK-8 assay after incubating NLCs with a dopaminergic cell culture. None of the concentrations for the nanoformulations tested in dopaminergic cell cultures were cytotoxic, showing percentages of cell viability >70%. Indeed, as shown in Figure 7B, at 48 h, cell viability for the cultures treated with DHAH-NLCs was slightly better at any of the tested concentrations compared to Mygliol-NLCs treated cells. The results of the viability assay for the microglia cell culture are, to some extent, different. As shown in Figure 7C,D, the tested concentrations of 100 and 75 µM for the Mygliol-NLC formulation decreased cell viability below 70% at both tested time points; this effect was not seen with DHAH-NLC for any of the tested time points. This beneficial effect for DHAH-NLC was seen in any of the tested conditions, being more notorious at 50, 25 and 12.5 µM concentrations (Figure 7C,D).

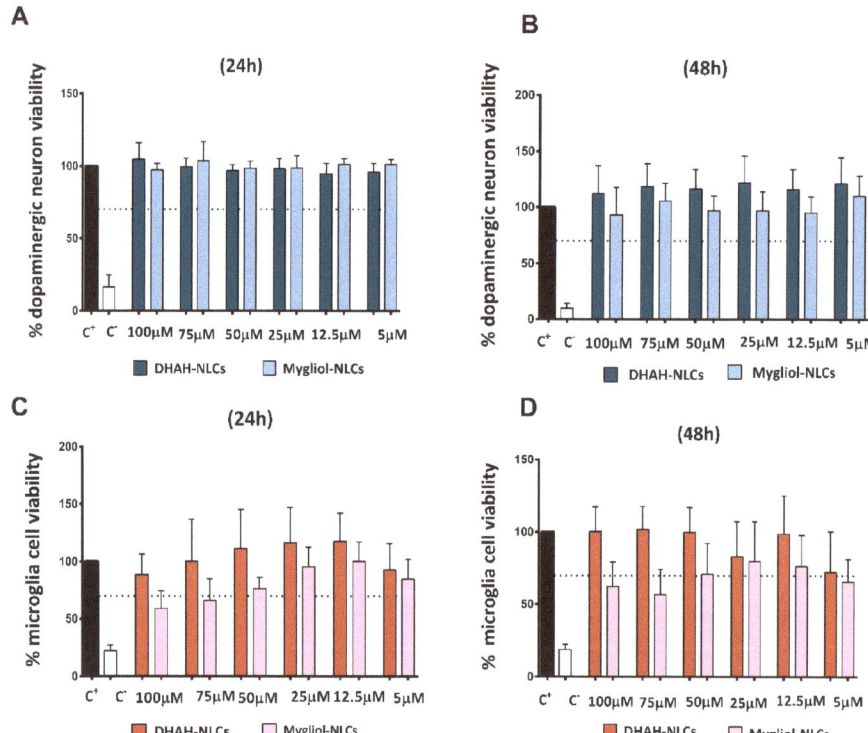

Figure 7. (**A**) Dopaminergic neuron viability at 24 h. (**B**) Dopaminergic neuron viability at 48 h. (**C**) Microglia cell viability at 24 h. (**D**) Microglia cell viability at 48 h. In all cases, different concentrations of DHAH-NLCs and Mygliol-NLCs were tested (the graphs show the results of three biological replicates media ± SD).

3.4. 6-OHDA Neurotoxin Effect on Dopaminergic Culture

The incubation of dopaminergic neurons with 6-OHDA decreased cell viability in a dose-dependent manner (Figure 2B). The incubation of cells with 500 µM of 6-OHDA resulted in only 6.78 ± 4.11 (**** $p < 0.0001$) remaining living cells, which is similar to the values obtained after the incubation with our C$^-$ (DMSO 10%) (5.45 ± 5.2, **** $p < 0.0001$). In the following test concentrations, the values for 100 and 50 µM were below 50% of the remaining living cells; more specifically, for 100 µM (13.82 ± 8.24, **** $p < 0.0001$) and for 50 µM (33.37 ± 11.87, **** $p < 0.0001$), the values were obtained. In the case of 25 µM, the remaining living cells were around 50% (49.05 ± 7.79, **** $p < 0.0001$), and, for 10 µM, it was slightly higher (60.37 ± 24.33, *** $p < 0.001$). Finally, the incubation of dopaminergic cells with 5 µM 6-OHDA neurotoxin led to no statistical difference when compared to the C^+ group, with 87.17 ± 18.02 remaining living cells.

3.5. DHAH-NLCs Exhibited A Neuroprotective Effect

After selecting the dose for generating a cell death of 50% after 24 h of incubation with 6-OHDA, 25 µM, we tried to demonstrate the neuroprotective effect of our DHAH-NLCs. The incubation of the dopaminergic neuron culture with DHAH-NLCs before and after 6-OHDA addition resulted in a neuroprotective effect in comparison to the neurotoxin itself (Figure 2C). The treatment with Mygliol-NLCs did not increase cell viability, with remaining living cell values similar to those obtained with just the neurotoxin incubation. The values for 50 µM Mygliol NLCs (38.35 ± 33.45), 25 µM Mygliol NLCs (49.49 ± 23.15) and 12.5 Mygliol NLCs (54.13 ± 19.11) were similar, without any neuroprotective effect. In contrast, for those cells treated with DHAH-NLCs, the values for the remaining living cells were similar to the control set as 100%. There were no statistical differences between the tested doses with the following values: 50 µM DHAH-NLCs (84.22 ± 10.58, ** $p < 0.01$), 25 µM DHAH-NLCs (82.70 ± 18.96, ** $p < 0.01$) and 12.5 µM DHAH-NLCs (79.92 ± 17.06, * $p < 0.05$). The images taken with fluorescence microscopy showed the difference in living cells, comparing the ones treated with DHAH-NLCs with those treated Mygliol-NLCs (Figure 2D).

3.6. DHAH-NLCs Decreased Cytokine Proinflammatory Release

In order to assess the antiinflammatory effect of our DHAH-enriched nanoparticles (DHAH-NLCs), we performed the ELISA technique from a cell culture supernatant, as described in the Materials and Methods section. The results obtained from the cell supernatants for TNF-α, IL-1β and IL-6 cytokines are summarized in Figure 3B–D.

Regarding TNF-α ELISA (Figure 2B), the basal levels of TNF-α, C^- (204.0 + 23.96) statically increased (**** $p < 0.0001$) after LPS treatment (50 ng/mL), named C^+ (879.4 ± 204.0). In addition, although DHAH-NLCs were not able to obtain control levels of this cytokine, it is noteworthy that the effect of this treatment decreases this proinflammatory cytokine release, as seen in Figure 3B. This effect can be seen in all DHAH-NLCs concentrations: 50 µM DHAH-NLCs (581.0 ± 100.1, *** $p < 0.001$), 25 µM DHAH-NLCs (532.1 ± 186.0, **** $p < 0.0001$) and 12.5 µM DHAH-NLCs (609.2 ± 55.1, ** $p < 0.01$), without any statistically significant differences between the different doses. In the case of Mygliol-NLCs, we could not see any positive effect decreasing cytokine levels for any of the tested concentrations ($p > 0.05$).

For the second tested cytokine, IL-6 (Figure 3C), we also observed the increase of basal levels (213.7 ± 47.3) up to almost double concentration (365.1 ± 125.9, *** $p < 0.001$) after the incubation with LPS. In this case, we could also see the decrease of this proinflammatory cytokine after the treatment with DHAH-NLCs. All the tested concentrations demonstrated a positive effect, decreasing IL-6 levels; indeed, 50 µM DHAH-NLCs (219.3 ± 29.3, ** $p < 0.01$), 25 µM DHAH-NLCs (232.7 ± 40.8, * $p < 0.05$) and 12.5 µM DHAH-NLCs (237.2 ± 15.4, * $p < 0.05$) were the obtained values. However, no statistically significant differences were observed between the different concentrations. Regarding Mygliol-NLCs, no antiinflammatory effect was obtained after the treatment with these nanoparticles for any of the tested concentrations ($p > 0.05$).

Finally, we analyzed the levels of IL-1β proinflammatory cytokine (Figure 3D). In this case, the LPS stimuli also increased the basal values (457.4 ± 125.8) more than three-fold, as we can see for the C^+ values (1495.0 ± 518.1, ** $p < 0.01$). As seen before with the other two proinflammatory cytokines, the treatment with DHAH-NLCs decreased IL-1β values. Actually, the values for DHAH-NLCs were the following: 50 µM DHAH-NLCs (726.2 ± 256.6, * $p < 0.05$), 25 µM DHAH-NLCs (948.7 ± 301.6) and 12.5 µM

DHAH-NLCs (985.6 ± 301.0). Although in this case only the group treated with 50 µM DHAH-NLCs showed a statistically significant difference, the trend to decrease this proinflammatory cytokine is notorious in all DHAH-NLCs concentrations. As in the previously analyzed proinflammatory cytokines, the levels of IL-1β remained elevated for the cells treated with Mygliol-NLCs, for any of the tested conditions, showing values similar to the positive control.

4. Discussion

NDs are one of the main problems of the public health system in the 21st century. Although they have different clinical manifestations and symptoms, they all share a complex mechanism of neurodegeneration, with aging as the main risk factor, and they are without an effective treatment [1,48]. In order to obtain an effective treatment for NDs, in the last few years, different therapeutic molecules have been raised as new clinical candidates. Among others, the use of functional lipids such as PUFAs and, more concretely, DHA and DHAH have been raised as a useful tool to treat NDs since they exhibit beneficial effects, decreasing neuroinflammation and protein deposit or increasing the release of neuroprotective agents [30,49]. However, no matter the treatment, one of the main issues with treating NDs is reaching the brain and passing through the BBB. That is why the use of nanotechnology and, more concretely, the NLCs, has exhibited promising results for targeting the brain, increasing bioavailability, protecting from oxidation and, therefore, maintaining the bioactivity of different molecules [19].

The main goal of this work was to combine both strategies to develop a new therapeutic nanocarrier enriched with PUFAs, more concretely, with DHAH, to generate a new type of NP that could target the brain and exhibit neuroprotective and antiinflammatory effects, therefore becoming a functional nanocarrier that could be combined with different molecules in the future to promote a synergistic therapy.

All the developed nanoformulations were 50–90 nm in size, with a PDI value below 0.5 indicating a homogenous suspension (Figure 4). The increment of the liquid lipid ratio led to a decrease in the size of the nanoparticles, as shown in previous publications (Table 2) [50,51]. Moreover, as seen in DSC thermograms (Figure A1), the addition of the liquid lipid to the solid lipid led to a slight reduction of the melting point of Precirol of 3–4 °C in all NLC thermograms, which is similar to previously conducted studies [50,52,53]. Anyway, the selected solid:liquid lipid ratio for the two different lipids, Mygliol and DHAH, was in the ratio normally used for NLC preparation [24]. After selecting the ratio and the lipid to constitute the new nanoformulation, the NPs' surface was modified with the addition of CS and TAT, resulting in two different formulations, named DHAH-NLCs and Mygliol-NLCs. The addition of CS and TAT peptide led to the conversion of Z potential from negative values to positive values (Tables 2 and 3), indicating that the undergoing process was successfully performed. Moreover, the presence of amide I in FTIR spectra (Figure A2) confirmed that the coating process with TAT was successfully performed. As we have previously demonstrated, the addition of CS and TAT increased in vivo brain targeting after intranasal administration [16,24]. Moreover, TAT is a well-known CPP, usually used to enhance the delivery of different cargos into different types of cells, such as neurons [54,55]. The resulting NPs were similar in size (around 100 nm) and exhibited positive zeta values due to the successful CS coating process (Table 3).

Among the different NDs, in this research paper, we aim to study the effect of our newly developed nanocarriers in a cell model of PD by adding 6-OHDA neurotoxin, one of the most widely used neurotoxins, to a dopaminergic cell culture to mimic the destruction of catecholaminergic neurons and the degeneration of the nigrostriatal pathway [56]. The addition of 25 µM 6-0HDA for 24 h led to a decrease in cell viability of 50%, as shown in Figure 2B. The dose and incubation time for this neurotoxin is variable, according to the scientific data available, varying from 5 to 100 µM and from 30 min to 48 h [57–60]. That is why we incubated the neuronal cells with different doses for 24 h, an intermediate time point in the published articles, and selected the dose that generated 50% cell death so we could really see the effect of the neurotoxin on cell viability. In order to check the safety and effectiveness of the DHAH incorporated into our NLCs, we incubated the nanoformulations for 24 and 48 h. All tested concentrations were shown to be safe (Figure 7A,B), with a viability up to 70% and showing better values for DHAH-NLCs at 48 h. Moreover, the effectiveness of DHAH-NLCs was also evaluated in dopaminergic cell cultures after the incubation with 6-OHDA. DHAH-NLCs were shown to be effective at protecting the cells from the neurotoxin compared to Mygliol-NLCs as the control group (Figure 2C,D). These data are in line with previous publications regarding the DHA neuroprotective effect shown in neuron cell cultures [61,62]. Moreover, it demonstrates the effectiveness of the DHAH functional lipid incorporated into the newly developed NLCs.

On the other hand, the neuroinflammatory process undergoing NDs and, more specifically, in PD is well known, being the consequence or the cause of the disease. Whatever the origin of the neuroinflammation, it is a fact that a therapeutic intervention downregulating this process could be great at halting the progression of the disease [63]. Although different cell types and molecules are involved in the neuroinflammation, microglia cells are the primary initiators of the central inflammatory response to acute and chronic disorders related to NDs [64]. In order to treat this inflammatory response, PUFAs and, more concretely, DHA and DHAH have been raised as emerging candidates to downregulate this process and become a new therapeutic approach [9,31]. The DHAH-NLCs developed in this study were shown to be safe at any of the tested concentrations, with a viability up to 70%, in contrast to Mygliol-NLCs, where higher concentrations decreased cell viability (Figure 7C,D). Thus, these results demonstrated that the newly developed formulation with DHAH can be used in high concentrations without affecting cell viability.

In order to mimic the neuroinflammatory process in primary microglia cells, different molecules can be used. Among them, the gold standard stimuli for generating reactive gliosis and activating the neuroinflammation cascade is LPS. LPS has been widely used to generate animal models of neuroinflammation or induce it in cell culture, both primary and microglia cell lines [65–67]. The addition of LPS at 50 ng/mL concentration in this study generated the production of proinflammatory cytokines in similar levels to those in previously published scientific articles for microglia primary cell cultures isolated after the shaking method [66]. Regarding the potential antiinflammatory effect of our NPs, we showed that the ability of DHAH to decrease neuroinflammation was maintained in DHAH-NLCs, obtaining proinflammatory cytokine levels similar to C− in IL-6 and IL-1β, and decreasing TNF-α almost by half for any of the tested concentrations (Figure 3B–D). The ability of PUFAs to decrease the cytokine proinflammatory levels has previously been described [68]; thus, this study enforces the use of these kinds of PUFAs formulated in NLCs as an emerging tool to treat the undergoing inflammatory process in NDs.

5. Conclusions

Altogether, these results highlight that the newly developed nanocarriers can constitute a new therapeutic tool for treating NDs. The DHAH-NLCs were similar to previously developed NLCs in size, PDI, zeta values and TEM morphology. Moreover, they exhibited neuroprotective effects in a cell culture model of dopaminergic neurons and antiinflammatory properties, decreasing proinflammatory cytokine levels in primary microglia cell cultures. Although future studies are needed to check its suitability in a different cell culture model or animal model of the disease, the results presented in this research article are promising for this new functional nanocarrier. Moreover, the combination of this new, safe and effective nanocarrier with different clinically approved or investigated therapeutic molecules could become in an emerging tool to treat, in a synergistic manner, the symptoms associated with NDs.

Author Contributions: Conceptualization, S.H., E.H., M.I. and R.M.H.; writing—original draft preparation, S.H.; writing—review and editing, S.H., E.H., M.I. and R.M.H.; visualization, S.H.; supervision, E.H., M.I. and R.M.H.; project administration, E.H., M.I. and R.M.H.; funding acquisition, M.I. and R.M.H. All authors have read and agreed to the published version of the manuscript.

Funding: This project was partially supported by the Spanish Ministry of Economy and Competitiveness (RTC-2015-3542-1) and the Basque Government (Consolidated Groups, IT 907-16).

Acknowledgments: The authors give thanks for the technical and human support provided by SGIker of UPV/EHU and European funding (ERDF and ESF). S. Hernando thanks the Basque Government for the fellowship grant.

Conflicts of Interest: The authors declare no conflict of interest.

Appendix A

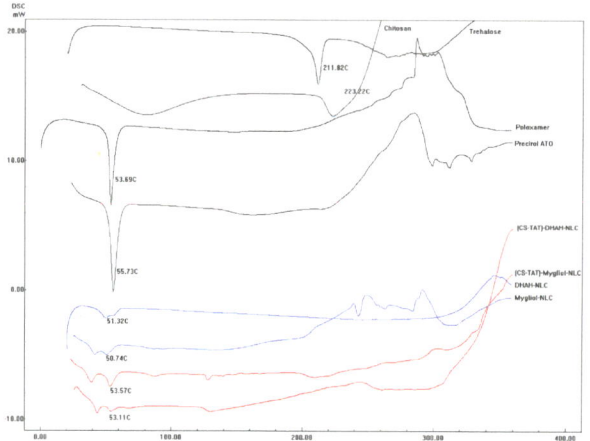

Figure A1. Differential scanning calorimetry (DSC) graphs of pure excipients (D-trehalose, Poloxamer 188, Precirol ATO 5, chitosan (CS) and the different developed nanoparticles).

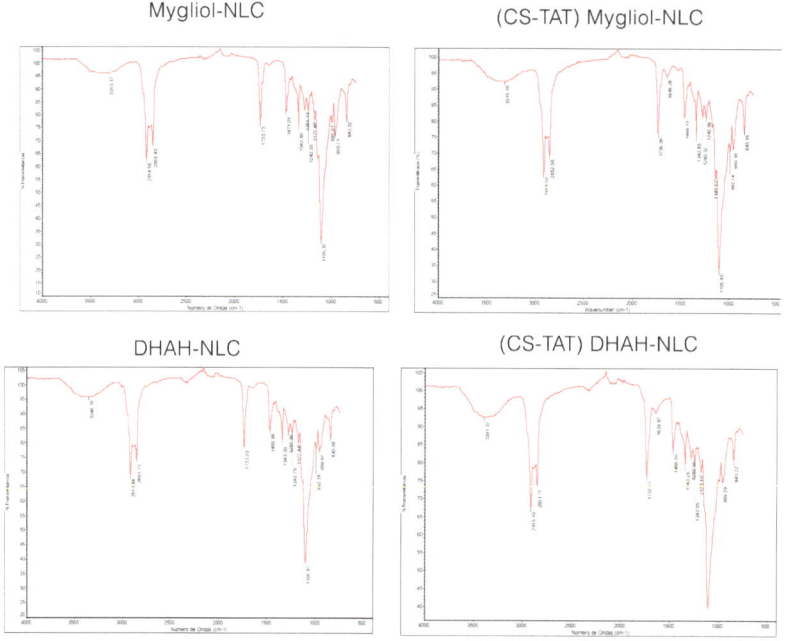

Figure A2. FTIR spectra of Mygliol-NLC, (CS-TAT) Mygliol-NLC, DHAH-NLC and (CS-TAT) DHAH-NL.

References

1. Hou, Y.; Dan, X.; Babbar, M.; Wei, Y.; Hasselbalch, S.G.; Croteau, D.L.; Bohr, V.A. Ageing as a risk factor for neurodegenerative disease. *Nat. Rev. Neurol.* **2019**, *15*, 565–581. [CrossRef] [PubMed]
2. Kalia, L.V.; Lang, A.E. Parkinson's disease. *Lancet* **2015**, *386*, 896–912. [CrossRef]
3. Scheltens, P.; Blennow, K.; Breteler, M.M.B.; de Strooper, B.; Frisoni, G.B.; Salloway, S.; Van der Flier, W.M. Alzheimer's disease. *Lancet* **2016**, *388*, 505–517. [CrossRef]
4. Kalia, L.V.; Kalia, S.K.; Lang, A.E. Disease-modifying strategies for Parkinson's disease. *Mov. Disord.* **2015**, *30*, 1442–1450. [CrossRef]
5. Xie, A.; Gao, J.; Xu, L.; Meng, D. Shared mechanisms of neurodegeneration in Alzheimer's disease and Parkinson's disease, Biomed. *Res. Int.* **2014**, *2014*, 648740.
6. Oertel, W.; Schulz, J.B. Current and experimental treatments of Parkinson disease: A guide for neuroscientists. *J. Neurochem.* **2016**, *139* (Suppl. 1), 325–337. [CrossRef]
7. Briggs, R.; Kennelly, S.P.; O'Neill, D. Drug treatments in Alzheimer's disease. *Clin. Med. (Lond).* **2016**, *16*, 247–253. [CrossRef]
8. Sarubbo, F.; Moranta, D.; Asensio, V.J.; Miralles, A.; Esteban, S. Effects of Resveratrol and Other Polyphenols on the Most Common Brain Age-Related Diseases. *Curr. Med. Chem.* **2017**, *24*, 4245–4266. [CrossRef]
9. Bazinet, R.P.; Laye, S. Polyunsaturated fatty acids and their metabolites in brain function and disease. *Nat. Rev. Neurosci.* **2014**, *15*, 771–785. [CrossRef]
10. Allen, S.J.; Watson, J.J.; Shoemark, D.K.; Barua, N.U.; Patel, N.K. GDNF, NGF and BDNF as therapeutic options for neurodegeneration. *Pharmacol. Ther.* **2013**, *138*, 155–175. [CrossRef]
11. Garbayo, E.; Estella-Hermoso de Mendoza, A.; Blanco-Prieto, M.J. Diagnostic and therapeutic uses of nanomaterials in the brain. *Curr. Med. Chem.* **2014**, *21*, 4100–4131. [CrossRef] [PubMed]
12. Hernando, S.; Herran, E.; Pedraz, J.L.; Igartua, M.; Hernandez, R.M. Nanotechnology Based Approaches for Neurodegenerative Disorders: Diagnosis and Treatment. In *Drug and Gene Delivery to the Central Nervous System for Neuroprotection*; Sharma, H.S., Muresanu, D.F., Sharma, A., Eds.; Springer International Publishing: Cham, Switzerland, 2017; pp. 57–87.
13. Meredith, M.E.; Salameh, T.S.; Banks, W.A. Intranasal Delivery of Proteins and Peptides in the Treatment of Neurodegenerative Diseases. *AAPS J.* **2015**, *17*, 780–787. [CrossRef] [PubMed]
14. Gambaryan, P.Y.; Kondrasheva, I.G.; Severin, E.S.; Guseva, A.A.; Kamensky, A.A. Increasing the Efficiency of Parkinson's Disease Treatment Using a poly(lactic-co-glycolic acid) (PLGA) Based L-DOPA Delivery System. *Exp Neurobiol.* **2014**, *23*, 246–252. [CrossRef] [PubMed]
15. Gartziandia, O.; Herrán, E.; Ruiz-Ortega, J.A.; Miguelez, C.; Igartua, M.; Lafuente, J.V.; Pedraz, J.L.; Ugedo, L.; Hernández, R.M. Intranasal administration of chitosan-coated nanostructured lipid carriers loaded with GDNF improves behavioral and histological recovery in a partial lesion model of Parkinson's disease. *J. Biomed. Nanotechnol.* **2016**, *12*, 1–11. [CrossRef]
16. Gartziandia, O.; Egusquiaguirre, S.P.; Bianco, J.; Pedraz, J.L.; Igartua, M.; Hernandez, R.M.; Préat, V.; Beloqui, A. Nanoparticle transport across in vitro olfactory cell monolayers. *Int. J. Pharm.* **2016**, *499*, 81–89. [CrossRef] [PubMed]
17. Kanazawa, T.; Akiyama, F.; Kakizaki, S.; Takashima, Y.; Seta, Y. Delivery of siRNA to the brain using a combination of nose-to-brain delivery and cell-penetrating peptide-modified nano-micelles. *Biomaterials* **2013**, *34*, 9220–9226. [CrossRef] [PubMed]
18. Hernando, S.; Gartziandia, O.; Herran, E.; Pedraz, J.L.; Igartua, M.; Hernandez, R.M. Advances in nanomedicine for the treatment of Alzheimer's and Parkinson's diseases. *Nanomedicine (Lond)* **2016**, *11*, 1267–1285. [CrossRef]
19. Re, F.; Gregori, M.; Masserini, M. Nanotechnology for neurodegenerative disorders. *Matur.* **2012**, *73*, 45–51. [CrossRef]
20. Srikanth, M.; Kessler, J.A. Nanotechnology-novel therapeutics for CNS disorders. *Nat. Rev. Neurol.* **2012**, *8*, 307–318. [CrossRef]
21. Da Rocha Lindner, G.; Bonfanti Santos, D.; Colle, D.; Gasnhar Moreira, E.L.; Daniel Prediger, R.; Farina, M.; Khalil, N.M.; Mara Mainardes, R. Improved neuroprotective effects of resveratrol-loaded polysorbate 80-coated poly(lactide) nanoparticles in MPTP-induced Parkinsonism. *Nanomedicine (Lond)* **2015**, *10*, 1127–1138. [CrossRef]

22. Sharma, S.; Lohan, S.; Murthy, R.S.R. Formulation and characterization of intranasal mucoadhesive nanoparticulates and thermo-reversible gel of levodopa for brain delivery. *Drug Dev. Ind. Pharm.* **2014**, *40*, 869–878. [CrossRef] [PubMed]
23. Shah, B.; Khunt, D.; Bhatt, H.; Misra, M.; Padh, H. Application of quality by design approach for intranasal delivery of rivastigmine loaded solid lipid nanoparticles: Effect on formulation and characterization parameters. *Eur. J. Pharm. Sci.* **2015**, *78*, 54–66. [CrossRef]
24. Hernando, S.; Herran, E.; Figueiro-Silva, J.; Pedraz, J.L.; Igartua, M.; Carro, E.; Hernandez, R.M. Intranasal Administration of TAT-Conjugated Lipid Nanocarriers Loading GDNF for Parkinson's Disease. *Mol. Neurobiol.* **2018**, *55*, 145–155. [CrossRef] [PubMed]
25. Beloqui, A.; Solinís, M.Á.; Rodríguez-Gascón, A.; Almeida, A.J.; Préat, V. Nanostructured lipid carriers: Promising drug delivery systems for future clinics. *Nanomedicine* **2016**, *12*, 143–161. [CrossRef] [PubMed]
26. Inês Teixeira, M.; Lopes, C.M.; Helena Amaral, M.; Costa, P.C. Current insights on lipid nanocarrier-assisted drug delivery in the treatment of neurodegenerative diseases. *Eur. J. Pharm. Biopharm.* **2020**, *149*, 192–217. [CrossRef]
27. Pedraz, J.L.; Igartua, M.; Maria, R.; Hernando, S. The role of lipid nanoparticles and its surface modification in reaching the brain: An approach for neurodegenerative diseases treatment. *Curr. Drug Deliv.* **2018**, *15*, 1218–1220.
28. Nanjwade, B.K.; Patel, D.J.; Udhani, R.A.; Manvi, F.V. Functions of lipids for enhancement of oral bioavailability of poorly water-soluble drugs. *Sci. Pharm.* **2011**, *79*, 705–727. [CrossRef]
29. Agrawal, Y.; Petkar, K.C.; Sawant, K.K. Development, evaluation and clinical studies of Acitretin loaded nanostructured lipid carriers for topical treatment of psoriasis. *Int. J. Pharm.* **2010**, *401*, 93–102. [CrossRef]
30. Hashimoto, M.; Hossain, S.; Mamun, A.A.; Matsuzaki, K.; Arai, H. Docosahexaenoic acid: One molecule diverse functions. *Crit. Rev. Biotechnol.* **2017**, *37*, 579–597. [CrossRef]
31. Hernando, S.; Requejo, C.; Herran, E.; Ruiz-Ortega, J.A.; Morera-Herreras, T.; Lafuente, J.V.; Ugedo, L.; Gainza, E.; Pedraz, J.L.; Igartua, M.; et al. Beneficial effects of n-3 polyunsaturated fatty acids administration in a partial lesion model of Parkinson's disease: The role of glia and NRf2 regulation. *Neurobiol. Dis.* **2019**, *121*, 252–262. [CrossRef]
32. Boudrault, C.; Bazinet, R.P.; Ma, D.W.L. Experimental models and mechanisms underlying the protective effects of n-3 polyunsaturated fatty acids in Alzheimer's disease. *J. Nutr. Biochem.* **2009**, *20*, 1–10. [CrossRef] [PubMed]
33. Hang, L.; Basil, A.H.; Lim, K.L. Nutraceuticals in Parkinson's Disease. *Neuromol. Med.* **2016**, *18*, 306–321. [CrossRef] [PubMed]
34. Avallone, R.; Vitale, G.; Bertolotti, M. Omega-3 Fatty Acids and Neurodegenerative Diseases: New Evidence in Clinical Trials. *Int. J. Mol. Sci.* **2019**, *20*, 4256. [CrossRef] [PubMed]
35. De Lau, L.M.; Bornebroek, M.; Witteman, J.C.; Hofman, A.; Koudstaal, P.J.; Breteler, M.M. Dietary fatty acids and the risk of Parkinson disease: The Rotterdam study. *Neurology* **2005**, *64*, 2040–2045. [CrossRef] [PubMed]
36. Morris, M.C.; Tangney, C.C.; Wang, Y.; Sacks, F.M.; Bennett, D.A.; Aggarwal, N.T. MIND diet associated with reduced incidence of Alzheimer's disease. *Alzheimers Dement.* **2015**, *11*, 1007–1014. [CrossRef]
37. Yadav, S.C.; Kumari, A.; Yadav, R. Development of peptide and protein nanotherapeutics by nanoencapsulation and nanobioconjugation. *Peptides* **2011**, *32*, 173–187. [CrossRef]
38. Layek, B.; Singh, J. Cell penetrating peptide conjugated polymeric micelles as a high performance versatile nonviral gene carrier. *Biomacromolecules* **2013**, *14*, 4071–4081. [CrossRef]
39. Costa, F.; Maia, S.; Gomes, J.; Gomes, P.; Martins, M.C. Characterization of hLF1-11 immobilization onto chitosan ultrathin films, and its effects on antimicrobial activity. *Acta Biomater.* **2014**, *10*, 3513–3521. [CrossRef]
40. Weinert, M.; Selvakumar, T.; Tierney, T.S.; Alavian, K.N. Isolation, culture and long-term maintenance of primary mesencephalic dopaminergic neurons from embryonic rodent brains. *J. Vis. Exp.* **2015**, *96*, 52475. [CrossRef]
41. Skaper, S.D.; Barbierato, M.; Ferrari, V.; Zusso, M.; Facci, L. Culture of Rat Mesencephalic Dopaminergic Neurons and Application to Neurotoxic and Neuroprotective Agents. *Methods Mol. Biol.* **2018**, *1727*, 107–118.
42. Gaven, F.; Marin, P.; Claeysen, S. Primary culture of mouse dopaminergic neurons. *J. Vis. Exp.* **2014**, *91*, e51751. [CrossRef] [PubMed]
43. Chen, X.; Zhang, Y.; Sadadcharam, G.; Cui, W.; Wang, J.H. Isolation, Purification, and Culture of Primary Murine Microglia Cells. *Bio-protocol* **2013**, *3*, e314. [CrossRef]

44. Gainza, G.; Pastor, M.; Aguirre, J.J.; Villullas, S.; Pedraz, J.L.; Hernandez, R.M.; Igartua, M. A novel strategy for the treatment of chronic wounds based on the topical administration of rhEGF-loaded lipid nanoparticles: In vitro bioactivity and in vivo effectiveness in healing-impaired db/db mice. *J. Controlled Release* **2014**, *185*, 51–61. [CrossRef] [PubMed]
45. Garcia-Orue, I.; Gainza, G.; Girbau, C.; Alonso, R.; Aguirre, J.J.; Pedraz, J.L.; Igartua, M.; Hernandez, R.M. LL37 loaded nanostructured lipid carriers (NLC): A new strategy for the topical treatment of chronic wounds. *Eur. J. Pharm. Biopharm.* **2016**, *108*, 310–316. [CrossRef]
46. Pastor, M.; Basas, J.; Vairo, C.; Gainza, G.; Moreno-Sastre, M.; Gomis, X.; Fleischer, A.; Palomino, E.; Bachiller, D.; Gutiérrez, F.B.; et al. Safety and effectiveness of sodium colistimethate-loaded nanostructured lipid carriers (SCM-NLC) against P. aeruginosa: In vitro and in vivo studies following pulmonary and intramuscular administration. *Nanomedicine* **2019**, *18*, 101–111. [CrossRef]
47. Gartziandia, O.; Herran, E.; Pedraz, J.L.; Carro, E.; Igartua, M.; Hernandez, R.M. Chitosan coated nanostructured lipid carriers for brain delivery of proteins by intranasal administration. *Colloids Surf. B Biointerfaces* **2015**, *134*, 304–313. [CrossRef]
48. Gan, L.; Cookson, M.R.; Petrucelli, L.; La Spada, A.R. Converging pathways in neurodegeneration, from genetics to mechanisms. *Nat. Neurosci.* **2018**, *21*, 1300–1309. [CrossRef]
49. Sun, G.Y.; Simonyi, A.; Fritsche, K.L.; Chuang, D.Y.; Hannink, M.; Gu, Z.; Greenlief, C.M.; Yao, J.K.; Lee, J.C.; Beversdorf, D.Q. Docosahexaenoic acid (DHA): An essential nutrient and a nutraceutical for brain health and diseases. *Prostaglandins Leukot Essent. Fatty Acids* **2017**, *136*, 3–13. [CrossRef]
50. Saedi, A.; Rostamizadeh, K.; Parsa, M.; Dalali, N.; Ahmadi, N. Preparation and characterization of nanostructured lipid carriers as drug delivery system: Influence of liquid lipid types on loading and cytotoxicity. *Chem. Phys. Lipids* **2018**, *216*, 65–72. [CrossRef]
51. Gokce, E.H.; Korkmaz, E.; Dellera, E.; Sandri, G.; Bonferoni, M.C.; Ozer, O. Resveratrol-loaded solid lipid nanoparticles versus nanostructured lipid carriers: Evaluation of antioxidant potential for dermal applications. *Int. J. Nanomed.* **2012**, *7*, 1841–1850. [CrossRef]
52. Thatipamula, R.; Palem, C.; Gannu, R.; Mudragada, S.; Yamsani, M. Formulation and in vitro characterization of domperidone loaded solid lipid nanoparticles and nanostructured lipid carriers. *DARU* **2011**, *19*, 23–32. [PubMed]
53. Huguet-Casquero, A.; Moreno-Sastre, M.; Lopez-Mendez, T.B.; Gainza, E.; Pedraz, J.L. Encapsulation of Oleuropein in Nanostructured Lipid Carriers: Biocompatibility and Antioxidant Efficacy in Lung Epithelial. *Cells. Pharm.* **2020**, *12*, 429. [CrossRef] [PubMed]
54. Suk, J.S.; Suh, J.; Choy, K.; Lai, S.K.; Fu, J.; Hanes, J. Gene delivery to differentiated neurotypic cells with RGD and HIV Tat peptide functionalized polymeric nanoparticles. *Biomaterials* **2006**, *27*, 5143–5150. [CrossRef]
55. Peng, L.; Niu, J.; Zhang, C.; Yu, W.; Wu, J.; Shan, Y.; Wang, X.; Shen, Y.; Mao, Z.; Liang, W.; et al. TAT conjugated cationic noble metal nanoparticles for gene delivery to epidermal stem cells. *Biomaterials* **2014**, *35*, 5605–5618. [CrossRef] [PubMed]
56. Schober, A. Classic toxin-induced animal models of Parkinson's disease: 6-OHDA and MPTP. *Cell Tissue Res.* **2004**, *318*, 215–224. [CrossRef] [PubMed]
57. Carrasco, E.; Werner, P. Selective destruction of dopaminergic neurons by low concentrations of 6-OHDA and MPP+: Protection by acetylsalicylic acid aspirin. *Parkinsonism Relat. Disord.* **2002**, *8*, 407–411. [CrossRef]
58. Wang, G.Q.; Li, D.D.; Huang, C.; Lu, D.S.; Zhang, C.; Zhou, S.Y.; Liu, J.; Zhang, F. Icariin Reduces Dopaminergic Neuronal Loss and Microglia-Mediated Inflammation in Vivo and in Vitro. *Front. Mol. Neurosci.* **2018**, *10*, 441. [CrossRef]
59. Yuan, W.J.; Yasuhara, T.; Shingo, T.; Muraoka, K.; Agari, T.; Kameda, M.; Uozumi, T.; Tajiri, N.; Morimoto, T.; Jing, M.; et al. Neuroprotective effects of edaravone-administration on 6-OHDA-treated dopaminergic neurons. *BMC Neurosci.* **2008**, *9*, 75.
60. Callizot, N.; Combes, M.; Henriques, A.; Poindron, P. Necrosis, apoptosis, necroptosis, three modes of action of dopaminergic neuron neurotoxins. *PLoS ONE* **2019**, *14*, e0215277. [CrossRef]
61. Cao, D.; Xue, R.; Xu, J.; Liu, Z. Effects of docosahexaenoic acid on the survival and neurite outgrowth of rat cortical neurons in primary cultures. *J. Nutr. Biochem.* **2005**, *16*, 538–546. [CrossRef]
62. Wang, P.-Y.; Chen, J.-J.; Su, H.-M. Docosahexaenoic acid supplementation of primary rat hippocampal neurons attenuates the neurotoxicity induced by aggregated amyloid beta protein (42) and up-regulates cytoskeletal protein expression. *J. Nutr. Biochem.* **2010**, *21*, 345–350. [CrossRef]

63. Hirsch, E.C.; Hunot, S. Neuroinflammation in Parkinson's disease: A target for neuroprotection? *Lancet Neurol.* **2009**, *8*, 382–397. [CrossRef]
64. Thurgur, H.; Pinteaux, E. Microglia in the Neurovascular Unit: Blood-Brain Barrier-microglia Interactions after Central Nervous System Disorders. *Neuroscience* **2019**, *405*, 55–67. [CrossRef] [PubMed]
65. Fourrier, C.; Remus-Borel, J.; Greenhalgh, A.D.; Guichardant, M.; Bernoud-Hubac, N.; Lagarde, M.; Joffre, C.; Laye, S. Docosahexaenoic acid-containing choline phospholipid modulates LPS-induced neuroinflammation in vivo and in microglia in vitro. *J. Neuroinflamm.* **2017**, *14*, 170. [CrossRef] [PubMed]
66. Lin, L.; Desai, R.; Wang, X.; Lo, E.H.; Xing, C. Characteristics of primary rat microglia isolated from mixed cultures using two different methods. *J. Neuroinflamm.* **2017**, *14*, 101. [CrossRef]
67. De Smedt-Peyrusse, V.; Sargueil, F.; Moranis, A.; Harizi, H.; Mongrand, S.; Laye, S. Docosahexaenoic acid prevents lipopolysaccharide-induced cytokine production in microglial cells by inhibiting lipopolysaccharide receptor presentation but not its membrane subdomain localization. *J. Neurochem.* **2008**, *105*, 296–307. [CrossRef]
68. Laye, S.; Nadjar, A.; Joffre, C.; Bazinet, R.P. Anti-Inflammatory Effects of Omega-3 Fatty Acids in the Brain: Physiological Mechanisms and Relevance to Pharmacology. *Pharmacol. Rev.* **2018**, *70*, 12–38. [CrossRef]

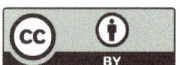

© 2020 by the authors. Licensee MDPI, Basel, Switzerland. This article is an open access article distributed under the terms and conditions of the Creative Commons Attribution (CC BY) license (http://creativecommons.org/licenses/by/4.0/).

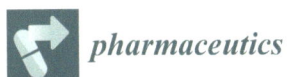 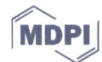

Article

Design, Optimization, Manufacture and Characterization of Efavirenz-Loaded Flaxseed Oil Nanoemulsions

Priveledge Mazonde, Sandile M. M. Khamanga and Roderick B. Walker

Department of Pharmaceutics, Faculty of Pharmacy, Rhodes University, Makhanda 6140, South Africa; pmazonde@live.com (P.M.); S.Khamanga@ru.ac.za (S.M.M.K.)
* Correspondence: r.b.walker@ru.ac.za; Tel.: +27-46-603-8412

Received: 20 July 2020; Accepted: 13 August 2020; Published: 23 August 2020

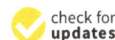

Abstract: The formation, manufacture and characterization of low energy water-in-oil (w/o) nanoemulsions prepared using cold pressed flaxseed oil containing efavirenz was investigated. Pseudo-ternary phase diagrams were constructed to identify the nanoemulsion region(s). Other potential lipid-based drug delivery phases containing flaxseed oil with 1:1 m/m surfactant mixture of Tween® 80, Span® 20 and different amounts of ethanol were tested to characterize the impact of surfactant mixture on emulsion formation. Flaxseed oil was used as the oil phase as efavirenz exhibited high solubility in the vehicle when compared to other vegetable oils tested. Optimization of surfactant mixtures was undertaken using design of experiments, specifically a D-optimal design with the flaxseed oil content set at 10% m/m. Two solutions from the desired optimization function were produced based on desirability and five nanoemulsion formulations were produced and characterized in terms of in vitro release of efavirenz, physical and chemical stability. Metastable nanoemulsions containing 10% m/m flaxseed oil were successfully manufactured and significant isotropic gel (semisolid) and o/w emulsions were observed during phase behavior studies. Droplet sizes ranged between 156 and 225 nm, zeta potential between −24 and −41 mV and all formulations were found to be monodisperse with polydispersity indices ≤ 0.487.

Keywords: nanoemulsion(s); phase-behavior; DoE; D-optimal design; vegetable oils; non-ionic surfactants; efavirenz; flaxseed oil

1. Introduction

The human immunodeficiency virus (HIV) is a global health burden. At the end of June 2019, approximately 24.5 million people were accessing antiretroviral therapy [1]. In efforts to improve access to HIV drugs, simplification of process chemistry, reformulation, dose reduction, inclusion of new drug classes and new therapeutic strategies have been developed and contributed to the reduction of the HIV burden [2]. Efavirenz (EFV) is a non-nucleoside reverse-transcriptase inhibitor (NNRTI) used, in combination, for first line treatment of HIV. EFV is a BCS Class II or poorly soluble and highly permeable compound with an aqueous solubility of <10 mg/mL and low bioavailability of approximately 40% [3]. Caco-2 and intestinal permeability studies suggest EFV is highly permeable [4] and the clinical efficacy may be limited by low solubility. The log P of 4.6 for EFV suggests it may be a good candidate for formulation into a lipid based drug delivery system [5,6].

Lipid-based drug delivery systems (LBDDS) specifically, self-nanoemulsifying drug delivery systems (SNEDDS) are a useful approach for overcoming poor solubility and low oral bioavailability of some drugs [7–9]. The different classes of LBDDS include micro and nanoemulsions, of which the latter are single optically isotropic and metastable liquid solutions with droplet sizes ranging between 20 nm and 600 nm with some published reports suggesting a maximum particle size of 300 nm and 1000 nm [10–12]. Microemulsions are mixtures of oil, water and surfactant which are single optically isotropic, transparent thermodynamically stable solutions which form spontaneously when thermodynamic variables such as temperature and composition are met with droplet sizes of up to 100 nm [13].

Crude edible vegetable oils are readily available, economic and green chemistry products with functional food properties that exhibit numerous health benefits for patients and have been used in LBDDS [14]. Grapeseed, flaxseed and soybean oil are rich in poly unsaturated fatty acid, such as α-linoleic acid, content which is positively associated with cardiovascular health due to down-regulation of low-density lipoprotein cholesterol production. Diets rich in α-linoleic acid inhibit lymphocyte proliferation and the immune response in healthy humans and thus may be beneficial to individuals that present with autoimmune disorders [15]. Nanoemulsions that require low-energy input are relatively simple and inexpensive to manufacture if an appropriate surfactant mixture for a specific oil phase is used however, research relating to the formation, phase behavior and microstructure of nanoemulsions produced using food grade materials has not been conducted. Crude edible oils are difficult to solubilize in o/w nanoemulsions [16] and low-energy production methods take advantage of the intrinsic physicochemical properties of the components in order to generate sub-micron droplets. The use of a co-surfactant and/or co-solvent may be required to solubilize multicomponent oil or crude cold pressed materials sufficiently, to ensure that single or isotropic phases are formed. Ethanol used in concentrations ranging between 10% and 20% v/v is acceptable for food applications and can be used as a co-solvent to produce nanoemulsions. Legislation about the use of ethanol as an excipient, particularly for pediatric medicines differs from country to country, consequently formulations should comply with the regulatory requirements in the country of origin [17]. Co-solvents may improve the solubility of the oil, surfactant, co-surfactant and active pharmaceutical compounds while also functioning as penetration enhancers or altering bulk properties such as viscosity, density, refractive index and interfacial tension of aqueous solutions [18].

Nanoemulsions have small droplet sizes that ensure a large interfacial surface area is available to facilitate drug absorption and nanoemulsions or lipid based nanoformulations can enhance intestinal lymphatic transport of drugs and therefore circumvent the hepatic first pass effect [19]. Mechanisms of transport include an increase in membrane fluidity that facilitates transcellular absorption and opening of tight junctions that facilitate paracellular transport [20].

Critical quality attributes (CQA) of nanoemulsions include droplet size (PS), polydispersity index (PDI), zeta potential (ZP) and drug loading capacity (DLC). In addition, there is a need to understand physiological processes such as hepatic uptake and accumulation, tissue diffusion, tissue extravasation and renal excretion as a function of droplet size. Nano carriers of diameter between 100 and 150 nm circulating in blood vessels do not easily leave the capillaries that perfuse tissues such as the kidney, lung, heart and brain. In contrast smaller droplets between 20 and 100 nm may distribute into the bone marrow, spleen and liver sinusoids and may leave the vasculature via fenestrated capillaries in the perfused organs [21,22]. In the case of efavirenz and associated central nervous system adverse effects, small droplet sizes < 100 nm may lead to more pronounced side effects due to the associated increase in blood brain barrier permeability and the pathophysiology of acute and/or chronic CNS disease [23,24]. The PDI describes the uniformity or lack thereof of the size distribution of particles and PDI values < 0.05 are only observed for monodisperse standards whereas PDI values > 0.7 indicate that the sample exhibits a broad size distribution. The ZP can influence the stability of products, cellular uptake and intracellular trafficking of emulsions [25]. Generally, nanoemulsions with a high positive or negative ZP are electrically stabilized while emulsions with a low ZP tend to coagulate or flocculate leading to poor physical stability. High positive values for ZP > 30 mV or negative values < −30 mV tend to exhibit enhanced physical stability. In contrast low values for ZP of <5 mV can lead to droplet agglomeration [26]. The optimization of mixtures to produce a product of predefined specifications through estimation of the effects of formulation components on the mixture can be achieved using design of experiments (DoE) such as box-Behnken or D-optimal mixture designs with the aid of response surface methodology (RSM). The D-optimal mixed design has been applied to product formulation in the food, pharmaceutical and cosmeceutical industries as a reduced number of experiments are used to generate data for which interactions between variables can be identified using statistical tools thereby avoiding the shortcomings of traditional "one factor at a time" experimental and/or manufacturing approaches [27–29].

2. Materials and Methods

Cold pressed flaxseed, soybean, sunflower, olive, grapeseed and macadamia oils were purchased from Escentia products (Johannesburg, Gauteng, South Africa). Span® 20 and Tween® 80 were purchased from Merck (Johannesburg, Gauteng, South Africa). HPLC grade acetonitrile from Burdick and Jackson™ and ethanol were purchased from Anatech (Olivedale, Gauteng, South Africa). EFV (Form 1) was donated by Adcock Ingram® Limited (Wadeville, Gauteng, South Africa). HPLC-grade water was produced using a RephiLe Bioscience Direct-Pure® Ultrapure RO Water system, (Boston, MA, USA). 600 mg EFV tablets produced by Adcock Ingram Limited (Midrand, South Africa), Cipla Medpro (Cape Town, South Africa), Aspen Pharmacare Limited (Port Elizabeth, Eastern Cape, South Africa) and Aurobindo Pharma Limited (Alberton, South Africa) were purchased from a local pharmacy. Unless otherwise indicated, all materials were at least of analytical grade and were used without further purification.

2.1. Quantitative Determination of Efavirenz

A reversed-phase high-performance liquid chromatographic (HPLC) method was developed and validated for the quantitation of EFV in solubility, loading capacity and in vitro release studies. The HPLC system consisted of a Waters® Alliance e2695 (Waters® Corporation, Milford, MA, USA) solvent delivery module, autosampler, an online degasser and a Waters® 2489 dual wavelength UV-vis detector (Waters® Corporation, Milford, MA, USA). The HPLC chromatographic separation was achieved using a Phenomenex Luna® C18 (2) 100 A 150 mm × 4.6 mm i.d. stationary phase (Separations, Johannesburg, Gauteng, South Africa) and a mobile phase flow rate of 0.8 mL/min at a wavelength of 247 nm. The injection volume was 10 µL and mobile phase was 85:15 v/v acetonitrile and 0.015-M acetate buffer of pH 4.5. The method was linear over the concentration range 1–350 µg/mL with a R^2 = 0.9958, precise with the % RSD < 0.79% for all samples tested. The LOQ was 0.15 µg/mL and LOD was 0.06 µg/mL.

2.2. Solubility

The solubility of EFV in different vegetable oils was determined by adding an excess amount of efavirenz to 5 mL of flaxseed, sunflower, soybean, macadamia, grapeseed and olive oil in Kimax® test tubes with Teflon®-lined crew caps (DWK Life Sciences, Hattenbergstr, Mainz, Germany). The tubes were agitated with the aid of cylindrical BRAND® (Wertheim, Germany) PTFE, length 5 mm, diameter 2-mm magnetic stirring bars at 100 rpm for 48 h at laboratory air-conditioned room temperature (22 ± 2 °C) using an FMH STR-MH magnetic stirring hot plate purchased from (Lasec® Group, Cape Town, South Africa). The samples were removed and centrifuged using a Damon IEC HN-SII centrifuge (Thermo Scientific, Waltham, MA, USA) at 3000 rpm for 15 min after which a 500-µL aliquot of the supernatant was collected and added to 50 mL ethanol and water in a ratio of 3:2 ratio prior to filtration through a Millipore® automation compatible 0.45-µm PVDF membrane syringe filter from (Merck Group, Darmstadt, Germany). The concentration of EFV in the oils was determined using the validated HPLC method described in Section 2.1.

2.3. Formulation Design and Optimization

2.3.1. Pseudo-Ternary Phase Diagrams and Emulsion Classification

The water titration method was used to construct phase diagrams to identify the type of structure that resulted following emulsification and to characterize the behavior of mixtures along dilution paths [30]. Preliminary studies were performed making mixtures of flaxseed oil and a surfactant mixture of (Tween® 80 and Span® 20) (1:1) m/m in ratios of 9:1, 4:1, 7:3, 3:2, 1:1, 2:3, 3:7, 1:4 m/m and Winsor I-type products with no isotropic regions were produced at 22 ± 2 °C and observed after 48 h of incubation Therefore, a surfactant, co-surfactant and co-solvent mixture was considered for further phase behavior investigations. Surfactants solutions of Tween® 80, Span® 20 and ethanol were mixed using a Genie two vortex mixer (Scientific Industries, Inc.™, Bohemia, NY, USA) at 800 rpm for 30 ± 2 s. Three surfactant mixtures $viz.$, S1, S2 and S3 comprised of combinations of ethanol: Tween® 80: Span® 20 in; 0.5:1:1, 1:1:1 and 1.5:1:1 m/m ratios, respectively. The surfactant mixtures were then added to flaxseed oil to produce pseudo-binary solutions in 9:1, 4:1, 7:3, 3:2, 1:1, 2:3, 3:7, 1:4, 1:9 m/m ratios to produce surfactant and oil mixtures in Kimax® test-tubes (DWK Life Sciences, Hattenbergstr, Mainz, Germany). The pseudo-binary pre-concentrates mixtures contained no additional water. To minimize this effect, 500 mL of >98% ethanol was poured in a Schott Duran bottle (DWK Life Sciences, Hattenbergstr, Mainz, Germany) containing 300 g of 3A and 4A (1:1) m/m molecular sieve pellets from (B & M Scientific, Cape Town, South Africa), sealed and kept under air-conditioned laboratory room temperature for 7 days for further dehydration [31,32]. The ethanol was then degassed under vacuum with the aid of a Model A-2S Eyela aspirator degasser (Rikakikai Co., Ltd., Tokyo, Japan) and filtered through a 0.45-μm HVLP Durapore® membrane filter (Millipore® Corporation, Bedford, MA, USA) prior to use. Each of the ratios tested represent a dilution line from one to nine on the Gibbs phase triangle depicted in Figure 1. Water was added in 5% ± 1% increments to each pseudo-binary mixture following the titration chart summarized in Table 1 and after a 48-h incubation at room temperature, 22 ± 2 °C the regions of the phase diagram were identified and characterized for Winsor behavior visually prior to further characterization of pre-defined and identified formulation attributes. The titration chart and Gibbs triangle plots were developed using Triplot version 4.1.2 software (Todd A. Thompson, LA, USA). Points that were located within the phase diagram were observed and evaluated against the Winsor phase behavior descriptions [33] as depicted in Figure 2 and the data were plotted as a phase diagram, a graphical plot using Triplot software spreadsheet (titration chart), example is shown in Table 1. The resultant pseudo-ternary phase diagrams for surfactant-mixtures S1, S2 and S3 have been reported to show a representative sample of the types of structures that form when different amounts of ethanol as used and these data are shown in the results. The mixtures for the eight pseudo-binary solutions produced were vortexed using a Genie two vortex mixer (Scientific Industries, Inc.™, Bohemia, NY, USA) and placed into Falcon® clear 24-well cell culture microplates with a lid from Corning®, Inc (Corning, NY, USA). The bottom surface was placed onto a Xerox WorkCenter 3655 scanner (Xerox™, Norwalk, CT, USA) with the top surface lid and sides covered with a clean white background paper. The transparency and turbidity of the phase diagram dilution-line ratio mixtures were visualized by the scanner, characterized for droplet size, PDI and zeta potential. The images for each of the pseudo-binary solutions and corresponding droplet size, PDI and ZP elucidated immediately (within 6 min) after vortex mixing are listed in Table S1 in the Supplementary Material, for the of analyses performed in triplicate. Conductivity of points P1 to P20, in Table 1, which represent each 5% w/w increment point from 0% water to 95% water approaching the water vertex along dilution-line 9 for surfactant-mixture 1 (S1) was measured using a FiveEasy™ F30 conductivity meter (Mettler Toledo, Greifensee, Switzerland). The electrical conductivity was used to classify the microstructure of the emulsions and establish if w/o or o/w emulsions had formed as o/w systems exhibit higher electrical conductivity than w/o emulsions and these data are reported in Table 1.

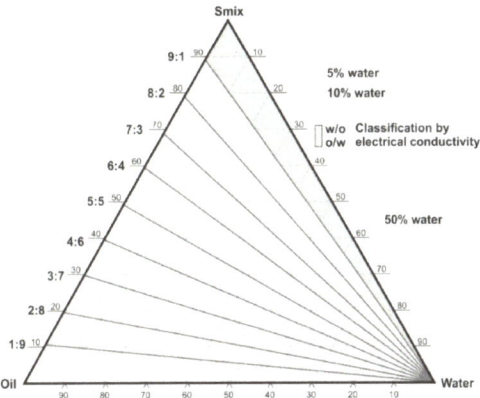

Figure 1. Pseudo-ternary phase diagram and scheme used for phase diagram plotting, showing dilution lines and areas in which electrical conductivity was tested. Adapted from [34].

Table 1. Titration chart for use along each dilution line to plot phase diagrams with proportions of each component in the nanoemulsion with conductivity along dilution-line 9 for surfactant-mixture 1.

Water Addition Points on Dilution Line	Oil mg	S1 mg	Water μL	Total mg	S 1 %	Oil %	Water %	Conductivity μScm^{-1}
P1	250	2250	0	2500	90.00	10.00	0.00	0.18
P2	250	2250	133	2633	85.45	9.49	5.05	0.2
P3	250	2250	280	2780	80.93	8.99	10.07	0.28
P4	250	2250	440	2940	76.53	8.50	14.96	0.45
P5	250	2250	625	3125	72.00	8.00	20.00	0.96
P6	250	2250	835	3335	67.46	7.49	25.03	1.67
P7	250	2250	1075	3575	62.93	6.99	30.06	7.76
P8	250	2250	1350	3850	58.44	6.49	35.06	11.43
P9	250	2250	1675	4175	53.89	5.98	40.11	25.3
P10	250	2250	2050	4550	49.45	5.49	45.05	119.6
P11	250	2250	2500	5000	45.00	5.00	50.00	142.2
P12	250	2250	3050	5550	40.54	4.504	54.95	147.6
P13	250	2250	3750	6250	36.00	4.00	60.00	173.6
P14	250	2250	4625	7125	31.57	3.50	64.91	173.9
P15	250	2250	5875	8375	26.86	2.98	70.14	202
P16	250	2250	7500	10,000	22.50	2.50	75.00	261
P17	250	2250	9950	12,450	18.07	2.00	79.91	278
P18	250	2250	14,275	16,775	13.41	1.49	85.09	356
P19	250	2250	22,500	25,000	9.00	1.00	90.00	389
P20	250	2250	46,600	49,100	4.58	0.50	94.90	433

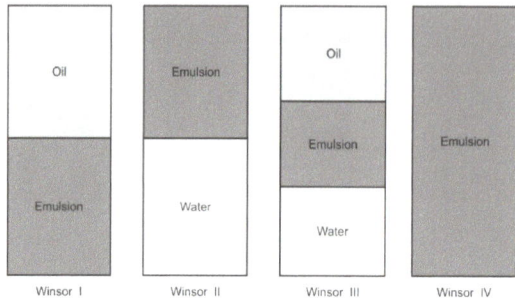

Figure 2. Winsor phase behavior used to assess phase diagram plots.

2.3.2. D-Optimal Design and Statistical Optimization

Surfactant-mixture optimization studies were performed using a D-optimal design to elucidate the effect(s) of the proportion of individual components of the surfactant mixture viz. Span® 20, Tween® 80 and ethanol content on droplet size, PDI and ZP. The D-optimal design studies were performed with the aid of Design-Expert version 12.0 software (Stat-Ease, Inc., Minneapolis, MN, USA). The proportion of oil in the nanoemulsion was maintained at 10% *v/v* for dilution-line 9, which falls in the nanoemulsion region. Span® 20, Tween® 80 and ethanol were independent variables and droplet size, PDI and ZP were the responses monitored. The oral route of delivery is proposed for these nanoemulsions, therefore the proportion of ethanol used was maintained at the permissible levels for food content with the largest concentrations at 20% *m/m* [35–37]. Legislation relating to the use of ethanol as an excipient in pediatric medicines or drugs is different in different countries and the American Academy of Pediatrics recommends that ethanol content in pediatric drugs should not produce a blood concentration >25 mg/100 mL following administration of a single recommended therapeutic dose. The dose size of EFV is 200 mg for pediatric patients and 600 mg for adults and as a nanoemulsion the dose unit is relatively small and is not expected to produce blood ethanol levels above regulated limits [38]. The European Medicines Agency (EMA) recommends a daily limit of 260.5 mg/kg/day of ethanol [39]. The levels for Span® 20 (A), Tween® 80 (B) and ethanol (C) used in the mixture fell in the range between the minimum and maximum levels listed in Table 2 with the sum of the components A, B and C always totaling 100%.

Table 2. Constraints for input variables for D-optimal design.

Lower Limit %		Compound		Upper Limit %
5	≤	Span® 20 (A)	≤	90
5	≤	Tween® 80 (B)	≤	90
5	≤	Ethanol (C)	≤	20
		Total: A + B + C	=	100

2.4. *Preparation of Nanoemulsions*

The nanoemulsion region was identified from the phase diagrams depicted in Figures 3–5. Excess EFV was placed into a test tube containing the nanoemulsion preconcentrate that was one of five different surfactant mixtures and 10% *m/m* flaxseed oil. Of the five surfactant mixtures evaluated three were identified from each phase diagram and two were numeric optimization solutions extracted using the D-optimal design. The nanoemulsion mixtures were stirred at 100 rpm at laboratory room temperature under air-conditioner at 22 ± 2 °C with the aid of an FMH-STR magnetic stirrer (Lasec®, Cape Town, South Africa) for 48 h. The saturated nanoemulsions were centrifuged at 3000 rpm for 15 min using a model HN-SII IEC centrifuge (Thermo Scientific, Waltham, MA, USA) to separate excess drug from the nanoemulsion. Aliquots (500 µL) of the supernatant were dispersed in 50 mL water for droplet size and ZP measurements. A further 500-µL aliquot of the supernatant was mixed with 50 mL of a 3:2 ratio ethanol: water solution, prior to quantitation of EFV.

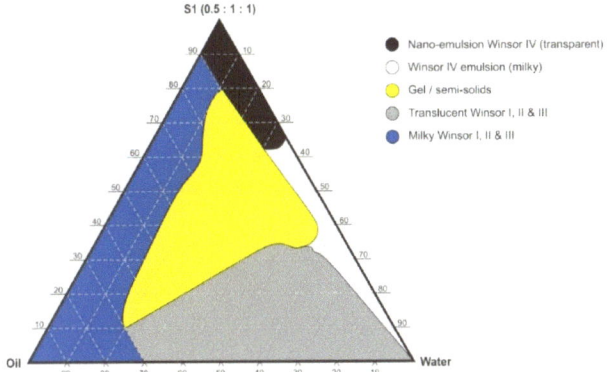

Figure 3. Pseudo-ternary phase diagram of flaxseed oil with surfactant-mixture S1 (0.5:1:1 *m/m* Ethanol: Tween® 80: Span® 20).

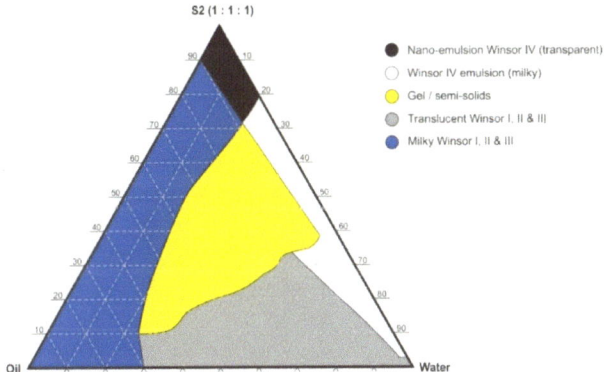

Figure 4. Pseudo-ternary phase diagram of flaxseed oil with surfactant-mixture S2 (1:1:1 *m/m* Ethanol: Tween® 80: Span® 20).

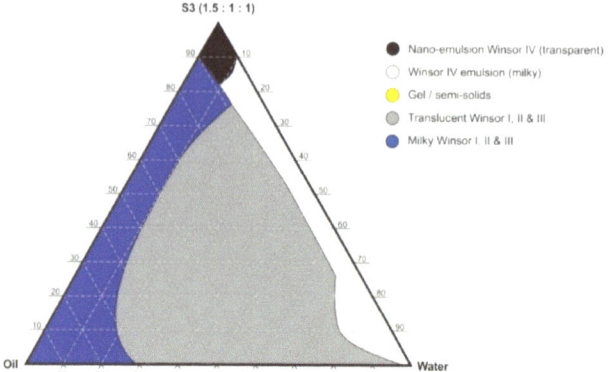

Figure 5. Pseudo-ternary phase diagram of flaxseed oil with surfactant-mixture S3 (1.5:1:1 *m/m* Ethanol: Tween® 80: Span® 20).

2.5. Characterization of Nanoemulsion Formulations

2.5.1. Zeta Potential

The ZP was determined using a Nano-ZS Malvern Zetasizer (Malvern Instruments, Worchester, UK). A folded capillary was used for zeta-potential determinations with the instrument set in the Laser Doppler Anemometry (LDA) mode. The sample was prepared by dispersing 500-µL aliquots of the saturated nanoemulsion in 50 mL HPLC grade water and placed into a folded capillary cell. All measurements ($n = 3$) were performed at an applied field strength of 20 V/cm and the Helmholtz-Smoluchowski equation used to calculate the ZP of each sample, in situ.

2.5.2. Polydispersity Index (PDI) and Droplet Size (PS)

The PDI and droplet size were determined using a Nano-ZS Malvern Zetasizer (Malvern Instruments, Worchester, UK) using the dynamic light scattering (DLS) mode. The sample was prepared by dispersing 500-µL aliquots of the saturated nanoemulsion in 50 mL HPLC grade water and placed into a 12.5 × 12.5 × 45 mm BRAND® disposable cuvette (BRAND GmbH + CO KG, Wertheim, Germany).

2.5.3. Transmission Electron Microscopy (TEM)

Transmission electron microscopy (TEM) was used to investigate the shape and surface morphology of the nanoemulsion and droplets in aqueous dispersions. Briefly, a drop of the aqueous nanoemulsion dispersion was placed onto a 3.05 mm copper grid fitted with a carbon film (FORMVAR/Carbon support 300 mesh) procured from TAAB Laboratories Equipment, Ltd., Alderson, Berks, RG7 8NA, UK. Excess liquid was removed using Whatman® 110 hydrophilic filter paper (Whatman® International, Ltd., Maidstone, UK) and the sample allowed to dry at room temperature (22 °C) for 24 h. The sample was visualized using a Zeiss® Libra Model 120 TEM (Zeiss, GmbH, Germany) operating at an accelerating voltage of 80 kV.

2.5.4. Raman Spectroscopy

Raman spectroscopy was used to identify all molecules present in the loaded and unloaded nanoemulsions to determine if new functional groups were evident sue to interaction of the components use in EFV loaded nanoemulsions. A Bruker Vertex 70-Ram II Raman spectrometer from (Bruker Optics, Inc., Billerica, MA, USA) equipped with a 1064 nm Nd: YAG laser for excitation in the region of 3400–80 cm^{-1} and liquid nitrogen cooled germanium detector was used to generate spectra that were acquired at 300 scans per minute. The instrument was set at 300 mW and the sample was placed in a hemispheric bore of an aluminum sample holder. The spectral resolution was 4 cm^{-1} and the spectra was processed using OPUS version 6.5 spectroscopy software (Bruker Optics, Inc., Billerica, MA, USA).

2.5.5. Fourier-Transform Infrared Spectroscopy (FT-IR)

The presence of EFV in the nanoemulsions was also investigated using FT-IR and infrared absorption spectra were recorded using attenuated total reflection with a PerkinElmer spectrum 100 FT-IR spectrometer (PerkinElmer® Pty, Ltd., Beaconsfield, UK) at 64 scans per minute over the frequency range 4000–650 cm^{-1}. Nanoemulsion samples were mounted onto a diamond crystal using an applied force of approximately 100 N. The spectral data were processed using software FT-IR spectrum version 10.5.4 software (PerkinElmer®, Inc. Pty, Ltd., Beaconsfield, UK).

2.5.6. In Vitro Release

A 300-µL aliquot of a saturated EFV nanoemulsion was placed into a size-00 hard gelatin capsule for in vitro EFV release studies. The dissolution time of the capsules ($n = 6$) in dissolution medium at 37 ± 1 °C was approximately 8 ± 1.03 min. In vitro dissolution studies were conducted using USP apparatus II with a Hanson Vision® G2 Elite 8 dissolution bath fitted with a Vision AutoPlus and DissoScan™ auto sampler (Teledyne Hanson Research, Chatsworth, LA, USA) operated at a rotation speed of 50 rpm in 900 mL 0.1-M hydrochloric acid pH 1.2 with 1% *w/v* SLS at a temperature maintained at 37 ± 1 °C. A 10-mL sample was withdrawn at 15, 30, 60, 120, 390 and 720 min and filtered under vacuum with a Model A-2S Eyela aspirator degasser (Rikakikai Co., Ltd., Tokyo, Japan) through a 0.45-µm HVLP Durapore® membrane filter (Millipore® Corporation, Bedford, MA, USA) and the EFV released ($n = 3$) determined using the HPLC method described in 2.1. Sink conditions were maintained by replacement of fresh dissolution medium after removal of each sample.

3. Results

3.1. Solubility

The highest solubility of 89.41 mg/mL for EFV was observed for flaxseed oil and the solubility data are summarized in Table 3. Flaxseed oil was therefore used as the oil phase for constructing pseudo-ternary phase diagrams for the self-emulsifying nanoemulsions. In addition to the physicochemical properties of the EFV the molecular volume, polarity of the oil, chain length and saturation or unsaturation of triglyceride chains of the vegetable oils also influence solubility (MCT) have due to their higher fluidity, better solubility properties [40]. Medium chain triglycerides (MCT) containing oils are best for LBDDS as they are resistant to oxidation and possess high solvent capacity when compared to long-chain triglycerides (LCT) oils because of the high effective concentration of ester functional groups in the oil [41]. However, most of the vegetable oils selected for this study (Table 3) are predominantly and commonly composed of LCT and C_{18} chains. It was observed that as the proportion of the unsaturated component $C_{18:3}$ component of the vegetable oils increases the solubility of EFV increased. Flaxseed oil has approximately 50% $C_{18:3}$, soybean oil approximately 9.5% $C_{18:3}$, grapeseed, sunflower and olive oil contain $C_{18:3}$ of <2% [42–44].

Table 3. Saturation solubility of efavirenz (EFV) in vegetable oils.

Oil	Mean EFV Solubility ($n = 3$) ± SD mg/mL
Flaxseed	89.41 ± 0.12
Soybean	81.53 ± 0.18
Macadamia	71.31 ± 0.12
Grapeseed	69.83 ± 0.16
Olive	69.55 ± 0.09
Sunflower	55.99 ± 0.87

3.2. Pseudo-Ternary Phase Diagrams

Pseudo-binary solutions of surfactant and oil in all ratios for the surfactant mixtures for dilution-line 1 to dilution-line 8 exhibited two phases of Winsor I-type phase behavior on standing for 30 min, but formed turbid mixtures following vortex mixing for 30 s at 800 rpm. Dilution-line 9 or ratio 9 resulted in a transparent and kinetically stable, isotropic system which exhibited Winsor IV-type behavior for up to 12 months at room temperature (22 °C). The droplet sizes of these ratio mixtures gradual increased as the proportion of flaxseed oil used increased while surfactant content decreased. The surfactant to oil ratio for the 9:1 pseudo-binary solution resulted in emulsions with the smallest droplet size and lowest PDI of all ratios tested. Both a nanoemulsion and microemulsion region was observed along dilution-line 9 for all three surfactant mixtures tested. Five distinct regions were formed viz., a nanoemulsion that is transparent Winsor IV, milky Winsor IV, i.e., cloudy isotropic mixture, translucent Winsor I, II and III, milky Winsor I, II and III in addition to a gel/semisolid region. Ratio 9 formed clear isotropic and transparent nanoemulsions with up to 35% *v/v* water addition for surfactant-mixture 1 as depicted in Figure 3, up to 20% *v/v* water for surfactant-mixture 2 as depicted in Figure 4 and only up to 5% *v/v* for surfactant-mixture 3 as depicted in Figure 5. While the nanoemulsion region area decreases as the ethanol content in the surfactant mixture increases, the milky isotropic and two or three-phase regions of the o/w emulsion also exhibit an increase in area whereas the gel region decreases in size with an increase in ethanol content, as the interfacial film is flexible, thereby solid structures are disrupted and the fluid phase areas increase in dimension. The dilute aqueous isotropic regions of cloudy o/w emulsions may be appropriate for an immediate release effect, due to the ease of dispersion of this phase in aqueous media [45]. Electrical conductivity measurements along dilution-line nine from the pseudo-binary solution of the surfactant/oil phase to the water vertex suggest that phase-inversion of system from a w/o to an o/w nano or microemulsion occurs at a specific point if not in a range of values as summarized in the titration chart followed in Table 1. The surfactant mixture for the S1 mixture exhibited the largest nanoemulsion region in the phase diagram and resulted in the production of the largest number of kinetically stable nanoemulsions following addition of water.

3.3. Statistical Analysis and Optimization

A single block D-optimal mixtures design was launched using the design constraints summarized in Table 2 on Design expert software version 12.0 software (Stat-Ease Inc., Minneapolis, MN, USA) to estimate the effects of the proportion of each of the surfactant-mixture components. To facilitate an understanding of the relationship(s) between one or more measured responses to input factors, a D-optimal design uses a sequential strategy that results in either first or second order polynomial mathematical relationships that can be best fit to statistical models such as quadratic, linear and cubic models for point prediction or optimization. The design produced was a simplex-lattice design with A + B + C = 1 or surfactant mixtures of 100% [46] which were then used for the manufacture of 10% *m/m* flaxseed oil containing nanoemulsions. A total of 16 runs with the compositions are summarized in Table 4 and the resulting droplet sizes, PDI and zeta potential. The most common empirical models fitted to experimental data include linear, quadratic or cubic models which increase in complexity of the polynomial from a 1st, 2nd, to 3rd degree, respectively. A 4th degree polynomial for systems involving composition, with the sum of the proportions by volume and weight has also been applied and reported [47]. Special quartic models are useful for modelling data generated from multicomponent mixtures and can be used to estimate multiple effects and the curvature of a response surface in the interior of a triangle to produce contour like effects [48,49]. All models were automatically fit by the design software for these data including linear, quadratic, cubic, special cubic, quartic and special quartic models were applied to the data then analyzed for the response variables monitored. The ANOVA analysis results are summarized in Table 5 for the suggested models and Table S2 in the Supplementary Material for all the models tested. The predicted residual sum of squares (PRESS) was used to establish the suitability of each model in respect of data fitting and the model with the lowest value for PRESS was identified as suitable for that response. The PRESS value is said to analyze the prediction ability of models and the model with the minimum PRESS is usually considered the best predictive model for a set of data [50]. ANOVA analysis following fitting of responses to each models are summarized in Table 5 to which droplet size and PDI were best fit to special quartic models while zeta potential was best fit to a linear model. Prior to predicting the optimized nanoemulsion formulation, composition residual analysis was undertaken to confirm that the assumptions for ANOVA analysis had been met. For this purpose, diagnostic plots viz., box Cox plots for residuals were plotted for all three responses and confirmed that data transformation was not required for droplet size and zeta potential and PDI. Diagnostic box Cox plots are depicted in Figures S3, S4 and S5 respectively in the Supplementary Material. When the statistical data are analyzed, input variables Span® 20 (A) Tween® 80 (B) and ethanol (C) are used to produce effects terms; A, B, C, AB, AC, BC, A^2BC, AB^2C, ABC^2 which are tested to asses which ones are significantly different from 0, i.e., >0 therefore estimated to give coefficient values of correlation for prediction of a specific response. The largest positive coefficient of model terms represents the model term with the largest effect on a specific response.

Table 4. Surfactant-mixture compositions generated by the D-optimal design and the experimental responses of 10% *m/m* flaxseed oil nanoemulsion in each run observed.

Run	Input Variables % m/m			Responses		
	Span® 20 A	Tween® 80 B	Ethanol C	Droplet Size nm	PDI	Zeta Potential mV
1	47.5	47.5	5	88.43	0.75	−23.85
2	66.875	24.375	8.75	408.25	0.332	−22.8
3	24.375	66.875	8.75	68.9	0.461	−21.9
4	5	82.5	12.5	173.4	0.176	−16.5
5	7.5	5	20	507.2	0.26	−23.2
6	7.5	5	20	404.4	0.324	−23
7	47.5	47.5	5	138.7	0.587	−18.8
8	5	75.0	20	180.56	0.481	−25.5
9	24.375	59.375	16.25	92.5	0.51	−18.6
10	5	90	5	70.5	0.12	−14.7
11	90.00	5	5	362.6	0.265	−21.4
12	5	75	20	58.1	0.412	−17.2
13	90	5	5	364.6	0.285	−21.9
14	43.75	43.75	12.5	441.1	0.365	−23.4
15	82.5	5	12.5	290.1	0.214	−23.4
16	5	90	5	70.75	0.119	−16.8

Table 5. ANOVA data for D-optimal responses and best-fit model.

Response	Predicted Model	f-Value	Degrees of Freedom	p-Value	R^2	Adjusted R^2	Predicted R^2	Adequate Precision
Droplet size	Special quartic	8.91	8	0.0046	0.910	0.908	−1.618	7.205
Polydispersity	Special quartic	86.11	8	0.0001	0.9899	0.9789	0.8335	29.195
Zeta potential	Linear	5.09	2	0.0233	0.439	0.353	0.115	5.982

3.3.1. Droplet Size

The droplet size ranged from 58.1 nm to 507.2 nm with the smallest droplet sizes observed when Tween® 80 was used at its maximum level of 0.9 in proportion in the surfactant-mixture design space whereas, the droplet size increased as Span® 20 content increased. A sharp increase in particle size was observed as ethanol content is increased in the region of the Span® 20 vertex as can be observed in the contour plot depicted in Figure 6. The model F-value of 8.91 indicated that the special quartic model for droplet size was significant and that there is only a 0.46% chance that a model F-value this large is due to noise. The p-value < 0.05 implied that the coefficients of the model terms were significantly different from zero, i.e., the effect of the model terms or combination of terms exerts an effect than can be estimated in the formulation composition. The model terms for the mixture A, B, C and A^2BC were significant. The terms AB, AC, BC, AB^2C and ABC^2 were not significant and the ANOVA data and results are summarized in the supplementary data. The lack of fit F-value of 3.59 implied that lack of fit was not significant. The predicted R^2 for droplet size was negative which implied that the mean data may be a better predictor for this response than using the model. However, adequate precision was >4 and was desirable showing that an adequate signal was observed and that the model could be used to navigate the design space and the model equation in terms of coded factors for droplet size is reported as Equation (1).

$$\text{Droplet size} = 342.00A + 90.75B + 3328.66C - 530.59AB - 2941.83AC - 3530.63BC + 52,488.71A^2BC - 11,742.82AB^2C - 32,873.13ABC^2 \quad (1)$$

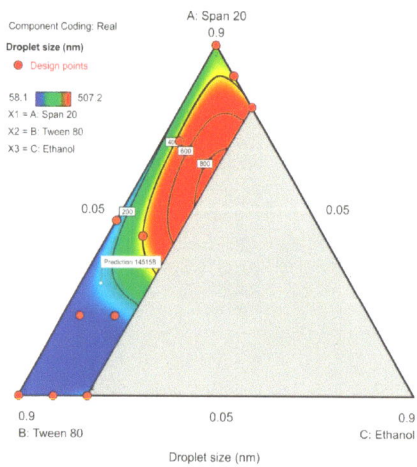

Figure 6. Contour plot for droplet size showing the characterized region where ethanol content is ≤20%.

3.3.2. Polydispersity Index

The PDI ranged between 0.119 to 0.75 in the design space with the highest PDI observed at the center-point for Tween® 80 and Span® 20 content with ethanol content used closest to the lower limit.

As the ethanol content was increased in the upper region of the contour plot towards the Span® 20 vertex, a general decrease in PDI is observed as depicted in (Figure 7). The model F-value of 86.11 indicates that the special quartic model for PDI was significant and that there is only a 0.01% chance that a model F-value this large was due to noise. A *p*-value of <0.05 implied that the coefficients of effect and relationship of the model terms A, B, C, AB, AC, BC, A²BC, AB²C and ABC² were significantly different from zero and could be estimated and the ANOVA data and results for this special quartic model are given in Table S4 of the Supplementary Material. The model equation in terms of coded factors for PDI is reported as Equation (2). The predicted R^2 0.8335 is in reasonable agreement with the adjusted R^2 0.9789. The lack of fit F-value 0.08 implies that lack of fit was not significant for the model and that there is a 56.02% chance that the lack of fit F-value this large is due to noise.

$$\text{Polydispersity index} = 0.2868A + 0.1155B + 10.85C + 2.19AB - 12.93AC - 10.78BC - 43.34A^2BC + 1.016AB^2C + 37.74ABC^2 \tag{2}$$

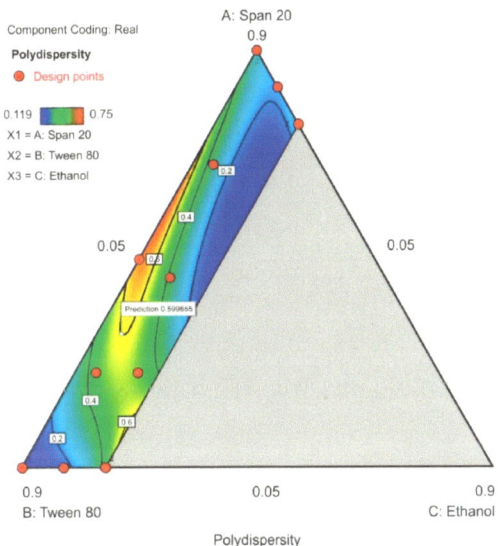

Figure 7. Contour plot for polydispersity index (PDI) showing point prediction when ethanol content is ≤20%.

3.3.3. Zeta Potential

All components of the surfactant mixture exhibited a combined effect on the zeta potential and a linear relationship for this model is reported in Equation (3). The ethanol content exhibited the greatest effect on the zeta potential as observed by the magnitude of the coefficient for the term C and in the contour plot where 20% ethanol (C) was used. The contour plot for ZP is depicted in Figure 8 in which a significant region (in blue) revealed that as the concentration of Span® 20 in the surfactant mixture was increased, the ZP decreased and became more negative with the lowest negative point occurring at the upper limit of ethanol and lower limit of Tween® 80 content. The model F-value of 5.09 for ZP indicated that the linear model for ZP was significant and that there was only a 2.33% chance that a model F-value this large was due to noise. The probability *p*-value of < 0.05 implied the model terms were significant, the coefficients of the effect of each model term was significantly different from zero and could be estimated for this linear model, thus therefore only model terms A, B and C were significant within the formulation composition of these nanoemulsions. The equation in terms of coded factors for ZP is reported as equation 3. The predicted R^2 of 0.1152 is not in close agreement with the adjusted R^2 of 0.3530 suggesting a large block effect or possible problem with the model although, the adequate precision > 4 which is desirable and the adequate signal indicates that the model could be used to navigate the design space. The lack of fit F-value 0.49 implies that lack of fit was not significant for the model and there is an 82.64% chance that a lack of fit F-value this large is due to noise.

$$\text{Zeta potential} = -23.10A - 17.08B - 29.48C \tag{3}$$

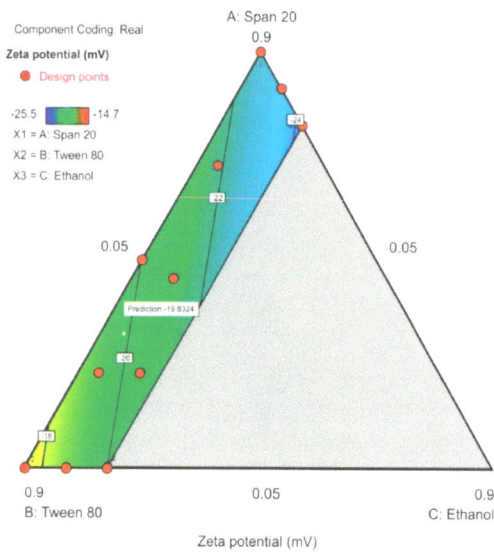

Figure 8. Contour plot for zeta potential (ZP) showing the point prediction when the ethanol content is ≤20%.

3.4. Optimization of Surfactant Mixtures and Assessment of Optimized Nanoemulsions

The optimization function was used to predict optimum levels for each for the components of the surfactant mixture. The primary criterion used was that the ethanol content should be minimized in the surfactant mixture. The second criterion required that a droplet size of between 100 and 200 nm was desired. Finally, the third and fourth criteria required minimization of the PDI and ZP. Two optimized solutions were produced based on the desirability function and the proportions of the formulation composition for the two solutions are reported as batches F4 and F5. Batches F1, F2 and F3 were nanoemulsion formulations made using arbitrary surfactant mixtures when assessing the phase behavior for the S1, S2 and S3 mixtures, respectively. The five formulations that were manufactured and assessed are listed in Table 6 with their respective compositions. The specified optimization criteria (constraints) in Table S6 and solutions produced are shown Table S7 with their associated desirability in the Supplementary Material. The prediction error was calculated against the experimental values obtained to give the prediction error of the D-optimal design. An overlay plot that depicts the area in which the desired optimization criteria is met is shown on Figure S6 in the Supplementary Materials.

Table 6. Composition of the surfactant mixtures used for the manufacture of 10% flaxseed nanoemulsions and assessed in in vitro release and characterization studies.

Formulation	Span® 20% m/m	Tween® 80% m/m	Ethanol% m/m	Droplet Size nm	PDI	Zeta Potential mV	Efavirenz Content mg/mL	Mass of 1 mL of Nanoemulsion g
F1	40	40	20	185.1 ± 0.7	0.444 ± 0.003	−35.4 ± 0.9	377 ± 4.9	0.989 ± 0.006
F2	33.3	33.3	33.3	190.3 ± 2.0	0.387 ± 0.016	−34.4 ± 0.7	437 ± 13.1	1.040 ± 0.009
F3	28.5	28.5	42.8	156.8 ± 23.4	0.342 ± 0.048	−41.0 ± 0.9	571 ± 18.7	1.040 ± 0.012
F4	58.1	36.0	6.0	225.6 ± 16.8	0.487 ± 0.003	−31.9 ± 3.12	329 ± 9.45	0.817 ± 0.007
F5	32.2	58.3	9.5	146.7 ± 25.3	0.402 ± 0.012	−24.1 ± 2.33	334 ± 11.2	0.833 ± 0.009

3.5. Characterization and Assessment of Nanoemulsions

Nanoemulsion F3 was able to incorporate the largest amount of EFV of 571 mg/mL suggesting that the high ethanol content improved the solubility of EFV and miscibility of flaxseed oil, Tween® 80 and Span® 20 in the nanoemulsion. A decrease in EFV loading was observed as the proportion of ethanol in the composition was decreased. The highest PDI of 0.487, although arguably monodisperse for batch F4, is bimodal (Figure 9). The droplet size distribution of F4 could be attributed to the high Span® 20 content due to a shift in HLB for these surfactant mixtures and the effect to thermodynamic stability [51]. A general decrease in the ZP was observed as the proportion of ethanol used was increased for batches F1 to F3 suggesting that the composition of F1, F2 and F3 would produce stable nanoemulsions over the long term. All five formulations exhibited ZP values < −20 mV suggesting the nanoemulsions that were produced were likely to be stable. The negative charge of nanoemulsion droplets may be useful for macrophage targeting since macrophages identify and take up negatively charged particles [52]. Macrophages are key factors in HIV infection and are significant cellular reservoirs of the HIV [53]. Emulsion droplets with a ZP of approximately ± 20 mV exhibit only short-term stability, with the tendency for the droplets to flocculate and coalesce [54]. To administer the recommended maximum adult dose of 600 mg formulation F3 would require a mass of 1.09 g of the nanoemulsion to be administered. The total mass is considerably lower and more convenient than the commercially available 600-mg EFV tablets manufactured by Cipla Medpro, Aurobindo, Adcock Ingram and Aspen Pharmacare for which tablets mass measured was 1.34 ± 0.09, 1.25 ± 0.11 g, 1.20 ± 0.08 g and 1.106 ± 0.045 g, respectively for (n = 20) suggesting that the nanoemulsion may produce a more convenient dosage form size for patients to use.

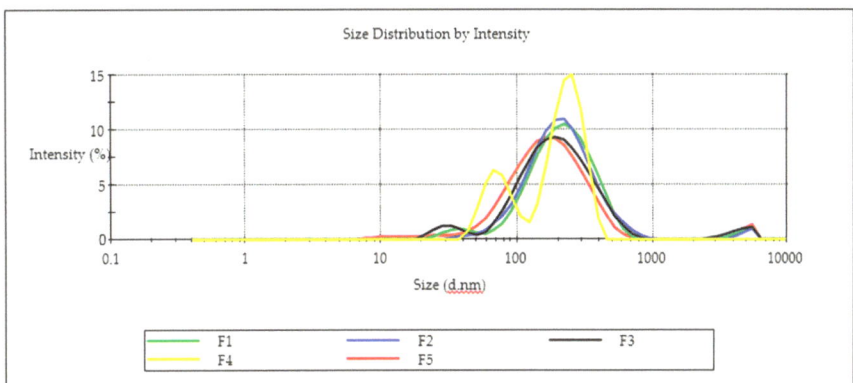

Figure 9. Particle-size distribution for batches F1, F2, F3, F4 and F5.

3.6. Transmission Electron Microscopy

Transmission electron microscopy revealed the presence of largely spherical droplets of lipid as depicted in Figure 10 with an average droplet size in close agreement with that determined using dynamic light scattering. Smaller droplets in the size range 20–100 nm were present in the nanoemulsion dispersion in lower numbers as reflected in the droplet size distribution in Figure 8. These small droplet sizes may add to therapeutic possibilities by reducing the viral load in reservoirs associated with CNS tissue by distributing and perfusion into such tissues [55,56]. The bimodal distribution observed for droplet size distribution for F4 can be explained by the differences in the surfactant composition of the formulation. Ethanol exhibited the largest effect on solvent capacity and miscibility of the mixture for both surfactants, the oil phase and EFV. Rigid interfacial films give rise to bimodal distributions [57] and the greater the ethanol content, the more flexible the interfacial film of the immiscible phase. The bimodal distribution for F4 can be explained by the solvent capacity of the system for the lipophilic phase, Tween® 80 and Span® 20 which become miscible with addition of ethanol. As formulation F4 includes only a small proportion of ethanol, some proportion of the lipophilic phase (span® 20 + 10% flaxseed oil) could possibly have been dispersed in agglomerates of a different size within the nanoemulsion mixture and larger than the small peaks of smaller particle sizes of F1, F2 and F3. Given the large concentration of ethanol in F3, the bimodal effects are seen to produce agglomerates within the nanoemulsion mixture of a smaller droplet size.

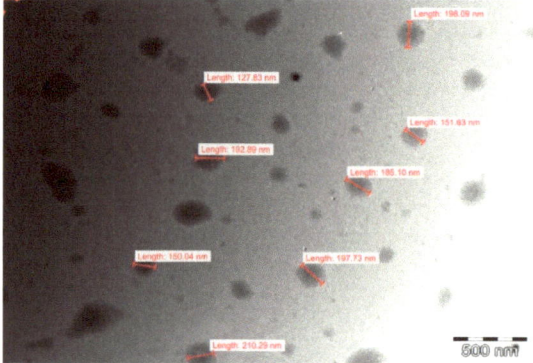

Figure 10. Transmission electron micrograph of nanoemulsion F5. The images for F1, F2, F3 and F4 are reported in the Supplementary Materials.

3.7. Raman Spectroscopy

The Raman spectra for EFV and EFV loaded nanoemulsions is reported in the Supplementary Materials (Figure S7). The EFV skeleton stretching vibrations were not affected by encapsulation of EFV in the nanoemulsion implying no interaction between EFV and lipids used in the formulation. The functional groups for EFV detected using Raman spectroscopy revealed that all expected signals observed for pure efavirenz and blank nanoemulsions were present and were in agreement with previously reported spectra [58]. The signal for the CH_2 (A) functional group at 3093 cm^{-1}, the C≡C (B) bond at 2250 cm^{-1}, the (C=O) (C) bond at 1750 cm^{-1} and the C–H stretch at approximately 1000 cm^{-1} reflect the presence of EFV [59]. A comparison of experimentally determined vibrational wavenumbers for EFV is listed in the Supplementary Materials (Table S8).

3.8. Fourier-Transform Infrared Spectroscopy (FT-IR)

To understand the possibility of chemical interactions between the drug and nanoemulsion mixture, blank nanoemulsion, pure EFV, EFV loaded nanoemulsions and EFV nanoemulsions after dissolution testing were harvested left to dry in an open petri dish under room temperature over 72 h and characterized by FT-IR. The FT-IR spectrum of EFV loaded nanoemulsion in Figure S8 (in the Supplementary Material) showed the characteristic peaks of alkyne at 2247.63 cm^{-1}, C–H stretch at 3000 cm^{-1}, C–F stretch at 1400 cm^{-1}, tertiary amide at 1602 cm^{-1} and C=O (D) at 1750 cm^{-1} [60].

A table of the comparison of the peaks reported in literature and those experimentally found are given in Table S8 in the Supplementary Material. The absorption band at approximately 3000 cm^{-1} was assigned to C–H stretching of the methylene group for Tween® 80 and Span® 20, the intensity of these peaks is diminished in the crystalline product harvested following dissolution testing and interaction of the EFV nanoemulsion with aqueous media resulting in conversion of electrons on carbon atoms changing from sp2 to sp3 [61]. The decrease in intensity of the O–H stretch detected as a broad band at 3500 cm^{-1} following dissolution testing may be due to the loss of ethanol from the nanoemulsion into the aqueous dissolution medium which results in an increase in the rate of nucleation and crystallization of EFV in solution.

3.9. In Vitro Efavirenz Release

In vitro release testing revealed burst release of EFV for batches F1, F2, F4, F5 and for pure EFV within the first two hours of commencement of testing. Dissolution testing was conducted for the formulations listed in Table 6 and the % EFV released was based on actual drug loading data generated following assay of the nanoemulsion formulations. The nanoemulsion for batch F5 exhibited the greatest extent of release at 12 h that decreased for batches F1, F4, F5 and F3 which exhibited a sustained release effect and the release profiles are depicted in Figure 11. The reduction in amount of EFV released from the nanoemulsions may be attributed to solubilization of EFV in droplets of the nanoemulsion and/or formation of the EFV solvate on crystallization. Drugs may precipitate in vitro and in vivo due to a rapid change in pH, dilution with body fluids or digestion of solubilizing excipients subsequently resulting in lower EFV concentrations within the aqueous phase and better entrapment of EFV within the crystal lattice structure. As the saturation method of manufacture was used to produce the nanoemulsions, following supersaturation the process of nucleation continues and promotes crystallization [62,63]. As the proportion of ethanol is increased, the percent efavirenz released at 12 h decreases. On interaction with 1% *m/v* SLS in 0.1-M HCl dissolution fluid, the nanoemulsion formulations crystallized and formed a white edged crystalline semisolid that sank to the bottom of the dissolution vessel. Nanoemulsions of batch F4 and F5 were prepared with the same amount of ethanol and different proportions of Tween® 80 and Span® 20 and batch F5 released a larger amount of EFV than batch F4 at 12 h possibly due to the different hydrophilic lipophilic balance (HLB) value of the surfactants used. Tween® 80 is soluble in an aqueous environment, whereas Span® 20 is not and therefore Tween® 80 interacts with the dissolution medium and contributed to better dissolution of EFV. Crystallization was observed for all batches and was greatest for batch F3. EFV precipitation is an undesirable outcome following administration of SNEDDS formulations. The loss of ethanol as observed with FT–IR analysis following dissolution testing may be the largest contributing factor to a reduced solubilization capacity and increased rate of nucleation in the supersaturated nanoemulsion formulations and hybridization of the C–H bond stretch that reduces the hydrophobicity of the formulation thereby affecting the interaction of EFV to form a solution.

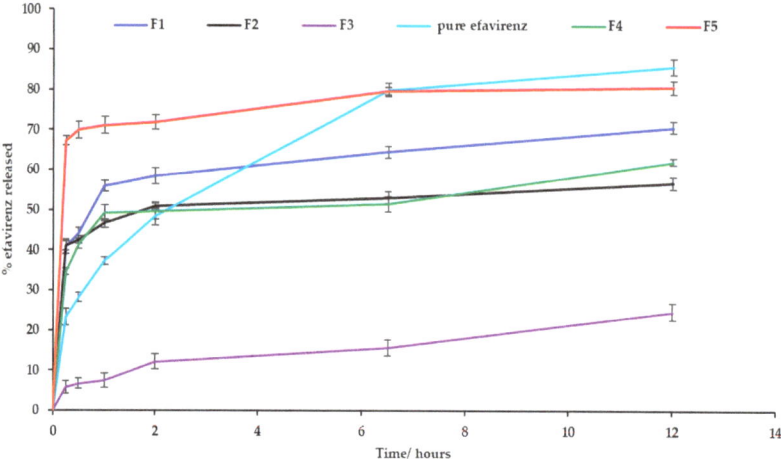

Figure 11. Dissolution profiles (mean ± SD (n = 3) for batches F1, F2, F3, F4 and F5 and EFV powder.

4. Conclusions

The recommended dose of efavirenz for adults is 600 mg taken once daily and the most common dosage form available is a tablet, which is inconveniently large in size that may negatively affect patient adherence. The design of LBDDS focused on making the release characteristics independent of the gastrointestinal physiology and the fed/fasted state of the patient [64,65] and in a dosage form size that is small and convenient for the patient to use would be an advantage. The administration of EFV using these SNEDD technology would require a small unit size of the dosage form due to the high drug loading capacities exhibited which may produce a more convenient sized dosage form. Co-solvents and co-surfactants maybe used to improve the thermodynamic stability of formulations that exhibit an increased solubilization capacity resulting in enhanced therapeutic performance. The negative ZP of nanoemulsion droplets would be useful for macrophage targeting since macrophages identify and take up negatively charged particles [52]. Macrophages are key cells in HIV infection and are significant reservoirs of the virus [53].

Investigation of phase behavior of LBDDS components is useful for optimization of formulations and pre-formulation studies assist in defining appropriate proportions of each component to use, in addition to facilitation of decisions in relation to manufacturing processes such as whether high pressure or high shear homogenization can be used. Such decisions are required to ensure that an optimum product with predefined quality attributes is produced. The phase behavior of crude cold pressed flaxseed oil with non-ionic surfactants revealed an area within pseudo-ternary phase diagrams for surfactant-mixtures S1 and S2 that formed gels/semisolid structures which can be exploited for other drug delivery strategies such as topical application. This research identified that optimization of mixture compositions to produce a product with the required characteristics through estimation of the effects of the formulation components. However, accurate optimization using a D-optimal design may not be possible to only a relatively good predictability in droplet size alone and therefore other designs should be explored for future optimization.

Kinetically stable low energy nanoemulsions of flaxseed oil, Tween® 80 and Span® 20 surfactant and co-surfactant with ethanol were successfully manufactured. On visual observation, different release profiles for efavirenz were observed from different nanoemulsions. These can be exploited for further optimization to produce formulations suitable for undertaking in vivo and pharmacokinetic studies. The side effects of EFV associated with dose dumping may be reduced by using nanoemulsions to modulate release. The nanoemulsion approach is promising however, stability of formulations in gelatin or other encapsulated forms in which crystallization of EFV from solution is minimized, should be explored. The use of flaxseed oil in dosage forms intended for oral delivery may be beneficial to patients as there are health benefits associated with use of polyunsaturated fatty acids in addition to flaxseed oil being a cheap renewable raw material for dosage forms. Flaxseed oil contains an abundant source of, viscous fiber components and phytochemicals, such as lignans and protein that have demonstrated clinical activity as one of the six plant materials in the study of cancer-preventive foods [66].

Supplementary Materials: The following are available online at http://www.mdpi.com/1999-4923/12/9/797/s1, Table S1: Scan images for investigation of turbidity and transparency during phase identification studies and results for selected critical quality attributes (CQA) viz., droplet size (DS), polydispersity index (PDI) and Zeta Potential (ZP), Table S2: PRESS statistic values and sum of squares for all models used to analyze the data, Table S3: ANOVA data for special quartic model for droplet size, df = degrees of freedom, Table S4: ANOVA data for special quartic model for polydispersity index, df = degrees of freedom, Table S5: ANOVA data for a linear model of Zeta Potential, df = degrees of freedom, Table S6: Constraints used for the target optimization criteria, Table S7: Solutions from Design Expert software for specified optimization criteria, Table S8: Theoretical (reported) and experimental wavenumbers characterized by FT-IR and Raman spectroscopy of efavirenz. Figure S1: Transmission electron micrograph of nanoemulsion F2, Figure S2: Transmission electron micrograph of nanoemulsion F4, Figure S3: (A) Diagnostic Box-Cox plot for power transforms and (B) predicted vs. actual plot for droplet size, Figure S4: (A) Diagnostic Box-Cox plot for power transforms and (B) predicted vs. actual plot for polydispersity index, Figure S5: (A) Diagnostic Box-Cox plot for power transforms and (B) predicted vs. actual plot for Zeta Potential, Figure S6: Overlay plot of the desirable area (yellow) derived using the specified criteria listed in Table S6, Figure S7: Raman Spectra of pure EFV, the control and EFV loaded nanoemulsions, Figure S8: FT-IR spectra of, pure EFV, Tween® 80, Span® 20, the control nanoemulsion, EFV loaded nanoemulsion and the nanoemulsion harvested following dissolution studies.

Author Contributions: R.B.W. conceptualized, supervised and contributed to writing and editing of the manuscript. P.M. performed the experiments, analyzed the data and wrote the article. S.M.M.K. contributed to the conceptualization, supervision, bibliographical research and proof reading of the manuscript. All authors have read and agreed to the published version of the manuscript.

Funding: This research received no external funding.

Acknowledgments: The authors acknowledge the National Research Foundation and the Research Committee of Rhodes University (R.B.W.). The authors acknowledge Bronwyn Tweedie for graphic assistance and Bwalya A. Witika for helpful research and experimental discussion.

Conflicts of Interest: The authors declare no conflict of interest.

References

1. UNAIDS. Global HIV & AIDS Statistics—2019 Fact Sheet. 2020. Available online: https://www.unaids.org/en/resources/fact-sheet (accessed on 8 March 2020).
2. Vitoria, M.; Rangaraj, A.; Ford, N.; Doherty, M. Current and future priorities for the development of optimal HIV drugs. *Curr. Opin. HIV AIDS* **2019**, *14*, 143–149. [CrossRef] [PubMed]
3. Taneja, S.; Shilpi, S.; Khatri, K. Formulation and optimization of efavirenz nanosuspensions using the precipitation-ultrasonication technique for solubility enhancement. *Artif. Cells Nanomed. Biotechnol.* **2016**, *44*, 978–984. [CrossRef] [PubMed]
4. Aungst, B.J. P-glycoprotein, secretory transport, and other barriers to the oral delivery of anti-HIV drugs. *Adv. Drug Deliv. Rev.* **1999**, *39*, 105–116. [CrossRef]
5. Persson, L.C.; Porter, C.J.H.; Charman, W.N.; Bergström, C.A.S. Computational prediction of drug solubility in lipid based formulation excipients. *Pharm. Res.* **2013**, *30*, 3225–3237. [CrossRef] [PubMed]
6. Rane, S.S.; Anderson, B.D. What determines drug solubility in lipid vehicles: Is it predictable? *Adv. Drug Deliv. Rev.* **2008**, *60*, 638–656. [CrossRef] [PubMed]
7. Kalepu, S.; Manthina, M.; Padavala, V. Oral lipid-based drug delivery systems—An overview. *Acta Pharm. Sin. B* **2013**, *3*, 361–372. [CrossRef]
8. Krstić, M.; Medarević, Đ.; Đuriš, J.; Ibrić, S. Self-nanoemulsifying drug delivery systems (SNEDDS) and self-microemulsifying drug delivery systems (SMEDDS) as lipid nanocarriers for improving dissolution rate and bioavailability of poorly soluble drugs. *Lipid Nanocarriers Drug Target.* **2018**, 473–508. [CrossRef]

9. Shahba, A.A.W.; Mohsin, K.; Alanazi, F.K. Novel self-nanoemulsifying drug delivery systems (SNEDDS) for oral delivery of cinnarizine: Design, optimization, and in-vitro assessment. *AAPS Pharmscitech* **2012**, *13*, 967–977. [CrossRef]
10. Saranya, J.S.; Elango, K.; Kumari, S.D.C.; Maheswari, A.U. Nose to brain direct delivery of levodopa from chitosan nano-particles–A novel approach. *IJPIs J. Pharm. Cosmetol.* **2012**, *2*, 30–39.
11. Solans, C.; Izquierdo, P.; Nolla, J.; Azemar, N.; Garcia-Celma, M.J. Nano-emulsions. *Curr. Opin. Colloid Interface Sci.* **2005**, *10*, 102–110. [CrossRef]
12. Jaiswal, M.; Dudhe, R.; Sharma, P.K. Nanoemulsion: An advanced mode of drug delivery system. *3 Biotech* **2015**, *5*, 123–127. [CrossRef] [PubMed]
13. Anton, N.; Vandamme, T.F. Nano-emulsions and micro-emulsions: Clarifications of the critical differences. *Pharm. Res.* **2011**, *28*, 978–985. [CrossRef] [PubMed]
14. Manea, A.M.; Ungureanu, C.; Meghea, A. Effect of vegetable oils on obtaining lipid nanocarriers for sea buckthorn extract encapsulation. *C. R. Chim.* **2014**, *17*, 934–943. [CrossRef]
15. Ander, B.P.; Dupasquier, C.M.C.; Prociuk, M.A.; Pierce, G.N. Polyunsaturated fatty acids and their effects on cardiovascular disease. *Exp. Clin. Cardiol.* **2003**, *8*, 164–172. [PubMed]
16. Salem, M.A.; Ezzat, S.M. Nanoemulsions in Food Industry. In *Some New Aspects of Colloidal Systems in Foods*; IntechOpen: London, UK, 2018. [CrossRef]
17. Garti, N.; Yaghmur, A.; Leser, M.E.; Clement, V.; Watzke, H.J. Improved oil solubilization in oil/water food grade microemulsions in the presence of polyols and ethanol. *J. Agric. Food Chem.* **2001**, *49*, 2552–2562. [CrossRef] [PubMed]
18. Flanagan, J.; Singh, H. Microemulsions: A potential delivery system for bioactives in food. *Crit. Rev. Food Sci. Nutr.* **2006**, *46*, 221–237. [CrossRef]
19. Komaiko, J.S.; Mcclements, D.J. Formation of Food-Grade Nanoemulsions Using Low-Energy Preparation Methods: A Review of Available Methods. *Compr. Rev. Food Sci. Food Saf.* **2016**, *15*, 331–352. [CrossRef]
20. Elfiyani, R.; Amalia, S.Y.P.A. Effect of Using the Combination of Tween 80 and Ethanol on the Forming and Physical Stability of Microemulsion of Eucalyptus Oil as Antibacterial. *J. Young Pharm.* **2017**, *9*, 118–121. [CrossRef]
21. Khan, A.A.; Mudassir, J.; Mohtar, N.; Darwis, Y. Advanced drug delivery to the lymphatic system: Lipid-based nanoformulations. *Int. J. Nanomed.* **2013**, *8*, 2733–2744. [CrossRef]
22. Humberstone, A.J.; Charman, W.N. Lipid-based vehicles for the oral delivery of poorly water soluble drugs. *Adv. Drug Deliv. Rev.* **1997**, *25*, 103–128. [CrossRef]
23. Bahari, L.A.S.; Hamishehkar, H. The impact of variables on particle size of solid lipid nanoparticles and nanostructured lipid carriers; A comparative literature review. *Adv. Pharm. Bull.* **2016**, *6*, 143–151. [CrossRef] [PubMed]
24. Danaei, M.; Dehghankhold, M.; Ataei, S.; Davarani, F.H.; Javanmard, R.; Dokhani, A.; Khorasani, S.; Mozafari, M.R. Impact of particle size and polydispersity index on the clinical applications of lipidic nanocarrier systems. *Pharmaceutics* **2018**, *10*, 57. [CrossRef] [PubMed]
25. Lamorde, M.; Byakika-Kibwika, P.; Tamale, W.S.; Kiweewa, F.; Ryan, M.; Amara, A.; Tjia, J.; Back, D.; Khoo, S.; Boffito, M.; et al. Effect of Food on the Steady-State Pharmacokinetics of Tenofovir and Emtricitabine plus Efavirenz in Ugandan Adults. *AIDS Res. Treat.* **2012**, *2012*, 1–6. [CrossRef] [PubMed]
26. Bertrand, L.; Dygert, L.; Toborek, M. Antiretroviral Treatment with Efavirenz Disrupts the Blood-Brain Barrier Integrity and Increases Stroke Severity. *Sci. Rep.* **2016**, *6*, 397838. [CrossRef]
27. Lu, G.W.; Gao, P. Emulsions and Microemulsions for Topical and Transdermal Drug Delivery. In *Handbook of Non-Invasive Drug Delivery Systems*; William Andrew Publishing: New York, NY, USA, 2010; pp. 59–94. [CrossRef]
28. Gumustas, M.; Sengel-Turk, C.T.; Gumustas, A.; Ozkan, S.A.; Uslu, B. Effect of Polymer-Based Nanoparticles on the Assay of Antimicrobial Drug Delivery Systems. In *Multifunctional Systems for Combined Delivery, Biosensing and Diagnostics*; Elsevier: Amsterdam, The Netherlands, 2017; pp. 67–108. ISBN 9780323527255. [CrossRef]
29. Kong, W.Y.; Salim, N.; Masoumi, H.R.F.; Basri, M.; da Costa, S.S.; Ahmad, N. Optimization of hydrocortisone-loaded nanoemulsion formulation using D-optimal mixture design. *Asian J. Chem.* **2018**, *30*, 853–858. [CrossRef]

30. Samson, S.; Basri, M.; Masoumi, H.R.F.; Karjiban, R.A.; Malek, E.A. Design and development of a nanoemulsion system containing copper peptide by D-optimal mixture design and evaluation of its physicochemical properties. *RSC Adv.* **2016**, *6*, 17845–17856. [CrossRef]
31. Chouhan, P.; Saini, T.R. D-optimal Design and Development of Microemulsion Based Transungual Drug Delivery Formulation of Ciclopirox Olamine for Treatment of Onychomycosis. *Indian J. Pharm. Sci.* **2016**, *78*, 498–511. [CrossRef]
32. Syed, H.K.; Peh, K.K. Identification of phases of various oil, surfactant/co-surfactants and water system by ternary phase diagram. *Acta Pol. Pharm. Drug Res.* **2014**, *71*, 301–309.
33. Cartón, A.; González, G.; De La Torre, A.I.; Cabezas, J.L. Separation of ethanol-water mixtures using 3A molecular sieve. *J. Chem. Technol. Biotechnol.* **1987**, *39*, 125–132. [CrossRef]
34. Banat, F.; Al-lagtah, N.; Al-sheh, S. Separation of ethanol–water mixtures using molecular sieves and biobased adsorbents. *Chem. Eng. Res. Des.* **2004**, *82*, 855–864. [CrossRef]
35. Winsor, P.A. Hydrotropy, solubilisation and related emulsification processes. Part I. *Trans. Faraday Soc.* **1947**, *44*, 376–398. [CrossRef]
36. Zeng, Z.; Zhou, G.; Wang, X.; Huang, E.Z.; Zhan, X.; Liu, J.; Wang, S.; Wang, A.; Li, H.; Pei, X.; et al. Preparation, characterization and relative bioavailability of oral elemene o/w microemulsion. *Int. J. Nanomed.* **2010**, *5*, 567–572. [CrossRef] [PubMed]
37. Flanagan, J.; Kortegaard, K.; Pinder, D.N.; Rades, T.; Singh, H. Solubilisation of soybean oil in microemulsions using various surfactants. In *Proceedings of the Food Hydrocolloids*; Elsevier: Amsterdam, The Netherlands, 2006; Volume 20, pp. 253–260. [CrossRef]
38. Zuccotti, G.V.; Fabiano, V. Safety issues with ethanol as an excipient in drugs intended for pediatric use. *Expert Opin. Drug Saf.* **2011**, *10*, 499–502. [CrossRef] [PubMed]
39. Valeur, K.S.; Hertel, S.A.; Lundstrøm, K.E.; Holst, H. The Cumulative Daily Tolerance Levels of Potentially Toxic Excipients Ethanol and Propylene Glycol Are Commonly Exceeded in Neonates and Infants. *Basic Clin. Pharmacol. Toxicol.* **2018**, *122*, 523–530. [CrossRef]
40. Chudasama, A.S.; Patel, V.V.; Nivsarkar, M.; Vasu, K.K.; Shishoo, C.J. In vivo Evaluation of Self Emulsifying Drug Delivery System for Oral Delivery of Nevirapine. *Indian J. Pharm. Sci.* **2014**, *76*, 218–224. Available online: https://pubmed.ncbi.nlm.nih.gov/25035533 (accessed on 8 August 2020).
41. Gurram, A.K.; Deshpande, P.B.; Kar, S.S.; Nayak, U.Y.; Udupa, N.; Reddy, M.S. Role of Components in the Formation of Self-microemulsifying Drug Delivery Systems. *Indian J. Pharm. Sci.* **2015**, *77*, 249–257. [CrossRef]
42. Bayrak, A.; Kiralan, M.; Ipek, A.; Arslan, N.; Cosge, B.; Khawar, K.M. Fatty acid compositions of linseed (*Linum Usitatissimum* L.) genotypes of different origin cultivated in Turkey. *Biotechnol. Biotechnol. Equip.* **2010**, *24*, 1836–1842. [CrossRef]
43. List, G.R. Oilseed Composition and Modification for Health and Nutrition. *Funct. Diet. Lipids* **2016**, 23–46. [CrossRef]
44. Garavaglia, J.; Markoski, M.M.; Oliveira, A.; Marcadenti, A. Grape Seed Oil Compounds: Biological and Chemical Actions for Health. *Nutr. Metab. Insights* **2016**, *9*, 59–64. [CrossRef]
45. Szumała, P. Structure of Microemulsion Formulated with Monoacylglycerols in the Presence of Polyols and Ethanol. *J. Surfactants Deterg.* **2015**, *18*, 97–106. [CrossRef]
46. Zen, N.I.M.; Abd Gani, S.S.; Shamsudin, R.; Masoumi, H.R.F. The use of D-optimal mixture design in optimizing development of okara tablet formulation as a dietary supplement. *Sci. World J.* **2015**. [CrossRef]
47. Gorman, J.W.; Hinman, J.E. Simplex Lattice Designs for Multicomponent Systems. *Technometrics* **1962**, *4*, 463–487. [CrossRef]
48. Hayati, I.N.; Man, Y.B.C.; Aini, I.N.; Tan, C.P. Dynamic rheological study on O/W emulsions as affected by polysaccharide interactions using a mixture design approach. In *Gums and Stabilisers for the Food Industry 15*; RSC Publishing: Istanbul, Turkey, 2010; pp. 267–274. [CrossRef]
49. U.S. Department of Commerce. *NIST/SEMATECH e-Handbook of Statistical Methods*; U.S. Department of Commerce: Washington, DC, USA, 2012. [CrossRef]
50. Sulaiman, I.S.C.; Basri, M.; Masoumi, H.R.F.; Ashari, S.E.; Ismail, M. Design and development of a nanoemulsion system containing extract of *Clinacanthus nutans* (L.) leaves for transdermal delivery system by D-optimal mixture design and evaluation of its physicochemical properties. *RSC Adv.* **2016**, *6*, 67378–67388. [CrossRef]

51. Koroleva, M.; Nagovitsina, T.; Yurtov, E. Nanoemulsions stabilized by non-ionic surfactants: Stability and degradation mechanisms. *Phys. Chem. Chem. Phys.* **2018**, *20*, 10369–10377. [CrossRef]
52. Kelly, C.; Jefferies, C.; Cryan, S.-A. Targeted Liposomal Drug Delivery to Monocytes and Macrophages. *J. Drug Deliv.* **2011**, *2011*, 1–11. [CrossRef] [PubMed]
53. Berger, E.; Breznan, D.; Stals, S.; Jasinghe, V.J.; Gonçalves, D.; Girard, D.; Faucher, S.; Vincent, R.; Thierry, A.R.; Lavigne, C. Cytotoxicity assessment, inflammatory properties, and cellular uptake of Neutraplex lipid-based nanoparticles in THP-1 monocyte-derived macrophages. *Nanobiomedicine* **2017**, *4*, 1–14. [CrossRef]
54. Li, P.H.; Lu, W.C. Effects of storage conditions on the physical stability of D-limonene nanoemulsion. *Food Hydrocoll.* **2016**, *53*, 218–224. [CrossRef]
55. Marban, C.; Forouzanfar, F.; Ait-Ammar, A.; Fahmi, F.; El Mekdad, H.; Daouad, F.; Rohr, O.; Schwartz, C. Targeting the brain reservoirs: Toward an HIV cure. *Front. Immunol.* **2016**, *7*, 1–13. [CrossRef]
56. Tojo, C.; de Dios, M.; Barroso, F. Surfactant effects on microemulsion-based nanoparticle synthesis. *Materials* **2010**, *4*, 55–72. [CrossRef]
57. Pokharkar, V.; Patil-Gadhe, A.; Palla, P. Efavirenz loaded nanostructured lipid carrier engineered for brain targeting through intranasal route: In-vivo pharmacokinetic and toxicity study. *Biomed. Pharmacother.* **2017**, *94*, 150–164. [CrossRef]
58. Marques, M.M.; Rezende, C.A.; Lima, G.C.; Marques, A.C.S.; Prado, L.D.; Leal, K.Z.; Rocha, H.V.A.; Ferreira, G.B.; Resende, J.A.L.C. New solid forms of efavirenz: Synthesis, vibrational spectroscopy and quantum chemical calculations. *J. Mol. Struct.* **2017**, *1137*, 476–484. [CrossRef]
59. Mishra, S.; Tandon, P.; Ayala, A.P. Study on the structure and vibrational spectra of efavirenz conformers using DFT: Comparison to experimental data. *Spectrochim. Acta Part. A Mol. Biomol. Spectrosc.* **2012**, *88*, 116–123. [CrossRef] [PubMed]
60. Reddy, N.P.; Padmavathi, Y.; Mounika, P.; Anjali, A. FTIR spectroscopy for estimation of efavirenz in raw material and tablet dosage form. *Int. Curr. Pharm. J.* **2015**, *4*, 390–395. [CrossRef]
61. Choudhury, S.R.; Mandal, A.; Chakravorty, D.; Gopal, M.; Goswami, A. Evaluation of physicochemical properties, and antimicrobial efficacy of monoclinic sulfur-nanocolloid. *J. Nanopart. Res.* **2013**, *15*. [CrossRef]
62. Dai, W.-G. In vitro methods to assess drug precipitation. *Int. J. Pharm.* **2010**, *393*, 1–16. [CrossRef] [PubMed]
63. Gao, P.; Shi, Y. Characterization of supersaturatable formulations for improved absorption of poorly soluble Drugs. *AAPS J.* **2012**, *14*, 703–713. [CrossRef] [PubMed]
64. Gursoy, R.N.; Benita, S. Self-emulsifying drug delivery systems (SEDDS) for improved oral delivery of lipophilic drugs. *Biomed. Pharmacother.* **2004**, *58*, 173–182. [CrossRef]
65. Lawrence, M.J.; Rees, G.D. Microemulsion-based media as novel drug delivery systems. *Adv. Drug Deliv. Rev.* **2012**, *64*, 175–193. [CrossRef]
66. Mazza, G. Health benefits of phytochemicals from selected Canadian crops. *Trends Food Sci. Technol.* **1999**, *10*, 193–198. [CrossRef]

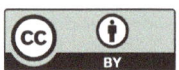

© 2020 by the authors. Licensee MDPI, Basel, Switzerland. This article is an open access article distributed under the terms and conditions of the Creative Commons Attribution (CC BY) license (http://creativecommons.org/licenses/by/4.0/).

30. Samson, S.; Basri, M.; Masoumi, H.R.F.; Karjiban, R.A.; Malek, E.A. Design and development of a nanoemulsion system containing copper peptide by D-optimal mixture design and evaluation of its physicochemical properties. *RSC Adv.* **2016**, *6*, 17845–17856. [CrossRef]
31. Chouhan, P.; Saini, T.R. D-optimal Design and Development of Microemulsion Based Transungual Drug Delivery Formulation of Ciclopirox Olamine for Treatment of Onychomycosis. *Indian J. Pharm. Sci.* **2016**, *78*, 498–511. [CrossRef]
32. Syed, H.K.; Peh, K.K. Identification of phases of various oil, surfactant/co-surfactants and water system by ternary phase diagram. *Acta Pol. Pharm. Drug Res.* **2014**, *71*, 301–309.
33. Cartón, A.; González, G.; De La Torre, A.I.; Cabezas, J.L. Separation of ethanol-water mixtures using 3A molecular sieve. *J. Chem. Technol. Biotechnol.* **1987**, *39*, 125–132. [CrossRef]
34. Banat, F.; Al-lagtah, N.; Al-sheh, S. Separation of ethanol–water mixtures using molecular sieves and biobased adsorbents. *Chem. Eng. Res. Des.* **2004**, *82*, 855–864. [CrossRef]
35. Winsor, P.A. Hydrotropy, solubilisation and related emulsification processes. Part I. *Trans. Faraday Soc.* **1947**, *44*, 376–398. [CrossRef]
36. Zeng, Z.; Zhou, G.; Wang, X.; Huang, E.Z.; Zhan, X.; Liu, J.; Wang, S.; Wang, A.; Li, H.; Pei, X.; et al. Preparation, characterization and relative bioavailability of oral elemene o/w microemulsion. *Int. J. Nanomed.* **2010**, *5*, 567–572. [CrossRef] [PubMed]
37. Flanagan, J.; Kortegaard, K.; Pinder, D.N.; Rades, T.; Singh, H. Solubilisation of soybean oil in microemulsions using various surfactants. In *Proceedings of the Food Hydrocolloids*; Elsevier: Amsterdam, The Netherlands, 2006; Volume 20, pp. 253–260. [CrossRef]
38. Zuccotti, G.V.; Fabiano, V. Safety issues with ethanol as an excipient in drugs intended for pediatric use. *Expert Opin. Drug Saf.* **2011**, *10*, 499–502. [CrossRef] [PubMed]
39. Valeur, K.S.; Hertel, S.A.; Lundstrøm, K.E.; Holst, H. The Cumulative Daily Tolerance Levels of Potentially Toxic Excipients Ethanol and Propylene Glycol Are Commonly Exceeded in Neonates and Infants. *Basic Clin. Pharmacol. Toxicol.* **2018**, *122*, 523–530. [CrossRef]
40. Chudasama, A.S.; Patel, V.V.; Nivsarkar, M.; Vasu, K.K.; Shishoo, C.J. In vivo Evaluation of Self Emulsifying Drug Delivery System for Oral Delivery of Nevirapine. *Indian J. Pharm. Sci.* **2014**, *76*, 218–224. Available online: https://pubmed.ncbi.nlm.nih.gov/25035533 (accessed on 8 August 2020).
41. Gurram, A.K.; Deshpande, P.B.; Kar, S.S.; Nayak, U.Y.; Udupa, N.; Reddy, M.S. Role of Components in the Formation of Self-microemulsifying Drug Delivery Systems. *Indian J. Pharm. Sci.* **2015**, *77*, 249–257. [CrossRef]
42. Bayrak, A.; Kiralan, M.; Ipek, A.; Arslan, N.; Cosge, B.; Khawar, K.M. Fatty acid compositions of linseed (*Linum Usitatissimum* L.) genotypes of different origin cultivated in Turkey. *Biotechnol. Biotechnol. Equip.* **2010**, *24*, 1836–1842. [CrossRef]
43. List, G.R. Oilseed Composition and Modification for Health and Nutrition. *Funct. Diet. Lipids* **2016**, 23–46. [CrossRef]
44. Garavaglia, J.; Markoski, M.M.; Oliveira, A.; Marcadenti, A. Grape Seed Oil Compounds: Biological and Chemical Actions for Health. *Nutr. Metab. Insights* **2016**, *9*, 59–64. [CrossRef]
45. Szumała, P. Structure of Microemulsion Formulated with Monoacylglycerols in the Presence of Polyols and Ethanol. *J. Surfactants Deterg.* **2015**, *18*, 97–106. [CrossRef]
46. Zen, N.I.M.; Abd Gani, S.S.; Shamsudin, R.; Masoumi, H.R.F. The use of D-optimal mixture design in optimizing development of okara tablet formulation as a dietary supplement. *Sci. World J.* **2015**. [CrossRef]
47. Gorman, J.W.; Hinman, J.E. Simplex Lattice Designs for Multicomponent Systems. *Technometrics* **1962**, *4*, 463–487. [CrossRef]
48. Hayati, I.N.; Man, Y.B.C.; Aini, I.N.; Tan, C.P. Dynamic rheological study on O/W emulsions as affected by polysaccharide interactions using a mixture design approach. In *Gums and Stabilisers for the Food Industry 15*; RSC Publishing: Istanbul, Turkey, 2010; pp. 267–274. [CrossRef]
49. U.S. Department of Commerce. *NIST/SEMATECH e-Handbook of Statistical Methods*; U.S. Department of Commerce: Washington, DC, USA, 2012. [CrossRef]
50. Sulaiman, I.S.C.; Basri, M.; Masoumi, H.R.F.; Ashari, S.E.; Ismail, M. Design and development of a nanoemulsion system containing extract of *Clinacanthus nutans* (L.) leaves for transdermal delivery system by D-optimal mixture design and evaluation of its physicochemical properties. *RSC Adv.* **2016**, *6*, 67378–67388. [CrossRef]

51. Koroleva, M.; Nagovitsina, T.; Yurtov, E. Nanoemulsions stabilized by non-ionic surfactants: Stability and degradation mechanisms. *Phys. Chem. Chem. Phys.* **2018**, *20*, 10369–10377. [CrossRef]
52. Kelly, C.; Jefferies, C.; Cryan, S.-A. Targeted Liposomal Drug Delivery to Monocytes and Macrophages. *J. Drug Deliv.* **2011**, *2011*, 1–11. [CrossRef] [PubMed]
53. Berger, E.; Breznan, D.; Stals, S.; Jasinghe, V.J.; Gonçalves, D.; Girard, D.; Faucher, S.; Vincent, R.; Thierry, A.R.; Lavigne, C. Cytotoxicity assessment, inflammatory properties, and cellular uptake of Neutraplex lipid-based nanoparticles in THP-1 monocyte-derived macrophages. *Nanobiomedicine* **2017**, *4*, 1–14. [CrossRef]
54. Li, P.H.; Lu, W.C. Effects of storage conditions on the physical stability of D-limonene nanoemulsion. *Food Hydrocoll.* **2016**, *53*, 218–224. [CrossRef]
55. Marban, C.; Forouzanfar, F.; Ait-Ammar, A.; Fahmi, F.; El Mekdad, H.; Daouad, F.; Rohr, O.; Schwartz, C. Targeting the brain reservoirs: Toward an HIV cure. *Front. Immunol.* **2016**, *7*, 1–13. [CrossRef]
56. Tojo, C.; de Dios, M.; Barroso, F. Surfactant effects on microemulsion-based nanoparticle synthesis. *Materials* **2010**, *4*, 55–72. [CrossRef]
57. Pokharkar, V.; Patil-Gadhe, A.; Palla, P. Efavirenz loaded nanostructured lipid carrier engineered for brain targeting through intranasal route: In-vivo pharmacokinetic and toxicity study. *Biomed. Pharmacother.* **2017**, *94*, 150–164. [CrossRef]
58. Marques, M.M.; Rezende, C.A.; Lima, G.C.; Marques, A.C.S.; Prado, L.D.; Leal, K.Z.; Rocha, H.V.A.; Ferreira, G.B.; Resende, J.A.L.C. New solid forms of efavirenz: Synthesis, vibrational spectroscopy and quantum chemical calculations. *J. Mol. Struct.* **2017**, *1137*, 476–484. [CrossRef]
59. Mishra, S.; Tandon, P.; Ayala, A.P. Study on the structure and vibrational spectra of efavirenz conformers using DFT: Comparison to experimental data. *Spectrochim. Acta Part. A Mol. Biomol. Spectrosc.* **2012**, *88*, 116–123. [CrossRef] [PubMed]
60. Reddy, N.P.; Padmavathi, Y.; Mounika, P.; Anjali, A. FTIR spectroscopy for estimation of efavirenz in raw material and tablet dosage form. *Int. Curr. Pharm. J.* **2015**, *4*, 390–395. [CrossRef]
61. Choudhury, S.R.; Mandal, A.; Chakravorty, D.; Gopal, M.; Goswami, A. Evaluation of physicochemical properties, and antimicrobial efficacy of monoclinic sulfur-nanocolloid. *J. Nanopart. Res.* **2013**, *15*. [CrossRef]
62. Dai, W.-G. In vitro methods to assess drug precipitation. *Int. J. Pharm.* **2010**, *393*, 1–16. [CrossRef] [PubMed]
63. Gao, P.; Shi, Y. Characterization of supersaturatable formulations for improved absorption of poorly soluble Drugs. *AAPS J.* **2012**, *14*, 703–713. [CrossRef] [PubMed]
64. Gursoy, R.N.; Benita, S. Self-emulsifying drug delivery systems (SEDDS) for improved oral delivery of lipophilic drugs. *Biomed. Pharmacother.* **2004**, *58*, 173–182. [CrossRef]
65. Lawrence, M.J.; Rees, G.D. Microemulsion-based media as novel drug delivery systems. *Adv. Drug Deliv. Rev.* **2012**, *64*, 175–193. [CrossRef]
66. Mazza, G. Health benefits of phytochemicals from selected Canadian crops. *Trends Food Sci. Technol.* **1999**, *10*, 193–198. [CrossRef]

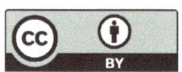

© 2020 by the authors. Licensee MDPI, Basel, Switzerland. This article is an open access article distributed under the terms and conditions of the Creative Commons Attribution (CC BY) license (http://creativecommons.org/licenses/by/4.0/).

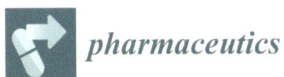

Article

Spontaneous In Situ Formation of Liposomes from Inert Porous Microparticles for Oral Drug Delivery

Maryam Farzan, Gabriela Québatte, Katrin Strittmatter, Florentine Marianne Hilty, Joachim Schoelkopf, Jörg Huwyler and Maxim Puchkov

[1] Division of Pharmaceutical Technology, Department of Pharmaceutical Sciences, University of Basel, Klingelbergstrasse 50, CH-4055 Basel, Switzerland; maryam.farzan@unibas.ch (M.F.); gabriela.quebatte@unibas.ch (G.Q.); katrin.strittmatter@gmx.de (K.S.); joerg.huwyler@unibas.ch (J.H.)

[2] Fundamental Research, Omya International AG, Baslerstrasse 42, CH-4665 Oftringen, Switzerland; florentine.hiltyvancura@omya.com (F.M.H.); joachim.schoelkopf@omya.com (J.S.)

* Correspondence: maxim.puchkov@unibas.ch

Received: 28 July 2020; Accepted: 13 August 2020; Published: 15 August 2020

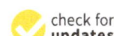

Abstract: Despite the wide-spread use of liposomal drug delivery systems, application of these systems for oral purposes is limited due to their large-scale formulation and storage issues. Proliposomes are one of the formulation approaches for achieving solid powders that readily form liposomes upon hydration. In this work, we investigated a dry powder formulation of a model low-soluble drug with phospholipids loaded in porous functionalized calcium carbonate microparticles. We characterized the liposome formation under conditions that mimic the different gastrointestinal stages and studied the factors that influence the dissolution rate of the model drug. The liposomes that formed upon direct contact with the simulated gastric environment had a capacity to directly encapsulate 25% of the drug in situ. The emerged liposomes allowed complete dissolution of the drug within 15 min. We identified a negative correlation between the phospholipid content and the rate of water uptake. This correlation corroborated the results obtained for the rate of dissolution and liposome encapsulation efficiency. This approach allows for the development of solid proliposomal dosage formulations, which can be scaled up with regular processes.

Keywords: oral drug delivery; dissolution enhancement; phospholipids; liposomes; solid dosage forms; porous microparticles

1. Introduction

Liposomes are one of the most studied drug delivery systems, owing to their ability to encapsulate various active substances of hydrophobic and hydrophilic nature, their biocompatibility, and design flexibility. Although liposomes were originally developed for parenteral drug delivery, their use for oral drug delivery has been a topic of research [1–4]. Liposomes are used for oral bioavailability enhancement of low-soluble or low-permeable active ingredients [4–7], as well as compounds with low stability in the gastrointestinal (GI) tract [2,8–11].

Compared to the widely used conventional solid dosage forms (i.e., tablets), production of liposomes is demanding due to production challenges, as well as physical and chemical stability issues. The production methods are optimized for small-scale production and are unlikely to qualify for oral dosage form production [12,13]. Moreover, liposomal dispersions that are stored in liquid form have a limited stability due to the risk of sedimentation, aggregation, and phospholipid hydrolysis [14]. It would also be beneficial to produce solid powders that can be processed using conventional tableting equipment.

Freeze-drying [15,16], spray-drying [17], spray freeze-drying [18], and supercritical fluid technology [19,20] are therefore used for producing solid liposomal formulations [21,22]. One of the methods for solidification of the oral liposomes is adsorption on solid inert carriers [23]. In 1986, Payne et al. [24] introduced dry and free-flowing liposomal formulations that could produce multi-lamellar liposomes upon hydration. These systems were given the name "proliposomal formulations" and have been a subject of various studies [5,25–29].

As adsorption carriers for dry liposomal formulations, water-soluble carriers such as sorbitol, mannitol, or cellulose derivatives have generally been used to enhance hydration of the phospholipids [27,30–34]. In this study, we propose the use of a pharmacologically inert porous carrier for a single-step production of solid proliposomal formulations. Porous materials offer various benefits for drug delivery, including their large surface area and large pore volumes that allow adsorption of materials and protection of the loaded material from harsh external conditions [35]. Additionally, porous media can facilitate the hydration of liposome-forming phospholipids by rapid water uptake due to the capillary action of the porous microstructure.

In the past years, we have focused on porous functionalized calcium carbonate (FCC) microparticles as a new carrier for drug delivery. FCC is a calcium carbonate that has undergone partial recrystallization to form a variable layer of lamellae of calcium phosphate (hydroxyapatite) on the surface of the particles. The particles have an average size of 10–20 µm and exhibit a specific surface area of 30–70 m^2/g and roughly 60% intra-particulate porosity [36]. The intra-particulate pore sizes range from 500 nm to less than 100 nm and the pores can be loaded with different materials [37]. We have harnessed the capabilities of the internal porosity of FCC particles to hold small molecular compounds [38,39] and peptides [35]. Drug loading into FCC particles allows for convenient handling and processing of compounds that would otherwise be challenging to formulate as conventional oral dosage forms. We have also studied the behavior of FCC in direct compaction and granulation processes that have resulted in FCC tablets with high tensile strength and fast disintegration [40]. Such unique mechanical characteristics of this novel porous material have allowed the production of orally disintegrating and gastro-retentive tablets from FCC [41–43].

The goal of the present study was to produce dry powder proliposomal formulations using the inert porous material FCC as a carrier. The feasibility of this approach was demonstrated on the basis of spontaneous formation of liposomes during hydration, drug encapsulation efficiency of the emerged liposomes, and their potential to improve the dissolution performance of nifedipine as a model low-soluble drug. Ultimately, the factors influencing the formation of liposomes and liposomal drug encapsulation were studied in different simulated gastrointestinal fluids.

2. Materials and Methods

FCC was kindly provided by Omya International AG (Oftringen, Switzerland), and 1,2-dimyristoyl-sn-glycero-3-phosphocholine (DMPC) was a contribution of Lipoid GmbH (Ludwigshafen, Germany). Nifedipine and methanol were supplied by Sigma-Aldrich (subsidiary of Merck KGaA, Darmstadt, Germany). Acetonitrile and fuming HCl were bought from Carl Roth GmbH (Karlsruhe, Germany). Fasted state-simulated intestinal fluid powder and buffer concentrate were purchased from Biorelevant.com Ltd. (London, United Kingdom). The solvents were of high-performance liquid chromatography (HPLC) grade, and all other materials were of analytical grade.

2.1. Loading of Nifedipine and DMPC in FCC

Nifedipine–DMPC–FCC formulations with various ratios of nifedipine and DMPC, as well as the corresponding control formulations, were produced by a one-step solvent evaporation method as follows: Required amounts of DMPC and nifedipine (Table 1) were dissolved in 20 mL methanol and in the final step, the sieved (355 µm) FCC powder was dispersed in this solution. The solvent was removed by evaporation in a rotary evaporator (Büchi, Switzerland). The initial pressure was set to 300 mbar and reduced by 100 mbar every 30 min. We kept the final pressure (20 mbar) for 60 min to ensure that most of the solvent was removed. The resulting drug-loaded FCC powders were then sieved through a 355 µm sieve.

Table 1. Expected drug and lipid composition of the sample formulations.

Formulation Code	DMPC (w/w%)	Nifedipine (w/w%)	FCC (w/w%)
D5N10	5	10	85
D5N15	5	15	80
D5N20	5	20	75
D10N10	10	10	80
D10N15	10	15	75
D10N20	10	20	70
D15N10	15	10	75
D15N15	15	15	70
D15N20	15	20	65
D20N10	20	10	70
D20N15	20	15	65
D20N20	20	20	60
Nif-FCC (control)	0	20	80
DMPC-Nif (control)	50	50	0
DMPC-FCC (control)	20	0	80
Physical mixture	20	20	60

Physical mixture was produced for reference purposes by manually blending the sieved (355 µm) amounts of individual components and mixing for 5 min.

2.2. Quantification of the Drug Content in Formulations

We quantified the nifedipine content in the formulations using a reverse-phase high-performance liquid chromatography (RP-HPLC) method. A C18 column, 90 Å, 5 µm, 3.9 × 150 mm (Resolve C18, Waters, Milford, MA, USA) was used as the stationary phase with a C18 guard column (Security Guard, Phenomenex, Torrance, CA, USA). A mobile phase composition of water/methanol/acetonitrile (50:25:25) was isocratically pumped at a flow rate of 1 mL/min. A high sensitivity flow cell for SPD-M30A diode array detector (Shimadzu, Kyoto, Japan) was used at 236 nm. The injection volume was 5 µL. Test solutions were prepared by dispersing 10 mg of the sample in 5 mL 0.1 M HCl to dissolve the calcium carbonate and calcium phosphate components of FCC. This was followed by sonicating the dispersions for 5 min to ensure complete dissolution of the carrier. A volume of 5 mL methanol was added in a subsequent step and the samples were sonicated again for 5 min. The solutions were diluted once more (1 mL to 10 mL) with the mobile phase and filtered through 0.45 µm syringe filters. All sample preparations were made in triplicate. The chromatographic measurements for each sample were carried out in triplicate. The absorbance was measured at a wavelength of 236 nm.

2.3. Screening for an Absence of External Crystallization

We investigated crystallization of nifedipine outside of the FCC particles by visual analysis of scanning electron microscopy (SEM) images (FEI Nova Nano SEM230, FEI, Hillsboro, OR, USA). Small amounts of the powders were placed on carbon adhesives and dedusted. The samples were sputtered with a 20 nm gold layer before imaging.

We used a focused ion beam scanning electron microscopy (FIB-SEM) method to visualize the internal structure of loaded FCC. To investigate the effect of phospholipid on nifedipine loading in FCC, we selected the formulations D5N20 and D20N20 as representative samples for lowest and highest phospholipid content, respectively, for FIB-SEM. Nif-FCC control formulation (without phospholipid) and pure FCC were used as reference material. To eliminate inter-particulate pores and visualize only the internal pore loading, we consolidated the powders with a compressive pressure of 50 MPa. Previous studies have shown that this pressure effectively eliminates inter-particulate pores without affecting the intra-particle structure [37,40]. The samples were sputtered with a 20 nm gold layer before visualization. Tilt angle of 52 degrees was used for ion beam processing and further imaging (FEI Helios Nano Lab 650, FEI, Hillsboro, OR, USA). To produce trenches with a size of 20 × 10 × 8 µm, we milled down the selected regions of the samples using a 21 nA gallium ion beam. Prior to the ion-milling step, a platinum protective layer with a thickness of 0.3 µm was deposited on the location of the trench to protect the surface of the sample from deformations during the ion beam application. After milling, the surface of the cross-section was polished with a 0.79 nA ion beam and sputtered with a 3 nm platinum layer, prior to SEM imaging, to enhance conductivity of the surface and reduce imaging artifacts.

2.4. Liposomal Size Measurement

Simulated gastric fluid without enzyme (SGF), pH 1.2, and phosphate buffer, pH 6.8, were produced as per United States Pharmacopeia and the National Formulary (USP-NF) [44]. The hydrodynamic size of the liposomes in SGF and phosphate buffer was measured by dynamic light scattering (DLS) using a Malvern Zetasizer Nano (Malvern Instruments, United Kingdom). For this measurement, aliquots of the powder formulations were added to the medium to result in a 5 mg/L concentration of nifedipine in the solution. The samples were stirred at 37 °C for 10 min to allow release of liposomes. The dispersions were then centrifuged at a 1000 relative centrifugal field (RCF) for 10 min at room temperature to separate FCC particles and undissolved drug from the liposomal dispersion. The DLS measurements were made on the supernatants for 10 measurement cycles.

2.5. Quantification of Nifedipine eEncapsulation in Liposomes

To quantify the nifedipine encapsulation efficiency of the liposomes, we dispersed the samples in the SGF and phosphate buffer and prepared them as described previously in Section 2.4. The total dissolved nifedipine in the supernatants was measured with HPLC. To separate the free drug from the liposomal-bound drug, we centrifuged the samples in 30 kDa cutoff Amicon Ultra Centrifugal Filter Units (Merck Millipore, Merck KGaA, Darmstadt, Germany) for 10 min at 4000 RCF at room temperature. The amount of the free drug and the encapsulated drug were measured by HPLC from the filtrate and the retentate, respectively, and the encapsulation efficiency of the liposomes in every formulation was calculated.

2.6. Liposome Imaging by Cryo-Electron Microscopy (Cryo-EM) and Fluorescent Microscopy

For cryo-EM imaging, the retentates from the centrifugal filtration were diluted with 500 µL of MilliQ water, loaded on holey carbon-coated grids (Lacey, Tedpella, Redding, CA, USA) and vitrified in liquid ethane at −180 °C using a vitrobot (FEI Company, Eindhoven, Netherlands). The frozen grids were transferred to a Talos Electron microscope (FEI, Hillsboro, OR, USA) and imaged at cryogenic temperatures using a Gatan 626 cryo-holder (Gatan, Pleasanton, CA, USA). The electron micrographs were recorded at an accelerating voltage of 200 V using a low-dose system (30 e$^-$/Å^2) and keeping the sample at −175 °C. Defocus values were −2 to −3 µm. Micrographs were recorded on a 4K × 4K Ceta CMOS camera.

For fluorescent imaging, formulations loaded with the 1,1′-dioctadecyl-3,3,3′,3′-tetramethylindocarbocyanine perchlorate (DiI) as a model hydrophobic substance were used. The samples were dispersed in a high concentration, suitable for imaging, as follows. A 20 mg aliquot of the sample was added to 50 mL of the solvent and the dispersion was shaken in a water bath at 37 °C. A droplet of the sample was visualized on a microscope slide with a cover glass using an Olympus CKX41 microscope (Olympus Ltd., Tokyo, Japan) at an excitation wavelength of 549 nm and an emission wavelength of 565 nm.

2.7. In Vitro Dissolution

Fasted state-simulated intestinal fluid (FaSSIF) was prepared according to the recommended recipe from the supplying company [45].

To determine the equilibrium solubility of the drug in SGF, we used phosphate buffer, pH 6.8, and FaSSIF, a saturation shake-flask method as follows: An excess amount (100 mg) of nifedipine was added to 5 mL of each buffer. The samples were protected from light and stirred in a water bath at 37 °C for 96 h. Samples were then centrifuged at 2000 RCF for 30 min and analyzed with HPLC. Each measurement was performed in triplicate.

For in vitro dissolution testing, aliquots of formulations were filled in hydroxypropyl methylcellulose capsules. The dosage of all formulations were selected to achieve a 5 mg/L concentration of nifedipine in the dissolution vessel. The dissolution experiments were carried out in a USP II apparatus (Sotax, Aesch, Switzerland) in 900 mL of medium [44] with stainless steel sinkers to prevent capsule floatation. The temperature was set to 37.1 ± 0.5 °C and the paddle speed was 100 rpm. Nifedipine concentration was measured by UV–VIS (Ultraspec 3100 pro, Amersham Biosciences, United Kingdom) at a 236 nm wavelength with 1-min software-controlled intervals (DissoControl v1.0, University of Basel, Basel, Switzerland). In parallel, to reduce errors introduced by possible phospholipid structures (i.e., lipid vesicles), for quantification of the dissolved nifedipine, we made manual samplings. Manual sampling was done after 5, 10, 15, 30, 60, 90, 120, and 150 min. To eliminate any undissolved nifedipine crystals in the dissolution aliquotes, we centrifuged an amount of 2 mL of the samples at 37 °C and 2000 RCF for 15 min. A volume of 500 µL of the supernatant was diluted with an equal volume of methanol to dissolve phospholipid vesicles. Removed volumes were replaced with fresh dissolution medium.

Assuming sink condition in the dissolution vessels, we fitted the dissolution profiles to Equation (1):

$$C_t = C_d - ae^{-kt} \tag{1}$$

where C_t (mg/L) is the concentration of nifedipine that is dissolved in the medium at time t (s), C_d (mg/L) is the concentration of the nifedipine after the dissolution reached a plateau, a is the scaling constant, and k is the dissolution rate constant. In order to obtain the dissolution rate constant value for all the tested formulations, we fitted the experimental dissolution curves to Equation (1). The fittings were done in Wolfram Mathematica software, version 12 (Wolfram, Oxfrodshire, UK, 2019). To measure the goodness of fit, we used the standard errors for parameter estimates from the default Non-linear Model Fit function of the Mathematica software [46]. Two-way ANOVA and Bonferroni post-hoc test were performed (OriginPro 2018, OriginLab, Northampton, MA, USA) on the obtained dissolution rate constants with significance levels of 0.05 and 0.005, respectively.

The dissolution efficiency (*DE*) of the formulations in the first 120 min of the in vitro dissolution was calculated according to Equation (2) [47]:

$$DE = \frac{\int_0^{120} D_{120}.dt}{D_{max}.120} \times 100 = \frac{AUC_{0-120}}{D_{max}} \times 100 \tag{2}$$

where D_{120} is the amount of drug dissolved at 120 min (%), D_{max} is the maximum drug dissolved at the end of the dissolution (%), and AUC_{0-120} is the area under the dissolution curve between the times of 0 and 120 min.

2.8. Differential Scanning Calorimetry

A differential scanning calorimeter (DSC3, Mettler Toledo, Columbus, OH, USA) was used for thermal analysis of the samples. The scans were carried out in the interval between 30 and 200 °C with a rate of 10 °C/min, followed by an isothermal step at 200 °C for 5 min. The amount of crystalline drug can be calculated on the basis of the melting enthalpy of the drug [48]. Here, a simplified method was used [49,50] to calculate the amount of crystalline drug in FCC-Nif and D5N20 formulations:

$$X_c(\%) = \frac{\Delta H_{load}}{\Delta H_{bulk}} \times 100 \tag{3}$$

where X_c is the amount of crystalline drug, ΔH_{load} is the melting enthalpy of the drug-loaded formulation, and ΔH_{bulk} is the melting enthalpy of the drug in bulk nifedipine.

2.9. X-ray Powder Diffraction

The solid state of the drug in the samples was investigated by X-ray powder diffraction (XRPD) with a Rigaku SmartLab diffractometer equipped with a 9 kW rotating anode and a HyPix-3000 detector (Rigaku Corporation, Tokyo, Japan). Bragg–Brentano optics were set as follows: 5.0 degree (deg) incident parallel Soller slit, 1/8 mm incident slit, 10 mm length limiting slit on the incident arm of the goniometer and 4 mm receiving slit #1, open parallel slit analyzer, 5.0 degree receiving parallel Soller slit, and 13 mm receiving slit #2 on the receiving arm of the goniometer.

The samples were exposed to X-rays of Cu wavelength (1.541 Å) and measured in 1D detection mode in a $\theta/2\theta$ range of 2–60 degree with a step size of 0.01 deg and a 1 deg/min scanning speed.

2.10. Surface Area Measurements

The specific surface area of the samples was measured using nitrogen sorption and a five-point Brunauer–Emmet–Teller (BET) method using a Nova 2000e surface area analyzer (Quantachrome Instruments, Boynton Beach, FL, USA). All measurements were carried out in triplicate. Prior to surface area measurements, the samples were evacuated and degassed for a minimum of 3 h at room temperature.

2.11. Water Sorption Measurements

The rate of the water uptake of the powder samples was measured using a Krüss K100 Force Tensiometer (KRÜSS GmbH, Hamburg, Germany). The powders were loosely packed in capillaries with an inner diameter of 1 mm. As soon as the samples came into contact with water, we recorded the increase in the mass. The Lucas–Washburn equation [51,52] was used to calculate the rate of water sorption:

$$\frac{l^2}{t} = \frac{(C \cdot \bar{r})\sigma \cos \theta}{4\eta} \tag{4}$$

where l (m) is the position of the wetting front, t (s) is the liquid sorption time, C is the quantity describing the orientation of the microcapillaries (*dimensionless*), $\bar{r}$ (m) is the average radius of the capillaries (assuming the powder porosity as a bundle of capillaries), σ (N/m) is the surface tension of the liquid, θ is the wetting angle (*deg*), and η (Pa × s) is the dynamic viscosity of the liquid [53]. The wetting constant $(C \times \bar{r})$ of each formulation was calculated by the LabDesk software (version 3.0, KRÜSS GmbH, Hamburg, Germany).

3. Results

3.1. Characteristics of the Liposomal System after Hydration of the Powder Formulations

Double chain phospholipids with a phosphatidylcholine head group have a packing parameter (ratio between the cross-sectional area of the hydrophobic region and the hydrophilic head-group) close to 1. Therefore, these lipids are likely to form bilayer structures as compared to micellar assemblies [54–56].

The DLS measurement, cryo-EM imaging, and fluorescent microscopy showed the size, morphology, and the formation dynamics of the liposomes after the hydration of the formulations in the acidic condition of SGF and the neutral condition of phosphate buffer (Figure 1, Figure S1).

The hydrodynamic diameter of the liposomes in SGF and phosphate buffer showed a population at 669 ± 169 nm and 490 ± 112 nm average size, respectively. However, in SGF, the liposomes additionally had a second population with an average size of 121 ± 36 nm (Figure 1, lower left panels). No difference was observed between the liposome sizes of different formulations (data not shown). Cumulant analysis of the samples obtained a z-average of 261 ± 83.07 (polydispersity index 0.56 ± 0.13) and 420 ± 86.86 nm (polydispersity index 0.60 ± 010) for the liposomes in SGF and phosphate buffer, respectively.

The cryo-EM imaging of the liposomes corroborated the DLS results by showing many uni-lamellar and a small number of multi-lamellar liposomes after dissolving in SGF. On the other hand, the liposomes in the phosphate buffer had larger sizes and mostly multi-lamellar and multi-vesicular morphologies.

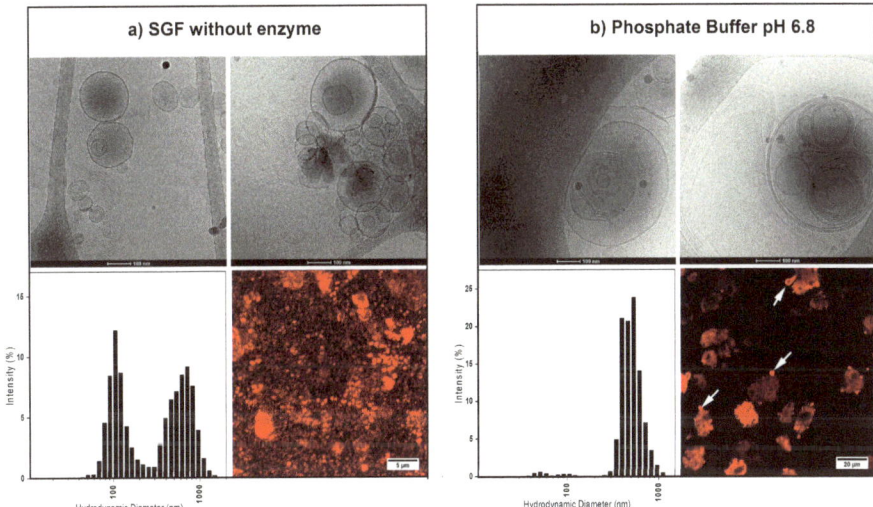

Figure 1. The morphology (i.e., uni-lamellar versus multi-lamellar) and size distribution of the liposomes after dispersing the powders in simulated gastric fluid without enzyme (SGF) (**a**) and phosphate buffer (**b**). For each sample, the top panels show the cryo-EM images of the resulting liposomes. The bottom left panels show the average hydrodynamic diameter of the liposomes in each medium, and the bottom right panels are the fluorescent microscopy images, showing the liposomes encapsulating a hydrophobic dye. In phosphate buffer, the liposomes can be seen emerging from the functionalized calcium carbonate (FCC) particles (white arrows).

Fluorescent imaging showed incorporation of the hydrophobic fluorescent dye (DiI) in the lipid bilayer of the liposomes. For samples prepared in SGF, almost no residuals of FCC particles could be observed. The supplementary optical microscopy video (Video S1) shows the dissolution process of FCC particles in SGF and formation of the liposomes. Formation of CO_2 bubbles resulting from the dissolution of calcium carbonate is clearly seen on the video. On the other hand, dispersion of the samples in phosphate buffer showed that FCC particles remain intact, while liposomes of various shapes and sizes slowly emerge out of the porous structure of the particles.

The encapsulation efficiency of nifedipine (Figure 2b) was significantly greater in the liposomes created in SGF, as compared to phosphate buffer. The encapsulation efficiency was generally higher in the formulations with lower phospholipid contents (5% and 10%) at a maximum average of 25% for D5N20. However, the encapsulation efficiency was not significantly different among the formulations in the same dissolution medium (p-value > 0.05).

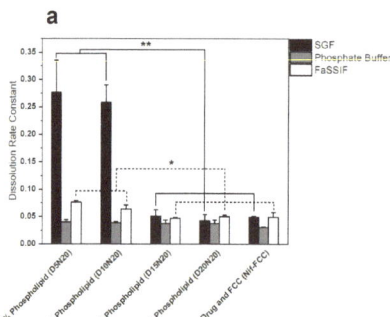 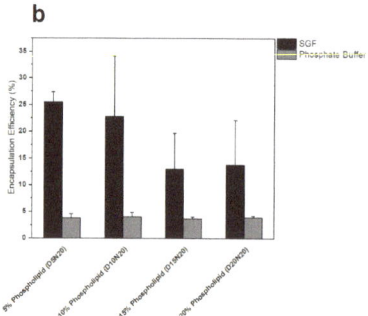

Figure 2. Comparison of the dissolution rate and liposomal encapsulation efficiency of nifedipine for different formulations. (**a**) The dissolution rate of formulations obtained from fitting the dissolution data to Equation (5), and (**b**) encapsulation efficiency of the liposomes after the hydration of powders in different media. Increasing the phospholipid content inversely affected both the dissolution rate and encapsulation efficiency. Single asterisk indicates a p-value < 0.05 and the double asterisk indicates a p-value < 0.005.

3.2. In Vitro Dissolution

Nifedipine equilibrium solubility in SGF, phosphate buffer, and FaSSIF were 17.94 ± 2.21 mg/L, 16.06 ± 1.71 mg/L, and 48.86 ± 25.26 mg/L, respectively. Therefore, the 5 mg/L drug concentration for in vitro dissolution tests was significantly below the saturation solubility of nifedipine in all three media, thus implying sink condition.

For all media, the dissolution rate of nifedipine was faster for the formulations with FCC than for the reference formulation without FCC (Nif-DMPC), as well as for the physical mixture (Figure 3).

The dissolution results in SGF showed that the rate of dissolution of nifedipine was inversely proportional to the phospholipid content. The changing ratio of drug to phospholipid did not have any influence on the rate of dissolution (Table S1). Therefore, all further analyses were carried out on the formulations with the highest drug load (20%) and with varying phospholipid content (i.e., D5N20, D10N20, D15N20, and D20N20).

The 5% and 10% phospholipid formulations showed significantly faster drug release in SGF, compared to the formulations with 15% and 20% phospholipid content, and Nif-FCC (Figures 2a and 3a). All formulations with DMPC and FCC reached at least 85% drug dissolution.

None of the formulations reached 85% dissolution (Figure 3b) in FaSSIF. However, the rate of dissolution was significantly faster for the formulations with 5% and 10% phospholipid content (Figure 2a).

Similar results were obtained in the phosphate buffer, where none of the formulations reached 85% dissolution (Figure 3c). The rate of dissolution in the phosphate buffer was not significantly different within the formulations with FCC (p-value > 0.05).

The dissolution efficiency (DE) of formulations, as a measure of the dissolution behavior of the formulations, are shown in Table 2.

The results show a reduction in the DE of Nif-DMPC in all media. In SGF, a trend of reduction in DE was seen with increasing phospholipid contents.

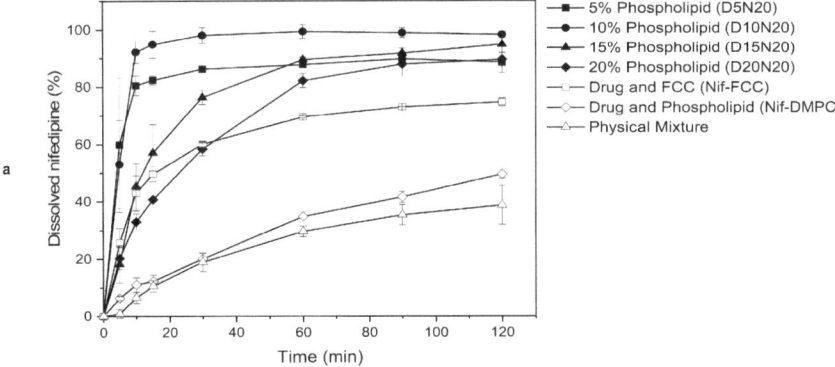

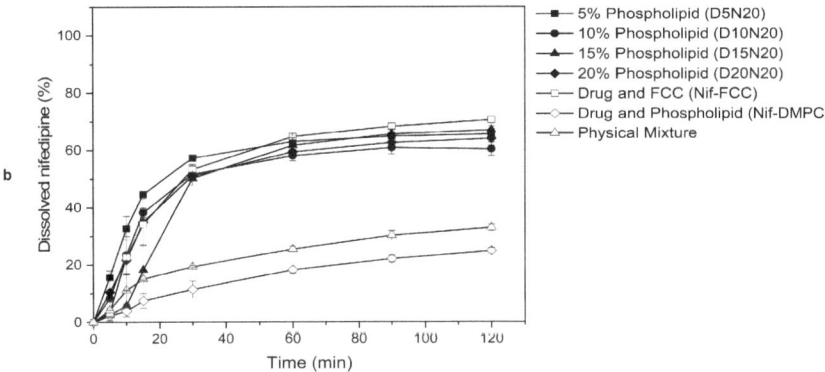

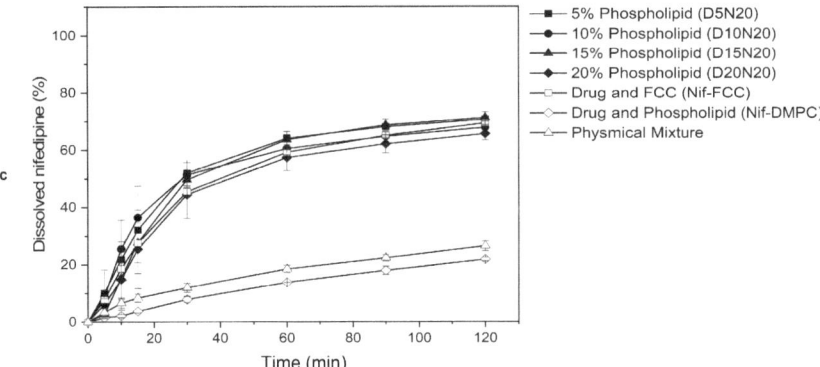

Figure 3. Selected FCC formulations (see Table 1) tested for dissolution in three different dissolution media: (**a**) SGF without enzyme, (**b**) fasted state-simulated intestinal fluid (FaSSIF), and (**c**) phosphate buffer, pH 6.8. Solid symbols represent formulations containing an increasing amount of phospholipid. Open symbols represent control formulations. Values are mean ± SD of n = 2 or 3 tests.

Table 2. Dissolution efficiency of formulations calculated based on Equation (2).

Formulation Code	SGF	Phosphate Buffer	FaSSIF
D5N20	91.53 ± 1.33	79.66 ± 4.33	86.40 ± 1.33
D10N20	89.74 ± 2.96	79.35 ± 1.31	84.88 ± 1.02
D15N20	84.23 ± 1.06	76.26 ± 2.19	78.09 ± 1.10
D20N20	77.45 ± 1.37	74.95 ± 6.76	80.34 ± 0.005
Nif-FCC	84.19 ± 1.13	73.66 ± 1.95	80.19 ± 2.01
Nif-DMPC	60.12 ± 9.79	57.23 ± 1.42	64.80 ± 3.25

3.3. Characterization of the Dry Powder Formulations

As an assessment of the loading efficiency, we visually investigated the appearance of the particles using SEM. The obtained images showed individual particles with neither agglomerates nor external drug crystallization (Figure 4b). There was no observable blocking or covering of the particle surfaces (Figure 4c). The images of the loaded samples were similar to the reference FCC material (Figure 4a).

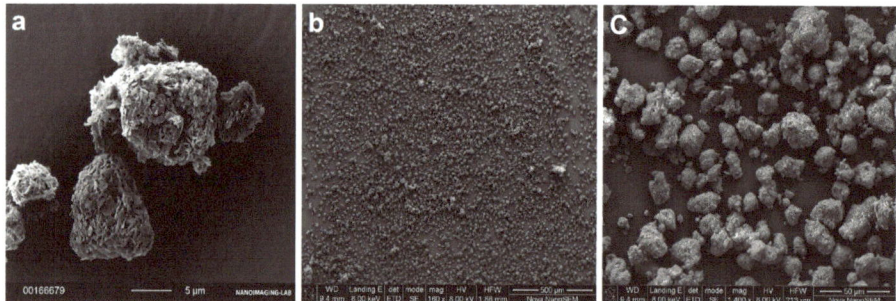

Figure 4. SEM images used for visual analysis of drug-loaded FCC. (**a**) The surface lamella of the unloaded FCC particles can be seen. (**b**) Representative overview of the powder formulation with highest loaded material (D20N20), showing the absence of agglomerates and external crystals. (**c**) Formulation D20N20 showing preserved lamellar structure of FCC after loading.

FIB-SEM images from the cross-section of the particles (Figure 5a) showed intra-particle larger pores evenly distributed throughout the entire FCC compact [40], while the drug-loaded formulations had smaller pores. The formulations Nif-FCC (Figure 5b) and D5N20 (Figure 5c) were not visually different, neither in pore sizes nor in pore shapes. On the contrary, the filled porous structure was seen for the formulation D20N20 (Figure 5d).

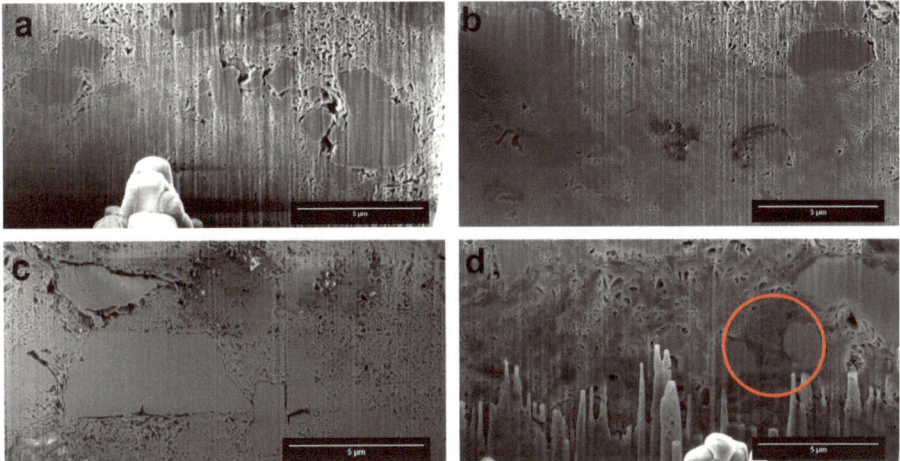

Figure 5. The focused ion beam scanning electron microscopy (FIB-SEM) images showed cross-sections of the formulations after consolidating the powder. (**a**) Pure FCC, (**b**) Nif-FCC without phospholipid, (**c**) D5N20, and (**d**) D20N20. The red circle shows an example of a region with blocked pores.

A loading efficiency of above 90% for the drug in all of the powder formulations was measured. On the basis of the results of BET surface area measurements, the specific surface area of the formulations decreased due to an increase in the phospholipid loading (Figure 6).

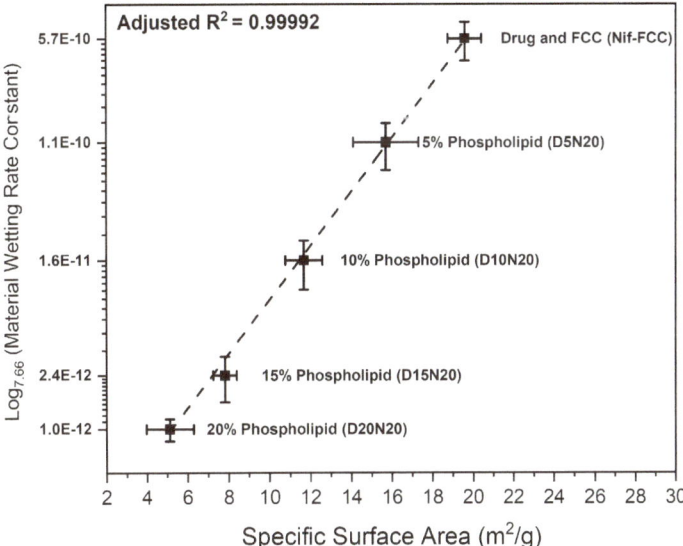

Figure 6. The semi-logarithmic plot (base 7.66) of the correlation between the wetting constants versus specific surface area of the powder samples.

The water sorption measurements showed an inverse correlation between the rate of water uptake and phospholipid content (Figure 6).

Figure 6 shows the correlation of the power law (represented as a semi-logarithmic plot) of the material wetting constant (obtained from Equation (4)) with the specific surface area of the formulations. For this correlation, the experimental data were fitted to Equation (5):

$$S = aC^n + b \qquad (5)$$

where S is the specific surface area (m^2); C is the wetting constant obtained from Equation (4); a is the scaling parameter, intercept $b \to 0$; and exponent $n = 7.66$ are the parameters obtained after fitting the experimental data to Equation (5). The two sets of results showed a strong positive power law correlation (adjusted $R^2 = 0.99992$).

X-Ray powder diffraction was used to exclude an effect of complete drug amorphization. The X-ray diffraction results of samples are presented in Figure 7. The control formulations in the absence of phospholipid or FCC both showed strong characteristic peaks of nifedipine at 8.11°, 11.76°, and 16.16°. The intensity of these peaks was lower in the formulations with DMPC and FCC.

The results of thermal analysis (Figure S2) showed the nifedipine melting peak at 172 °C. However, the samples with 5% phospholipid (D5N20) and without phospholipid (Nif-FCC) showed a reduced melting enthalpy for nifedipine. On the basis of calculations according to Equation (3), we detected crystallinity ratios of 60.76 ± 0.69% and 57 ± 9.91% for the D5N20 and Nif-FCC samples, respectively. The nifedipine melting peak was not present in the samples prepared with higher content of phospholipid.

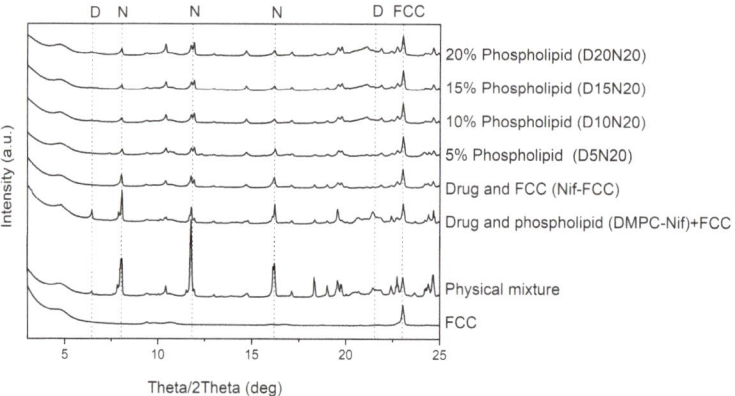

Figure 7. XRPD results of the formulations and physical mixture. The model drug was present in partial crystalline form in all formulations. The reference peaks of nifedipine (N) (8.11°, 11.76°, and 16.16°) and 1,2-dimyristoyl-sn-glycero-3-phosphocholine (DMPC) (D) (6.65° and 20.98°) are marked with dashed lines. A reference peak for FCC at 23.01° is also marked. The sample DMPC-Nif was physically mixed with FCC to keep the ratio of the components constant for all samples.

4. Discussion

The results of the present study showed massive spontaneous in situ formation of liposomes from a porous inorganic drug carrier combined with phospholipids. This effect was observed in media simulating the conditions of the different regions of the GI tract. As a consequence, this effect led to dissolution rate enhancement of a model low soluble drug.

A successful drug loading in the internal pores of the carrier is essential for effective porous structure exploitation. In this study, the loading efficiency was visually controlled. Absence of external deposition of drug crystals and phospholipid material was confirmed by visual image analysis for every formulation (excluding physical mixtures), as shown in Figure 4. The results suggest that the phospholipid and nifedipine were loaded in the internal structure of the porous FCC particles.

This result was corroborated by FIB cross-sectioning of the consolidated and loaded FCC, as shown in Figure 5. By visual analysis of internal porosity reduction, as clearly seen on the FIB-SEM images (Figure 5d), we could confirm the loading of drug and phospholipid into internal carrier structures. The results of BET measurements (Figure 6) showed a reduction in specific surface area, which further confirmed the hypothesis of internal (i.e., intraparticulate) deposition of the loaded material.

Both calcium carbonate and calcium phosphate, the main constituents of FCC, readily dissolve in the low pH of the gastric medium, which triggers an immediate release of liposomes (Video S1). On the other hand, in neutral pH media, the formation of liposomes from FCC particle followed a different mechanism. Since the carrier was not immediately dissolved in the neutral pH, the liquid was taken up into the particles by the carrier's micro-capillaries. This observation suggests a capillary pump action for the porous microstructure of FCC. The capillary pump effect supposedly drives the hydrated phospholipids out of the pores and promotes self-assembly of liposomes. This process can be seen in the confocal microscopy images, revealing the liposomes emerging (budding) out of the pores of FCC (Figure 1).

In SGF (i.e., medium with a low pH), a significantly large population of the liposomes had a size of 121 ± 36 nm and were observed as uni-lamellar structures in cryo-EM images. This size range was possibly due to fast release of liposomes from FCC, aided by the eddy currents created as a result of CO_2 formation from calcium carbonate dissolution in the acidic pH. The liposomes formed in this process were able to encapsulate up to 25% of the nifedipine, resulting in a faster dissolution of the drug compared to the drug release rate from the formulation without phospholipids. The different liposome formation mechanism in neutral pH produced large multi-lamellar liposomes (490 ± 112 nm) as seen in the cryo-EM images. These liposomes had a lower encapsulation efficiency, as compared to the uni-lamellar liposomes in SGF. This finding was surprising since the multi-lamellar liposomes were expected to have a higher encapsulation efficiency for hydrophobic drugs compared to uni-lamellar liposomes. The low encapsulation efficiency in neutral media was explained by the slow rate of formation and release of the liposomes from FCC particles, which allowed enough time for the drug to escape from the liposomes before their detachment from the carrier. This assumption was further confirmed by the results that showed a similar rate of dissolution of nifedipine from FCC phospholipid formulations and the Nif-FCC (the formulation without phospholipid) in neutral pH. In other words, in neutral pH, nifedipine dissolution takes place independently of the liposome formation, and the dissolution rate is enhanced solely by the large specific surface area of the carrier.

Due to the surface-active properties of phospholipids, faster dissolution rates are expected from formulations with higher DMPC content. Despite the latter, an increased phospholipid content resulted in slower dissolution rates in SGF (Figures 2 and 3). The higher phospholipid amounts in FCC reduce the overall surface area available for drug release by blocking out the carrier's porous meshwork, which leads to a reduction in the surface available for dissolution. This effect was confirmed by the results of BET surface area experiments, where a reduction of specific surface area with an increase in the phospholipid content was measured. For example, the D5N20 sample with 5% phospholipid content had a threefold larger specific surface area and an almost sevenfold faster dissolution as compared to D20N20.

The importance of the available medium-to-solid contact surface is emphasized since FCC itself dissolves in the low pH dissolution medium. This is forcing single particles to disintegrate, which leads to a faster release of the liposomes that can better encapsulate the drug (i.e., not letting sufficient time for the drug to escape the forming liposomes) and results in a faster rate of dissolution. Additions of more phospholipid lead to a slower wetting, confirmed by the water sorption studies, and therefore slower reaction of FCC with the medium. This makes the drug release dependent on the diffusion of the drug from the carrier's pores. A complete dissolution of calcium carbonate in SGF results in disappearance of the carrier particles; therefore, the only microclimate pH change may be expected within the formed liposomes. In theory, a change in the dissolution kinetics of the drug is expected to be negligible due to close proximity of undissolved drug crystals to the lipophilic layer of the phospholipids.

The high surface area of FCC itself effectively exposes the deposited drug to the medium and, even without phospholipids, leads to a faster dissolution of nifedipine from the FCC formulations compared to the physical mixture (Figure 3, Nif-FCC vs. physical mixture).

The X-ray diffraction and DSC results did not exclude the fact that the nifedipine might be partially deposited in a non-crystalline form in the carrier. The DSC thermograms of FCC formulations showed a reduced melting enthalpy, which was possibly a result of partial amorphization of the drug (Figure S2). Moreover, the X-ray diffractograms clearly indicated the crystalline state of nifedipine in all formulations (Figure 7); therefore, an enhanced dissolution cannot be solely attributed to the drug amorphization by phospholipids.

The wetting constant and the specific surface area depend on each other according to Equation (5), which represents the power law function (Figure 6). The reduction of the individual area of a pore's cross section depends on squared diameter of remaining pore opening as follows from simple geometric considerations. Thus, under an assumption of constant rate of capillary transport, there is a quadratic dependency of the porous cross-section area on the rate of material deposition in a material with idealized equisized pore geometries. However, for different pore size distributions in real materials, the power exponent is expected to be significantly different from two. Therefore, due to loading of materials into the FCC particles, the smaller pores are filled first and the total liquid throughput (i.e., water uptake) through the particle meshwork changes according to power law with exponents greater than two. The applicability of the power law correlation can be extended to the dissolution rate and liposomal encapsulation efficiency as a function of the phospholipid content in the FCC-based formulations. The latter suggests a guidance for the design or section of porous carriers for such formulations.

On the basis of the results, we could show that the combination of porous FCC microparticles and phospholipids can be used to produce solid formulations oral liposomal delivery. This method is suitable for classical scale-up. We demonstrated that the fast water uptake and dissolution of the carrier is essential for achieving the highest encapsulation efficiency and the fastest drug dissolution rate.

5. Conclusions

As a general principle, the in situ formation of liposomes from a combination of phospholipids and porous carriers in the simulated GI conditions is an effective approach for formulating liposomes for oral delivery. We propose that a single-step loading of phospholipids and drug substances can be used as a simple and effective method for the production of proliposomal formulations. This method is suitable for scale-up. We showed the mechanism of the spontaneous in situ formation of liposomes in different dissolution media and demonstrated drug encapsulation in the emerging liposomes. To enhance the encapsulation efficiency and reduce drug leakage from the liposomes, other types of phospholipids and their combinations with amphiphilic polymers can be used with porous microparticulate carriers, such as FCC.

Supplementary Materials: The following are available online at http://www.mdpi.com/1999-4923/12/8/777/s1, Figure S1: Cryo-EM images of liposomes. Figure S2: Differential scanning calorimeter (DSC) spectra of the formulations and physical mixture. Table S1: The time required for 80% of the drug content to dissolve in SGF. Video S1: Formation of liposomes in SGF.

Author Contributions: M.F.: conceptualization, methodology, formal analysis, investigation, writing—original draft, visualization. G.Q.: conceptualization, methodology, investigation, writing—review and editing, funding acquisition. K.S.: methodology, investigation. F.M.H.: writing—review and editing, resources, funding acquisition. J.S.: writing—review and editing, resources, funding acquisition. J.H.: conceptualization, resources, writing—review and editing, supervision, funding acquisition. M.P.: conceptualization, formal analysis, writing—review and editing, supervision, project administration, funding acquisition. All authors have read and agreed to the published version of the manuscript.

Funding: This research was co-funded by Omya International AG and Phospholipid Research Center.

Acknowledgments: We express deep gratitude to Darryl Borland for his remarkable job regarding technical support of the experimental set ups and for proofreading the manuscript, as well as Peter van Hoogevest for the helpful discussions throughout the execution of the project and for the valuable comments on the manuscript.

Conflicts of Interest: The authors declare the following financial interests/personal relationships that may be considered as potential competing interests: two of the authors (F.H. and J.S.) are employees of Omya International AG, the supplier of the material used in this study. Omya International AG had no role in the design of the study; in the collection, analyses or interpretation of data; in the writing of the manuscript, nor in the decision to publish the results. Other authors declare no conflict of interest.

References

1. Dapergolas, G.; Gregoriadis, G. Hypoglycqmic effect of liposome-entrapped insulin administered intragastrically into rats. *Lancet* **1976**, *308*, 824–827. [CrossRef]
2. Patel, H.; Ryman, B.E. Oral administration of insulin by encapsulation within liposomes. *FEBS Lett.* **1976**, *62*, 60–63. [CrossRef]
3. Tang, W.-L.; Chen, W.C.; Diako, C.; Ross, C.; Li, S.-D.; Tang, W.-H. Development of a rapidly dissolvable oral pediatric formulation for mefloquine using liposomes. *Mol. Pharm.* **2017**, *14*, 1969–1979. [CrossRef]
4. Uhl, P.; Pantze, S.; Storck, P.; Parmentier, J.; Witzigmann, D.; Hofhaus, G.; Huwyler, J.; Mier, W.; Fricker, G. Oral delivery of vancomycin by tetraether lipid liposomes. *Eur. J. Pharm. Sci.* **2017**, *108*, 111–118. [CrossRef]
5. Song, K.-H.; Chung, S.-J.; Shim, C.-K. Enhanced intestinal absorption of salmon calcitonin (sCT) from proliposomes containing bile salts. *J. Control. Release* **2005**, *106*, 298–308. [CrossRef]
6. Lee, M.-K. Liposomes for enhanced bioavailability of water-insoluble drugs: In Vivo evidence and recent approaches. *Pharmaceutics* **2020**, *12*, 264. [CrossRef] [PubMed]
7. Zidan, A.S.; Spinks, C.B.; Habib, M.J.; Khan, M.A. Formulation and transport properties of tenofovir loaded liposomes through Caco-2 cell model. *J. Liposome Res.* **2013**, *23*, 318–326. [CrossRef] [PubMed]
8. Uhl, P.; Helm, F.; Hofhaus, G.; Brings, S.; Kaufman, C.; Leotta, K.; Urban, S.; Haberkorn, U.; Mier, W.; Fricker, G. A liposomal formulation for the oral application of the investigational hepatitis B drug Myrcludex B. *Eur. J. Pharm. Biopharm.* **2016**, *103*, 159–166. [CrossRef] [PubMed]
9. Hashimoto, A.; Kawada, J. Effects of oral administration of positively charged insulin liposomes on alloxan diabetic rats: Preliminary study. *Endocrinol. Jpn.* **1979**, *26*, 337–344. [CrossRef] [PubMed]
10. Li, H. Polyethylene glycol-coated liposomes for oral delivery of recombinant human epidermal growth factor. *Int. J. Pharm.* **2003**, *258*, 11–19. [CrossRef]
11. Liu, W.; Ye, A.; Liu, W.; Liu, C.; Han, J.; Singh, H. Behaviour of liposomes loaded with bovine serum albumin during in vitro digestion. *Food Chem.* **2015**, *175*, 16–24. [CrossRef] [PubMed]
12. He, H.; Lu, Y.; Qi, J.; Zhu, Q.; Chen, Z.; Wu, W. Adapting liposomes for oral drug delivery. *Acta Pharm. Sin. B* **2018**, *9*, 36–48. [CrossRef] [PubMed]
13. Wu, W.; Lu, Y.; Qi, J. Oral delivery of liposomes. *Ther. Deliv.* **2015**, *6*, 1239–1241. [CrossRef] [PubMed]
14. Van Hoogevest, P. Review—An update on the use of oral phospholipid excipients. *Eur. J. Pharm. Sci.* **2017**, *108*, 1–12. [CrossRef] [PubMed]
15. Franze, S.; Selmin, F.; Samaritani, E.; Minghetti, P.; Cilurzo, F. Lyophilization of liposomal formulations: Still necessary, still challenging. *Pharmaceutics* **2018**, *10*, 139. [CrossRef]
16. Chen, C.; Han, D.; Cai, C.; Tang, X. An overview of liposome lyophilization and its future potential. *J. Control. Release* **2010**, *142*, 299–311. [CrossRef]
17. Brinkmann-Trettenes, U.; Bauer-Brandl, A. Solid phospholipid nano-particles: Investigations into formulation and dissolution properties of griseofulvin. *Int. J. Pharm.* **2014**, *467*, 42–47. [CrossRef]
18. Sweeney, L.G.; Wang, Z.; Loebenberg, R.; Wong, J.P.; Lange, C.F.; Finlay, W.H. Spray-freeze-dried liposomal ciprofloxacin powder for inhaled aerosol drug delivery. *Int. J. Pharm.* **2005**, *305*, 180–185. [CrossRef]
19. Otake, K.; Imura, T.; Sakai, H.; Abe, M. Development of a new preparation method of liposomes using supercritical carbon dioxide. *Langmuir* **2001**, *17*, 3898–3901. [CrossRef]
20. Imura, T.; Otake, K.; Hashimoto, S.; Gotoh, T.; Yuasa, M.; Yokoyama, S.; Sakai, H.; Rathman, J.F.; Abe, M. Preparation and physicochemical properties of various soybean lecithin liposomes using supercritical reverse phase evaporation method. *Colloids Surf. B Biointerfaces* **2003**, *27*, 133–140. [CrossRef]
21. Misra, A.; Jinturkar, K.; Patel, D.; Lalani, J.; Chougule, M. Recent advances in liposomal dry powder formulations: Preparation and evaluation. *Expert Opin. Drug Deliv.* **2009**, *6*, 71–89. [CrossRef] [PubMed]
22. Ingvarsson, P.T.; Yang, M.; Nielsen, H.M.; Rantanen, J.; Foged, C. Stabilization of liposomes during drying. *Expert Opin. Drug Deliv.* **2011**, *8*, 375–388. [CrossRef] [PubMed]

23. Jannin, V.; Musakhanian, J.; Marchaud, D. Approaches for the development of solid and semi-solid lipid-based formulations. *Adv. Drug Deliv. Rev.* **2008**, *60*, 734–746. [CrossRef] [PubMed]
24. Payne, N.I.; Timmins, P.; Ambrose, C.V.; Ward, M.D.; Ridgway, F. Proliposomes: A Novel solution to an old problem. *J. Pharm. Sci.* **1986**, *75*, 325–329. [CrossRef]
25. Jia, J.; Zhang, K.; Zhou, X.; Ma, J.; Liu, X.; Xiang, A.; Ge, F. Berberine-loaded solid proliposomes prepared using solution enhanced dispersion by supercritical CO2: Sustained release and bioavailability enhancement. *J. Drug Deliv. Sci. Technol.* **2019**, *51*, 356–363. [CrossRef]
26. Khan, I.; Yousaf, S.; Subramanian, S.; Alhnan, M.A.; Ahmed, W.; Elhissi, A. Proliposome tablets manufactured using a slurry-driven lipid-enriched powders: Development, characterization and stability evaluation. *Int. J. Pharm.* **2018**, *538*, 250–262. [CrossRef]
27. Weng, W.; Wang, Q.; Wei, C.; Man, N.; Zhang, K.; Wei, Q.; Adu-Frimpong, M.; Toreniyazov, E.; Ji, H.; Yu, J.-N.; et al. Preparation, characterization, pharmacokinetics and anti-hyperuricemia activity studies of myricitrin-loaded proliposomes. *Int. J. Pharm.* **2019**, *572*, 118735. [CrossRef]
28. Fong, S.Y.K.; Brandl, M.; Bauer-Brandl, A. Phospholipid-based solid drug formulations for oral bioavailability enhancement: A meta-analysis. *Eur. J. Pharm. Sci.* **2015**, *80*, 89–110. [CrossRef]
29. Vanić, Ž.; Planinšek, O.; Škalko-Basnet, N.; Tho, I. Tablets of pre-liposomes govern In Situ formation of liposomes: Concept and potential of the novel drug delivery system. *Eur. J. Pharm. Biopharm.* **2014**, *88*, 443–454. [CrossRef]
30. Chu, C.; Tong, S.-S.; Xu, Y.; Wang, L.; Fu, M.; Ge, Y.-R.; Yu, J.-N.; Xu, X.-M. Proliposomes for oral delivery of dehydrosilymarin: Preparation and evaluation In Vitro and In Vivo. *Acta Pharmacol. Sin.* **2011**, *32*, 973–980. [CrossRef]
31. Bobbala, S.K.R.; Veerareddy, P.R. Formulation, evaluation, and pharmacokinetics of isradipine proliposomes for oral delivery. *J. Liposome Res.* **2012**, *22*, 285–294. [CrossRef] [PubMed]
32. Xu, H.; He, L.; Nie, S.; Guan, J.; Zhang, X.; Yang, X.; Pan, W. Optimized preparation of vinpocetine proliposomes by a novel method and In Vivo evaluation of its pharmacokinetics in New Zealand rabbits. *J. Control. Release* **2009**, *140*, 61–68. [CrossRef] [PubMed]
33. Janga, K.Y.; Jukanti, R.; Velpula, A.; Sunkavalli, S.; Bandari, S.; Kandadi, P.; Veerareddy, P.R. Bioavailability enhancement of zaleplon via proliposomes: Role of surface charge. *Eur. J. Pharm. Biopharm.* **2012**, *80*, 347–357. [CrossRef] [PubMed]
34. Velpula, A.; Jukanti, R.; Janga, K.Y.; Sunkavalli, S.; Bandari, S.; Kandadi, P.; Veerareddy, P.R. Proliposome powders for enhanced intestinal absorption and bioavailability of raloxifene hydrochloride: Effect of surface charge. *Drug Dev. Ind. Pharm.* **2012**, *39*, 1895–1906. [CrossRef] [PubMed]
35. Roth, R.; Schoelkopf, J.; Huwyler, J.; Puchkov, M. Functionalized calcium carbonate microparticles for the delivery of proteins. *Eur. J. Pharm. Biopharm.* **2018**, *122*, 96–103. [CrossRef] [PubMed]
36. Ridgway, C.; Gane, P.A.; Schoelkopf, J. Modified calcium carbonate coatings with rapid absorption and extensive liquid uptake capacity. *Colloids Surf. A Physicochem. Eng. Asp.* **2004**, *236*, 91–102. [CrossRef]
37. Farzan, M.; Roth, R.; Québatte, G.; Schoelkopf, J.; Huwyler, J.; Puchkov, M. Loading of porous functionalized calcium carbonate microparticles: Distribution analysis with focused ion beam electron microscopy and mercury porosimetry. *Pharmaceutics* **2019**, *11*, 32. [CrossRef]
38. Preisig, D.; Haid, D.; Varum, F.J.; Bravo, R.; Alles, R.; Huwyler, J.; Puchkov, M. Drug loading into porous calcium carbonate microparticles by solvent evaporation. *Eur. J. Pharm. Biopharm.* **2014**, *87*, 548–558. [CrossRef]
39. Preisig, D.; Roth, R.; Tognola, S.; Varum, F.J.; Bravo, R.; Cetinkaya, Y.; Huwyler, J.; Puchkov, M. Mucoadhesive microparticles for local treatment of gastrointestinal diseases. *Eur. J. Pharm. Biopharm.* **2016**, *105*, 156–165. [CrossRef]
40. Stirnimann, T.; Atria, S.; Schoelkopf, J.; Gane, P.; Alles, R.; Huwyler, J.; Puchkov, M. Compaction of functionalized calcium carbonate, a porous and crystalline microparticulate material with a lamellar surface. *Int. J. Pharm.* **2014**, *466*, 266–275. [CrossRef]
41. Stirnimann, T.; Di Maiuta, N.; Gerard, D.E.; Alles, R.; Huwyler, J.; Puchkov, M. Functionalized calcium carbonate as a novel pharmaceutical excipient for the preparation of orally dispersible tablets. *Pharm. Res.* **2013**, *30*, 1915–1925. [CrossRef] [PubMed]

42. Wagner-Hattler, L.; Wyss, K.; Schoelkopf, J.; Huwyler, J.; Puchkov, M. In Vitro characterization and mouthfeel study of functionalized calcium carbonate in orally disintegrating tablets. *Int. J. Pharm.* **2017**, *534*, 50–59. [CrossRef] [PubMed]
43. Eberle, V.A.; Schoelkopf, J.; Gane, P.A.; Alles, R.; Huwyler, J.; Puchkov, M. Floating gastroretentive drug delivery systems: Comparison of experimental and simulated dissolution profiles and floatation behavior. *Eur. J. Pharm. Sci.* **2014**, *58*, 34–43. [CrossRef] [PubMed]
44. The United States Pharmacopeial Convention. *The United States Pharmacopeia 2018*; United States Pharmacopeial Convention: Rockville, MD, USA, 2017.
45. FaSSIF/FeSSIF/FaSSGF Biorelevant Dissolution Media. Biorelevant. Available online: https://biorelevant.com/fassif-fessif-fassgf/buy/ (accessed on 22 June 2020).
46. Wolfram Language Documentation, Numerical Operations on Data. Available online: https://reference.wolfram.com/language/tutorial/NumericalOperationsOnData.html#19037 (accessed on 22 April 2020).
47. Khan, K.A.; Rhodes, C.T. Effect of compaction pressure on the dissolution efficiency of some direct compression systems. *Pharm. Acta Helv.* **1972**, *47*, 594–607. [PubMed]
48. Ting, J.; Navale, T.S.; Bates, F.S.; Reineke, T.M. Design of tunable multicomponent polymers as modular vehicles to solubilize highly lipophilic drugs. *Macromolecules* **2014**, *47*, 6554–6565. [CrossRef]
49. Vitez, I.M. Utilization of DSC for pharmaceutical crystal form quantitation. *J. Therm. Anal. Calorim.* **2004**, *78*, 33–45. [CrossRef]
50. Shah, B.; Kakumanu, V.K.; Bansal, A.K. Analytical techniques for quantification of amorphous/crystalline phases in pharmaceutical solids. *J. Pharm. Sci.* **2006**, *95*, 1641–1665. [CrossRef]
51. Washburn, E.W. The dynamics of capillary flow. *Phys. Rev.* **1921**, *17*, 273–283. [CrossRef]
52. Lucas, R. Ueber das zeitgesetz des kapillaren aufstiegs von flüssigkeiten. *Colloid Polym. Sci.* **1918**, *23*, 15–22. [CrossRef]
53. *Krüss Tensiometer K100 Instruction Manual*; Krüss GmbH: Hamburg, Germany, 2005.
54. Stuart, M.C.A.; Boekema, E.J. Two distinct mechanisms of vesicle-to-micelle and micelle-to-vesicle transition are mediated by the packing parameter of phospholipid–detergent systems. *Biochim. Biophys. Acta (BBA) Biomembr.* **2007**, *1768*, 2681–2689. [CrossRef]
55. Marsh, D. *Handbook of Lipid Bilayers*, 2nd ed.; CRC Press, Taylor & Francis Group: Boca Raton, FL, USA, 2013.
56. Israelachvili, J.N. Soft and biological structures. In *Intermolecular and Surface Forces*, 3rd ed.; Israelachvili, J.N., Ed.; Academic Press: San Diego, CA, USA, 2011; pp. 535–576.

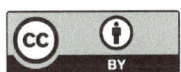

© 2020 by the authors. Licensee MDPI, Basel, Switzerland. This article is an open access article distributed under the terms and conditions of the Creative Commons Attribution (CC BY) license (http://creativecommons.org/licenses/by/4.0/).

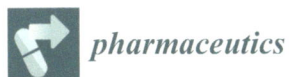

Article

Light-Activated Liposomes Coated with Hyaluronic Acid as a Potential Drug Delivery System

Otto K. Kari, Shirin Tavakoli, Petteri Parkkila, Simone Baan, Roosa Savolainen, Teemu Ruoslahti, Niklas G. Johansson, Joseph Ndika, Harri Alenius, Tapani Viitala, Arto Urtti and Tatu Lajunen

1. Drug Research Program, Division of Pharmaceutical Biosciences, Faculty of Pharmacy, University of Helsinki, Viikinkaari 5 E, FI-00790 Helsinki, Finland; otto.kari@helsinki.fi (O.K.K.); shirin.tavakoli@helsinki.fi (S.T.); petteri.parkkila@helsinki.fi (P.P.); s.d.baan@uu.nl (S.B.); roosa.pp.savolainen@helsinki.fi (R.S.); teemu.ruoslahti@aalto.fi (T.R.); tapani.viitala@helsinki.fi (T.V.); arto.urtti@helsinki.fi (A.U.)
2. Pharmaceutics, Utrecht Institute for Pharmaceutical Sciences, Utrecht University, P.O. Box 80.082, 3508 TB Utrecht, The Netherlands
3. Drug Research Program, Division of Pharmaceutical Chemistry and Technology, Faculty of Pharmacy, University of Helsinki, Viikinkaari 5 E, FI-00790 Helsinki, Finland; niklas.johansson@helsinki.fi
4. Human Microbiome Research, Faculty of Medicine, University of Helsinki, Haartmaninkatu 3, FI-00290 Helsinki, Finland; joseph.ndika@helsinki.fi (J.N.); harri.alenius@helsinki.fi (H.A.)
5. Institute of Environmental Medicine, Karolinska Institutet, 171 77 Stockholm, Sweden
6. School of Pharmacy, Faculty of Health Sciences, University of Eastern Finland, Yliopistonranta 1, 70210 Kuopio, Finland
7. Institute of Chemistry, St. Petersburg State University, Petergof, Universitetskii pr. 26, 198504 St. Petersburg, Russia
8. Laboratory of Pharmaceutical Technology, Department of Pharmaceutical Science, Tokyo University of Pharmacy & Life Sciences, 1432-1 Hachioji, Tokyo 192-0392, Japan
* Correspondence: tatu.lajunen@helsinki.fi; Tel.: +81-7044-589-511

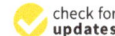

Received: 6 July 2020; Accepted: 9 August 2020; Published: 12 August 2020

Abstract: Light-activated liposomes permit site and time-specific drug delivery to ocular and systemic targets. We combined a light activation technology based on indocyanine green with a hyaluronic acid (HA) coating by synthesizing HA–lipid conjugates. HA is an endogenous vitreal polysaccharide and a potential targeting moiety to cluster of differentiation 44 (CD44)-expressing cells. Light-activated drug release from 100 nm HA-coated liposomes was functional in buffer, plasma, and vitreous samples. The HA-coating improved stability in plasma compared to polyethylene glycol (PEG)-coated liposomes. Liposomal protein coronas on HA- and PEG-coated liposomes after dynamic exposure to undiluted human plasma and porcine vitreous samples were hydrophilic and negatively charged, thicker in plasma (~5 nm hard, ~10 nm soft coronas) than in vitreous (~2 nm hard, ~3 nm soft coronas) samples. Their compositions were dependent on liposome formulation and surface charge in plasma but not in vitreous samples. Compared to the PEG coating, the HA-coated liposomes bound more proteins in vitreous samples and enriched proteins related to collagen interactions, possibly explaining their slightly reduced vitreal mobility. The properties of the most abundant proteins did not correlate with liposome size or charge, but included proteins with surfactant and immune system functions in plasma and vitreous samples. The HA-coated light-activated liposomes are a functional and promising alternative for intravenous and ocular drug delivery.

Keywords: hyaluronic acid; liposome; drug release; light activation; stability; mobility; biocorona

1. Introduction

Liposomes are a well-accepted drug delivery system and still the most common nanomedicines in clinical trials [1]. Most liposomal carriers are coated with polyethylene glycol (PEG) to prolong their residence times in blood circulation [2,3], but there are still problems related to reduced uptake into the target cells [3,4], immunogenicity [5,6], and undesired protein interactions [7]. Therefore, alternatives for PEG were proposed, including polyvinylpyrrolidone (PVP) [8], polycarbonates [9], pullulan [10], polyoxazolines [11], and hyaluronic acid (HA) or hyaluronan [12].

HA is a negatively charged natural polysaccharide of D-glucuronic acid and N-acetyl-D-glucosamine disaccharide units that are connected via alternating β-1,4 and β-1,3 glycosidic bonds. HA contains carboxyl, hydroxyl, and amino groups that can be derivatized. HA is biocompatible, biodegradable, non-toxic, and less immunogenic than PEG [12,13]. In addition, HA binds the CD44 receptors that are overexpressed in melanomas, lymphomas, breast cancer, lung, and rectal tumor cells [12] and present in the retinal pigment epithelium [14]. Thus, the HA coating combines steric stabilization ("stealth") and active targeting functions. Furthermore, HA improves liposomal stability in freeze-drying due to its high water-binding capacity [15].

Passive drug release from liposomes is often erratic and inadequate [16], but this can be improved by external triggers such as light [17,18]. Light activation is feasible for drug release in superficial organs (eye and skin), as well as in deeper tissues with light guides, and light parameters can be optimized for treatment (e.g., wavelength, light intensity, exposure time, and beam size) [19]. We developed light-activated PEG-coated liposomes using indocyanine green (ICG) as the light-sensitizing compound [20–22]. Light-activated release of small and large compounds was achieved with near-infrared (NIR) light with only five-second light exposures [22–24]. Amphiphilic ICG can be integrated into the liposomal bilayers or clustered with the hydrophilic coating on the liposome surface (e.g., PEG). ICG is a fluorescent dye approved by the European Medicines Agency (EMA) [23] and the United States (US) Food and Drug Administration (FDA) [24] for angiographic and lymphatic system imaging in the clinics [25].

The acquired protein corona determines the "biological identity" and fate of liposomes in a biological environment [26,27]. We demonstrated that ICG clustered with PEG on the liposome surface influenced the structure and composition of the protein corona, including the beneficial enrichment of "dysopsonin" molecules such as clusterin and apolipoprotein E [28]. Even though the liposomal protein coronas were characterized in plasma, their formation in the vitreous humor of the eye was studied only in our recent publication [29]. The structure and contents of the vitreal liposome corona were not dependent on the composition of 50 nm anionic light-activated liposomes [28]. This is in line with earlier observations with silica and gold nanoparticles in dilute dog vitreous samples [30]. The slight increase (10–12%) in liposomal diameter due to corona formation did not affect the mobility of the liposomes in the vitreous humor [29].

HA is an endogenous component in the vitreous humor and, in that respect, an interesting coating material for ocular liposomes. This report describes the development of light-activated liposomes with HA coating. We produced HA–lipid conjugates in-house and characterized the HA-coated liposomes for drug release, stability, protein corona formation, and mobility in the vitreous humor.

2. Materials and Methods

2.1. Materials

Dipalmitoylphosphatidylcholine (DPPC), 1,2-distearoyl-*sn*-glycero-3-phosphocholine (DSPC), lysophosphatidylcholine (LysoPC), 1,2-distearoyl-*sn*-glycero-3-phosphorylethanolamine (DSPE), 1,2-distearoyl-*sn*-glycero-3-phosphoethanolamine-*N*-[amino(polyethylene glycol)-2000] (DSPE-PEG), 1,2-distearoyl-*sn*-glycero-3-phosphoglycerol (DSPG), and the 1,2-dioleoyl-*sn*-glycero-3-phosphoethanolamine-*N*-(Cyanine 5) lipid dye were purchased from Avanti Polar Lipids, Inc. (Alabaster, AL, USA). Citrate-phosphate-dextrose (CPD)-anticoagulated human plasma frozen within 24 h was bought from the Finnish Red Cross Blood Service (Helsinki, Finland), which is provided as an anonymized blood product for research use only that constitutes non-identifiable human material under the Declaration of Helsinki. Vitreous humour for proteomics experiments was isolated from porcine eyes supplied by HKScan

Finland Oyj (Forssa, Finland) and homogenized as described previously [29,31]. Triton X-100 was from MP Biomedicals (Santa Ana, CA, USA). Hyaluronic acid (HA; 8–15 kDa) and all other chemicals were bought from Sigma-Aldrich (St. Louis, MO, USA). Buffer and calcein solutions were made in advance of the liposome preparations. The buffer contained 20 mM 4-(2-hydroxyethyl)-1-piperazineethanesulfonic acid (HEPES) and 140 mM sodium chloride (NaCl) in purified water, and the calcein solution for release studies had 60 mM calcein and 29 mM NaCl in purified water, both adjusted to pH 7.4 with sodium hydroxide (NaOH). Microwell dishes were from MatTek Corporation (Ashland, MA, USA).

2.2. DSPE–HA Conjugate

The DSPE–HA conjugate was produced with the protocol described by Yao et al. with a few modifications [32]. Briefly, 50 mg of HA sodium salt (8–15 kDa) was added to 20 mL of purified water. The solution was dialyzed (2 kDa cut-off) against 1 L of 0.01 M hydrochloric acid (HCl) for 24 h to acidify the HA, and then against 1 L of purified water for 24 h. After the dialysis, the solution pH was increased to 9 with a few drops of 20% tetrabutylammonium hydroxide (TBA-OH). The mixture was then stirred for 2 h at room temperature and thereafter dialyzed against an excess of purified water. Water was removed from the final dialysis product by lyophilization with SCANVAC CoolSafe 110 (LaboGene ApS, Allerød, Denmark).

The freeze-dried HA–TBA powder was dissolved in 3.5 mL of anhydrous dimethyl sulfoxide (DMSO) under an argon atmosphere, and the solution was stirred at 60 °C until the powder dissolved completely. Then, 16.3 mg of DSPE and 6.1 µL of dry triethylamine were mixed with 0.87 mL of anhydrous chloroform, and the solution was sonicated for a short period until all the particles visibly dissolved. The HA and DSPE solutions were combined and stirred for 2 h at 60 °C. Thereafter, a solution containing 9.2 mg of sodium triacetoxyborohydride (NaBH(OAc)$_3$) and 0.87 mL of anhydrous DMSO was added dropwise to the DSPE–HA–TBA solution. This mixture was allowed to react for 72 h at 60 °C and then cooled to room temperature.

Chloroform was evaporated from the suspension under a constant nitrogen gas flow. Then, 30 mL of purified water was added to the suspension, which was then centrifuged at 10,000× g for 30 min. The supernatant was dialyzed against 0.01 M HCl for 24 h and under purified water for an additional 24 h to remove the acidic form of the TBA salt. Finally, the product was freeze-dried with the SCANVAC CoolSafe 110 (LaboGene ApS) over the duration of two days.

2.3. DSPE–HA Conjugate Analysis

The conjugation products were analyzed with nuclear magnetic resonance spectroscopy (NMR) and Fourier-transform infrared spectroscopy (FT-IR). The ^{1}H-NMR analysis was performed with a 400 MHz NMR Bruker AVANCE-III HD spectrometer (Bruker BioSpin, Rheinstetten, Germany). For the measurement, DSPE was dissolved in deuterated chloroform (CDCl$_3$), whereas the DSPE–HA conjugate was dissolved in deuterated dimethyl sulfoxide (DMSO-d_6).

A Vertex 70 FT-IR spectrometer (Bruker Optics, Ettlingen, Germany) equipped with a MIRacle attenuated total reflectance attachment was used in the FT-IR analysis, so that a tiny amount of either DSPE or DSPE–HA conjugate was placed on a diamond single-bounce crystal (Pike Technologies, Fitchburg, WI, USA). The scan was performed in the 650–4000 cm^{-1} wavelength range, while the spectral resolution was 4 cm^{-1}. The background signal measured from a blank crystal was deducted from the average of 256 scans with Opus software.

2.4. Light-Activated Liposomes

ICG liposomes were prepared via the thin film hydration method followed by an extrusion and purification, as described previously with a few modifications [20,29]. Three formulations were prepared, uncoated (F1), PEG-coated (F2), and HA-coated (F4) liposomes with a basic lipid composition of DPPC/DSPC/(18:0)LysoPC at molar ratios of 75/15/10, supplemented with either 4 mol DSPE, 4 mol DSPE-PEG2000, or 1 mol DSPE–HA. The molar ratio of the DSPE–HA was chosen to correspond with the coating polymer mass of traditional PEG-coated liposomes. The thin lipid layer was hydrated with 0.322 mg/mL of ICG in 500 µL of HEPES buffer or calcein solution. In the case of the HA-coated liposomes, DSPE–HA was added during the hydration step instead of the initial mixture in chloroform. Prior to the thin film hydration step, the hydration solution with DSPE–HA was vortexed and heated to 64 °C until the lipid conjugate dissolved. The liposomes were extruded 11 times at 60 °C through a polycarbonate membrane with 100 nm diameter pores (unless otherwise specified) with a syringe-type extrusion device (Avanti Polar Lipids). Thereafter, the liposomes were quickly cooled and stored in a refrigerator. The unencapsulated calcein and ICG were removed by gel filtration through a Sephadex G-50 (Sigma-Aldrich) column with HEPES buffer elution. The final lipid and ICG concentration of the purified samples was 1.5 mM and 30 µM, respectively. For protein corona studies, similar liposomes with PEG (F3) and HA coating (F5), but without ICG, were also prepared. Additionally, anionic 50 nm liposomes with a lipid composition of DPPC/DSPC/DSPG/(18:0)LysoPC/DSPE (F6) or DSPE-PEG2000 (F7) at molar ratios of 75/5/10/10/4 were prepared as described by Tavakoli et al. [29].

2.5. Size and Zeta Potential Analysis in Buffer

The hydrodynamic diameters of the liposomes were analyzed with a Zetasizer APS dynamic light scattering (DLS) automated plate sampler (Malvern Instruments, Malvern, United Kingdom) and reported as size distributions by particle number and polydispersity index (PdI). The zeta potential was measured with a Zetasizer ZS (Malvern Instruments) using DTS1070 cuvettes. All samples were diluted 1:10 (*v/v*) with buffer and measured in triplicate with 10 subruns at room temperature.

2.6. Size Analysis by Flow Cytometry in Vitreous and Plasma Samples

Flow cytometry (Apogee Flow Systems, Hertfordshire, UK) was used to differentiate between the liposomes and other possible porcine vitreous and human plasma components of the same size by large-angle light scattering (LALS) and by detecting the calcein fluorescence to separate the liposome population. The LALS measurements returned the relative size and coefficient of variation (CV) of the liposome population. A calibration line for the liposome size was produced by measuring liposomes of different size in buffer with DLS, as described earlier, and then measuring the same samples with Apogee flow cytometry (Figure S4A). The generated calibration line had the following equation ($R^2 = 0.96$):

$$\text{LALS} = 21.666 \times \text{DLS(nm)} - 888.11. \quad (1)$$

The flow cytometry signal from bulk vitreous and plasma without liposomes was analyzed separately, and only the liposome population was gated into the final data (Figure S4B–E, Supplementary Materials).

2.7. Differential Scanning Calorimetry

The phase transition temperature (T_m) was analyzed using 20 µL of the unpurified sample with differential scanning calorimetry (Mettler Toledo DSC 823e, Mettler-Toledo GmbH, Greifensee, Switzerland). The sample and reference pans were heated using a linear temperature gradient from 25 °C to 80 °C in a nitrogen environment. The phase transitions were detected as negative endothermic peaks in the baseline-corrected thermographs following analysis with STARe software (Mettler Toledo).

2.8. ICG Stability

ICG degrades quickly in aqueous solutions and loses its absorbance peak at the 800 nm wavelength [33]. Thus, the absorbance can be used to measure ICG leakage from liposomes. The ICG amounts were measured in black clear-bottom well plates (Corning Inc., Corning, NY, USA) using a Varioskan LUX multimode plate reader (Thermo Fisher Scientific Inc., Waltham, MA, USA). The 100 µL sample absorbances were measured at 800 nm, and the amount of intact ICG (ICG_i) compared to the initial concentration was calculated using Equation (2).

$$ICG_i = \frac{ICG_t}{ICG_0} \times 100\%, \qquad (2)$$

where ICG_t is the absorbance at the specific time point, and ICG_0 is the absorbance at the start of the experiment.

2.9. Temperature-Induced Release

The release of calcein caused by heating was measured at 35, 37, 38, 39, 40, 41, 42, and 44 °C. Firstly, 490 µL of HEPES buffer was warmed to the desired temperature in an Eppendorf ThermoMixer C (Eppendorf AG, Hamburg, Germany). Once the target temperature was reached, 10 µL of the liposome solution was added into the pre-warmed buffer in the incubator, and the mixture was stirred for 10 min at 300 rpm. The sample was then rapidly cooled in a bucket of ice. The cold control that contained only 490 µL of buffer was kept in the fridge until the addition of 10 µL of the liposomes just before the measurements. Finally, the calcein fluorescence (excitation 493 nm, emission 518 nm) was measured with Varioskan LUX (Thermo Fisher Scientific). The calcein release (R) was calculated as percentages using Equation (3).

$$R = \frac{F - F_0}{F_{100} - F_0} \times 100\%, \qquad (3)$$

where F is the fluorescence of the sample, F_0 denotes the background fluorescence measured from the control, and F_{100} is the maximum fluorescence when the content is completely released from the liposomes (addition of 10 µL of 1% Triton X-100 solution for total decomposition).

2.10. Light-Activated Release

Photothermal calcein release was triggered using a compact single-mode laser module ML6700 (Modulight Inc., Tampere, Finland). Then, 500 µL of liposomes were incubated in HEPES buffer (37 °C), porcine vitreous (35 °C), or human plasma (37 °C) samples in Eppendorf ThermoMixer C (Eppendorf AG). After a sufficient incubation period, the sample was exposed to 800 nm laser for 5 or 15 s with the intensity of 3.2 W/cm^2, based on our previous studies [18,21]. During the light exposure, the control tube was shielded from the laser. Right after the laser irradiation, the sample and the control were immediately cooled down in ice. The calcein fluorescence was measured with Varioskan LUX as described earlier and the release was calculated using Equation (3).

2.11. Liposome Stability in Vitreous and Plasma

The storage stability of the PEG- and HA-coated liposomes was studied for one week in porcine vitreous and human plasma (25% liposome solution/75% biological fluid) samples. The mixtures were stored in the ThermoMixer C (Eppendorf AG) under 300 rpm shaking in tubes at 35 °C for the vitreous and 37 °C for the plasma samples, respectively. Samples were collected at time points of 0, 1, 3, 6, 48, 96, and 168 h, and their calcein leakage, ICG stability, and liposome size were determined as described above. Light-activated release was performed at the 3 h time point for vitreous (35 °C) and plasma (37 °C) samples, as well as at the 24 h time point for the vitreous samples.

2.12. Diffusion of Liposomes in Intact Porcine Vitreous

Vitreal diffusion of uncoated, PEG-coated, and HA-coated liposomes in the porcine eye was investigated as reported previously [29]. In brief, fresh porcine eyes (age: six months) enucleated with a transconjunctival incision 15 min after sacrificing the animal were obtained from the slaughterhouse (HKScan Finland Oyj). After cutting out the extraocular tissues, the eyes were shortly immersed in 70% ethanol and then kept in phosphate buffered saline (PBS) buffer at 4 °C. The anterior segment of the eye was cut circumferentially 2 mm below the limbus, and the lens was removed. Then, 50 µL of 0.25 mg/mL fluorescently labeled liposomes was injected into the center of the exposed vitreous humor at a depth of 0.5 cm using a 30 G insulin syringe (BD, Franklin Lakes, NJ, USA). Next, a 35 mm microwell dish with a 14 mm diameter glass window (MatTek Corporation) was placed on top of the cut eyecup, while avoiding air bubble formation between the glass window and the vitreous humor. In order to prepare the eye for imaging, the dish-covered eyecup was carefully flipped over, and the edges of the eye were fixed to the dish using Loctite Precision super glue (Henkel Corp., NJ, USA). Imaging was carried out at 37 °C with a spinning disc confocal microscope (Marianas, Intelligent Imaging Innovation (3i) Colorado, USA) and 50 ms temporal-resolution movies were recorded using Slidebook® Software v. 6 (Intelligent Imaging Innovation). Movement of the Cy5-labeled liposomes was tracked using the single-particle tracking technique, and the trajectories were analyzed with Imaris v. 9.2 software (Bitplane AG, Zurich, Switzerland). Finally, the particle mean square displacement (MSD) was computed using the @msdanalyzer MATLAB plug-in (MathWorks Inc., Massachusetts, USA), and the vitreal diffusion coefficient of liposomes (D_V) was calculated using Equation (4).

$$D_V = \frac{MSD}{2d\tau}, \qquad (4)$$

where MSD is derived from the slope of the MSD curve, d is defined as dimensionality of the movement ($d = 2$ for 2D tracks), and τ is the lag time of the calculated displacement. The results are reported as D_W/D_V, which indicates how many times more rapidly the liposomes diffuse in water compared to the more viscous vitreous gel. The theoretical diffusion in water (D_W) was calculated according to the Stokes–Einstein equation at 37 °C, and the radii of liposome particles were obtained from DLS measurements as described above.

2.13. Protein Corona Structure and Composition

The two-wavelength surface plasmon resonance (SPR) measurements and calculations, LC–MS/MS data acquisition, and sample preparation were conducted as described previously [28,29]. The LC gradients used for human plasma and porcine vitreous samples were 1 h and 3 h, respectively. The 500 µL liposome injection volume per replicate corresponds to ~16 × 10^{12} particles, with ~13.2 × 10^9 immobilized liposomes on the sensor with ~55 nm^2 of active surface area. Each SPR replicate run accounts for the measured number of immobilized liposomes on the sensor before the determination of corona thicknesses, which assumes random sequential adsorption [28,29]. Raw data from earlier publications in human plasma with neutral 100 nm ICG liposomes (F1–F3) [28] were integrated with new data for 100 nm HA liposomes with and without ICG (F4–F5) and 50 nm ICG liposomes with and without PEG. Raw data from porcine vitreous studies with the 50 nm ICG liposomes (F6–F7) [29] were integrated with new data for the optimized pegylated formulation F2 and the HA liposome F4 in porcine vitreous humor. The non-functional liposomes without ICG were not tested in vitreous humor.

Upon integration of the two datasets, principal component analysis excluded the presence of significant batch effects. As such, LC–MS/MS raw data were processed and median-normalized without additional batch effect corrections. Protein identification and quantification of protein groups (LC–MS/MS data processing) were carried out with the MaxQuant v. 1.6.1.0 [34], with the UniProtKB FASTA file either for *Sus scrofa* (40,701 protein and 23,223 gene entries) or for *Homo sapiens* (86,725 protein and 20,605 gene entries), to which 245 commonly observed contaminants and all reverse sequences were added. Differential abundance and hierarchical clustering analyses for relative enrichment were carried out with Perseus v. 1.6.5.0 [35]. Protein identifications with non-zero intensity values in at least three samples in plasma and vitreous humor were retained for comparisons and annotated with pI, gene names, and sequences. Abundances were log_2-transformed, and protein identifications were classified as "only identified by site". Reverse sequences and potential contaminants were filtered out. When applicable, a protein's median intensity (after normalization) across all samples where it was identified was used to rank and select high abundance (physiological expression or corona-enriched) proteins. Missing intensity values of unidentified protein groups were replaced with random numbers to mimic low abundance measurements, using the input from the normal distribution function in Perseus. After removal of outliers, 2–4 replicates of all formulations were retained for multiple sample testing.

ANOVA with a Benjamini–Hochberg false discovery rate (FDR) of 0.05 on the top 20 proteins from the assigned groups (source, HC, SC) was followed by two-sample Student's t-tests with Benjamini–Hochberg FDR correction. To determine the protein physicochemical properties, gene names for the majority protein within each mass spec-identified protein group and their default protein sequences were obtained from UniProtKB. Unmapped identifications were excluded, and the same protein name was consistently retained for genes that encode multiple proteins. The same sequences were used to calculate the theoretical pI, molecular weight, and grand average of hydropathy (GRAVY) using the the ExPASy server ProtParam tool (https://web.expasy.org/protparam/) or the GRAVY Calculator (http://www.gravy-calculator.de/). The sums of the aromatic residues (phenylalanine, tyrosine, tryptophan, with and without histidine) were calculated from the sequences using the LEN function in MS Excel that returns the number of characters in a text string. For analysis of common gene subsets without accounting for enrichment, the HC Intersection in plasma and the HC Union in vitreous humor were used. Additional comparisons between gene sets were conducted using Venn diagram software (http://bioinformatics.psb.ugent.be/webtools/Venn/), followed by GeneMANIA (http://genemania.org) for functional analysis.

2.14. Statistical Analysis

All stability experiments were carried out in triplicate, and the data are presented as mean ± standard deviation (S.D.). The analysis consisted of a Student's t-test to evaluate the significance between the groups ($p < 0.05$). Outliers were detected and excluded using Grubb's outlier test ($p < 0.05$). Additional statistics were conducted with Prism 8.2.1 (GraphPad Software Inc., La Jolla, CA, USA).

3. Results

3.1. Analysis of the DSPE–HA Conjugate

The DSPE–HA conjugate was analyzed with ^{1}H-NMR and FT-IR spectroscopy (Figure S1, Supplementary Materials). The ^{1}H-NMR spectra showed the typical peaks for DSPE–HA sugar rings (3–4 ppm), N-acetate (1.7–2 ppm), methylene (~1.2 ppm), and terminal methyl (~0.9 ppm) as reported by other groups [32,36]. DSPE and DSPE–HA were analyzed with FT-IR. The DSPE–HA spectra showed comparable peaks (3366, 2918, 2853, 1730, and 1643 cm^{-1}) with both the HA and the DSPE spectra in accordance with a previous report by Yao et al. [32]. The analysis confirmed the successful production of the DSPE–HA conjugate.

3.2. Properties of the HA-Coated Liposomes

The physicochemical properties of the four different liposome formulations produced for the experiments are displayed in Table 1. The lipid composition of all liposomes is based on an optimized formulation for light-activated ICG liposomes reported earlier [18,20]. Depending on the liposome coating, the ICG is either located within the lipid bilayer or bound by the surface polymers [21]. HA-coated liposomes were produced at different sizes (~70 nm and ~100 nm), demonstrating their robust size control. Polydispersity indexes were in the range of 0.05–0.08. The HA-coated liposomes showed lower zeta potential than the uncoated and PEG-coated liposomes. The PEG- and HA-coated liposomes had comparable ICG absorbances, suggesting that the polymer coating did not affect ICG binding on the liposomes, but the uncoated liposomes bound less ICG (Table 1).

Table 1. Physico-chemical properties of the liposome formulations produced for the experiments (mean of triplicate measurements with SD). ICG—indocyanine green; PEG—polyethylene glycol; HA—hyaluronic acid; n.a.—not available.

	Size (nm)	Zeta Potential (mV)	ICG Absorbance (a.u.)
Uncoated	102 ± 24	−0.44 ± 1.32	0.72 ± 0.08
PEG	119 ± 30	−2.94 ± 0.69	0.90 ± 0.13
HA	104 ± 25	−11.27 ± 0.21	0.88 ± 0.12
HA (30 nm extrusion)	68 ± 16	n.a.	0.86 ± 0.03

The coating had no significant effect on the lipid phase transition in the liposomes (Figure 1A). The transition to the liquid-disordered phase began at ~42 °C and reached its peak at ~44 °C. On the other hand, temperature-induced calcein release from small HA-coated liposomes took place at 39–41 °C, while the 100 nm liposomes released their contents at 38–40 °C (Figure 1B). Light activation in buffer for 15 s was sufficient to induce complete content release from all liposomes, while, at 5 s exposure, the small HA-coated liposomes showed lower content release than the 100 nm liposomes (Figure 1B). Differences in content release between light-activated and normal liposomes were significant ($p < 0.01$) (Figure 1C).

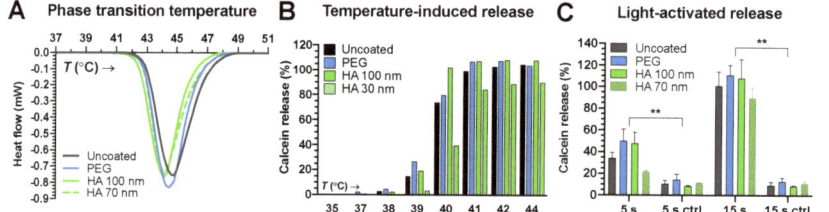

Figure 1. (**A**) Calorimetric analysis of liposomes. Heat flow as a function of temperature (T) is shown. (**B**) Calcein release from liposomes at different temperatures. (**C**) Light-activated content release from liposomes after 5 s or 15 s exposures (800 nm laser at 3.2 W/cm^2) was significant compared to controls (ctrl) absent the light exposure (** $p < 0.01$).

Liposomes with a doubled amount of HA (molar ratio = 2) did not show significant differences compared to the liposomes with lower HA content (Figure S2, Supplementary Materials). In order to determine the ICG binding capacity of the HA coating, we successfully doubled the amount of ICG (Figure S3, Supplementary Materials). The ICG was bound to the liposomes at higher quantities (ICG absorbance of 1.61 ± 0.04 a.u., as compared to 0.88 ± 0.12 a.u. for the regular HA-coated liposomes). However, if the ICG content was doubled at normal HA levels (molar ratio = 1), significant calcein leakage was observed below 37 °C, which rendered these liposomes unsuitable for in vivo use. Due to the suboptimal stability and pharmacokinetics of the uncoated liposomes, they were excluded from the stability studies.

3.3. Stability Studies

3.3.1. ICG Stability and Passive Content Leakage

Light-activated liposomes should stay intact and avoid passive content leakage for sufficient duration. The stability of the PEG- and HA-coated liposomes was assessed in porcine vitreous and human plasma samples at 35 °C and 37 °C, respectively (Figure 2). The ICG absorbance and calcein leakage were measured for one week. Significant changes in ICG absorbance were not seen in vitreous or plasma samples.

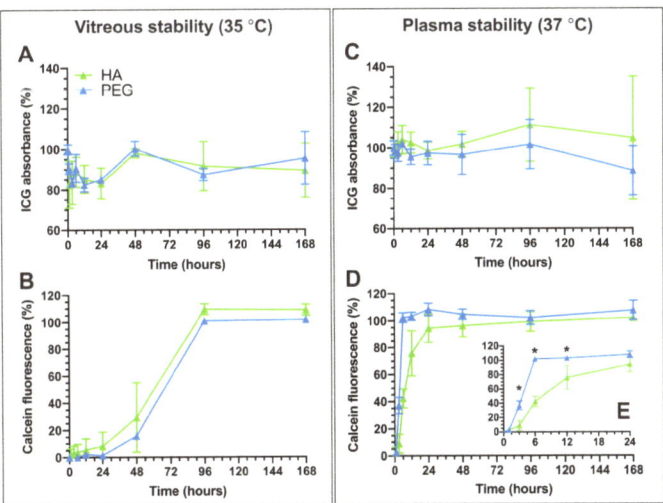

Figure 2. Stability of the HA- and PEG-coated liposomes at physiological temperatures monitored for 168 h (one week) based on ICG absorbance (**A,C**) and calcein fluorescence (**B,D**) in porcine vitreous (**A,B**) and human plasma (**B,D**) samples. Liposome solution (25%) was mixed with the biological fluids (75%). The snapshot (**E**) shows the time-points during the first 12 h of calcein release (* $p < 0.05$).

Both PEG- and HA-coated liposomes showed significant calcein leakage in 2–4 days in the vitreous sample (Figure 2B). Leakage of the liposomal contents was faster in plasma than in vitreous samples, as complete leakage was observed within 24 h (Figure 2E). However, the content release in plasma from the HA-coated liposomes was significantly slower than from the PEG-coated liposomes.

3.3.2. Light-Activated Content Release in Vitreous and Plasma Samples

The light-triggered content release mechanism should be functional in biological media. Light-activated calcein release from HA-coated liposomes was studied at 3 h and 24 h in the vitreous (35 °C) and at 3 h in plasma (37 °C) samples (Figure 3). The longer light exposure (15 s vs. 5 s) significantly increased the calcein release in the vitreous sample at 3 h and 24 h (* $p < 0.05$). Even more pronounced triggered release was observed in plasma (Figure 3).

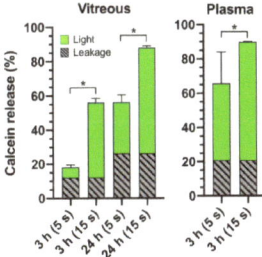

Figure 3. Light-activated release from HA-coated liposomes with 5 s and 15 s light exposures (800 nm laser at 3.2 W/cm^2) and passive content release (leakage) following a 3 h or 24 h incubation of the liposomes in 75% porcine vitreous (35 °C) or human plasma (37 °C) samples. Significant differences in calcein release were observed between different exposure times (* $p < 0.05$).

3.3.3. Liposome Size Change

Flow cytometry was used to analyze the liposomal size change during the stability study (Section 3.3.1), because the large number of natural particles in biological solutions prevents reliable measurements with DLS. The large-angle light scattering (LALS) measurements of the liposome populations in vitreous and plasma samples with Apogee flow cytometry were converted into hydrodynamic diameters using a calibration curve (Figure 4B; Figure S4A, Supplementary Materials). Only the liposome population was gated based on the fluorescence, removing the naturally occurring particle aggregates from the signal (Figure S4B–E, Supplementary Materials). The coefficients of variance were 70–100 for all samples throughout the experiment without showing a clear tendency for increase or decrease.

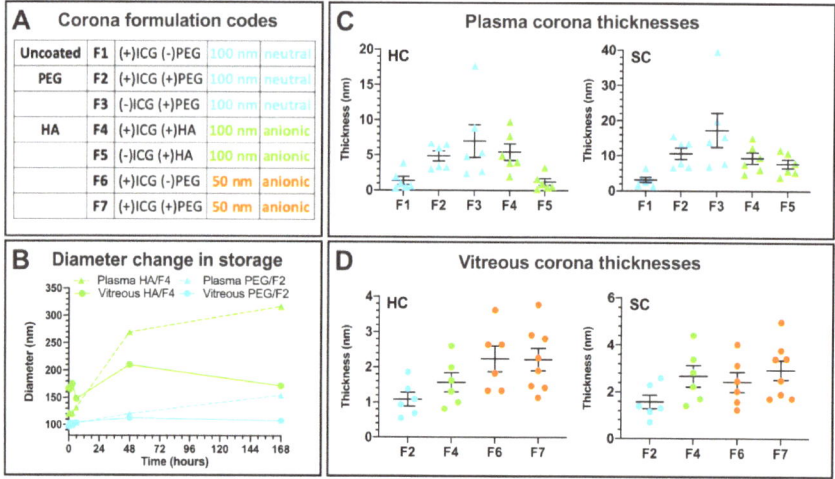

Figure 4. (**A**) Liposome formulations and their color-coded groups in corona experiments, combined with data from earlier studies [28,29]. (**B**) Large-angle light scattering measurements (LALS) for size change during storage in plasma and vitreous samples. (**C**) Surface plasmon resonance (SPR) measurements for hard (HC) and soft corona (SC) thickness in undiluted plasma with individual data points, mean, and SD. (**D**) Corona thicknesses in undiluted vitreous.

The diameter of the PEG-coated liposomes remained unchanged throughout the one-week exposure period in vitreous. In plasma, a gradual size increase up to a diameter of 155 nm was observed. The relative size increase was even higher for the HA-coated liposomes in plasma (270 nm at two days, 318 nm at one week), whereas, in the vitreous sample, the HA-coated liposomes reached a diameter of 150 nm in the beginning and remained at that level until the end of the experiment.

3.4. Protein Corona Formation

3.4.1. Hard and Soft Corona Thickness

Surface plasmon resonance (SPR) measurements under dynamic conditions in undiluted human plasma and porcine vitreous samples were carried out to determine the hard (HC) and soft corona (SC) thicknesses and separate these fractions for proteomics analysis of their composition [28]. Due to the higher number of the samples as a result of data integration from earlier studies, additional formulation numbers (F1–7) and color codes based on charge and size are used (Figure 4A). In plasma, the HA liposomes formed a 5.4 ± 1.2 nm hard corona and a 9.3 ± 1.6 nm soft corona, which is on par with the 4.9 ± 0.7 and 10.6 ± 1.6 nm SC obtained for the PEG liposome (Figure 4C). The uncoated 50 nm anionic liposome without PEG (F6) formed a very thin HC and SC in a consistent trend with the uncoated

100 nm neutral liposome (F1). The HA liposome without ICG (F5) formed a thinner corona than its ICG-containing counterpart.

In the vitreous sample, the HA liposome formed a thicker 1.6 ± 0.3 nm HC and 2.7 ± 0.5 nm SC than the PEG liposome (1.1 ± 0.2 nm and 1.6 ± 0.3 nm, respectively). Both 100 nm formulations formed thinner coronas than the 50 nm anionic liposomes regardless of surface charge or polymer coating, and the SC thickness suggests that it comprised only a few additional loosely interacting proteins in addition to the HC. The protein concentrations of the undiluted porcine vitreous and human plasma samples determined using the bicinchonic acid (BCA) assay were 1.5 mg/mL and 75.8 mg/mL, respectively. These correspond to dynamic exposures of 0.25 mL at 375 μg of protein per replicate in the vitreous sample (1.4 pg/nm^2/min) and at least 0.75 mL at 57 mg if protein per replicate in plasma (57 pg/nm^2/min). The unfunctional formulations without ICG were not tested in the vitreous sample.

3.4.2. Hard and Soft Corona Composition

The HC and SC corona fractions from Figure 4C,D were eluted for high-resolution proteomics analysis with nanoliquid chromatography tandem mass spectrometry. Sufficient chromatographic separation was obtained with a one-hour linear gradient for plasma, while the vitreous samples required three-hour gradients. Figure 5 shows the relative enrichment and hierarchical clustering of the top 60 most abundant proteins in human plasma after median normalization. A list and a heatmap of the 178 proteins identified in at least three samples are provided in Figure S5 (Supplementary Materials).

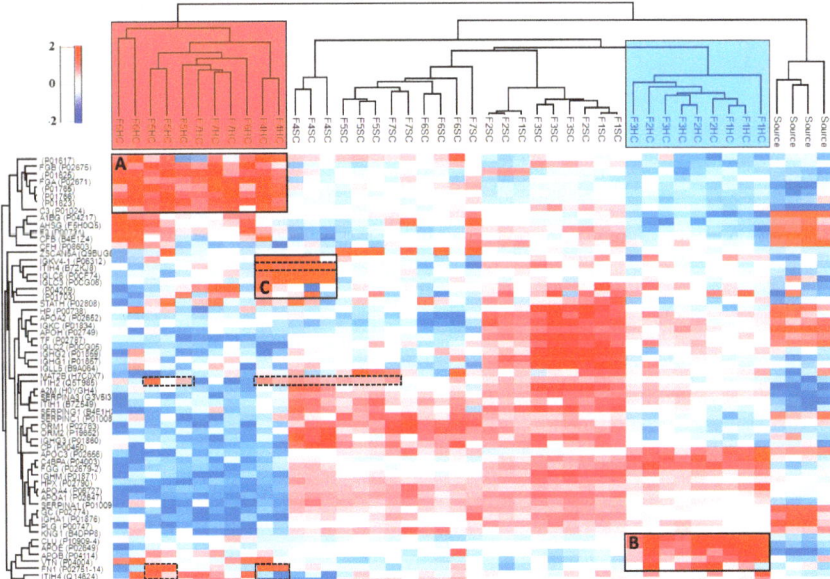

Figure 5. Heatmap of the top 60 most abundant proteins in at least three samples in human plasma after median normalization (178 proteins). Distinct clusters are observed for the HC, SC, and plasma source (including 1× and 7× diluted, surface plasmon resonance (SPR) instrument flow-through, and untreated). The HC subsections of the tested formulations cluster based on their anionic (*light-red box*) or neutral (*light-blue box*) surface charge. The corresponding significantly enriched proteins are highlighted with black boxes (**A–C**). The *dashed boxes* indicate the enrichment of hyaluronic acid-binding inter-alpha-trypsin inhibitor heavy chain proteins (ITIH2, ITIH4) and fibronectin (FN1). The range for relative enrichment (*red*) and depletion (*blue*) is two standard deviations from the mean on the log$_2$ scale.

The HC, SC, and source plasma cluster into distinct groups (Figure 5). In addition, the anionic and neutral liposome groups cluster regardless of liposome size. The notably enriched proteins in the *anionic* HC intersection are fibrinogen alpha and beta (FGA and FGB), complement component C3, thrombin (F2), and immunoglobulin variable regions (Figure 5A). *Neutral* liposomes were enriched with fibrinogen gamma (FGG), complement component C4, fibronectin (FN1), and apolipoproteins B (APOB) and E (APOE), as well as clusterin (CLU) (Figure 5B). The HA-coated liposomes were also enriched with the extracellular matrix component fibronectin (FN1) and the hyaluronic acid-binding proteins inter alpha trypsin inhibitors (ITIH2 and ITIH4) (dashed boxes in Figure 5). In addition, the HA-coated liposome with ICG (F4) was enriched with additional immunoglobulin light-chain regions, which was not observed in the absence of ICG (F5; Figure 5C).

The vitreous corona samples had 728 proteins that were identified in at least three samples (Figure S6; Supplementary Materials). The relative enrichment and hierarchical clustering of the top 60 most abundant proteins after median normalization are shown in Figure 6. In the vitreous sample, the corona subsections do not cluster based on charge or formulation. The relatively enriched HC proteins on the 50 nm anionic liposomes (F6–F7) and to a lesser extent on the 100 nm PEG-coated liposome (F2) include the cytoskeletal protein tubulin alpha (TUBA1B) and the glucose metabolism-associated glyceraldehyde-3-phosphate dehydrogenase (GAPDH) (Figure 6A). Enrichment of tubulin beta chain variants (P02554; A0A287A275) was more pronounced in the PEG-coated liposome HCs (Figure 6B). These formulations were also enriched with clusterin (CLU) and hemoglobin subunit zeta (HBZ) in their HCs in addition to beta-crystallin (CRYBB1), which were mostly depleted on the HA-coated liposome (F4). The enrichment of the Dickkopf Wnt signaling pathway inhibitor 3 (A0A286ZNN6; DKK3) and an uncharacterized Ig-like protein (A0A286ZJL9) was less pronounced in these groups (Figure 6A,B), both of which were depleted on the HA-coated liposome (Figure 6C). Although GAPDH and TUBA1B were also enriched on replicates of the HA-coated liposome, their variants GADPHS and tubulin alpha chain (TUBA1A) showed higher enrichment (Figure 6d). The 50 nm anionic liposomes were also enriched with the retinol-binding protein 3 (RBP3) and albumin (ALB) in their HCs, which were mostly abundant in the SCs of the other formulations. One biological replicate of the PEG-coated liposome was an outlier, with a high abundance of immunoglobulins (Figure 6b,e,f). Both the HA-coated (F4) and PEG-coated liposomes (F2) with ICG were enriched with A0A286ZTT9, which is a 14-kDa immunoglobulin subtype deleted from the UniProt repository as obsolete in December 2019 (Figure 6f). Many of the other protein identifications that were not mapped into genes in Figure 6 are also immunoglobulins. Some of these proteins were found highly enriched in the SC of the HA-coated liposome with ICG (F4) and in some individual SC replicates (Figure 6e). The commonality between the source controls with different treatments (undiluted, diluted, SPR instrument flow-through) was 70% for plasma and 42% for vitreous samples.

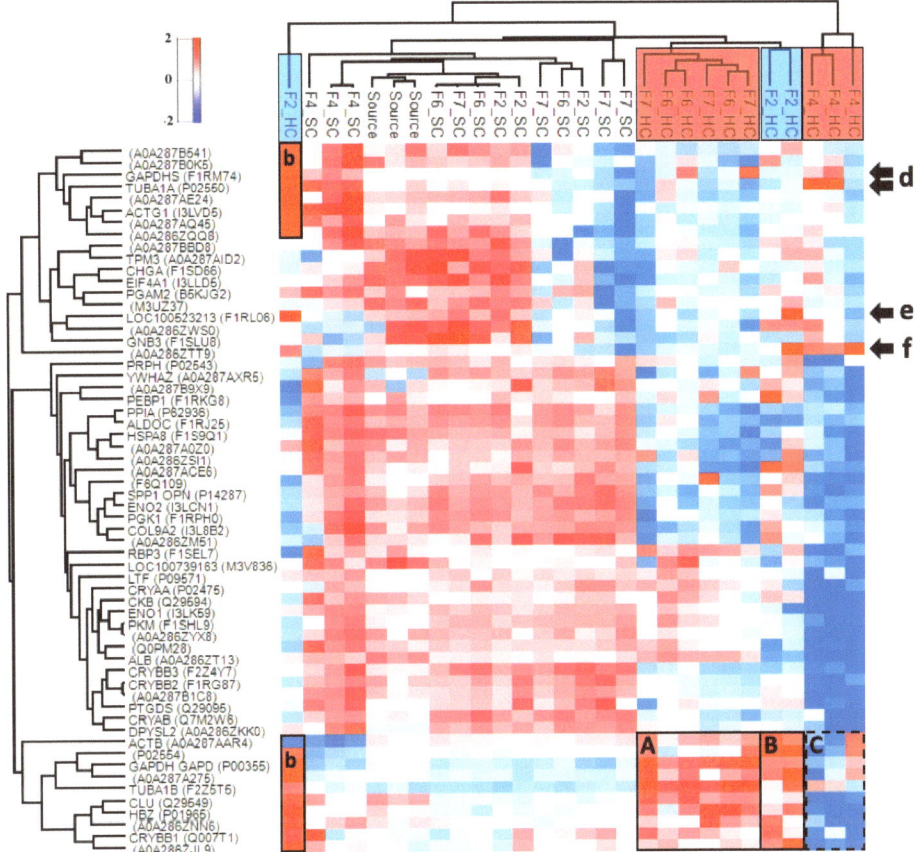

Figure 6. Heatmap of the top 60 most abundant proteins in porcine vitreous humor in at least three samples after median normalization (728 proteins). Distinct clusters are observed for the HC, SC, and plasma source. The HC subsections of the tested formulations do not cluster based on their anionic or neutral surface charge. The boxes (**A–B**) indicate the enrichment of tubulins, glyceraldehyde phosphate dehydrogenase (GAPDH), hemoglobin (HBZ), Dickkopf-related protein 3 (A0A286ZNN6), and clusterin (CLU) on the 50 nm anionic and 100 nm PEG-coated liposomes, which were depleted or less enriched on the HA-coated liposome (dashed box (**C**)). Interestingly, variants of glyceraldehyde phosphate dehydrogenase (GAPDHS) and tubulin (TUBA1A) were enriched on the HA-coated liposomes (**d**). One replicate of the PEG-coated 100-nm liposome showed high enrichment of these variants along with immunoglobulin family proteins (boxes (**b**,**e**)), which also enriched on the HA-coated liposome (**d**,**f**). An obsolete immunoglobulin subtype was enriched on the HA-coated liposome (**e**). The range for relative enrichment (*red*) and depletion (*blue*) is two standard deviations from the mean on the $\log_2$ scale.

3.4.3. Properties of the Corona-Enriched Proteins

The HC and SC subsections in plasma were enriched with 17–47 proteins per formulation, while some vitreous corona samples had up to 620 enriched proteins per formulation ($\log_2$ fold-change ≥ 1.00). Notably, the HA-coated formulation with ICG (F4) and the 50 nm PEG-liposome (F7) were enriched with only 17 proteins in plasma. The HA liposome with ICG also had the smallest number of enriched proteins in its vitreous HC (102). The smaller dynamic concentration range of proteins in the vitreous sample is reflected in the narrower range of fold-changes, suggesting that the abundances of adsorbed proteins are also lower in vitreous than in plasma samples (Supplementary File 2). To ensure comparability between samples and biological matrices, the top 20 most abundant proteins after median normalization were selected for the analysis of protein physicochemical properties (Supplementary Files 3 and 4). Their protein sequences were used to calculate the grand average of hydropathy (GRAVY), the theoretical isoelectric point (pI), the molecular weight (MW), and the number of the aromatic residues phenylalanine, tyrosine, tryptophan, and histidine (Ar (+His)) for the top 20 corona proteins in the corona subsections and the plasma or vitreous sources. The results for HC are displayed in Figure 7, while the corresponding figure for SC is shown in Figure S7 (Supplementary Materials). Summary data for both corona subsections in plasma and vitreous samples are provided as Supplementary File 5.

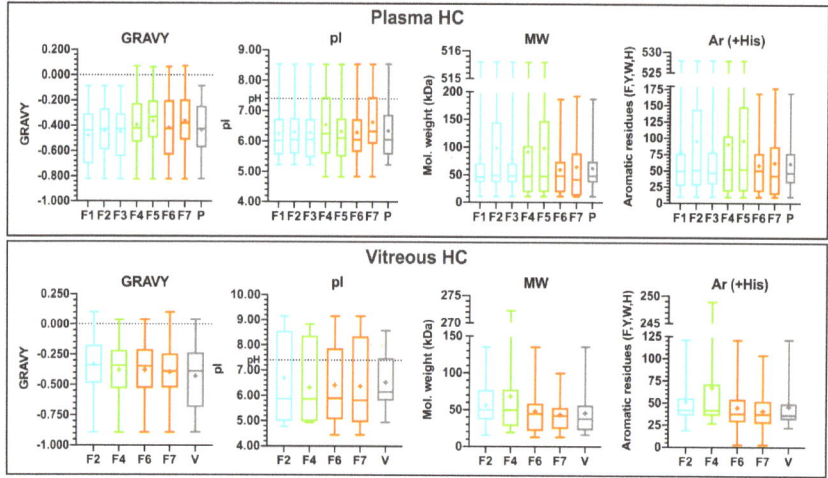

Figure 7. Properties of the top 20 enriched proteins in the hard coronas (HC) and the plasma or vitreous sources (P or V) with the max–min range, first and second quartiles, median, and mean (+). The color-coded groups are neutral 100 nm (*blue*), anionic 100 nm HA-coated (*green*), and small 50 nm anionic (*orange*) liposomes. GRAVY: grand average of hydropathy (positive score indicates hydrophobicity); pI: theoretical isoelectric point (pI under pH indicates net negative charge); MW: molecular weight; Ar (+His): aromatic residues phenylalanine, tyrosine, tryptophan, and histidine. Note the different y-axis ranges.

There are no statistically significant correlations between liposome size or surface charge and the protein physicochemical properties. However, the anionic formulations had individual hydrophobic proteins in their HCs in plasma. The contributors of these positive hydropathicity values in plasma are immunoglobulin heavy chain V-III regions BRO and TIL. The median molecular weight of HC proteins is ~50 kDa in both plasma and vitreous samples, while the corresponding means are ~87 kDa and ~54 kDa, respectively, with higher variance in plasma. The anionic 50 nm liposomes (F6–F7) did not bind proteins with molecular weights above 200 kDa in their plasma HCs. The trend with aromatic residues mirrors that of the molecular weight in plasma. In vitreous humor, the second quartile of the pI is above the pH, indicating a higher abundance of proteins with a positive charge, while the majority of proteins in plasma and vitreous samples hold a negative charge at physiological pH. The top-range high-molecular-weight protein on the HA-coated liposome with ICG (F4) in vitreous is fibronectin (FN1). The protein properties for the top 20 proteins in SCs largely mirror the plasma and vitreous sources (Figure S7, Supplementary Materials).

3.4.4. Common Subsets of Hard Corona Proteins in Plasma and Vitreous Samples

There were 22 common species among all the enriched proteins found in the plasma HCs of more than one liposome (Supplementary File 6). Among the seven proteins enriched in the HCs of all formulations, in addition to FGA and FGB, C3, and immunoglobulin constant fragments, were serotransferrin (TF) and alpha-2-macroglobulin (A2M), an iron transfer protein and protease inhibitor that are both highly abundant in plasma. In vitreous humor, only three proteins were common to the four formulations, including two structural crystallins and lactotransferrin (LTF), which is involved in iron transfer and immune functions (Supplementary File 6). Overall, the vitreous common subset included 14 proteins, such as glyceraldehyde-3-phosphate dehydrogenase (GADPH), clusterin (CLU), albumin (ALB), and alpha-enolase (ENO1), the latter being associated with glucose metabolism and a number of functions including coagulation and immune stimulation.

Figure 8 displays the commonality between plasma and vitreous for the common subsets for the four liposomes tested in both biological matrices. It demonstrates that the liposomes interact with 30–34 common proteins across the matrices, 74% of which are common to all formulations tested in both plasma and vitreous samples. These 28 proteins are listed in Figure 8B along with the corresponding top enriched biological functions in Figure 8C. Plasma HC common subset proteins carry a negative charge at physiological pH and are dominantly hydrophilic, similar to the top 20 most abundant proteins (Supplementary File 6). The same holds for the vitreous common subset, which was composed of smaller-molecular-weight proteins with fewer hydrophobic residues on average. Among both common subsets, the retinol-binding protein 3 (RBP3) in the vitreous subset was the only one with a positive hydropathicity value. It is a visual cycle glycoprotein with a significantly higher molecular weight at 135 kDa compared to the 49 kDa mean. Although it also had the lowest pI, it was highly enriched on the 50 nm anionic liposome HCs, despite being mostly present in the source and SCs of the other formulations (Figure 6).

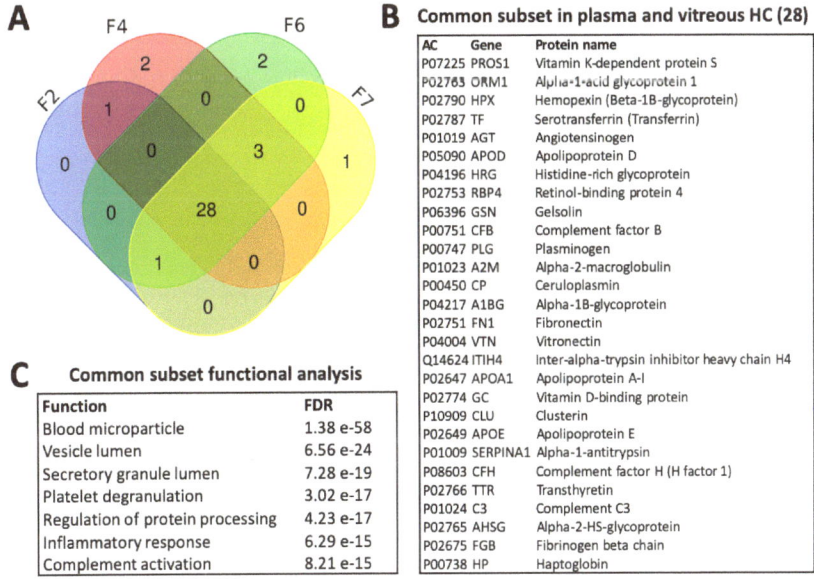

Figure 8. (**A**) Venn diagram of the commonalities between all proteins identified in the plasma and vitreous HCs of liposome formulations F2, F4, F6, and F7 without accounting for relative enrichment. (**B**) Proteins of the common subset. (**C**) Enriched biological functions in the common subset. AC: protein accession code; FDR: false discovery rate.

All of the common subset proteins were also among the top 20 most abundant proteins in plasma and vitreous samples (Figure 9). A list of the proteins and their properties in plasma and vitreous is provided in Supplementary Files 3 and 4. There is a high overlap between HC and SC identifications (Figure 9). Interestingly, an analysis of the *outlier* proteins that were specific to HA-coated liposomes with ICG (F4) in plasma showed the enrichment of collagen binding and extracellular matrix organization, with 67% of the predicted network explained by physical interactions (Figure S8; Table S3, Supplementary Materials). The small anionic liposomes were enriched with glycerolipid metabolism and actin filament organization functions, whereas the top enriched functions on neutral liposomes in plasma were related to glucose metabolism and immune activation. Overall, the top 20 HC enrichment patterns in plasma are mainly associated with blood microparticle and plasma lipoprotein particle-related functions, suggesting that they are secreted proteins that interact with lipid membranes (Figure S9; Table S4, Supplementary Materials). While complement activation did not rank highly, many of the proteins present in the common subset are associated with blood microparticle or plasma lipoprotein particles, or both, in addition to their immune system role (e.g., clusterin, CLU). Many of these proteins are also physical interaction partners. Glycolysis, visual perception, and blood microparticle were among the highest ranked functions in vitreous humor (Tables S5 and S10, Supplementary Materials).

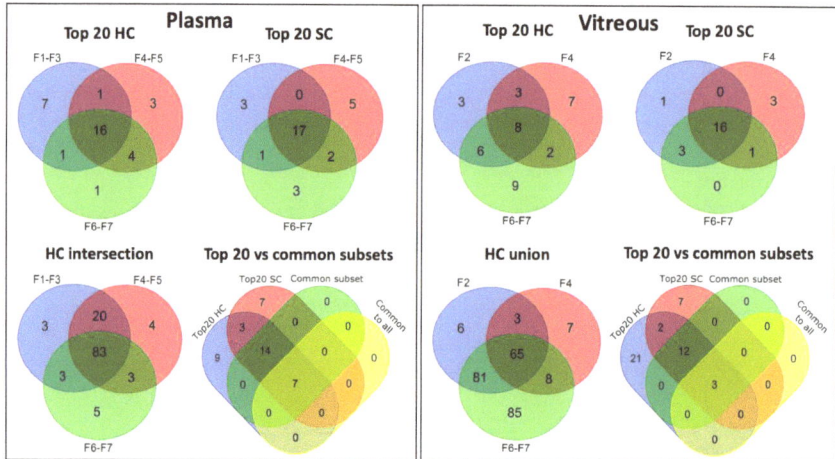

Figure 9. Venn diagrams of the commonalities between the neutral 100 nm (F1–F3 or F2), anionic 100 nm HA-coated (F4–F5 or F4), and anionic 50 nm (F6–F7) groups. Plasma: the top 20 most abundant proteins in the plasma HC (Top 20 HC) and SC (Top 20 SC), and their comparison with the common subsets (Top 20 vs common subsets), and for all HC proteins in found in plasma samples (HC intersection). Vitreous: the top 20 most abundant proteins in the vitreous HC (Top 20 HC) and SC (Top 20 SC), and their comparison with the common subsets (Top 20 vs common subsets), and for all HC proteins in found in vitreous samples (HC union).

3.5. Vitreal Mobility

The vitreal mobility of HA-coated liposomes was compared against their PEGylated counterparts (Table 2) [29]. While there were no significant differences in the mean track speeds between the PEG- and HA-coated liposomes, both formulations had higher overall speeds than the uncoated liposome ($p < 0.05$; Figure 10B). The vitreal diffusion coefficient (D_v), determined based on the mean square displacement by single-particle tracking analysis, showed that the HA-coated liposome diffused 1.5 times less than the PEG-coated liposomes despite their negative surface charge (Figure 10A). The diffusivity of the HA-coated liposomes was reduced 20-fold compared to their theoretical diffusion in water (D_w), indicating that they encounter more resistance in the vitreous humor compared to the

PEGylated and uncoated liposomes (D_w/D_v = 13 and 16, respectively). Nonetheless, the mobility hindrance observed with the HA-coated liposome was minimal, as evident by the representative Brownian trajectories (Figure 10C).

Table 2. Comparison of the vitreal diffusion of HA-coated, PEG-coated, and uncoated liposome formulations. D_v was obtained experimentally by single-particle tracking for 1 s, and the D_w was calculated based on the Stoke–Einstein equation (N = 3). * Data from Reference [29].

Formulation	Mean Diameter (nm)	PdI	D_v (µm²/s)	D_w (µm²/s)	D_w/D_v
HA	116.1	0.008	0.28 ± 0.14	5.68	20.2
PEG *	107.6	0.086	0.47 ± 0.25	6.12	13.0
Uncoated *	125.8	0.035	0.33 ± 0.17	5.27	16.0

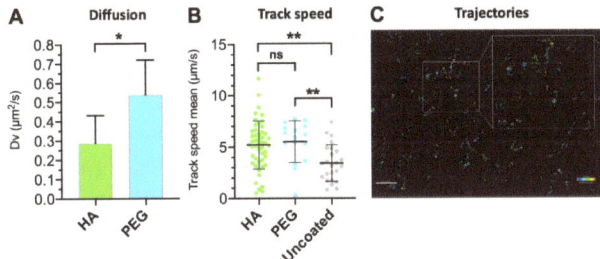

Figure 10. Comparison between (**A**) vitreal diffusion of HA- and PEG-coated light-triggered liposomes, analyzed by unpaired *t*-test (* p < 0.05); (**B**) ensemble-average speed of HA-coated, PEGylated, and uncoated light-activated liposomes (τ = 1 s). Means with significant differences are shown as analyzed by ordinary one-way ANOVA with Tukey's multiple comparison test (** p < 0.01). Error bars indicate SD. (**C**) Representative trajectories of the HA-coated liposome in the intact porcine vitreous. Inset shows the zoomed-in view of tracks obtained using the single-particle tracking technique.

4. Discussion

DSPE was conjugated with HA in-house to prepare hyaluronated liposomes, since there was no pre-existing conjugate available commercially. The successful reductive amination method was based on the work of Yao et al. [32]. The HA-coating on the liposomes did not significantly change the size, ICG encapsulation efficiency, or phase transition temperature of the liposomes (Table 1; Figure 1A). In the presence of hydrophilic coatings such as PEG, the ICG is stabilized by polymer clusters on the external side of the lipid bilayer [21]. Doubling the amount of both HA and ICG doubled the encapsulated amount of ICG without affecting the bilayer stability, while doubling ICG alone destabilized the membrane, causing passive leakage at 37 °C. This is in accordance with our previous results with PEG-coated ICG liposomes and suggests that HA is at least as efficient as PEG in stabilizing ICG [20]. The change in the surface coating of the 100 nm liposomes did not affect the temperature-induced release of calcein, although the small liposomes (~70 nm) had slightly higher release temperatures compared to the larger HA-coated liposomes (Figure 1B). A similar observation was previously made with PEG-coated ICG liposomes, which may be caused by curvature-modulated phase separation in the lipid bilayer [18]. This observation is supported by the light-activated release study, where small (~70 nm) HA-coated liposomes released less of their contents than the larger ones in response to a 5 s light exposure (Figure 1C).

Notably, while light-activated drug release from 100 nm HA-coated liposomes was comparable to the PEGylated liposomes in buffer, plasma, and vitreous samples, the HA coating improved liposomal stability in plasma at 37 °C (Figure 2C,D). Vitreal stability was comparable for both formulations over the period of one week. Following a 3-h incubation period in vitreous and plasma samples, the 15 s light exposure increased release by as much as 44% and 69% compared to passive leakage. The light-activated release was more pronounced in plasma, possibly due to the lipid bilayer-destabilizing effect of the biocorona on thermosensitive liposomes [37]. Therefore, the better plasma stability of the HA-coating especially within the first 12 h permits longer delays between intravenous (i.v.) administration and light activation, which is a beneficial property from a therapeutic perspective. The HA coating also made the liposomes significantly anionic (−11 mV), caused by the deprotonation of disaccharide carboxyl groups in an aqueous environment [38]. The analysis of the top 20 most abundant corona protein properties showed that the HA-coated liposomes were predominantly enriched with proteins that carry a negative charge in both plasma and vitreous pH, suggesting that the liposome anionic charge is also retained after coronation (Figure 7). This may partly explain the improvement in the stealth properties of HA-coated liposomes compared to their PEGylated counterparts [13,39].

In human plasma, ~5 nm HCs and ~10 nm SCs formed on the HA and PEG-coated liposomes, which correspond to sparse monolayers [28,40]. The formulation-dependent compositions also clustered based on liposomal surface charge (Figure 5). The influence of nanoparticle surface charge on the HC composition and the enrichment of fibrinogens under in vitro conditions were reported [41,42]. ICG also influences corona composition, as evidenced by the higher relative enrichment of complement and immunoglobulin proteins on the 8–15 kDa HA-coated liposome with ICG (F4) than without ICG (F5). This is likely due to trace endotoxins, since <400-kDa HA is not immunogenic [43]. The enrichment of immunoglobulin variable regions may be due to the particular epitope repertoire of the plasma donors [44].

In undiluted vitreous, the thinner ~2 nm HCs and ~3 nm SCs had formulation-independent compositions (Figure 4C,D). The slightly higher SC thicknesses but significantly different composition compared to the HCs suggest that it consists of only a few loosely interacting molecules. Interestingly, the 100 nm HA-coated formulation bound more proteins than the PEG-coated liposome in vitreous humor, while the reverse was seen in plasma. Interactions with the structural HA–collagen meshwork of the eye involve alpha and beta-crystallins, both abundant in vitreal coronas, as well as fibronectin and the inter-alpha trypsin inhibitors found in both plasma and vitreous HCs (Figure 8B). In plasma, the proteins that were only found on the HA-coated liposomes interact with fibrillar collagen type I and cell-adhesion protein collagen type XIV (Figure S8; Table S3, Supplementary Materials). These functions were not enriched in vitreous humor, possibly due to the low number of identified proteins on the HA-coated liposomes (Figure S10, Table S5, Supplementary Materials). Therefore, the "biological identity" ensuing from the HA coating may result in physical interactions with the structural collagen of the eye [45].

Consequently, these interactions may explain the slightly slower vitreal mobility of the HA-coated liposomes compared to PEG-coated liposomes. Since the increase in liposome diameter as a result of corona formation did not influence the diffusion of 50 nm anionic pegylated liposomes [29], it is inconsequential for neutral 100 nm liposomes at similar corona thicknesses. Although anionic nanoparticles diffuse freely in the vitreous humor [46], PEG-coated nanoparticles diffuse faster, possibly as a result of a "shielding" effect against charge-mediated interactions with the meshwork [47]. The HA- and PEG-coated liposomes diffused at comparable speeds, but significantly faster than the uncoated formulation (Figure 10). The random walk diffusion patterns indicate that particles with higher speeds do not necessarily relocate longer distances (Figure 10C). This is evident based on the comparable diffusion coefficients of the HA-coated and uncoated liposomes, despite the faster mean track speed of HA-coated liposomes. The more heterogeneous track speed distribution of the HA-coated liposomes may be explained by vitreous meshwork interactions.

The HA-coated liposomes had a low number of identified proteins with a narrow range of fold-changes in vitreous humor (Supplementary File 2). However, as a result of median normalization, proteins with high abundances in individual replicates could be identified. The consistency (36–38% of the highest number of identifications) suggests that this is a consequence of physical interactions, such as protein complex binding to the liposomes. Stable physical interactions between proteins are needed for cellular processes, and evolutionarily conserved soluble complexes are abundant in the human proteome [48]. The vitreous humor is abundant in energy metabolism-related proteins, such as GAPDH, which interact with other proteins to exert their functions [49]. Earlier, we found that 20–22% of the highly enriched vitreal corona proteins on 50 nm anionic liposomes were physical interaction partners of GAPDH [29]. These showed a preference for the PEGylated formulation, as can also be seen in Figure 6A (F7). It is, therefore, possible that some of the less enriched proteins interact with GAPDH or other HC proteins instead of the nanoparticle surface, as demonstrated with complement protein C3 [50]. Protein complexes should be considered a factor that influences corona composition and structure.

It was proposed that protein complexity of the HC increases with nanoparticle size, and small nanoparticles bind proteins with more aromatic residues [51]. In our study, the 50 nm liposomes did not bind proteins above 200 kDa, which may reflect the effect of surface curvature, but this also decreased the number of aromatic residues. In vitreous humor, the uncoated anionic 50 nm liposome (F6) had the most distinct HC (50% unique protein identifications), and the small anionic liposome group had slightly more outliers than the other groups in plasma and vitreous samples (Figure 9). Therefore, our findings suggest an inverse relationship with HC complexity and liposome size. In addition, the properties of the top 20 most abundant proteins in HC or SC did not correlate with liposome size or charge (Figure 7 and Figure S7, Supplementary Materials). As expected based on earlier studies [29,30], there was also no correlation with liposome properties and the corona composition in vitreous, although these liposomes had formulation-dependent coronas in plasma. However, our analysis confirmed that the HC and SC proteins are predominantly hydrophilic and carry an anionic charge in both plasma and vitreous samples. Similar observations were made in diluted plasma [42], as well as in diluted and undiluted vitreous humor with more limited sample sets [29,30]. Our results indicate that this trend is more universal than previously known.

Biocorona formation is influenced by nanoparticle-related and experimental factors [27,44] together with the biological environment, such as the nature and amount of its constituents and ionic strength [52]. However, the volume available to proteins influences all aspects of their behavior, including adsorption processes [53]. As a result, incubation in diluted and undiluted solutions results in different corona compositions and thicknesses [54]. Except for Digiacomo et al. [54], molecular crowding received little attention in the context of biocorona formation. Since there is a significant difference in plasma (~76 mg/mL) and vitreous (~1.5 mg/mL) protein concentrations, crowding agents such as structural HA are important modulators of ocular protein interactions [52,53,55]. Molecular crowding directly influences thermodynamics and diffusion, the drivers of protein adsorption and corona formation [56,57]. It is, therefore, likely that the differences in corona formation between plasma and vitreous samples, at physiological concentrations due to the use of undiluted fluids, are explained partly by structural HA. This would also explain the need for longer LC separation gradients and the lower number of protein identifications on HA-coated liposomes in vitreous humor. It should be noted that porcine vitreous humor is the best substitute to human vitreous humor in terms of its protein and HA concentrations [29] and viscoelastic properties [58].

The most abundant corona proteins most likely determine the ensuing biological responses, due to the higher probability of encountering cellular receptors in the correct orientation [26,59]. It is noteworthy that there is a common subset of 30–34 proteins in both plasma and vitreous samples, 74% of which were found in all of the HCs, including on 100 nm PEG-coated and HA-coated liposomes and on 50 nm uncoated and PEG-coated liposomes (Figure 8). Functional analysis showed an association with blood microparticle and immune activation functions (Figure 8C), which are also among the enriched functions for the top 20 HC proteins in plasma (Figure S9; Table S4, Supplementary Materials). Considering that nanoparticle aggregation and protein adsorption are driven by surface free energy, it is interesting to note the "double role" of lung surfactant proteins, where they participate in immune surveillance in addition to reducing alveolar surface tension [52]. The common subset, therefore, labels the liposomes "non-self" lipid particles regardless of the biological environment (plasma or vitreous), a possible consequence of combined surfactant and immune activity in response to the "abnormally" high surface energy of cell-mimetic lipid bilayers. This may also explain why the lipid corona is insensitive to nanoparticle properties [60,61].

The two-fold increases in hydrodynamic diameters measured with LALS results indicate aggregation (Figure 4B) [57]. Although the HA-coated liposomes showed comparable or improved stability in vitreous and plasma samples, respectively (Figure 2), they may be more susceptible to clustering and aggregation than the PEG-coated liposomes. This may also be influenced by the higher abundance of immunoglobulins [52,62]. However, protein adsorption did not influence the liposome stability or mobility in vitreous humor, regardless of the formulation. Future studies should explore the mechanism of biocorona formation in the ocular environment together with the ensuing biological responses, including elimination by ocular phagocytes and retinal cell uptake [63].

5. Conclusions

A novel HA–lipid conjugate was successfully synthesized for the preparation of light-activated indocyanine green liposomes. HA-coated liposomes were functional in light-triggered drug release in vitreous and plasma samples. The HA-coated liposomes showed adequate stability and mobility in the vitreous humor. Protein corona formation on the HA-coated liposomes was characterized in the vitreous and plasma samples, and its properties were compared to PEG-coated and uncoated liposomes. Suitable stability and pharmacokinetic properties are vital for triggered release delivery systems that rely on controlled phase changes. The results showed the significance of nanoparticle coating materials on the stability, as well as on the interactions with vitreal and plasma components. These in turn may affect the immunological reactions to the drug delivery system, the implications of which are essential for intravitreal therapy due to the immunoprivilege of the eye. Future studies should further elucidate the mechanisms and consequences of corona formation in vitreous humor, taking into consideration the molecular crowding activity of structural HA. In conclusion, the HA-coated light-activated liposomes are a promising drug delivery system for intravenous and ocular applications.

Supplementary Materials: The following are available online at http://www.mdpi.com/1999-4923/12/8/763/s1: Figure S1. ^{1}H-NMR and FT-IR spectra of the synthetized DSPE–HA conjugate; Figure S2. Size, T_m profiles, heat- and light-triggered calcein releases, and ICG absorbances; Figure S3. Size, T_m profiles, heat-triggered calcein releases, and ICG absorbances; Figure S4. Dynamic light scattering and large-angle light scattering; Figure S5. Heatmap of the 178 proteins identified in human plasma; Figure S6. Heatmap of the 728 proteins identified in porcine vitreous humor; Figure S7. Properties of the top 20 enriched proteins; Figure S8. Enriched functions and gene interaction network of HC proteins only enriched on HA-coated liposomes in plasma; Figure S9. Enriched biological functions and gene interaction network based on top 20 most abundant HC proteins in plasma; Figure S10. Enriched biological functions and gene interaction network based on top 20 most abundant HC proteins in vitreous humor; Table S1. Venn diagram of the protein-encoding genes in the plasma HC intersection; Table S2. Venn diagram of the protein-encoding genes in the vitreous HC union; Table S3. Enriched biological functions in the HC-enriched outlier sets per liposome group in plasma; Table S4. Top 100 enriched biological functions of the top 20 most abundant HC proteins in plasma; Table S5. Enriched biological functions based on the top 20 most abundant HC proteins in vitreous humor; Supplementary File 1. Plasma matrix and enriched (MS Excel); Supplementary File 2. Vitreous full matrix and enriched (MS Excel); Supplementary File 3. Top 20 plasma (PDF); Supplementary File 4. Top 20 vitreous (PDF); Supplementary File 5. Top 20 plasma vs. vitreous (PDF); Supplementary File 6. Common gene subsets plasma and vitreous (PDF).

Author Contributions: Conceptualization, O.K.K., A.U., and T.L.; methodology, O.K.K., S.T., P.P., N.G.J., T.V., and T.L.; software, P.P., J.N., and H.A.; formal analysis, O.K.K., S.T., S.B., and T.L.; investigation, O.K.K., S.T., S.B., R.S., T.R., N.G.J., J.N., and T.L.; resources, H.A., T.V., A.U., and T.L.; data curation, O.K.K. and T.L.; writing—original draft preparation, O.K.K., R.S., and T.L.; writing—review and editing, O.K.K., S.T., J.N., H.A., T.V., A.U., and T.L.; visualization, O.K.K., S.T., and T.L.; supervision, A.U. and T.L.; project administration, T.L.; funding acquisition, O.K.K., A.U., and T.L. All authors read and agree to the published version of the manuscript.

Funding: This research was funded by the Academy of Finland (#311122, #317336), Business Finland (#4208/31/2015), EU Horizon 2020 Marie Skłodowska-Curie Innovative Training Networks NANOMED project (#676137), Orion Research Foundation (#9-8214-9), Phospholipid Research Center, Emil Aaltonen Foundation, Instrumentarium Science Foundation, Mary and Georg C. Ehrnrooth Foundation, Evald and Hilda Nissi Foundation, Inkeri and Mauri Vänskä Foundation, Paulo Foundation, and Päivikki and Sakari Sohlberg Foundation. Open access funding provided by University of Helsinki.

Acknowledgments: Marja Hagström is acknowledged for her assistance with sample preparation for proteomics analysis. The University of Helsinki EV core is acknowledged for the flow cytometry support.

Conflicts of Interest: The authors declare no conflicts of interest.

References

1. Etheridge, M.L.; Campbell, S.A.; Erdman, A.G.; Haynes, C.L.; Wolf, S.M.; McCullough, J. The big picture on nanomedicine: The state of investigational and approved nanomedicine products. *Nanomed. Nanotechnol. Biol. Med.* **2013**, *9*, 1–14. [CrossRef]
2. Vonarbourg, A.; Passirani, C.; Saulnier, P.; Simard, P.; Leroux, J.-C.; Benoit, J.-P. Evaluation of pegylated lipid nanocapsules versus complement system activation and macrophage uptake. *J. Biomed. Mater. Res. Part A* **2006**, *78A*, 620–628. [CrossRef]
3. Amoozgar, Z.; Yeo, Y. Recent advances in stealth coating of nanoparticle drug delivery systems. *Wiley Interdiscip. Rev. Nanomed. Nanobiotechnol.* **2012**, *4*, 219–233. [CrossRef]
4. Romberg, B.; Metselaar, J.M.; Baranyi, L.; Snel, C.J.; Bünger, R.; Hennink, W.E.; Szebeni, J.; Storm, G. Poly(amino acid)s: Promising enzymatically degradable stealth coatings for liposomes. *Int. J. Pharm.* **2007**, *331*, 186–189. [CrossRef]
5. Sroda, K.; Rydlewski, J.; Langner, M.; Kozubek, A.; Grzybek, M.; Sikorski, A.F. Repeated injections of PEG-PE liposomes generate anti-PEG antibodies. *Cell. Mol. Biol. Lett.* **2005**, *10*, 37–47.
6. Yang, Q.; Lai, S.K. Anti-PEG immunity: Emergence, characteristics, and unaddressed questions. *Wiley Interdiscip. Rev. Nanomed. Nanobiotechnol.* **2015**, *7*, 655–677. [CrossRef]
7. Knop, K.; Hoogenboom, R.; Fischer, D.; Schubert, U.S. Poly(ethylene glycol) in drug delivery: Pros and cons as well as potential alternatives. *Angew. Chemie Int. Ed.* **2010**, *49*, 6288–6308. [CrossRef] [PubMed]
8. Kaneda, Y.; Tsutsumi, Y.; Yoshioka, Y.; Kamada, H.; Yamamoto, Y.; Kodaira, H.; Tsunoda, S.I.; Okamoto, T.; Mukai, Y.; Shibata, H.; et al. The use of PVP as a polymeric carrier to improve the plasma half-life of drugs. *Biomaterials* **2004**, *25*, 3259–3266. [CrossRef] [PubMed]
9. Engler, A.C.; Ke, X.; Gao, S.; Chan, J.M.W.; Coady, D.J.; Ono, R.J.; Lubbers, R.; Nelson, A.; Yang, Y.Y.; Hedrick, J.L. Hydrophilic polycarbonates: Promising degradable alternatives to poly(ethylene glycol)-based stealth materials. *Macromolecules* **2015**, *48*, 1673–1678. [CrossRef]
10. Kang, E.; Akiyoshi, K.; Sunamoto, J. Surface coating of liposomes with hydrophobized polysaccharides. *J. Bioact. Compat. Polym.* **1997**, *12*, 14–26. [CrossRef]
11. Magarkar, A.; Róg, T.; Bunker, A. A computational study suggests that replacing PEG with PMOZ may increase exposure of hydrophobic targeting moiety. *Eur. J. Pharm. Sci.* **2017**, *103*, 128–135. [CrossRef]
12. Wickens, J.M.; Alsaab, H.O.; Kesharwani, P.; Bhise, K.; Amin, M.C.I.M.; Tekade, R.K.; Gupta, U.; Iyer, A.K. Recent advances in hyaluronic acid-decorated nanocarriers for targeted cancer therapy. *Drug Discov. Today* **2017**, *22*, 665–680. [CrossRef]
13. Zhang, Q.; Deng, C.; Fu, Y.; Sun, X.; Gong, T.; Zhang, Z. Repeated Administration of Hyaluronic Acid Coated Liposomes with Improved Pharmacokinetics and Reduced Immune Response. *Mol. Pharm.* **2016**, *13*, 1800–1808. [CrossRef] [PubMed]
14. Eliaz, R.E.; Szoka, J. Liposome-encapsulated doxorubicin targeted to CD44: A strategy to kill CD44-overexpressing tumor cells. *Cancer Res.* **2001**, *61*, 2592–2601.
15. Peer, D.; Florentin, A.; Margalit, R. Hyaluronan is a key component in cryoprotection and formulation of targeted unilamellar liposomes. *Biochim. Biophys. Acta Biomembr.* **2003**, *1612*, 76–82. [CrossRef]
16. Torchilin, V.P. Recent advances with liposomes as pharmaceutical carriers. *Nat. Rev. Drug Discov.* **2005**, *4*, 145–160. [CrossRef]
17. Gómez-Hens, A.; Fernández-Romero, J.M. Analytical methods for the control of liposomal delivery systems. *TrAC Trends Anal. Chem.* **2006**, *25*, 167–178. [CrossRef]
18. Lajunen, T.; Nurmi, R.; Kontturi, L.-S.; Viitala, L.; Yliperttula, M.; Murtomäki, L.; Urtti, A. Light activated liposomes: Functionality and prospects in ocular drug delivery. *J. Control. Release* **2016**, *244*, 157–166. [CrossRef]
19. Alvarez-Lorenzo, C.; Bromberg, L.; Concheiro, A. Light-sensitive intelligent drug delivery systems. *Photochem. Photobiol.* **2009**, *85*, 848–860. [CrossRef] [PubMed]

20. Lajunen, T.; Kontturi, L.-S.; Viitala, L.; Manna, M.; Cramariuc, O.; Róg, T.; Bunker, A.; Laaksonen, T.; Viitala, T.; Murtomäki, L.; et al. Indocyanine green-loaded liposomes for light-triggered drug release. *Mol. Pharm.* **2016**, *13*, 2095–2107. [CrossRef] [PubMed]
21. Lajunen, T.; Nurmi, R.; Wilbie, D.; Ruoslahti, T.; Johansson, N.G.; Korhonen, O.; Rog, T.; Bunker, A.; Ruponen, M.; Urtti, A. The effect of light sensitizer localization on the stability of indocyanine green liposomes. *J. Control. Release* **2018**, *284*, 213–223. [CrossRef] [PubMed]
22. Viitala, L.; Pajari, S.; Lajunen, T.; Kontturi, L.S.; Laaksonen, T.; Kuosmanen, P.; Viitala, T.; Urtti, A.; Murtoma-ki, L. Photothermally triggered lipid bilayer phase transition and drug release from gold nanorod and indocyanine green encapsulated liposomes. *Langmuir* **2016**, *32*, 4554–4563. [CrossRef] [PubMed]
23. European Medicines Agency. *Guideline on the Evaluation of the Pharmacokinetics of Medicinal Products in Patients with Impaired Hepatic Function*; European Medicines Agency: London, UK, 2005.
24. U.S. Food and Drug Administration. *Product insert NDA 11-525-S-017: IC-Green^{TM}, Indocyanine Green for Injection*; Silver Springs: Rockville, MD, USA, 2006.
25. Kraft, J.C.; Ho, R.J.Y. Interactions of indocyanine green and lipid in enhancing near-infrared fluorescence properties: The basis for near-infrared imaging in vivo. *Biochemistry* **2014**, *53*, 1275–1283. [CrossRef] [PubMed]
26. Monopoli, M.P.; Åberg, C.; Salvati, A.; Dawson, K.A.; Åberg, C.; Salvati, A.; Dawson, K.A.; Aberg, C.; Salvati, A.; Dawson, K.A. Biomolecular coronas provide the biological identity of nanosized materials. *Nat. Nanotechnol.* **2012**, *7*, 779–786. [CrossRef] [PubMed]
27. Ke, P.C.; Lin, S.; Parak, W.J.; Davis, T.P.; Caruso, F. A Decade of the Protein Corona. *ACS Nano* **2017**, *11*, 11773–11776. [CrossRef]
28. Kari, O.K.; Ndika, J.; Parkkila, P.; Louna, A.; Lajunen, T.; Puustinen, A.; Viitala, T.; Alenius, H.; Urtti, A. In situ analysis of liposome hard and soft protein corona structure and composition in a single label-free workflow. *Nanoscale* **2020**, *12*, 1728–1741. [CrossRef]
29. Tavakoli, S.; Kari, O.K.; Turunen, T.; Lajunen, T.; Schmitt, M.; Lehtinen, J.; Tasaka, F.; Parkkila, P.; Ndika, J.; Viitala, T.; et al. Diffusion and protein corona formation of lipid-based nanoparticles in vitreous humor: Profiling and pharmacokinetic considerations. *Mol. Pharm.* **2020**. [CrossRef]
30. Jo, D.H.; Kim, J.H.; Son, J.G.; Dan, K.S.; Song, S.H.; Lee, T.G.; Kim, J.H. Nanoparticle-protein complexes mimicking corona formation in ocular environment. *Biomaterials* **2016**, *109*, 23–31. [CrossRef]
31. Rimpelä, A.-K.; Schmitt, M.; Latonen, S.; Hagström, M.; Antopolsky, M.; Manzanares, J.A.; Kidron, H.; Urtti, A. Drug Distribution to Retinal Pigment Epithelium: Studies on Melanin Binding, Cellular Kinetics, and Single Photon Emission Computed Tomography/Computed Tomography Imaging. *Mol. Pharm.* **2016**. [CrossRef]
32. Yao, H.J.; Sun, L.; Liu, Y.; Jiang, S.; Pu, Y.; Li, J.; Zhang, Y. Monodistearoylphosphatidylethanolamine-hyaluronic acid functionalization of single-walled carbon nanotubes for targeting intracellular drug delivery to overcome multidrug resistance of cancer cells. *Carbon N. Y.* **2016**, *96*, 362–376. [CrossRef]
33. Saxena, V.; Sadoqi, M.; Shao, J. Degradation Kinetics of Indocyanine Green in Aqueous Solution. *J. Pharm. Sci.* **2003**, *92*, 2090–2097. [CrossRef] [PubMed]
34. Cox, J.; Hein, M.Y.; Luber, C.A.; Paron, I.; Nagaraj, N.; Mann, M. Accurate Proteome-wide Label-free Quantification by Delayed Normalization and Maximal Peptide Ratio Extraction, Termed MaxLFQ. *Mol. Cell. Proteomics* **2014**, *13*, 2513–2526. [CrossRef] [PubMed]
35. Tyanova, S.; Temu, T.; Sinitcyn, P.; Carlson, A.; Hein, M.Y.; Geiger, T.; Mann, M.; Cox, J. The Perseus computational platform for comprehensive analysis of (prote)omics data. *Nat. Methods* **2016**, *13*, 731–740. [CrossRef] [PubMed]
36. Saadat, E.; Amini, M.; Dinarvand, R.; Dorkoosh, F.A. Polymeric micelles based on hyaluronic acid and phospholipids: Design, characterization, and cytotoxicity. *J. Appl. Polym. Sci.* **2014**, *131*, 1–8. [CrossRef]
37. Al-Ahmady, Z.S.; Hadjidemetriou, M.; Gubbins, J.; Kostarelos, K. Formation of protein corona in vivo affects drug release from temperature-sensitive liposomes. *J. Control. Release* **2018**, *276*, 157–167. [CrossRef]
38. Choi, K.Y.; Min, K.H.; Yoon, H.Y.; Kim, K.; Park, J.H.; Kwon, I.C.; Choi, K.; Jeong, S.Y. PEGylation of hyaluronic acid nanoparticles improves tumor targetability in vivo. *Biomaterials* **2011**, *32*, 1880–1889. [CrossRef]
39. Rege, K.; Medintz, I.L. *Methods in Bioengineering: Nanoscale Bioengineering and Nanomedicine*; Artech House: Norwood, MA, USA, 2009; ISBN 9781596934115.

40. Soo Choi, H.; Liu, W.; Misra, P.; Tanaka, E.; Zimmer, J.P.; Itty Ipe, B.; Bawendi, M.G.; Frangioni, J.V. Renal clearance of quantum dots. *Nat. Biotechnol.* **2007**, *25*, 1165–1170. [CrossRef]
41. Hadjidemetriou, M.; Al-Ahmady, Z.; Mazza, M.; Collins, R.F.; Dawson, K.; Kostarelos, K. In Vivo Biomolecule Corona around Blood-Circulating, Clinically Used and Antibody-Targeted Lipid Bilayer Nanoscale Vesicles. *ACS Nano* **2015**, *9*, 8142–8156. [CrossRef]
42. Tenzer, S.; Docter, D.; Kuharev, J.; Musyanovych, A.; Fetz, V.; Hecht, R.; Schlenk, F.; Fischer, D.; Kiouptsi, K.; Reinhardt, C.; et al. Rapid formation of plasma protein corona critically affects nanoparticle pathophysiology. *Nat. Nanotechnol.* **2013**, *8*, 772–781. [CrossRef]
43. Dong, Y.; Arif, A.; Olsson, M.; Cali, V.; Hardman, B.; Dosanjh, M.; Lauer, M.; Midura, R.J.; Hascall, V.C.; Brown, K.L.; et al. Endotoxin free hyaluronan and hyaluronan fragments do not stimulate TNF-α, interleukin-12 or upregulate co-stimulatory molecules in dendritic cells or macrophages. *Sci. Rep.* **2016**, *6*, 1–15. [CrossRef]
44. Mahmoudi, M. Debugging Nano–Bio Interfaces: Systematic Strategies to Accelerate Clinical Translation of Nanotechnologies. *Trends Biotechnol.* **2018**, *36*, 755–769. [CrossRef] [PubMed]
45. Bishop, P. Structural Macromolecules and Supramolecular Organisation of the Vitreous Gel. *Prog. Retin. Eye Res.* **2000**, *19*, 323–344. [CrossRef]
46. Xu, Q.; Boylan, N.J.; Suk, J.S.; Wang, Y.-Y.; Nance, E.A.; Yang, J.-C.; McDonnell, P.J.; Cone, R.A.; Duh, E.J.; Hanes, J. Nanoparticle diffusion in, and microrheology of, the bovine vitreous ex vivo. *J. Control. Release* **2013**, *167*, 76–84. [CrossRef] [PubMed]
47. Käsdorf, B.T.; Arends, F.; Lieleg, O. Diffusion Regulation in the Vitreous Humor. *Biophys. J.* **2015**, *109*, 2171–2181. [CrossRef] [PubMed]
48. Havugimana, P.C.; Hart, G.T.; Nepusz, T.; Yang, H.; Turinsky, A.L.; Li, Z.; Wang, P.I.; Boutz, D.R.; Fong, V.; Phanse, S.; et al. A census of human soluble protein complexes. *Cell* **2012**, *150*, 1068–1081. [CrossRef]
49. Skeie, J.M.; Roybal, C.N.; Mahajan, V.B. Proteomic insight into the molecular function of the vitreous. *PLoS ONE* **2015**, *10*, 1–19. [CrossRef]
50. Bertrand, N.; Grenier, P.; Mahmoudi, M.; Lima, E.M.; Appel, E.A.; Dormont, F.; Lim, J.-M.; Karnik, R.; Langer, R.; Farokhzad, O.C. Mechanistic understanding of in vivo protein corona formation on polymeric nanoparticles and impact on pharmacokinetics. *Nat. Commun.* **2017**, *8*, 777. [CrossRef]
51. Shannahan, J.H.; Lai, X.; Ke, P.C.; Podila, R.; Brown, J.M.; Witzmann, F.A. Silver Nanoparticle Protein Corona Composition in Cell Culture Media. *PLoS ONE* **2013**, *8*. [CrossRef]
52. Tsuda, A.; Konduru, N.V. The role of natural processes and surface energy of inhaled engineered nanoparticles on aggregation and corona formation. *NanoImpact* **2016**, *2*, 38–44. [CrossRef]
53. Kuznetsova, I.M.; Turoverov, K.K.; Uversky, V.N. What macromolecular crowding can do to a protein. *Int. J. Mol. Sci.* **2014**, *15*, 23090–23140. [CrossRef]
54. Digiacomo, L.; Giulimondi, F.; Mahmoudi, M.; Caracciolo, G. Effect of molecular crowding on the biological identity of liposomes: An overlooked factor at the bio-nano interface. *Nanoscale Adv.* **2019**, *1*, 2518–2522. [CrossRef]
55. Dewavrin, J.; Hamzavi, N.; Shim, V.P.W.; Raghunath, M. Tuning the architecture of three-dimensional collagen hydrogels by physiological macromolecular crowding. *Acta Biomater.* **2014**, *10*, 4351–4359. [CrossRef] [PubMed]
56. Nel, A.E.; Mädler, L.; Velegol, D.; Xia, T.; Hoek, E.M.V.; Somasundaran, P.; Klaessig, F.; Castranova, V.; Thompson, M. Understanding biophysicochemical interactions at the nano-bio interface. *Nat. Mater.* **2009**, *8*, 543–557. [CrossRef] [PubMed]
57. Walkey, C.D.; Chan, W.C.W. Understanding and controlling the interaction of nanomaterials with proteins in a physiological environment. *Chem. Soc. Rev.* **2012**, *41*, 2780–2799. [CrossRef]
58. Swindle, K.E.; Hamilton, P.D.; Ravi, N. In situ formation of hydrogels as vitreous substitutes: Viscoelastic comparison to porcine vitreous. *J. Biomed. Mater. Res. Part A* **2008**, *87*, 656–665. [CrossRef]
59. Kelly, P.M.; Åberg, C.; Polo, E.; O'Connell, A.; Cookman, J.; Fallon, J.; Krpetić, Ž.; Dawson, K.A. Mapping protein binding sites on the biomolecular corona of nanoparticles. *Nat. Nanotechnol.* **2015**, *10*, 472–479. [CrossRef]
60. Raesch, S.S.; Tenzer, S.; Storck, W.; Rurainski, A.; Selzer, D.; Ruge, C.A.; Perez-Gil, J.; Schaefer, U.F.; Lehr, C.M. Proteomic and Lipidomic Analysis of Nanoparticle Corona upon Contact with Lung Surfactant Reveals Differences in Protein, but Not Lipid Composition. *ACS Nano* **2015**, *9*, 11872–11885. [CrossRef]

61. Müller, J.; Prozeller, D.; Ghazaryan, A.; Kokkinopoulou, M.; Mailänder, V.; Morsbach, S.; Landfester, K. Beyond the protein corona – lipids matter for biological response of nanocarriers. *Acta Biomater.* **2018**, *71*, 420–431. [CrossRef]
62. Simon, J.; Müller, L.K.; Kokkinopoulou, M.; Lieberwirth, I.; Morsbach, S.; Landfester, K.; Mailänder, V. Exploiting the biomolecular corona: Pre-coating of nanoparticles enables controlled cellular interactions. *Nanoscale* **2018**, *10*, 10731–10739. [CrossRef]
63. del Amo, E.M.; Rimpelä, A.-K.; Heikkinen, E.; Kari, O.K.; Ramsay, E.; Lajunen, T.; Schmitt, M.; Pelkonen, L.; Bhattacharya, M.; Richardson, D.; et al. Pharmacokinetic aspects of retinal drug delivery. *Prog. Retin. Eye Res.* **2016**, 1–52. [CrossRef]

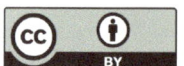

© 2020 by the authors. Licensee MDPI, Basel, Switzerland. This article is an open access article distributed under the terms and conditions of the Creative Commons Attribution (CC BY) license (http://creativecommons.org/licenses/by/4.0/).

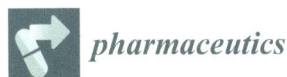

Article

Porous Nanostructure, Lipid Composition, and Degree of Drug Supersaturation Modulate In Vitro Fenofibrate Solubilization in Silica-Lipid Hybrids

Ruba Almasri, Paul Joyce, Hayley B. Schultz, Nicky Thomas, Kristen E. Bremmell and Clive A. Prestidge

1. UniSA Clinical and Health Sciences, University of South Australia, Adelaide 5000, Australia; Ruba.Almasri@mymail.unisa.edu.au (R.A.); Paul.Joyce@unisa.edu.au (P.J.); Hayley.Schultz@unisa.edu.au (H.B.S.); Nicky.Thomas@unisa.edu.au (N.T.); Kristen.Bremmell@unisa.edu.au (K.E.B.)
2. ARC Centre of Excellence in Convergent Bio-Nano Science and Technology, University of South Australia, Adelaide 5000, Australia
* Correspondence: Clive.Prestidge@unisa.edu.au; Tel.: +61-8830-22438

Received: 3 July 2020; Accepted: 20 July 2020; Published: 21 July 2020

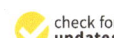

Abstract: The unique nanostructured matrix obtained by silica-lipid hybrids (SLHs) is well known to improve the dissolution, absorption, and bioavailability of poorly water-soluble drugs (PWSDs). The aim of this study was to investigate the impact of: (i) drug load: 3–22.7% w/w, (ii) lipid type: medium-chain triglyceride (Captex 300) and mono and diester of caprylic acid (Capmul PG8), and (iii) silica nanostructure: spray dried fumed silica (FS) and mesoporous silica (MPS), on the in vitro dissolution, solubilization, and solid-state stability of the model drug fenofibrate (FEN). Greater FEN crystallinity was detected at higher drug loads and within the MPS formulations. Furthermore, an increased rate and extent of dissolution was achieved by FS formulations when compared to crystalline FEN (5–10-fold), a commercial product; APO-fenofibrate (2.4–4-fold) and corresponding MPS formulations (2–4-fold). Precipitation of FEN during in vitro lipolysis restricted data interpretation, however a synergistic effect between MPS and Captex 300 in enhancing FEN aqueous solubilization was attained. It was concluded that a balance between in vitro performance and drug loading is key, and the optimum drug load was determined to be between 7–16% w/w, which corresponds to (200–400% equilibrium solubility in lipid S_{eq}). This study provides valuable insight into the impact of key characteristics of SLHs, in constructing optimized solid-state lipid-based formulations for the oral delivery of PWSDs.

Keywords: supersaturation; silica-lipid hybrid; spray drying; lipolysis; lipid-based formulation; fenofibrate; mesoporous silica; oral drug delivery

1. Introduction

Due to the staggering number of new drug entities with poor physicochemical properties under development, formulation scientists are challenged to design innovative formulations that successfully overcome these molecules' inherent slow dissolution and poor oral absorption [1]. Amongst novel drug delivery systems, lipid-based formulations (LBFs) present opportunities for successfully delivering poorly water-soluble drugs (PWSDs), owing to their ability to mimic the postprandial effect [2]. Upon ingestion, the lipid content within these formulations triggers the release of digestive pancreatic and gallbladder enzymes and a sequence of digestive processes that result in the dynamic formation of a range of colloidal systems (e.g., micelles) [3,4]. This naturally occurring phenomenon maintains the drug in the solubilized state and creates a concentration gradient that acts as a driving force for absorption, thus reducing the food effect for lipophilic drugs. Furthermore, such formulations deliver the drug to the gastrointestinal tract (GIT) in a pre-solubilized form, eliminating the requirement for dissolution as a rate limiting step for absorption [5]. As such, LBFs present promising benefits for poorly water-soluble, highly permeable, BCS (Biopharmaceutics Classification System) class II drugs [6,7].

Numerous studies have shown that, by manipulating the lipids and excipients used, enhancements in permeability, intestinal solubilization and absorption through the lymphatic system can be achieved, along with benefits in bypassing first-pass metabolism, inhibition of efflux transporters, and prevention of pre-systemic metabolism [4,8,9]. Although considerable research has been devoted to examining and refining formulation approaches to enhance the biopharmaceutical performance of LBFs, the number of successful products on the market are limited [5]. This is mainly due to their low stability, tendency to recrystallize and precipitate in vivo and costly manufacturing processes. In addition, several studies have reported poor correlation between in vitro and in vivo results [10,11].

Solidification represents an effective solution to overcome challenges associated with liquid LBFs, while optimizing the advantages related to lipids [6,12,13]. Solid-state LBFs are fabricated by adsorbing the liquid-state LBFs onto a solid carrier material. This can be achieved using various solid carriers (silica and silicate materials, polysaccharide, polymeric, and protein) and/or by adapting different techniques, including spray drying, lyophilization, rotary evaporation, melt extrusion, and melt granulation [14–16]. Silica-based adsorbents are commonly used as solid carriers for LBFs due to their biocompatibility, inert nature and highly porous structure [17,18], which provides increased surface area for adsorption of liquid lipids [19,20]. Furthermore, the high degree of versatility afforded by silica materials introduces the ability to manipulate the biopharmaceutical performance of silica lipid hybrids (SLHs) through changes in particle size, nanostructure and porosity [17,21,22]. For example, several studies have verified the ability to control both the rate and extent of lipid digestion, and the subsequent rate of drug release and absorption in SLHs through changes in nanostructure and surface chemistry [23–26]. Therefore, careful examination of the physiochemical properties of the silica carrier and composition should be considered during the fabrication of solid-state LBFs in order to seize their full therapeutic potential.

For most LBFs, typical drug loads are ≤5% w/w [24,27]. The drug loads are further reduced when LBFs are solidified by adsorption onto a solid carrier [16,19], such as for SLH, which in turn limits their potential commercial application to low dose, highly potent drugs. Thus, despite their success in stabilizing precursor liquid LBFs and significantly enhancing dissolution and solubilization of model drugs, low drug loading levels limit the commercial translation of SLHs. In addition to understanding the structure-activity relationships between porous silica properties and drug solubilization, recent attention has been afforded to improving the drug loading within SLHs through a supersaturation approach, which has led to the creation of supersaturated SLHs (super-SLH) [28–31].

Super-SLH, defined as drug dissolved in lipid above its equilibrium solubility (S_{eq}) at room temperature, were fabricated by dissolving quantities of drug in a lipid using heat, followed by solidification employing preformed mesoporous silica microparticles, which upon cooling, generated supersaturated powders [30]. The lipid-drug solution was imbibed into the nanopores of the silica and/or stabilized on the surface of the silica particles to maintain the drug in a molecular state [31]. The method has demonstrated high drug loading, increased stability of the supersaturated drug, enhanced dissolution, and improved oral bioavailability of the PWSDs ibuprofen (IBU) [29,30] and abiraterone acetate (AbA) [28,31]. However, there is a fine balance between increasing the drug loading/supersaturation level and achieving enhanced biopharmaceutical performance, as the drug can recrystallize in the solid state, resulting in reduced dissolution. For IBU super-SLH, the ideal supersaturation level was 227% S_{eq}, which achieved a 2.2-fold enhancement in oral bioavailability in Sprague-Dawley rats when compared to the commercial product, Nurofen [30]. In contrast, for AbA super-SLH, despite the supersaturated formulations significantly enhancing in vitro solubilization, only the unsaturated SLH (at 90% S_{eq}) achieved an oral bioavailability that exceeded the commercial product Zytiga (1.4-fold) in Sprague-Dawley rats [28]. Furthermore, when AbA super-SLH contained different lipids (Capmul PG8 or Capmul MCM), there were significant differences between their loading and in vitro and in vivo performances.

The published literature on super-SLH highlights that their performance is highly drug- and lipid-dependent, with only two drugs and two lipids being investigated thus far. Furthermore, only one type of silica has been applied to super-SLH. Therefore, there is significant opportunity for further investigation into the influence of these excipients to develop improved super-SLH formulations and exploit their full potential. On this basis, the focus of this study was to investigate the impact of (i) porous silica nanostructure, (ii) lipid type, and (iii) drug loading on the in vitro solubilization, dissolution, and solid-state stability of super-SLH [26]. To investigate silica nanostructure, preformed mesoporous silica microparticles were compared to a bottom-up approach to prepare porous silica microparticles that could be loaded with liquid lipid through spray drying fumed silica (FS). The lipids Capmul PG8 (monoester of caprylic acid) and Captex 300 (medium chain triglyceride) were investigated, with drug loads corresponding to 80, 200, 400, and 600% S_{eq}. Fenofibrate (FEN), an antilipemic agent and BCS class II compound, was selected as the model drug to be applied to super-SLH for this study. It was chosen due to its poor water solubility (<3 µg/mL at 37 °C), its extensive use as a model drug, well documented application to LBFs, and as the first neutral compound to be applied to super-SLH [27–31]. Furthermore, this study marks the first application of FS as a solid carrier that can be loaded with supersaturated liquid lipid in super-SLH. The key findings of this study provide a valuable insight into the role of porous silica nanostructure, lipid type, and drug loading, for constructing optimized solid-state LBFs for the oral delivery of PWSDs.

2. Materials and Methods

2.1. Materials

Fenofibrate (FEN) (≥99%, powder) was purchased from Sigma-Aldrich (Castle Hill, Australia). Commercially available standard APO-fenofibrate tablets (Apotex, Macquarie Park, Australia) were purchased from local suppliers and crushed into a powder before use. The lipids, Capmul PG8, Captex 300 and Capmul MCM, were sourced from Abitec (Columbus, OH, USA). Fumed hydrophilic silica nanoparticles (Aerosil 300 Pharma), with a surface area of 300 ± 30 m^2/g were donated by Evonik (Melbourne, Australia). Mesoporous silica microparticles (Parteck SLC 500), with a particle size of 9–11 µm and pore size of 6 nm, and sodium lauryl sulfate (SLS) (used to prepare dissolution medium) were donated and purchased from Merck (Melbourne, Australia), respectively. Fasted state simulated intestinal fluid/fed state simulated intestinal fluid/fasted state simulated gastric fluid (FaSSIF/FeSSIF/FaSSGF) biorelevant powder, to prepare biorelevant media for gastrointestinal lipolysis, was obtained from Biorelevant (Biorelevant.com, London, UK). Porcine pancreatin extract was supplied by MP Biomedicals (Seven Hills, Australia). 4-bromophenylboronic acid (4-BBA) and lipase from *Candida antarctica* were purchased from Sigma-Aldrich (Castle Hill, Australia). HPLC-grade methanol was purchased from local suppliers. High purity Milli Q water (Merck Millipore, Bayswater, Australia) was used throughout the study.

2.2. HPLC Assay for Fenofibrate Quantification

Fenofibrate was analyzed using a Shimadzu high-performance liquid chromatograph (HPLC) system (Kyoto, Japan) equipped with a Phenomenex Kinetex® 2.6 µm PS C18 column (250 × 4.6 mm) maintained at 40 °C. The mobile phase contained 90% methanol and 10% water and was eluted at a flow rate of 0.7 mL/min. The effluents were analyzed by a UV detector at 288 nm, and the retention time for FEN was approximately 5.8 min. The concentration of FEN in each sample was determined using calibration curves generated over the range of 0.05–10 µg/mL with R^2 values > 0.999.

2.3. Lipid Solubility Studies

The equilibrium solubility (S_{eq}) of FEN in Capmul PG8, Captex 300, and Capmul MCM was determined in triplicate at 25, 40, and 60 °C. An excess of FEN was added to centrifuge tubes containing approximately 0.5 g lipid. The tubes were vortex mixed for 10–20 s to aid drug dissolution and placed on a rotator in an oven at the required temperature. After 24 h, samples were centrifuged at 44,800 rcf for 30 min at the required temperature to precipitate any undissolved drug. Methanol was used to extract the dissolved drug from the supernatant and was appropriately diluted with mobile phase prior to HPLC analysis. Samples were vortexed and returned to the rotator in the oven and analyzed every 24 h until equilibrium solubility was reached. This was indicated by <10% change in consecutive solubility measurements.

Due to a temperature limit on the centrifuge, centrifugation was not possible at 60 °C. Therefore, samples were left in the oven to allow for undissolved drug to settle as a pellet, and aliquots were carefully taken from supernatant. This method was previously validated [29], and an acceptable standard deviation was attained.

2.4. Fabrication of FEN Loaded Super-SLH

2.4.1. Preparation of Spray Dried Microparticles

In order to obtain porous silica microparticles, a suspension of fumed silica nanoparticles (5% *w/w*) was sonicated overnight to allow effective hydration and separation of the silica nanoparticles prior to spray drying with a Büchi Mini Spray Dryer B290 apparatus (Büchi, Flawil, Switzerland). Spray drying was performed under the following conditions: inlet temperature 160 °C, outlet temperature 90 °C, aspirator setting 100, pump set at 20%, and product flow rate 6 mL/min. Fumed silica nanoparticles were successfully spray dried to form porous silica microparticles (80% yield).

2.4.2. Preparation of Super-SLH

This method was adapted from the previously established methods [29,30]. FEN was weighed into glass vials with 0.5 g of lipid to achieve concentrations equivalent to 80, 200, 400, and 600% S_{eq} at room temperature. The glass vials were placed in the oven at 60 °C for approximately 10–30 min with intermittent shaking to dissolve the drug. Half a gram of silica microparticles (either FS or MPS) was added into the glass vial and immediately physically mixed to allow the mixture to form a white free flowing powder and allowed to cool. A ratio of 1:1 *w/w* silica: lipid was maintained throughout the study. Formulations were freshly prepared and were tested within 24 h.

2.5. Physicochemical Characterization

2.5.1. Solid-State Characterization

Crystallinity of encapsulated FEN was investigated using X-ray powder diffraction (XRPD) and differential scanning calorimetry (DSC) (TA instrument, Rydalmere, Australia). XRPD data was obtained using a Malvern Panalytical Empyrean XRPD (Malvern, UK). Samples were scanned between 5° and 90° (2θ) at a rate of 5 s/point and step size of 0.02°. For DSC analysis, samples were accurately weighed into aluminum pans and hermetically sealed with an aluminum lids and heated at a rate of 10 °C/min over a temperature range of 25–120 °C. XRPD and DSC measurements were taken 1 day after formulations were fabricated.

2.5.2. Scanning Electron Microscopy (SEM)

The surface morphology of SLH was examined using scanning electron microscopy (SEM) (Zeiss Merlin, Oberkochen, Germany). Samples were applied to double-faced adhesive carbon tape and sputter coated with 10 nm platinum prior to imaging at an accelerating voltage of 1 kV.

2.5.3. Confocal Laser Scanning Microscopy

A Zeiss Elyra PS-1 microscope (Jena, Germany) was used to perform confocal laser scanning microscopy on blank SLH. Silica microparticles were labeled with rhodamine B and lipids were labeled with coumarin 6. Confocal images were captured at the emission wavelength of 488 nm for coumarin 6 (excitation wavelength 497 nm) and 625 nm for rhodamine B (excitation wavelength 540 nm).

2.5.4. Drug Load Determination

FEN content was determined by solvent extraction. Approximately 10 mg of formulation was weighed into a glass vial, followed by the addition of 10 mL of methanol. Vials were sonicated for 45 min to extract FEN. Aliquots were centrifuged (44,800 rcf for 20 min) to sediment undissolved solids. Then, the supernatants were appropriately diluted and analyzed using HPLC.

2.6. Aqeous Media Solubility Studies

The equilibrium solubility of FEN in 0.0125 M SLS, FaSSGF, and FaSSIF was determined by the addition of excess FEN to 1 mL of media in 1.5 mL centrifuge tubes. The tubes were vortexed for 10–20 s to aid drug dissolution and placed on a rotator in the oven at 37 °C. After 48 h, samples were centrifuged at 44,800 rcf for 30 min at 37 °C to precipitate any undissolved drug. Methanol was used to extract dissolved drug from the supernatant, prior to dilution with mobile phase and quantification of FEN content by HPLC.

2.7. In Vitro Dissolution Studies

FEN dissolution studies were performed to compare the dissolution kinetics of various SLH formulations, crystalline FEN and APO-fenofibrate. The studies were performed in 0.0125 M SLS solution, as FEN is a neutral drug and practically insoluble in aqueous media [32]. However, using SLS significantly enhances its solubility, and its use as a dissolution media has been evaluated for multiple FEN-containing formulations in order to achieve sink conditions [33–36]. Dissolution was performed using a Vankel USP II apparatus (Agilent Technologies, Santa Clara, CA, USA), 450 mL of media was maintained at 37 °C and rotating at 50 rpm. An equivalent of 10 mg of FEN of formulation was added to the dissolution vessel. Three-milliliter aliquots were removed at 1, 5, 10, 15, 30, 45, 60, and 90 min, replaced by fresh media, and filtered using 0.45 µm syringe filter prior to appropriate dilution with mobile phase and analysis with HPLC.

2.8. In Vitro Gastrointestinal Lipolysis Studies

For the present study, a combined gastrointestinal (GI) in vitro lipolysis model adapted from [37] was employed to test solubilization of FEN under digesting conditions. FaSSIF/FeSSIF/FaSSGF powder was used to prepare gastric (FaSSGF) and intestinal (FaSSIF) media, according to manufacturer's protocol (biorelevant.com, London, UK). Media were freshly prepared before each experiment and used within 48 h, according to manufacturer's recommendations.

2.8.1. Preparation of Simulated Gastric Lipolysis Media

FaSSGF buffer (pH 1.6 ± 0.01) was prepared by dissolving 2.00 g NaCl in 1 L Milli Q water and adjusting the pH with 0.2 M HCl, prior to the addition of 0.06 g biorelevant powder to prepare biorelevant FaSSGF.

2.8.2. Preparation of Simulated Intestinal Lipolysis Media

FaSSIF was prepared by dissolving 2.240 g FaSSIF/FeSSIF/FaSSGF powder in 1L pH 6.5 ± 0.01 buffer (0.42 g NaOH, 3.4 g NaH_2PO_4, 6.2 g NaCl, 1L MilliQ). NaOH (1 M) and HCl (1 M) were used to adjust the pH of the intestinal buffer. Following preparation and before use, intestinal lipolysis media was left standing for 2 h to allow equilibrium of buffer excipients and micelles formation. On the day of the experimental procedure, pancreatin extracts were prepared by stirring 2 g of pancreatin powder in 10 mL of intestinal lipolysis buffer (pH 6.5) for 15 min, followed by centrifugation (2268 rcf, 20 min, 4 °C). The supernatant was collected in a glass vial and kept refrigerated.

2.8.3. Gastrointestinal Digestion Experimental Procedure

Lipid digestion kinetics were monitored for a total of 90 min (30 min gastric step followed by 60 min intestinal step). A Metrohm 902 Titrando pH-stat titration apparatus equipped with a Dosino 800 dosing apparatus (Herisau, Switzerland) was used for the studies. The experimental procedure was initiated with the addition of an amount of formulation corresponding to 3 mg of FEN into a temperature-controlled reaction vessel containing 10 mL of freshly prepared FaSSGF (37 °C, pH 1.6). Gastric lipolysis was carried out for 30 min and was initiated by the addition of 100 µL *Candida* lipase (600 tributyrin units lipase activity). Following gastric lipolysis, 18 mL of FaSSIF media was added (pH 6.5) to the reaction vessel, and the pH was automatically adjusted by the pH-stat apparatus to maintain pH at 6.5 ± 0.01. Following a pH-equilibration time of 3–5 min, intestinal lipolysis was initiated by the addition of 2 mL freshly prepared pancreatin extract, bringing the total volume to 30 mL. Fatty acids (FA) produced as a result of digestion were instantly titrated with 0.6 M NaOH to maintain a constant pH of 6.50 ± 0.01. The cumulative volume of NaOH was converted to the number of moles of NaOH consumed, which in turn corresponded to the number of moles of FA released. Data obtained from NaOH titration were used to compare the rate and extent of lipid digestion for the different formulations. It is important to note that NaOH titration during the gastric step does not reflect extent of lipolysis since the FA produced are protonated at pH 1.6 and could therefore not be recorded during gastric lipolysis [37].

2.8.4. Drug Phase Partitioning During In Vitro Lipolysis

The solubilization of FEN in the aqueous phase during in vitro gastrointestinal lipolysis was measured. Aliquots (1 mL) were withdrawn at 1, 15, and 30 min (gastric phase) and 1, 5, 10, 15, 30, 45, and 60 min (intestinal phase) and transferred into 1.5 mL centrifuge tubes prefilled with 10 µL of 4-BBA (0.5 M in methanol) as a lipase inhibitor. Samples were centrifuged (32,760 rcf, 10 min, 25 °C) to separate the aqueous phase, containing solubilized FEN, and precipitated pellet. The supernatant was appropriately diluted prior to analysis by HPLC. The supernatant was discarded to leave the pellet and was re-dispersed through addition of 1 mL methanol, vortex mixed for 30 s, followed by sonication for 45 min. The tube was centrifuged (32,760 rcf, 10 min, 25 °C), and the supernatant was diluted and analyzed by HPLC.

2.9. Statistical Analysis

All statistical analyses of experimental data were performed using GraphPad Prism Version 8.0. Statistically significant differences were determined by one-way ANOVA followed by Tukey's post-test for multiple comparisons. Values are reported as the mean ± standard deviation (SD), and the data were considered statistically significant when $p < 0.05$.

3. Results

3.1. Influence of Temperature on FEN Solubility in Lipids

In order to select the optimum lipids for supersaturating FEN, solubility studies were performed at 25, 40, and 60 °C in Capmul PG8 (PG8), Captex 300 (C300) and Capmul MCM (MCM). It was evident that FEN solubility in all lipids increased considerably with temperature, achieving 4.4- to 7.7-fold greater FEN solubility at 60 °C compared to 25 °C (Figure 1). Regardless of temperature, FEN displayed greatest solubility in PG8, achieving a solubility of 98 ± 3.5 mg/g at 25 °C and 516 ± 29.5 mg/g at 60 °C. PG8 and C300 were chosen for the fabrication of FEN-loaded SLH due to both lipids exerting the highest drug loading at 60 °C. MCM was excluded due to its inferior drug loading capacity.

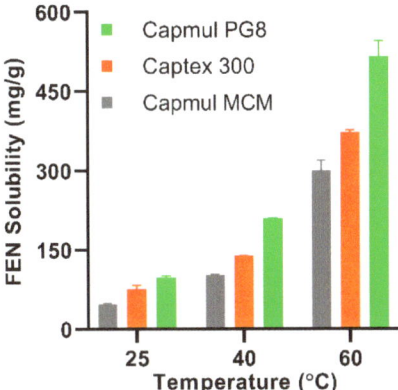

Figure 1. The temperature-dependent solubility of fenofibrate (FEN) in Capmul MCM (grey bars), Captex 300 (orange bars), and Capmul PG8 (green bars). Values represent mean ± SD, $n = 3$.

3.2. Super-SLH Preparation and Characterization

FEN-loaded SLH were fabricated with varying (i) lipid types, (ii) silica types, and (iii) drug loads. The compositions and drug loads of the fabricated formulations are summarized in Table 1. Subsequently, fabricated SLH formulations were identified and categorized according to type of lipid used to dissolve FEN (PG8 or C300), type of silica microparticles used to stabilize precursor liquid lipid (FS or MPS), and drug load based on % S_{eq} ranging from 80% S_{eq} (unsaturated) to 600% S_{eq} (highly supersaturated). Furthermore, liquid lipid formulations were prepared at 80% S_{eq} in both lipids, in order to compare the influence of solidification on drug release and solubilization. Drug loads ranging from 3.8 to 22.7% w/w were attained for PG8-containing formulations and 3 to 18.8 % w/w for C300-containing formulations. Furthermore, three formulations were randomly selected to evaluate the homogeneity of FEN throughout the formulation and to assess the drug loading efficiency (Table S1). All tested formulations displayed high drug loading efficiency of at least 94 ± 2.8% w/w with small standard deviation.

Table 1. The calculated composition of the fabricated FEN-loaded liquid and silica-lipid hybrid (SLH) formulations.

Lipid Type	Silica Type	Formulation Name	Saturation Level (% S_{eq})	Drug Load (% w/w)	Lipid Load (% w/w)	Silica Load (% w/w)
Capmul PG8	-	80% Liquid PG8 *	80	7.3	92.7	-
	FS	80% FS PG8	80	3.8	48.1	48.1
		200% FS PG8	200	8.9	45.5	45.5
		400% FS PG8	400	16.4	41.8	41.8
		600% FS PG8	600	22.7	38.6	38.6
	MPS	80% MPS PG8	80	3.8	48.1	48.1
		200% MPS PG8	200	8.9	45.5	45.5
		400% MPS PG8	400	16.4	41.8	41.8
		600% MPS PG8	600	22.7	38.6	38.6

Table 1. Cont.

Lipid Type	Silica Type	Formulation Name	Saturation Level (% S_{eq})	Drug Load (% w/w)	Lipid Load (% w/w)	Silica Load (% w/w)
Captex 300	-	80% Liquid C300 *	80	5.8	94.2	-
	FS	80% FS C300	80	3	48.5	48.5
		200% FS C300	200	7.1	46.4	46.4
		400% FS C300	400	13.4	43.3	43.3
		600% FS C300	600	18.8	40.6	40.6
	MPS	80% MPS C300	80	3	48.5	48.5
		200% MPS C300	200	7.2	46.4	46.4
		400% MPS C300	400	13.4	43.3	43.3
		600% MPS C300	600	18.8	40.6	40.6

* Liquid formulations do not contain any silica (solid carrier).

3.2.1. Drug Crystallinity

DSC and XRPD were utilized for the qualitative, solid-state characterization of FEN in the SLH formulations. The DSC thermograms of a physical mixture (5% w/w crystalline FEN with FS), crystalline FEN, FS, and MPS formulations are displayed in Figure 2. Crystalline FEN exhibited a sharp endothermic peak at 80 °C, corresponding to its melting point [38], whereas the FS physical mixture exhibited a small endothermic peak (Figure 2A). Furthermore, this thermogram suggests that crystalline FEN could be detected at concentrations ~5% w/w when present within silica particles. Regardless of the silica type or lipid used, endothermic peaks were absent for all 80% and 200% SLH formulations, suggesting that the drug was in a non-crystalline state. However, all other formulations of higher drug loads demonstrated shifted endothermic peaks varying in size and stretching between 45–60 °C. The shifted endothermic peaks for all 400% formulations were smaller than for the 600% formulations, which suggests the presence of higher concentrations of crystalline FEN at higher saturation levels (Figure 2B,C). No apparent difference in DSC thermograms was observed between PG8 or C300 SLH formulations, whether loaded in FS or MPS. Therefore, XRPD patterns were only obtained for SLH formulations containing PG8, since higher drug loads were achieved in comparison to the SLH C300 formulations.

Crystalline FEN demonstrated characteristic XRPD patterns as previously reported (Figure 2D) [39]. For the 5% w/w physical mixture, characteristic crystalline FEN patterns can be observed but differ in intensity between FS and MPS (Figure 2E,F). XRP diffractograms indicate that the method can detect as low as 5% w/w crystalline FEN. In SLH formulations fabricated with FS PG8, no crystalline FEN was detected at drug loads of 80% and 200%. However, at 400% and 600% FS PG8, intense peaks were observed, suggesting the presence of crystalline FEN. These findings correspond with data obtained with DSC analysis. However, all supersaturated MPS PG8 formulations (200, 400, and 600% S_{eq}) displayed characteristic peaks of varying intensities, suggesting the presence of crystalline FEN (Figure 2F), and no crystalline drug was detected with unsaturated 80% P PG8 formulation. It is important to note that some characteristic peaks where absent from XRPD pattern obtained from 200% P PG8, suggesting the presence of a FEN polymorph [38]. For both FS and MPS systems, XRPD patterns obtained from 600% S_{eq} formulations displayed peaks with higher intensities than corresponding 400% S_{eq} formulations, displaying an ~2-fold increased intensity, suggesting the presence of higher amounts of crystalline FEN in SLH prepared at 600% S_{eq}. Furthermore, MPS formulations exhibited peaks with higher relative intensities compared to corresponding FS formulations that were ~1.6-fold higher at

400% and 600% S_{eq}. This was evident when the peak intensities obtained at 22.3° (2θ) were plotted against % S_{eq}, as displayed in Figure S1.

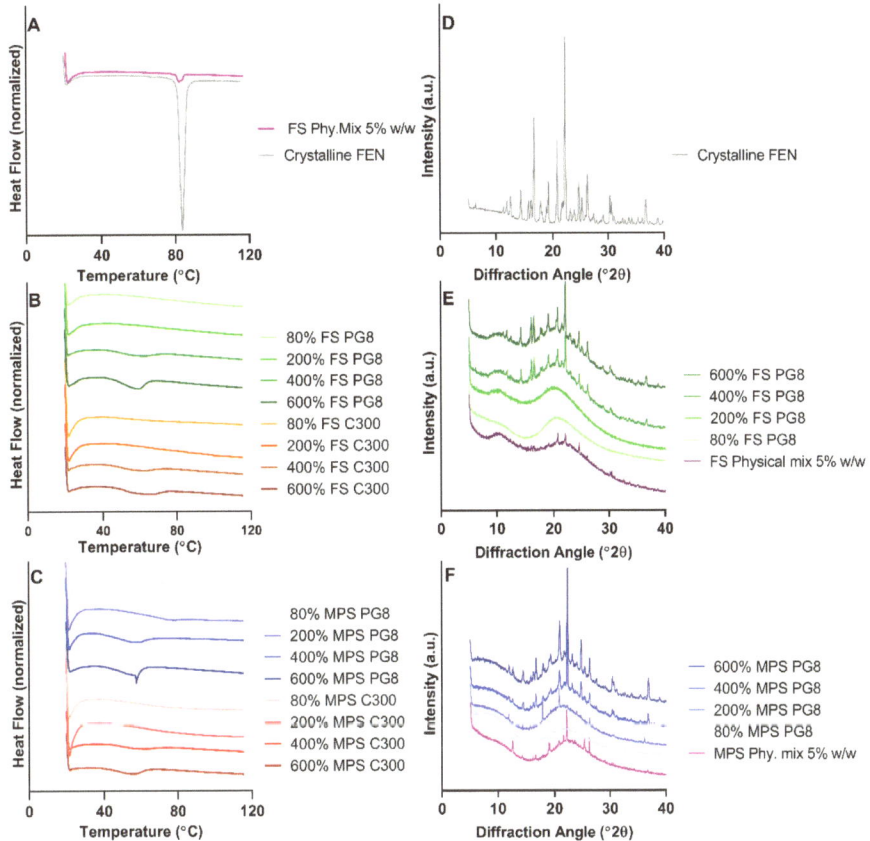

Figure 2. Differential scanning calorimetry (DSC) thermograms of (**A**) crystalline FEN and fumed silica (FS) physical mix 5% *w/w*, (**B**) FEN-loaded FS formulations and (**C**) FEN-loaded mesoporous silica (MPS) formulations. The X-ray powder diffraction (XRPD) diffractograms of (**D**) crystalline FEN, (**E**) FS PG8 formulations and (**F**) MPS PG8 formulations.

3.2.2. Surface Morphology and Lipid Distribution

Surface morphology, internal structure, and lipid distribution within fabricated SLH formulations were examined using SEM and confocal laser scanning micriscopy (Figures 3 and 4). Blank FS particles formed semi-spherical shapes of varying particle sizes with distinct concave-like structures (Figure 3A). No difference in appearance was observed between blank FS and 80% FS PG8 (Figure 3B). However, at 200% saturation level, regardless of the lipid used, FS particles appeared to form clusters and large aggregates (Figure 3C). In contrast, MPS appeared as angular structures and formed aggregates irrespective of the lipid used or FEN saturation level (Figure 3E,F). No difference in appearance was observed between SLH prepared with either lipid types; therefore, only SEM images of SLH prepared with PG8 are shown.

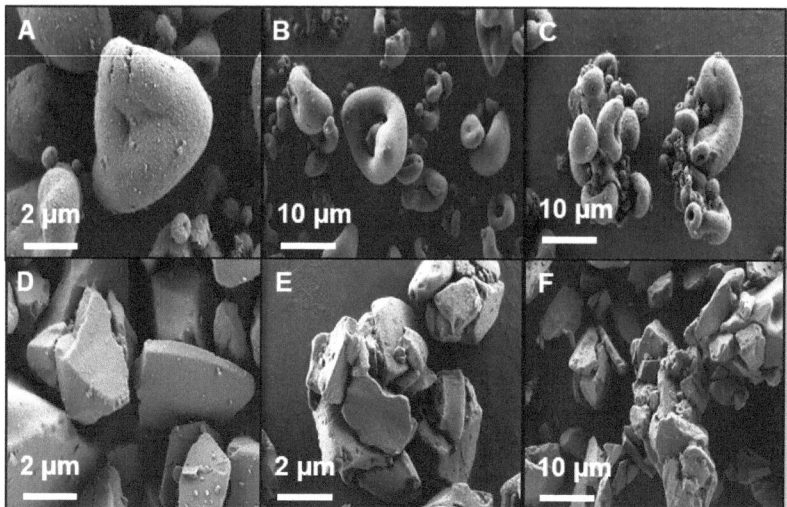

Figure 3. SEM images of (**A**) blank FS, (**B**) 80% FS PG8, (**C**) 200% FS PG8, (**D**) blank MPS, (**E**) 80% MPS PG8, and (**F**) 200% MPS PG8.

Confocal imaging revealed that the lipid distribution within the silica microparticles was dependent on the type of silica and lipid used. More lipid was observed within the internal structure of FS particles than MPS, evidenced by the intensity of the fluorescently labeled lipid within the pores of the silica microparticles (Figure 4). However, it was evident that PG8 was less prone to imbibe into the porous matrix compared to C300, with lipid droplets tending to reside between inter-particle cavities, irrespective of the silica type. In contrast, C300 homogeneously distributed throughout the internal structure, with the presence of additional lipid droplets between the particles.

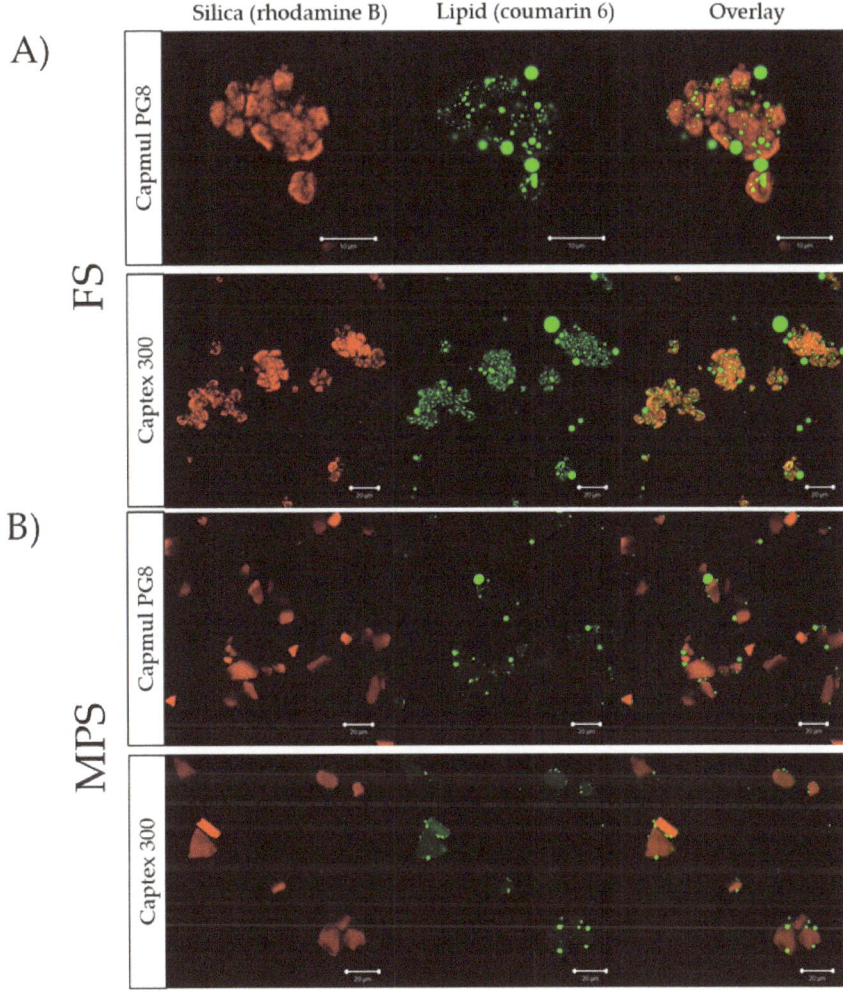

Figure 4. Confocal images of: (**A**) SLH prepared with FS and (**B**) SLH prepared with MPS. Rhodamine B (red) was used to label silica, and coumarin 6 (green) was used to label lipid.

3.3. In Vitro Dissolution

The dissolution performance of various SLH prepared with FS and MPS, APO-fenofibrate, and crystalline FEN is reported in Figure 5. The equilibrium solubility of FEN in 0.0125 M SLS (0.36%) was 128 ± 0.01 µg/mL; thus, the study was performed under sink conditions. Crystalline FEN and APO-fenofibrate displayed 7.8% and 25.1% solubilization after 90 min, respectively. At 80% saturation level, all SLH formulations, irrespective of type of silica or lipid, exhibited significantly enhanced FEN dissolution, with FS formulations achieving 70.9–98.1% after 90 min and displaying slightly improved performance compared to MPS formulations ($p > 0.05$). FEN dissolution from FS formulations at 80% S_{eq} corresponded to 8- to 10-fold and 2.6- to 3.2-fold increase in dissolution compared to crystalline FEN and APO-fenofibrate, respectively ($p < 0.05$). However, FEN dissolution from supersaturated SLH formulations was dependent on type of lipid and silica utilized. FS PG8 formulations at all saturation levels (80%, 200%, 400%, 600% S_{eq}) achieved a comparable extent of FEN dissolution of ~80% after

90 min, despite 600% FS PG8 displaying slower release kinetics ($p > 0.05$) (Figure 5B). In contrast, FEN dissolution was significantly hindered in supersaturated MPS PG8 formulations, with 200% MPS PG8 achieving 43.9% FEN dissolution after 90 min, and was further reduced for 400% and 600% S_{eq} with no significant difference compared to crystalline FEN and APO-fenofibrate ($p > 0.05$).

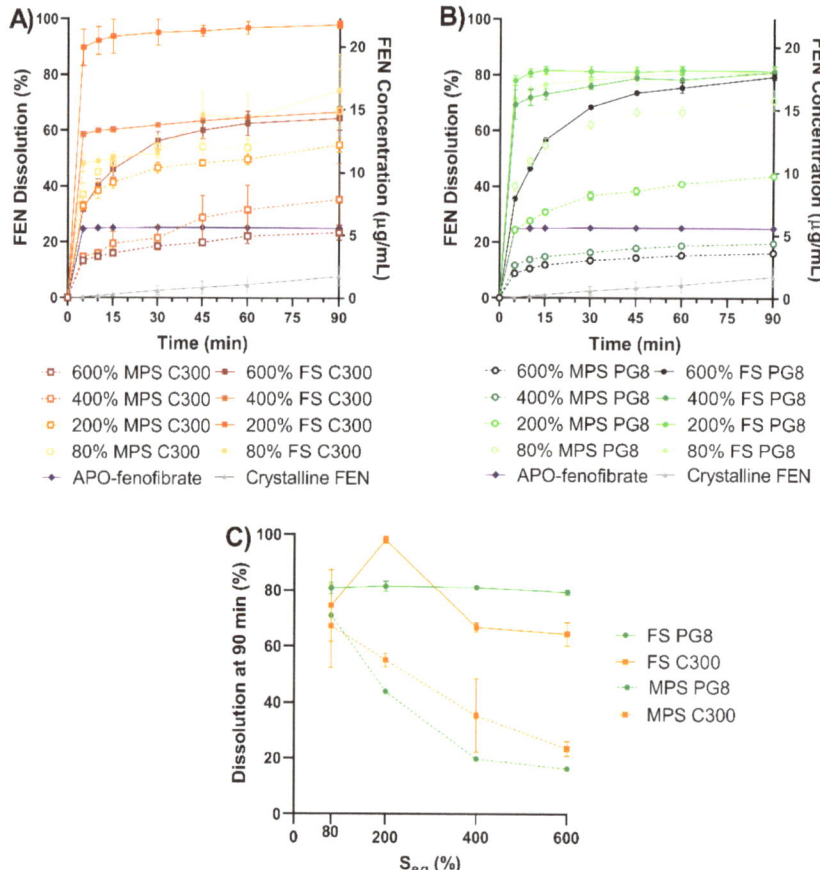

Figure 5. The in vitro dissolution profiles of crystalline FEN, APO-fenofibrate and FEN-loaded SLH formulations (at different saturation levels) in 0.0125 M SLS, dosed at 10 mg of FEN over 90 min at sink conditions. (mean ± SD, $n = 3$). (**A**) SLH C300 formulations, (**B**) SLH PG8 formulations, and (**C**) FEN % dissolution at 90 min vs % S_{eq}.

The 200% FS C300 formulation achieved the highest FEN dissolution of 98.1%, which corresponds to approximately 4- and 14-fold increased dissolution compared to APO-fenofibrate and crystalline FEN, respectively ($p < 0.05$). However, this was not statistically significant when compared to 200% FS PG8 ($p > 0.05$). Only 66.8% and 64.6% FEN dissolution was observed from 400% and 600% S_{eq} for FS C300 formulations, respectively. When MPS was utilized to solidify supersaturated C300 LBFs, a similar pattern was observed to supersaturated MPS PG8 formulations (Figure 5C), where the dissolution was significantly reduced with increased supersaturation. 200% MPS C300 achieved 55.2% FEN dissolution, whereas FEN dissolution of only 35.4% and 23.5% was attained from 400% and 600% MPS C300 formulations, respectively, with no significant difference compared to crystalline FEN and APO-fenofibrate ($p > 0.05$). The influence of silica type and saturation level on FEN dissolution was evident when FEN dissolution at 90 min was plotted against saturation level (S_{eq}). As displayed in Figure 5C, SLH prepared with FS, irrespective of type of lipid or % S_{eq}, achieved similar extent of dissolution ($p > 0.05$). In contrast, MPS stabilized SLH formulations displayed significant linear reduction in FEN dissolution with an increase in % S_{eq}. The decrease in performance was more profound for MPS PG8 formulations ($R^2 = 0.86$) than MPS C300 formulations ($R^2 = 0.80$); however, it was not statistically significant ($p > 0.05$).

3.4. In Vitro Lipolysis and Aqueous Solubilization

3.4.1. Aqueous Solubilization

The partitioning of FEN between the aqueous phase and the pellet was measured over 90 min during two-phase gastrointestinal lipolysis. The total percentage of FEN recovered ranged between 70 to 98% for all formulations (Figures S2 and S3). Difficulty in isolating the pellet and possible pellet loss during the separation of the aqueous phase and pellet have contributed to having less than 100% total recovered FEN. This issue has been previously reported and was attributed to either drug loss during the separation process or inability to analyze drug retained in the undigested oil phase [28].

The aqueous concentration-time profiles of solubilized FEN during in vitro gastrointestinal lipolysis are displayed in Figure 6A,B. Crystalline FEN displayed negligible solubilization during the gastric phase, while achieving only 3.5% solubilization after complete intestinal lipolysis. For APO-fenofibrate, once re-dispersed in simulated intestinal digesting media, 5% of total FEN was immediately solubilized with no further changes in solubilization over the entirety of the lipolysis period. The characteristic precipitation of FEN from LBFs caused difficulties in data interpretation and distinguishing enabling formulations. However, the extent and occurrence of FEN precipitation was influenced by the silica nanostructure, type of lipid and drug load evident in patterns observed from the aqueous solubilization-time profiles and area under the intestinal solubilization-time curve (AUC) reported in Figure 6. It is important to note that SLH formulations prepared at 400% and 600% S_{eq} did not improve FEN dissolution (Figure 5); therefore, these formulations were not pursued further in aqueous solubilization studies.

When comparing solidified formulations to 80% liquid lipid, enhanced performance was observed with 80% liquid PG8 during the gastric step, achieving the highest FEN solubilization of 25%, after 30 min ($p < 0.05$). Despite FEN precipitation during the intestinal phase between 1–5 min, FEN solubilization gradually increased to reach 18%, after 90 min, which was significantly higher than all SLH PG8 formulations ($p < 0.05$). However, 80% liquid C300 formulation displayed an enhanced FEN aqueous solubilization profile during the intestinal phase compared to corresponding solidified 80% FS C300 but lower performance than corresponding 80% MPS C300 ($p < 0.05$) (Figure 6A,C).

For FEN solubilization from SLH formulations prepared at 80% S_{eq}, FEN precipitation was triggered by the transition into the intestinal phase at time points ranging between 1–5 min and was followed by a period of slightly enhanced solubilization prior to another decrease in solubilization after 15 min. During the gastric step, 80% FS PG8, 80% MPS PG8, 80% FS C300, and 80% MPS C300 formulations displayed enhanced FEN solubilization of 15%, 16%, 19%, and 12.4%, after 30 min, respectively ($p > 0.05$). This corresponds to 3.5- to 5-fold and 3- to 3.7-fold significantly enhanced solubilization compared to crystalline FEN and APO-fenofibrate, respectively ($p < 0.05$) (Figure 6A,B). Transition into the intestinal phase triggered FEN precipitation where the percentage FEN solubilized decreased to 13% and 6.7% from 80% MPS PG8 and 80% MPS C300, respectively. However, a more dramatic drop in FEN solubilization to 9% and 5.9% was observed from 80% FS PG8 and 80% FS C300 formulations, respectively, at 1 min of the intestinal phase. Furthermore, 80% MPS C300 was able to gradually enhance FEN solubilization and prevent its precipitation, achieving 16% FEN solubilization, after 90 min which was significantly greater than FEN solubilization achieved by corresponding 80% FS C300 formulation ($p < 0.05$).

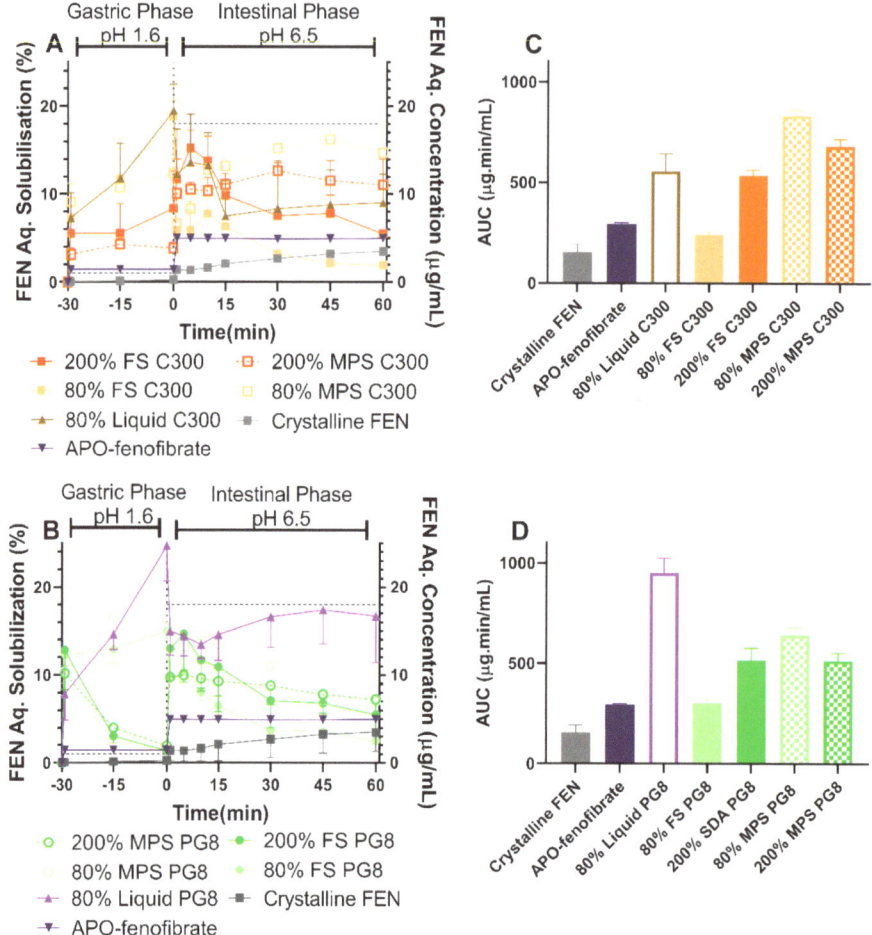

Figure 6. FEN aqueous concentration-time profiles from crystalline FEN, APO-fenofibrate, and FEN-loaded SLH formulations, in fasted state simulated gastric fluid (FaSSGF) (30 min) and fed state simulated intestinal fluid (FaSSIF) (60 min) under digesting conditions, dosed at 3 mg of FEN (mean ± SD, n = 3). (**A**) SLH C300 formulations and (**B**) SLH PG8 formulations. Dotted line represents the FEN S_{eq} in biorelevant media. The area under the curve (AUC) of FEN aqueous solubilization-time profile measured during the intestinal phase from (**C**) crystalline FEN, APO-fenofibrate, and SLH C300 formulations and (**D**) crystalline FEN, APO-fenofibrate, and SLH PG8 formulations.

In contrast, FEN solubilization behavior from super-SLH (200% S_{eq}) was dependent on the type of lipid utilized, where a decrease in FEN solubilization was attained in the gastric phase for 200% FS PG8 and 200% MPS PG8 followed by enhanced solubilization in the intestinal phase achieving 15% and 10% solubilization, respectively (Figure 6C). FEN solubilization was maintained at 4–5% during the gastric phase by 200% FS C300 and 200% MPS C300 formulations followed by enhanced FEN solubilization in the intestinal phase, achieving 15.3% and 10.4%, after 5 min, respectively, prior to FEN precipitation by only 200% FS C300, at 15 min, dropping FEN solubilization to less than 10%. In contrast, FEN solubilization from 200% MPS C300 gradually increased during the intestinal phase achieving 12.7%, after 90 min. This corresponds to 3.6- and 2-fold enhanced solubilization compared to crystalline FEN and APO-fenofibrate, respectively.

All SLH formulations achieved FEN solubilization above FEN equilibrium solubility in FaSSGF (1.1 ± 0.4 μg/mL) during the gastric phase and below its equilibrium solubility in FaSSIF during the intestinal phase (18.1 ± 0.8 μg/mL). Regardless of lipid type, a pattern of enhanced FEN solubilization with increased drug load in FS formulations was clearly evident in data obtained from AUC of FEN solubilization-time profile during the intestinal phase (Figure 6C,D), whereas a decrease in performance with supersaturation was observed for MPS formulations. It was evident that 80% MPS C300 improved the aqueous solubilization of FEN when compared to the 80% liquid C300. In contrast, for PG8 formulations, the presence of both silica types reduced FEN aqueous solubilization when compared to 80% liquid PG8.

3.4.2. Lipid Digestion

The lipid digestion profiles during the intestinal phase of the gastrointestinal lipolysis of all investigated LBF are displayed in Figure 7. Crystalline FEN and APO-fenofibrate did not display any lipid digestion as they did not contain lipid (data not shown). The fabricated formulations differed in their lipid content per dose, as dosing was based on the amount of formulation equivalent to 3 mg of FEN. The amount of lipid dosed ranged from 19.5–48.7 mg (Table S2). The 80% liquid PG8 formulation exhibited the lowest extent of digestion compared to its corresponding solidified SLH formulation (FS or MPS). In contrast, 80% liquid C300 displayed a slow gradual increase in lipolysis over 60 min, but the final extent of lipolysis was lower than corresponding SLH formulations. The amount of digestion decreased as a function of increasing drug load, since all 80% SLH formulations displayed significantly higher extent of digestion when compared to their corresponding 200% formulations, regardless of the type of lipid ($p < 0.05$). FA released from C300 SLH formulations were 5-fold greater than corresponding SLH PG8 formulations, regardless of the type of silica or drug load. At the same saturation level and lipid type, FS facilitated greater extent of lipolysis when compared to corresponding MPS formulations; however, the difference was not statistically significant ($p > 0.05$).

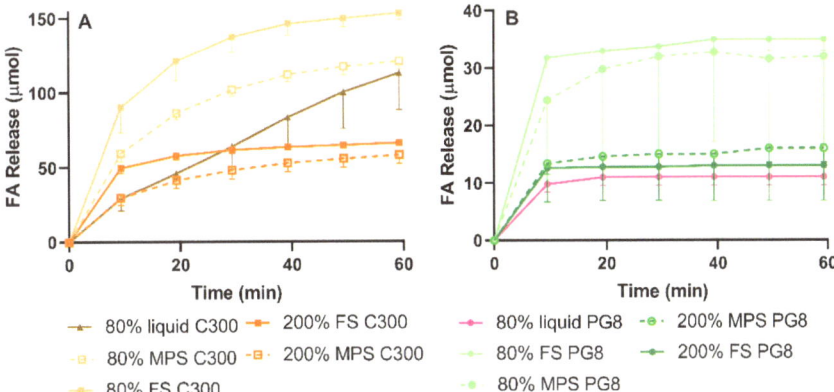

Figure 7. Fatty acid (FA) release-time profile from: (**A**) C300 formulations and (**B**) PG8 formulations, during the intestinal phase of in vitro gastrointestinal (GI) lipolysis in FaSSIF for 60 min, dosed at 3 mg of FEN (mean − SD, $n = 3$).

4. Discussion

Numerous studies have shown that small changes in the nanostructure, surface chemistry and composition of SLH particles can significantly impact lipid digestion dynamics, which in turn influences drug solubilization and release kinetics [23,40]. Therefore, the aim here was to examine the influence of

(i) silica nanostructure, (ii) type of lipid, and (iii) drug load on the in vitro solubilization and solid-state stability of the model drug FEN when incorporated into an SLH formulation.

It is well known that spray drying is amongst the techniques commonly employed to solidify liquid-state LBFs and is recognized to generate highly porous three-dimensional nanostructured matrices with superior physicochemical properties [14]. Here, spray drying was employed to generate porous silica microparticles (FS) from precursor fumed silica nanoparticles suspensions, prior to drug/lipid encapsulation via adapting the simple mixing technique [29]. Supersaturation was achieved by adding drug above its equilibrium saturation level in either of two lipids (PG8 or C300) using heat (≤60 °C) [29]. The generated, thermodynamically unstable, supersaturated liquid lipids were adsorbed into the nanopores or onto the surface of FS or MPS to allow for direct comparison.

4.1. Impact of Drug Loading

All synthesized formulations were found to be homogeneous and achieved high FEN loading efficiency regardless of the type of silica or lipid. Thus, this validates the efficiency of the simple mixing technique in minimizing drug/lipid loss during the fabrication process. The small amount of drug loss (<6% *w/w*) (Table S1) can be attributed to lipid solution of the drug sticking to the vial and not being adsorbed into the nanopores.

Both FS and MPS, silica microparticles were able to maintain FEN in a non-crystalline state at a sub-saturation level of 80% S_{eq}, regardless of the lipid type. DSC and XRPD data confirmed the presence of a greater extent of FEN crystallinity in all 600% S_{eq} formulations, compared to 400% S_{eq} (Figure 2). This correlated with reduced in vitro dissolution performance (Figure 5). Furthermore, FEN dissolution and aqueous solubilization from unsaturated (80% S_{eq}) and super-SLH (200, 400 and 600% S_{eq}) was dependent on the type of silica and lipid utilized. The overall trend was that an increase in drug load resulted in an increase in FEN crystallization and aggregation of the silica microparticles.

It is important to note that, for FEN-SLH formulations, the endothermic peak observed in DSC thermographs were at a lower temperature than the melting point of crystalline FEN. The depression in melting point was previously reported in IBU-loaded super-SLH formulations and was attributed to the confinement of the drug crystallites in the nanopores [29]. The authors postulated that the presence of the drug outside of the pores and on the surface on the silica will not cause any depression in melting point, which implies the successful imbibition of drug and lipid into the nanopores of the silica microparticles. Based on this hypothesis and supported by XRPD data, it was confirmed that crystalline FEN is present in the formulations where display shifted endothermic peaks at 45–60 °C. Furthermore, it was hypothesized that the heating process during DSC analysis caused crystalline FEN present to re-dissolve in the lipid component of the SLH formulations displaying a shifted endothermic peak. However, further investigations are required to fully validate this hypothesis.

4.2. Impact of Silica Nanostructure

FS exhibited superior stabilization capacity and was able to stabilize a FEN saturation level of 200% S_{eq}. It was evident that saturation levels greater than 400% S_{eq} surpassed silica's stabilization capability and was reflected in DSC thermograms and XRP diffractograms. The relative intensities of XRPD patterns of MPS and FS formulations propose the presence of greater amounts of crystalline FEN in MPS compared to FS formulations, suggesting the nanostructured matrix of silica microparticles influences the physical state of the drug. XRPD is highly sensitive to molecular packing; therefore, any changes in the internal structure of the drug can be reflected in the patterns obtained [39]. This was evident in the XRPD pattern of 200% MPS PG8 formulation, suggesting the presence of FEN in a polymorphic form. However, the identification and confirmation of the presence and stability of FEN in any polymorphic form needs to be further investigated. Therefore, 200% S_{eq} was considered optimal in combination with FS as a solid carrier to maximize drug load while maintaining FEN in a solubilized non-crystalline state. These findings were in agreement with previous studies where super-SLH containing IBU and AbA displayed an increased amount of crystalline drug with increase in drug loading and optimum drug loading, which was 227% for IBU and 150% for AbA [28,31].

During in vitro dissolution studies (Figure 5), unsaturated (at 80% S_{eq}) MPS and FS formulations had a comparable performance, regardless type of lipid used. In contrast, both the rate and extent of dissolution from super-SLH (200%, 400%, and 600% S_{eq}) were significantly enhanced when using FS compared to corresponding MPS formulations. At higher saturation levels (400% and 600% Seq), it was evident that FS was able to maintain excellent FEN dissolution despite the presence of "crystalline" FEN and less amount of lipid in the formulations. However, the relatively larger amount of crystalline FEN present at 600% FS PG8 and 600% FS C300 resulted in slower release kinetics. In contrast, a reduction in dissolution performance was observed by MPS formulations with an increase in drug load. These findings were consistent with data obtained from FEN aqueous solubilization during in vitro lipolysis, despite the complexity of the data generated due to FEN precipitation.

FEN is a commonly used model PWSD in LBFs, and its tendency to precipitate from LBFs has been previously reported in multiple studies [11,41–43]. In these studies, authors proposed that, as digestion proceeds, formulations lose their solubilization capacity along with dilution of formulation triggered by the transition into intestinal digestion, where FEN precipitates with increasing FA concentration [41]. However, in these studies, FEN precipitation during in vitro lipolysis did not correlate with poor in vivo performance. Thomas et al. observed more extensive in vitro FEN precipitation from supersaturated self-nanoemulsifying drug delivery systems (super-SNNEDS) than from unsaturated SNEDDS [11]. Nevertheless, all SNEDDS formulations displayed enhanced in vivo bioavailability. FEN was shown to precipitate in a crystalline form in vitro but the extent of FEN precipitation in vitro was not known. These studies indicate that in vitro lipolysis models are not predictive of in vitro performance of FEN in a LBFs and should be used carefully to interpret such data [42].

In a previous study, in order to understand the underlying mechanism of FEN absorption and possible precipitation in vivo, orlistat as a lipase inhibitor was co-administered with SNEDDS containing FEN [43]. The study showed that lipase inhibition did not influence FEN bioavailability from SNEDDS, therefore digestion does not impact FEN absorption but can be beneficial when FEN is present in crystalline form in the formulation. However, it was still not known whether FEN precipitation occurs in vivo and to what extent. Recently, Tanaka et al. [44] found that FEN precipitated in the stomach of rats in an amorphous form with 20% microemulsion (ME) and crystalline form with 90% ME. In both cases, rapid redissolution was attained in the duodenum and 90% ME achieved significantly enhanced bioavailability. It is important to note that precipitation was more pronounced in the closed in vitro lipolysis system, which implies the importance of adding an absorption mimicking step [45]. The authors concluded that precipitation from the supersaturated state in the gastrointestinal environment was suppressed by the rapid absorption process for a highly permeable drug, like FEN, creating an absorption sink that acts as a driving force for absorption. In addition, the authors suggested the possibility of enhanced solubilization capacity of GI fluid caused by the formation of colloidal species upon digestion of the lipid. Therefore, formulations that cause higher supersaturation in the GI fluid [46] and the inclusion of medium chain triglycerides might result in enhanced bioavailability, despite their tendency to precipitate in vitro. However, such conclusions cannot be made for this study as further in vitro studies are required to validate the full potential of the fabricated SLH formulations.

In the present study, a higher extent of lipid digestion, as reflected in FA release, correlated with more pronounced FEN precipitation. This was evidenced by the 80% liquid PG8 formulation exerting the greatest FEN solubilization but reduced FA release. Liquid lipid formulations investigated in this study formed large emulsion droplets during in vitro lipolysis, providing less surface area for lipase action. However, when lipid was internalized within a porous silica matrix, a high surface area for lipase-mediated digestion was provided [40], which led to a more pronounced FA release and subsequent FEN precipitation. In the case of SLH prepared by FS, supersaturation resulted in enhanced FEN solubilization. In contrast, SLH prepared with MPS achieved the best performance when unsaturated. This was in agreement with solubilization data and previous studies where AbA-loaded super-SLH (prepared with MPS) compromised its solubilization performance during lipolysis when compared to unsaturated SLH [25]. However, this was not the case for IBU (dissolution studies), which implies that the benefits of super-SLH are drug dependent and require further investigation and optimization.

The difference in performance achieved by FS and MPS formulations can be attributed to their unique structure and resulting dynamic microenvironment when re-dispersed in biorelevant media (Figure 8). It is hypothesized that SLH microparticles prepared with FS de-aggregate and dissociate to their precursor silica nanoparticles upon dispersion in aqueous media, providing high surface area for lipase mediated digestion, dynamic mixed micelle formation, and subsequent drug release. For FEN, this results in a more profound precipitation in the closed in vitro digestion model, which lacks an absorption step. In contrast, FEN-loaded lipid droplets need to diffuse out of the 6 nm [29] structured nanopores of the MPS particles. This slows the kinetics of lipid/drug release, hindering lipolysis, which in turn leads to less pronounced FEN precipitation. In addition, MPS formulations were aggregated at all FEN saturation levels, suggesting poor lipid encapsulation which further reduced the surface area available for lipase action.

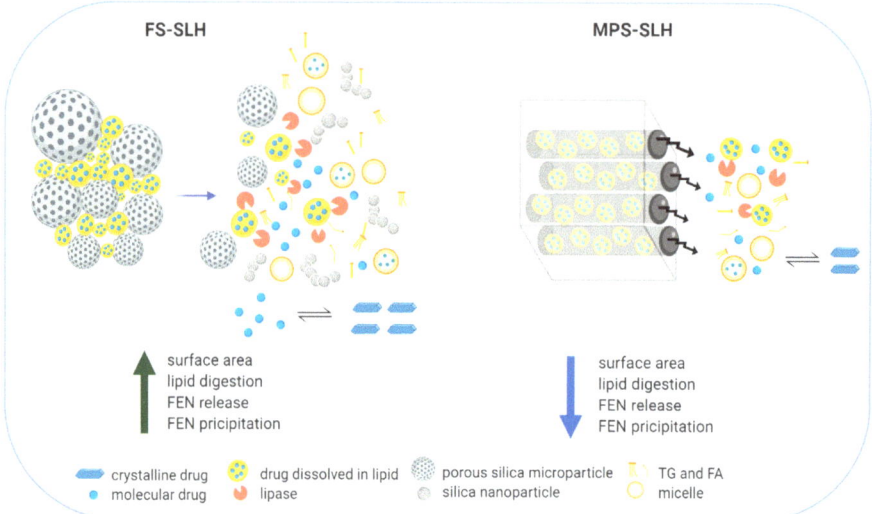

Figure 8. A schematic representation of the proposed mechanism of FEN release and precipitation from SLH made with FS and MPS, during in vitro lipolysis. Created with BioRender.com.

4.3. Impact of Lipid Type

FEN precipitation from SLH formulations occurred either during the gastric phase or during the intestinal phase depending on drug load and type of lipid used. Unlike dissolution, this made discrimination between formulations challenging. However, data generated display the benefits provided by super-SLH evident in the enhanced performance of all SLH formulations when compared to crystalline drug and APO-fenofibrate.

Lipids utilized in this study differ in their chemical composition and the physical interaction when imbibed into the silica nanopores. PG8 consists of propylene glycol (PG) mono (>90%)- and di (<10%)-esters of caprylic acid, while C300 is a medium-chain triglyceride manufactured by the esterification of glycerin and fatty acids, mainly caprylic (≈70%) and capric acid [47]. This impacts their physical encapsulation within the silica nanopores, lipolysis kinetics, digestibility, and the arrangement of digestion products [40]. Subsequently, influencing drug release and solubilization. Therefore, at the same lipid dose, C300 can generate greater FA release when digested compared to

PG8. This was reflected in the FA release-time profiles. Conversely, the greater extent of digestion observed in C300 formulations did not correlate with enhanced FEN solubilization as no significant differences in solubilization capacity between SLH C300 and corresponding SLH PG8 formulations were observed.

Lipid distribution within the particles was different for each lipid. As evidenced in the confocal images (Figure 4), more PG8, compared to C300, was adsorbed on the surface of the silica microparticles than the pores with large droplets in between the particles, suggesting incomplete lipid loading that, in turn, can lead to aggregation, as observed in SEM images (Figure 3) and more evident with supersaturated FEN formulations. The distribution profile of PG8 within the SLH was similar to what was previously reported by Schultz et al. [31]. However, unlike findings in this study, the solubilization capacity of all SLH prepared with PG8 was much greater than those prepared with Capmul MCM, despite its even distribution within the silica matrix. In addition, it is important to highlight the synergistic effect obtained by the slow release kinetics of MPS along with higher amount of digestion products produced from the digestion of C300 in 80% and 200% MPS C300 formulations. As evidenced by the enhanced solubilization of FEN, these were the only SLH formulations to significantly enhance FEN solubilization between 15–60 min during the intestinal phase of in vitro GI lipolysis (Figure 6).

In the present work, we were able to highlight the importance of understanding the nanostructured matrix and composition of SLH microparticles in order to seize their full potential in enhancing the biopharmaceutical performance in delivering PWSDs, such as FEN. Each type of silica provides competitive advantages that can be tailored according to the outcome desired from the formulation. It has become evident that changes in the nanostructure and surface chemistry of SLH particles, even if small, can have significant impact on lipase activity which, in turn, influences drug release kinetics and absorption. Therefore, Future work will be directed toward understanding the influence of internal silica particles nanostructure, microporosity, and surface area on drug solubilization.

5. Conclusions

The role of key SLH characteristics on in vitro performance of FEN-loaded SLHs and super-SLH were investigated and compared. It was evident that the silica's internal nanostructure influences lipase accessibility, which, in turn, affects the mechanism of drug release and FEN precipitation behavior. The crystalline FEN present at higher drug loads correlated with poor in vitro performance. Furthermore, the type of lipid utilized to dissolve the drug can impact its encapsulation within silica microparticles and the extent of digestion. When supersaturated, all FS formulations significantly enhanced FEN in vitro dissolution and aqueous solubilization compared to corresponding MPS formulations, crystalline FEN, and APO-fenofibrate. The implications of the main findings suggest that balance between high drug load and performance is key. Therefore, we can conclude that the optimum FEN loading is between 7–16% w/w, which corresponds to 200–400% S_{eq}. GI lipolysis served as an important test to investigate FEN precipitation in vitro; therefore, future studies with absorption capabilities will be of great benefit to improve the understanding of this trend. Furthermore, the use of C300, a medium chain triglyceride, has proven to be beneficial in enhancing the aqueous solubilization of FEN and demonstrated synergistic action with MPS displaying best aqueous solubilization at 80% S_{eq}, under digesting conditions. This was attributed to C300's ability to generate a larger amount of digestion species along with the slow release kinetics from the restricted pores of MPS, resulting in enhanced FEN solubilization and less precipitation. However, further in vivo investigations are required to validate its full potential. The findings of this research demonstrate the impact of SLH structure and composition in fabricating optimized solid-state LBFs for the oral delivery of PWSDs; since the various silica and lipid types provide competitive advantages, formulations can be tailored depending on the release profile or outcome desired.

Supplementary Materials: The following are available online at http://www.mdpi.com/1999-4923/12/7/687/s1, Table S1: Drug loading efficiencies of 3 FEN-loaded formulations (values represent mean ± SD, $n = 3$), Table S2:

The lipid content of the formulations and lipid dosed to lipolysis vessel. Figure S1. The relationship between XRPD peak intensity at 22.3° (2θ) and supersaturated drug loading (Seq) for FS PG8 formulations and MPS PG8 formulations, Figure S2. The % phase partitioning of FEN between the aqueous phase and pellet over 90 min after a 3 mg FEN dose of 80% formulations, Crystalline FEN and APO-fenofibrate, under biorelevant gastric and intestinal conditions. Values represent mean ± SD, n = 3 and Figure S3. The % phase partitioning of FEN between the aqueous phase and pellet over 90 min after a 3 mg FEN dose of supersaturated formulations, under biorelevant gastric and intestinal conditions. Values represent mean ± SD, n = 3.

Author Contributions: Conceptualization, R.A., H.B.S. and C.A.P.; Formal analysis, R.A. and P.J.; Funding acquisition, C.A.P.; Investigation, R.A.; Methodology, R.A. and P.J.; Supervision, N.T., K.E.B. and C.A.P.; Validation, R.A.; Writing—original draft, R.A.; Writing—review & editing, P.J., H.B.S., N.T., K.E.B. and C.A.P. All authors have read and agreed to the published version of the manuscript.

Funding: This research was funded by the Australian Research Council Centre of Excellence in Bio-Nano Science and Technology, grant number ARC CE140100036.

Acknowledgments: The Australian Government Research Training Program is acknowledged for the master's Scholarship of Ruba Almasri.

Conflicts of Interest: The authors declare no conflict of interest.

References

1. Williams, H.D.; Trevaskis, N.L.; Charman, S.A.; Shanker, R.M.; Charman, W.N.; Pouton, C.W.; Porter, C.J.H. Strategies to address low drug solubility in discovery and development. *Pharmacol. Rev.* **2013**, *65*, 315–499. [CrossRef] [PubMed]
2. Feeney, O.M.; Crum, M.F.; McEvoy, C.L.; Trevaskis, N.L.; Williams, H.D.; Pouton, C.W.; Charman, W.N.; Bergstrom, C.A.S.; Porter, C.J.H. 50 years of oral lipid-based formulations: Provenance, progress and future perspectives. *Adv. Drug Deliv. Rev.* **2016**, *101*, 167–194. [CrossRef] [PubMed]
3. Fricker, G.; Kromp, T.; Wendel, A.; Blume, A.; Zirkel, J.; Rebmann, H.; Setzer, C.; Quinkert, R.-O.; Martin, F.; Müller-Goymann, C. Phospholipids and lipid-based formulations in oral drug delivery. *Pharm. Res.* **2010**, *27*, 1469–1486. [CrossRef] [PubMed]
4. Porter, C.J.H.; Trevaskis, N.L.; Charman, W.N. Lipids and lipid-based formulations: Optimizing the oral delivery of lipophilic drugs. *Nat. Rev. Drug Discov.* **2007**, *6*, 231–248. [CrossRef]
5. Porter, C.J.H.; Pouton, C.W.; Cuine, J.F.; Charman, W.N. Enhancing intestinal drug solubilisation using lipid-based delivery systems. *Adv. Drug Deliv. Rev.* **2008**, *60*, 673–691. [CrossRef]
6. Joyce, P.; Dening, T.J.; Meola, T.R.; Schultz, H.B.; Holm, R.; Thomas, N.; Prestidge, C.A. Solidification to improve the biopharmaceutical performance of SEDDS: Opportunities and challenges. *Adv. Drug Deliv. Rev.* **2018**. [CrossRef]
7. Savla, R.; Browne, J.; Plassat, V.; Wasan, K.M.; Wasan, E.K. Review and analysis of FDA approved drugs using lipid-based formulations. *Drug Dev. Ind. Pharm.* **2017**, *43*, 1743–1758. [CrossRef]
8. Chen, X.-Q.; Gudmundsson, O.S.; Hageman, M.J. Application of lipid-based formulations in drug discovery. *J. Med. Chem.* **2012**, *55*, 7945–7956. [CrossRef]
9. Trevaskis, N.L.; Kaminskas, L.M.; Porter, C.J.H. From sewer to saviour—Targeting the lymphatic system to promote drug exposure and activity. *Nat. Rev. Drug Discov.* **2015**, *14*, 781–803. [CrossRef]
10. Kollipara, S.; Gandhi, R.K. Pharmacokinetic aspects and in vitro–in vivo correlation potential for lipid-based formulations. *Acta Pharm. Sin. B.* **2014**, *4*, 333–349. [CrossRef]
11. Thomas, N.; Richter, K.; Pedersen, T.B.; Holm, R.; Müllertz, A.; Rades, T. In vitro lipolysis data does not adequately predict the in vivo performance of lipid-based drug delivery systems containing fenofibrate. *AAPS J.* **2014**, *16*, 539–549. [CrossRef]
12. Jannin, V.; Musakhanian, J.; Marchaud, D. Approaches for the development of solid and semi-solid lipid-based formulations. *Adv. Drug Deliv. Rev.* **2008**, *60*, 734–746. [CrossRef] [PubMed]
13. Tang, B.; Cheng, G.; Gu, J.-C.; Xu, C.-H. Development of solid self-emulsifying drug delivery systems: Preparation techniques and dosage forms. *Drug Discov. Today* **2008**, *13*, 606–612. [CrossRef] [PubMed]
14. Tan, A.; Rao, S.; Prestidge, C.A. Transforming lipid-based oral drug delivery systems into solid dosage forms: An overview of solid carriers, physicochemical properties, and biopharmaceutical performance. *Pharm. Res.* **2013**, *30*, 2993–3017. [CrossRef]

15. Mandić, J.; Zvonar Pobirk, A.; Vrečer, F.; Gašperlin, M. Overview of solidification techniques for self-emulsifying drug delivery systems from industrial perspective. *Int. J. Pharm.* **2017**, *533*, 335–345. [CrossRef]
16. Kang, J.H.; Oh, D.H.; Oh, Y.-K.; Yong, C.S.; Choi, H.-G. Effects of solid carriers on the crystalline properties, dissolution and bioavailability of flurbiprofen in solid self-nanoemulsifying drug delivery system (solid SNEDDS). *Eur. J. Pharm. Biopharm.* **2012**, *80*, 289–297. [CrossRef]
17. Dening, T.J.; Rao, S.; Thomas, N.; Prestidge, C.A. Novel nanostructured solid materials for modulating oral drug delivery from solid-state lipid-based drug delivery systems. *AAPS J.* **2016**, *18*, 23–40. [CrossRef] [PubMed]
18. Barbé, C.; Bartlett, J.; Kong, L.; Finnie, K.; Lin, H.Q.; Larkin, M.; Calleja, S.; Bush, A.; Calleja, G. Silica Particles: A Novel Drug-Delivery System. *Adv. Mater.* **2004**, *16*, 1959–1966. [CrossRef]
19. Bremmell, K.E.; Tan, A.; Martin, A.; Prestidge, C.A. Tableting lipid-based formulations for oral drug delivery: A case study with silica nanoparticle-lipid-mannitol hybrid microparticles. *J. Pharm. Sci.* **2013**, *102*, 684–693. [CrossRef]
20. Yang, P.; Gai, S.; Lin, J. Functionalized mesoporous silica materials for controlled drug delivery. *Chem. Soc. Rev.* **2012**, *41*, 3679–3698. [CrossRef]
21. Simovic, S.; Heard, P.; Hui, H.; Song, Y.; Peddie, F.; Davey, A.K.; Lewis, A.; Rades, T.; Prestidge, C.A. Dry Hybrid Lipid–Silica Microcapsules Engineered from Submicron Lipid Droplets and Nanoparticles as a Novel Delivery System for Poorly Soluble Drugs. *Mol. Pharm.* **2009**, *6*, 861–872. [CrossRef]
22. Williams, H.D.; Speybroeck, M.V.; Augustijns, P.; Porter, C.J.H. Lipid-Based Formulations Solidified Via Adsorption onto the Mesoporous Carrier Neusilin® US2: Effect of Drug Type and Formulation Composition on In Vitro Pharmaceutical Performance. *J. Pharm. Sci.* **2014**, *103*, 1734–1746. [CrossRef]
23. Tan, A.; Davey, A.K.; Prestidge, C.A. Silica-Lipid Hybrid (SLH) versus non-lipid formulations for optimising the dose-dependent oral absorption of celecoxib. *Pharm. Res.* **2011**, *28*, 2273–2287. [CrossRef] [PubMed]
24. Dening, T.J.; Rao, S.; Thomas, N.; Prestidge, C.A. Silica encapsulated lipid-based drug delivery systems for reducing the fed/fasted variations of ziprasidone in vitro. *Eur. J. Pharm. Biopharm.* **2016**, *101*, 33–42. [CrossRef]
25. Joyce, P.; Whitby, C.P.; Prestidge, C.A. Interfacial processes that modulate the kinetics of lipase-mediated catalysis using porous silica host particles. *RSC Adv.* **2016**, *6*, 43802–43813. [CrossRef]
26. Joyce, P.; Tan, A.; Whitby, C.P.; Prestidge, C.A. The role of porous nanostructure in controlling lipase mediated digestion of lipid loaded into silica particles. *Langmuir* **2014**, *30*, 2779–2788. [CrossRef]
27. Tan, A.; Simovic, S.; Davey, A.K.; Rades, T.; Prestidge, C.A. Silica-lipid hybrid (SLH) microcapsules: A novel oral delivery system for poorly soluble drugs. *J. Control Release* **2009**, *134*, 62–70. [CrossRef] [PubMed]
28. Schultz, H.B.; Wignall, A.D.; Thomas, N.; Prestidge, C.A. Enhancement of abiraterone acetate oral bioavailability by supersaturated-silica lipid hybrids. *Int. J. Pharm.* **2020**, *582*, 119264. [CrossRef] [PubMed]
29. Schultz, H.B.; Thomas, N.; Rao, S.; Prestidge, C.A. Supersaturated silica-lipid hybrids (super-SLH): An improved solid-state lipid-based oral drug delivery system with enhanced drug loading. *Eur. J. Pharm. Biopharm.* **2018**, *125*, 13–20. [CrossRef]
30. Schultz, H.B.; Kovalainen, M.; Peressin, K.F.; Thomas, N.; Prestidge, C.A. Supersaturated silica-lipid hybrid (super-SLH) oral drug delivery systems: Balancing drug loading and in vivo performance. *J. Pharmacol. Exp. Ther.* **2018**. [CrossRef]
31. Schultz, H.B.; Joyce, P.; Thomas, N.; Prestidge, C.A. Supersaturated-silica lipid hybrids improve in vitro solubilization of abiraterone acetate. *Pharm. Res.* **2020**, *37*, 77. [CrossRef] [PubMed]
32. CLing, H.; Luoma, J.T.; Hilleman, D. A Review of currently available fenofibrate and fenofibric acid formulations. *Cardiol. Res.* **2013**, *4*, 47–55. [CrossRef]
33. Granero, G.E.; Ramachandran, C.; Amidon, G.L. Dissolution and solubility behavior of fenofibrate in sodium lauryl sulfate solutions. *Drug Dev. Ind. Pharm.* **2005**, *31*, 917–922. [CrossRef] [PubMed]
34. Sanganwar, G.P.; Gupta, R.B. Dissolution-rate enhancement of fenofibrate by adsorption onto silica using supercritical carbon dioxide. *Int. J. Pharm.* **2008**, *360*, 213–218. [CrossRef] [PubMed]
35. Kumar, R.; Siril, P.F. Enhancing the solubility of fenofibrate by nanocrystal formation and encapsulation. *AAPS PharmSciTech* **2018**, *19*, 284–292. [CrossRef] [PubMed]

36. Pestieau, A.; Krier, F.; Brouwers, A.; Streel, B.; Evrard, B. Selection of a discriminant and biorelevant in vitro dissolution test for the development of fenofibrate self-emulsifying lipid-based formulations. *Eur. J. Pharm. Sci.* **2016**, *92*, 212–219. [CrossRef]
37. Joyce, P.; Gustafsson, H.; Prestidge, C.A. Enhancing the lipase-mediated bioaccessibility of omega-3 fatty acids by microencapsulation of fish oil droplets within porous silica particles. *J. Funct. Foods* **2018**, *47*, 491–502. [CrossRef]
38. Shi, X.; Shao, Y.; Sheng, X. A new polymorph of fenofibrate prepared by polymer-mediated crystallization. *J. Cryst. Growth* **2018**, *498*, 93–102. [CrossRef]
39. Tipduangta, P.; Takieddin, K.; Fábián, L.; Belton, P.; Qi, S. A new low melting-point polymorph of fenofibrate prepared via talc induced heterogeneous nucleation. *Cryst. Growth Des.* **2015**, *15*, 5011–5020. [CrossRef]
40. Joyce, P.; Gustafsson, H.; Prestidge, C.A. Engineering intelligent particle-lipid composites that control lipase-mediated digestion. *Adv. Colloid Interface Sci.* **2018**, *260*, 1–23. [CrossRef]
41. Khan, J.; Rades, T.; Boyd, B. The Precipitation Behavior of Poorly Water-Soluble Drugs with an Emphasis on the Digestion of Lipid Based Formulations. *Pharm. Res.* **2016**, *33*, 548–562. [CrossRef] [PubMed]
42. Griffin, B.T.; Kuentz, M.; Vertzoni, M.; Kostewicz, E.S.; Fei, Y.; Faisal, W.; Stillhart, C.; O'Driscoll, C.M.; Reppas, C.; Dressman, J.B. Comparison of in vitro tests at various levels of complexity for the prediction of in vivo performance of lipid-based formulations: Case studies with fenofibrate. *Eur. J. Pharm. Biopharm.* **2014**, *86*, 427–437. [CrossRef] [PubMed]
43. Hotoft Michaelsen, M.; Siqueira Jorgensen, S.D.; Mahad Abdi, I.; Wasan, K.M.; Rades, T.; Mullertz, A. Fenofibrate oral absorption from SNEDDS and super-SNEDDS is not significantly affected by lipase inhibition in rats. *Eur. J. Pharm. Biopharm.* **2019**. [CrossRef]
44. Tanaka, Y.; Tay, E.; Nguyen, T.H.; Porter, C.J.H. Quantifying in vivo luminal drug solubilization-supersaturation-precipitation profiles to explain the performance of lipid based formulations. *Pharm. Res.* **2020**, *37*, 47. [CrossRef]
45. Crum, M.F.; Trevaskis, N.L.; Williams, H.D.; Pouton, C.W.; Porter, C.J. A new in vitro lipid digestion—In vivo absorption model to evaluate the mechanisms of drug absorption from lipid-based formulations. *Pharm. Res.* **2016**, *33*, 970–982. [CrossRef] [PubMed]
46. Williams, H.D.; Sassene, P.; Kleberg, K.; Calderone, M.; Igonin, A.; Jule, E.; Vertommen, J.; Blundell, R.; Benameur, H.; Müllertz, A.; et al. Toward the establishment of standardized in vitro tests for lipid-based formulations, part 3: Understanding supersaturation versus precipitation potential during the in vitro digestion of type I, II, IIIA, IIIB and IV lipid-based formulations. *Pharm. Res.* **2013**, *30*, 3059–3076. [CrossRef]
47. Tran, T.; Siqueira, S.D.V.S.; Amenitsch, H.; Rades, T.; Müllertz, A. Monoacyl phosphatidylcholine inhibits the formation of lipid multilamellar structures during in vitro lipolysis of self-emulsifying drug delivery systems. *Eur. J. Pharm. Sci.* **2017**, *108*, 62–70. [CrossRef]

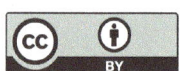

© 2020 by the authors. Licensee MDPI, Basel, Switzerland. This article is an open access article distributed under the terms and conditions of the Creative Commons Attribution (CC BY) license (http://creativecommons.org/licenses/by/4.0/).

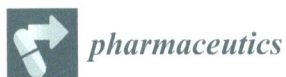

Article

Effectiveness of a Controlled 5-FU Delivery Based on FZD10 Antibody-Conjugated Liposomes in Colorectal Cancer In vitro Models

Maria Principia Scavo, Annalisa Cutrignelli, Nicoletta Depalo, Elisabetta Fanizza, Valentino Laquintana, Giampietro Gasparini, Gianluigi Giannelli and Nunzio Denora

1. Personalized Medicine Laboratory, National Institute of Gastroenterology "S. deBellis", Via Turi 26 Castellana Grotte, 70125 Bari, Italy
2. Department of Pharmacy-Drug Science, University of Bari, Via E. Orabona 4, 70125 Bari, Italy; annalisa.cutrignelli@uniba.it (A.C.); valentino.laquintana@uniba.it (V.L.); nunzio.denora@uniba.it (N.D.)
3. Institute for Chemical and Physical Processes (IPCF)-CNR SS Bari, Via Orabona 4, 70125 Bari, Italy; n.depalo@ba.ipcf.cnr.it (N.D.); e.fanizza@ba.ipcf.cnr.it (E.F.)
4. Department of Chemistry, University of Bari, Via E. Orabona 4, 70125 Bari, Italy
5. Oncology Unit, Hospital San Filippo Neri, 00135 Rome, Italy; giampietro.gasparini@hotmail.it
6. Scientific Direction, National Institute of Gastroenterology "de Bellis", Via Turi 26 Castellana Grotte, 70125 Bari, Italy; gianluigi.giannelli@irccsdebellis.it
* Correspondence: maria.scavo@irccsdebellis.it; Tel.: +39-080-4994697

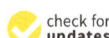

Received: 11 June 2020; Accepted: 6 July 2020; Published: 10 July 2020

Abstract: The use of controlled delivery therapy in colorectal cancer (CRC) reduces toxicity and side effects. Recently, we have suggested that the Frizzled 10 (FZD10) protein, a cell surface receptor belonging to the FZD protein family that is overexpressed in CRC cells, is a novel candidate for targeting and treatment of CRC. Here, the anticancer effect of novel immuno-liposomes loaded with 5-Fluorouracil (5-FU), decorated with an antibody against FZD10 (anti-FZD10/5-FU/LPs), was evaluated in vitro on two different CRC cell lines, namely metastatic CoLo-205 and nonmetastatic CaCo-2 cells, that were found to overexpress FZD10. The anti-FZD10/5-FU/LPs obtained were extensively characterized and their preclinical therapeutic efficacy was evaluated with the MTS cell proliferation assay based on reduction of tetrazolium compound, scratch test, Field Emission Scanning Electron Microscopes (FE-SEM) investigation and immunofluorescence analysis. The results highlighted that the cytotoxic activity of 5-FU was enhanced when encapsulated in the anti-FZD10 /5-FU/LPs at the lowest tested concentrations, as compared to the free 5-FU counterparts. The immuno-liposomes proposed herein possess a great potential for selective treatment of CRC because, in future clinical applications, they can be encapsulated in gastro-resistant capsules or suppositories for oral or rectal delivery, thereby successfully reaching the intestinal tract in a minimally invasive manner.

Keywords: liposomes; target delivery nanosystem; FZD10 protein; colon cancer therapy

1. Introduction

Colorectal cancer (CRC) is the second leading cause of cancer death worldwide [1]. Cytotoxic drugs-based chemotherapy is the main treatment in cancer management, in addition to surgery, radiation, and biological therapies [2]. 5-Fluorouracil (5-FU) is widely used in CRC chemotherapy, as also other different drugs employed to interfere with cell replication by acting as nucleoside analogs and leading to S-phase arrest, or by damaging deoxyribonucleic acid (DNA) [3]. Unfortunately, owing to the short half-life (5–14 min), poor membrane permeability and rapid metabolism in the body, continuous administration of high doses of 5-FU is required to maintain the minimum therapeutic serum concentration; this is usually associated with numerous side effects and severe toxicity [4]. Nanostructured carriers have been proposed as an alternative therapeutic approach, since they can be properly surface-functionalized and consequently reach a specific target on pathological cells. Therefore, targeted drug delivery nanosystems can ensure the specific release of drugs in tumor areas, at lower and more efficient doses than conventional treatments, thus maximizing the bioavailability of anticancer agents and their uptake into the cancer tissue, while reducing side effects and drug distribution to healthy tissues. Drug-loaded nanovectors have also been demonstrated to be able to overcome the canonical drug-resistance pathways, e.g., membrane pumps, for cellular internalization that usually occurs when using small therapeutic molecules [5,6]. Furthermore, drug delivery nanocarriers can be protected by using pH-dependent polymer coatings or pH-dependent encapsulation systems, to prevent their degradation in the gastric tract [7,8].

Liposomes (LPs) are lipid-based nanostructures with a hydrophilic core and a lipophilic shell, where different types of drugs can be encapsulated [9,10]. The small size of LPs is fundamental to promote extravasation and accumulation phenomena in tumor sites. In the literature, several examples of liposomes have been proposed for CRC treatment, by intravenous, oral or rectal administration [11,12]. The coupling of the LPs surface with selected antibodies, as ligands able to recognize and bind specific plasma membrane proteins that are overexpressed in cancer tissues, allows immuno-LPs to be created, taking a further step forward in the development of efficient targeted drug delivery nanosystems [13,14].

The FZD proteins (FZDs) are the main cell surface receptors for the WNT family of ligands and include ten members (FZD1–FZD10). FZDs are involved in the regulation of several cell processes, which occur not only in normal development of different body systems, but also in various cancers. Indeed, numerous studies proved that FZDs play a crucial role in different cancer functions, thus promoting proliferation, migration, invasion, angiogenesis, and also chemoresistance. Furthermore, modulation of expression levels for specific FZD depending on up- or downregulation of the corresponding messenger RNA (mRNA) was observed in different cancers tissues [15–20]. Among the FZD proteins, FZD10 was suggested to be one of the most promising receptors for the development of targeted therapy of CRC. Indeed, a study by S. Nagayama et al. evaluated the immunohistochemical expression patterns of FZD-10 in tissue samples of patients affected by CRCs. Interestingly, their study indicated that FZD10 was expressed only in cancer cells and it was absent in adjacent normal cells [21,22]. Furthermore, we have reported a study performed on tissues of three different cancers, namely CRC, melanoma and gastric cancer, demonstrating a strong correlation between the expression levels of FZD10 and different tumor stages. In the colon, a significant increase of FZD10 expression in membrane and cytoplasm and, concomitantly, a significant reduction in nuclei expression were observed, passing from nondysplastic to malignant tissue [22,23]. Based on these premises, FZD10 can be effectively exploited as a novel candidate target with a good potential in the development of selective therapeutic approaches for CRC.

The aim of the study will be to create stealth LPs functionalized with FZD 10 antibody and loaded with 5-FU (anti-FZD10/5-FU/LPs), towards the development of efficacious nanostructured formulations for the selective delivery and sustained release of anticancer drug to CRC sites by exploiting active targeting. A deep in vitro investigation on their preclinical therapeutic efficacy in CRC treatment will be performed.

2. Material and Methods

5-fluorouracil (5-FU, MW = 130.077 g/mol) was purchased from Sigma-Aldrich (Milan, Italy) and used as stock solution in ethanol (380 mM). The Liposomes Kit, composed of cholesterol (Chol, 9 µmol/package), L-α-Phosphatidylcholine (egg yolk, 63 µmol/package) and stearylamine (18 µmol/package), N-(3-dimethylamino-propyl)-N′-ethylcarbodiimide hydrochloride (EDC), N-hydroxysulfosuccinimide (sulfo-NHS) and phosphotungstic acid (99.995%) were purchased from Sigma-Aldrich (Milan, Italy). 1,2-stearoyl-sn-glycero-3-phosphoethanolamine-N-[carboxy(poly(ethylene glycol)-2000)] (DSPE-PEG2000-COOH) and 1,2-distearoyl-sn-glycero-3-

phosphoethanolamine-N-[methoxy(polyethylene glycerol)-2000] (DSPE-PEG2000) were purchased from Avanti Polar Lipids (Alabaster, AL, USA). Fetal bovine serum, penicillin/streptomycin and glutamine were purchased from Thermo-Fisher Scientific (Waltham, MA, USA). Polyclonal antibody against FZD10 was purchased from ABCAM (Cambridge, UK). Mouse monoclonal anti-human vimentin and rabbit polyclonal anti-human phospho-Paxillin were purchased from Cell Signaling Technology (Beverly, MA, USA) Goat anti-Mouse IgG (H + L), Superclonal™ Recombinant Secondary Antibody, Alexa Fluor 488 and goat anti-Rabbit IgG (H + L) Cross-Adsorbed Secondary Antibody, Alexa Fluor 555 were purchased from Thermo Fisher Scientific (Waltham, MA, USA) Prolong gold antifade reagent containing the nuclear staining 4′,6-diamidino-2-phenylindole dichloride (DAPI) was purchased from Invitrogen (Carlsbad, CA, USA). CellTiter 96 AQueous One Solution Cell Proliferation Assay (MTS) was purchased from Promega (Madison, WI, USA). All aqueous solutions were prepared using water obtained from a Milli-Q Gradient A-10 system (Millipore, 18.2 MΩcm, organic carbon content ≥ 4 µg/L). All other solvents and reagents were of analytical grade.

2.1. Preparation of Liposomes

Nude LPs loaded with 5-FU (5-FU/LPs) were prepared using the ether injection method [24]. Briefly, 2.738 mL of an ether/chloroform (1:1, *v/v*) solution, 0.274 mL of a chloroform solution of lipid mix containing cholesterol, phosphatidylcholine and stearylamine (7:3:1 molar ratio) and 11 µL of a chloroform solution of DSPE-PEG2000 were mixed in a glass vial using a magnetic stirrer, brought to a lipid mix/DSPE-PEG2000 molar ratio of 3:0.3. Then, 3 mL of aqueous solution 5-FU (38 mM) were rapidly injected into the organic lipid solution using a sterile glass syringe. LPs were then obtained according to the previously reported experimental procedure [24]. Empty LPs were prepared following the same protocol, but without 5-FU addition.

For the preparation of 5-FU/LPs conjugated with FZD10 antibody (anti-FZD10/5-FU/LPs), 5-FU/LPs were previously surface-functionalized with carboxylic groups (5-FU/LPs-COOH). For this purpose, the above-described experimental protocol was followed, using as starting lipid mixture, 2.738 mL of an ether/chloroform (1:1, *v/v*) solution, 0.274 mL of a chloroform solution of lipid mix, 3 µL of a chloroform solution of DSPE-PEG2000 and 8 µL of a chloroform solution of DSPE-PEG2000-COOH. The final total lipid concentration in all the liposomal formulations was kept constant at 3 mM. After the purification procedure, 5-FU/LPs-COOH (300 µL) dispersed in ultrapure distilled water were activated by adding sulfo-NHS (11 mg) and EDC (9 mg). The reaction mixture was left under gentle stirring overnight at room temperature. Then, the samples were ultracentrifuged at 10,000× *g* for 40 min at 4 °C to remove excess crosslinking reagents. The activated 5-FU/LPs-COOH were recovered as pellets, dispersed in 300 µL of PBS and incubated with 5 µg of anti-FZD10 antibody. The mixture was gently stirred overnight at room temperature. Finally, the anti-FZD10/5-FU/LPs were purified by ultracentrifugation at 10,000× *g* at 4 °C for 40 min to remove unbound antibody. All the liposomal formulations were lyophilized (Christal freeze dryer alpha 1-4 LSC) and then reconstituted in PBS or water prior to their use or characterization. The experimental details on the indirect detection of FZD10-antibody bound onto the surface of LPs are reported in Supplementary Materials.

2.2. Evaluation of Encapsulation Efficiency (EE%)

The encapsulation efficiency (EE%) of 5-FU encapsulated in 5-FU/LPs or anti-FZD10/5-FU/LPs was evaluated according to the following formula:

$$EE\% = W_t/W_i \times 100 \qquad (1)$$

where W_t is the amount of drug effectively incorporated into the liposomal formulation and W_i the total quantity of 5-FU initially added during the preparation. To evaluate the drug content, samples were lyophilized and treated with methanol (1:100 dilution) and then the absorbance spectra (Perkin Elmer Double beam UV-Visible Spectrophotometer Lambda Bio 20) were recorded at 265 nm versus a methanol solution containing the same lipid mixture used for liposome preparation (baseline) [20]. Three measurements were performed on three different batches for each liposomes formulation. A calibration curve of 5-FU was generated by measuring the drug absorbance at 265 nm of standard methanol solutions at concentrations ranging from 0.25 mM to 0.05 mM.

2.3. In vitro Drug Release Study

1 mL of FZD10-anti/5-FU/LPs was introduced into dialysis tubing (cut-off 3.5 kDa, Spectrapore) and dialyzed against 50 mL of PBS (10 mM and pH=7.4, outer medium). The dialysis was conducted at 37 °C in a water bath shaker. At defined time intervals, over 48 h, 100 µL of outer medium were collected, removed and replaced with fresh PBS. Each collected aliquot was lyophilized and solubilized in methanol; the drug concentration was determined by measuring the UV-Vis absorbance at 265 nm. The calibration curve described in the previous paragraph was used for the quantitative evaluation of the released drug. Measurements were conducted three times per sample.

2.4. Cell Culture

The CaCo-2 cell line is originally derived from a primary colon adenocarcinoma (Cancer Coli-2) and was established by Jorgen Fogh at the Sloan Kettering Cancer Research Institute, from a Caucasian male (ATCC). The CoLo-205 cell line has been established from ascites fluid obtained from a male patient with metastatic adenocarcinoma of the colon (ATCC). CaCo-2 cells were cultured in Eagle's Minimum Essential Medium, (GibCo), which was added with 10% of fetal bovine serum, 1% of penicillin/streptomycin and 1% of glutamine. For the CoLo-205 cell line, ATCC-formulated Roswell Park Memorial Institute (RPMI)-1640 Medium was employed, with the addition of 10% of fetal bovine serum (10%), 1% of penicillin/streptomycin (1%) and 1% of glutamine (1%). When the cell lines confluence was about 70%, the cell layer was rinsed with PBS, and trypsinized, for the subsequent in vitro experiments.

2.5. Cells Proliferation Assay

The MTS cell proliferation assay (CellTiter 96® AQueous One Solution Cell Proliferation Assay, Promega) was used to determine metabolic activity in CaCo-2, CoLo-205 cell lines. Briefly, cells were seeded into 96-well plates at a density of 2×10^3 cells/well. After 24 h, the cells were treated with free drug (5-FU), empty LPs, 5-FU/LPs and anti-FZD10/5-FU/LPs, at 5-FU concentrations ranging from 1 µmol to 10 µmol (5-50 µM, in terms of total lipid concentration for the liposomal formulations), for 24, 48 or 72 h. After cell incubation with the different samples, cells were treated with the MTS tetrazolium compound for three additional hours and the absorbance was measured at a wavelength of 490 nm using a Perkin Elmer Victor Plate Reader (Mechelen, Belgium).

2.6. In vitro Investigation by Field Emission Scanning Electron Microscopy

CaCo-2 and CoLo-205 cells were seeded on silicon wafers (Ted Pella Inc., Redding, CA, USA) at a density of 2×10^3/well in 24-wells plates and at a subconfluent density, exposed to 5-FU/LPs and anti-FZD10/5-FU/LPs at a drug concentration of 2 µM for 6, 24 and 96 h. After cell washing with PBS, all cell lines were fixed with 3% glutaraldehyde in PBS for 1 h at 4 °C and incubated in 1% OsO_4 for 1 h. The samples were washed five times with aqueous solution of sodium cacodylate (0.005 M, pH 7.2). Then, sequential cell treatment steps with water/acetone mixtures, gradually increasing the acetone volume from 20% to 100%, were carried out to accomplish the complete dehydration process of the cells. The same fixation procedure was carried out after deposition on silicon chips also for the untreated cell lines. The fixed and dried cells were coated with a uniform Au metal film, a few nanometers thick, that was deposited on the samples placed on silicon chips using a turbomolecular pump SC7620 Mini Sputter/Glow Discharge System, Quorum Technologies, and imaged using a Zeiss Sigma FE-SEM. A constant Extra-High Tension (EHT) value of 3.00 kV and a working distance (WD) ranging from 1.8 to 3 mm were set for the FE-SEM observation. For each experiment and sample,

2.7. In vitro Scratch Assay

CaCo-2 and CoLo-205 cells were plated in six-well plates to create a cell monolayer, following the protocol described by C. Liang et al [25]. Briefly, a "scratch" with a p200 pipette tip was created on the cell monolayer, for each sample and experiment. After removal of the debris by washing with 1 mL of culture medium, an ultrafine tip marker was used to create markings on the outer bottom of the plate that represent reference points close to the scratch. For the scratch assay, each cell line was incubated with 3 mL of medium containing free 5-FU, 5-FU/LPs or anti-FZD10/5-FU/LPs at a 5-FU concentration of 2 µmol for 24 or 48 h. The experiments were conducted at 37 °C. Untreated cells were used as control for each tested cell line. At 0, 24 and 48 h, the plates were placed under a confocal microscope Nikon Eclipse Ti2, for phase-contrast assessment to acquire the images of the scratch before and after cell incubation with the different samples.

2.8. Immunofluorescence Analysis

CaCo-2 and CoLo-205 cells were seeded into four-well slides chambers at a density of 10×10^3 cells per well at 37 °C and treated with free 5-FU, 5-FU/LPs or anti-FZD10/5-FU/LPs, respectively, for 24 or 48 h. Untreated cells were used as control. Subsequently, treated and untreated cells were washed three times with PBS, fixed with cold ethanol (96°) for 25 min and permeabilized with an aqueous solution of Triton X-100 (0.5%) in PBS for 15 min. Then cells were blocked with an aqueous solution of normal serum (5%) in PBS for 1 h and incubated at 4 °C over-night with the two primary antibodies mix. The protocol applied has been previously described [19], with the following antibodies: mouse monoclonal anti human Vimentin (diluted 1:250 in Blocking) and rabbit polyclonal anti human phospho-Paxillin (Tyr118) (diluted 1:200 in Blocking). Then, cells were washed twice with PBS and incubated with a specific green-fluorescent (goat anti-mouse IgG (H + L) secondary antibody Alexa Fluor 488 conjugate) and red-fluorescent (goat anti-rabbit IgG (H + L) superclonal secondary antibody, Alexa Fluor 555) secondary antibodies for 1 h, at room temperature, in the dark. After washing with PBS, the cells were mounted using prolonged gold antifade reagent containing DAPI (blue). Images were acquired using the Nikon confocal microscope Eclipse Ti2 and the fluorescence intensity was quantified using Image J software (number of pixels/area). Five different areas from the single well for each single independent experiment performed in triplicate were randomly selected [26].

2.9. Dynamic Light Scattering Analysis and ζ-Potential Investigation

The hydrodynamic diameter (size), the size distribution and the colloidal stability of the liposomal formulations were detected using a Zetasizer Nano ZS, Malvern Instruments Ltd., Worcestershire, UK (DTS 5.00), as previously reported [20]. Three measurements were performed on at least three different batches of each vesicles formulation, and results are reported together with the corresponding standard deviation.

2.10. Morphological Characterization by Transmission Electron Microscopy (TEM)

For TEM investigation, liposomal formulations deposition was made onto 400 mesh amorphous carbon-coated Cu grids. For each sample, 5 µL of aqueous dispersion of LPs were dropped on the grid and the solvent was left to evaporate. Then, the grid was placed in contact with the top surface of a drop composed of an aqueous phosphotungstic acid solution (2%, v/v) for 30 s. Finally, ultrapure free water was used to wash the grid. TEM measurements were carried out using a Jeol JEM-1011 microscope, working at an accelerating voltage of 100 kV and fitted with an Olympus Quemesa Camera (11 Mpx).

2.11. Statistical Analysis

All the experiments were performed three times and all results are presented as mean ± standard deviation. Data were analyzed by one-way ANOVA followed by Bonferroni test using GraphPad Prism version 5 for Windows (GraphPad Software, San Diego, CA, USA) and statistical significance was set at $p < 0.001$.

3. Results

3.1. Liposomes Formulation and Characterization

Poly ethylene glycol (PEG)-stabilized and 5-FU-loaded LPs (5-FU/LPs) were decorated with anti-FZD10 and in vitro tested to evaluate their effectiveness for selective CRC treatment (Figure 1A). A schematic illustration of active targeting of CRC by molecular recognition between anti-FZD10/5-FU/LPs and FZD10, expressed at the plasma membrane surface of CRC cells, is shown in Figure 1B.

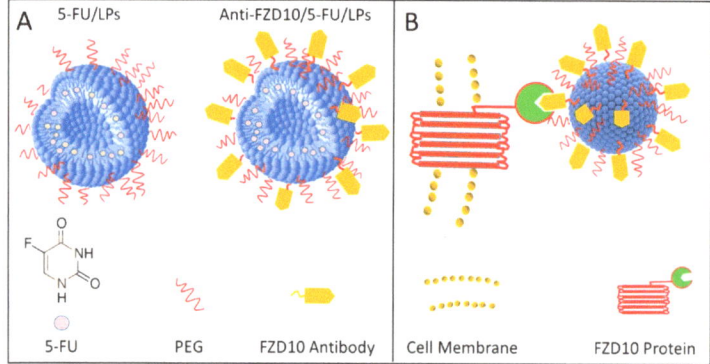

Figure 1. Pictorial sketch of PEG (Poly ethylene glycol) stabilized and 5-Fluorouracil (5-FU)-loaded liposomes (LPs) before (5-FU/LPs) and after (anti-FZD10/5-FU/LPs) conjugation with FZD10 antibody, according to the corresponding legend (**A**). Schematic representation of molecular recognition between anti-FZD10/5-FU/LPs and FZD10 protein expressed on the colorectal cancer (CRC) cell membrane surface. Drawings not to scale. (**B**).

For the preparation of anti-FZD10/5-FU/LPs, 5-FU/LPs bearing carboxylic groups were covalently conjugated with the primary amine groups of anti-FZD10 antibody by crosslinking chemistry. The effective occurrence of the conjugation reaction between FZD10-antibody and 5-FU/LPs was assessed by labeling the surface of anti-FZD10/5-FU/LPs with a specific secondary antibody-Alexa Fluor 555. The indirect detection of FZD10-antibody on anti-FZD10/5-FU/LPs was demonstrated by UV-Vis absorbance spectroscopy analysis, as described in the Supplementary Materials. In particular, the presence of a peak centered at 555 nm, due to the covalent binding of the dye conjugated secondary antibody to the surface of anti-FZD10/5-FU/LPs, can be observed in the absorption spectrum of anti-FZD10/5-FU/LPs, after their incubation with labelled secondary antibody (Figure S1B, Supplementary Materials), while the same peak does not appear in the absorbance spectrum of untreated anti-FZD10/5-FU/LPs (Figure S1A, Supplementary Materials).

The formulated LPs, namely 5-FU/LPs and anti-FZD10/5-FU/LPs, were characterized in terms of size, morphology and colloidal stability by performing DLS investigation, TEM analysis and ζ-potential measurements (Table 1). DLS investigation revealed that the mean hydrodynamic diameter of bare 5-FU/LPs was equal to (155 ± 47) nm, and this domain size was a consequence of the porosity of the polycarbonate membrane used for the extrusion. Anti-FZD10/5-FU/LPs exhibited a larger average size

(193 ± 12) nm, as expected when the surface functionalization of liposomes is carried out. The values of polydispersion index (PDI) denoted the presence of a fairly uniform LPs population in dimensional terms for both the formulations (Table 1).

Table 1. Intensity-average hydrodynamic diameter and corresponding polydispersity index (PDI) determined by Dynamic Light Scattering (DLS), ζ-potential, and encapsulation efficiency (EE%) of 5-FU/LPs and anti-FZD10/5-FU/LPs.

Samples	D_h (nm)	PDI	ζ-Potential (mV)	Drug EE (%)
5-FU/LPs	155 ± 47	0.32 ± 0.05	−37.73 ± 5.38	65.9 ± 2.9
Anti-FZD10/5FU/LPs	193 ± 12	0.33 ± 0.15	−43.43 ± 4.75	45.7 ± 5.9

The representative TEM micrographs of 5-FU/LPs (Figure 2A,A1) and FZD10-anti/5-FU/LPs (Figure 2B,B1) proved the formation of nanostructures with quite round shape for both the liposomal formulations. In the TEM micrographs of 5-FU/LPs (Figure 2A,A1) and anti-FZD10/5-FU/LPs (Figure 2B,B1), nanostructures with a rounded shape can be observed for both the formulated LPs, having size ranging from 30 to 110 nm and from 40 to 195 nm for 5-FU/LPs and FZD10-anti/5-FU/LPs, respectively. Furthermore, for both the bare and the engineered LPs, some nano-objects revealing a darker, circular bilayer and a brighter interior space, as typically ascribed to LP structures, can be appreciated, as highlighted in the two high magnification close-ups (Figure 2A1,B1).

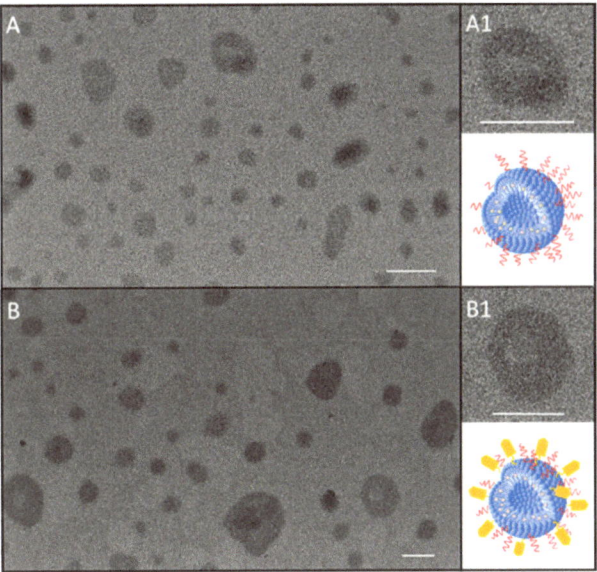

Figure 2. Representative transmission electron microscopy (TEM) micrograph of 5-FU/LPs (**A,A1**) and anti-FZD10/5-FU/LPs (**B,B1**). High magnification close-up of 5-FU/LPs (**A1**) and anti-FZD10/5-FU/LPs (**B1**) along with the corresponding sketch. Scale bar 100 nm.

The TEM observations resulted in a good agreement with the data obtained by DLS investigation, also considering that the deposition procedure of samples on the TEM grid, performed before TEM analysis, induced a drying process and consequently a shrinking of the soft organic matter based LPs.

The ζ-potential measurements highlighted the presence of an overall negative charge at the surface of both investigated formulations, as the phosphate moieties of the phospholipids used for the preparation of 5-FU/LPs and anti-FZD10/5-FU/LPs are expected to be exposed onto their surface (Table 1).

The decrease in drug EE% recorded for anti-FZD10/5-FU/LPs can be reasonably explained by taking into account the different steps required for the conjugation reaction, starting from bare 5-FU/LPs: the first incubation with the crosslinking agents, the subsequent centrifugation to remove the excess of reagents, the second incubation with the FZD10 antibody and the final centrifugation to remove the unbound antibody molecules.

The drug release study for FZD10-anti/5-FU/LPs, monitored by UV-Vis absorption spectroscopy, is reported in Figure S2 of Supplementary Materials.

3.2. Effectiveness of Formulated Liposomes on Cell Viability

CoLo-205 and CaCo-2 cells were selected as FZD10-positive CRC cell lines (Figure S3, Supplementary Materials). The effect of 5-FU and anti-FZD10/LPs on CoLo-205 and CaCo-2 cells viability was evaluated by MTS proliferation assay. For comparison, free 5-FU and nontargeted LPs were tested. The effect of the empty LPs (having a ζ-potential value of (-32.84 ± 3.42) mV) on cell viability was also assessed, in order to investigate on the cytotoxicity of liposomal vectors. In particular, the two cell lines were treated with free 5-FU, 5-FU/LPs and anti-FZD10/5-FU/LPs at drug concentrations ranging from 1 to 10 μM (in the range from 5 to 50 μM, in terms of total lipid concentration for the liposomal formulations), at 24, 48, and 96 h. CoLo-205 and CaCo-2 cell viability is reported in Section 3.3. The viability of both colon cancer cell lines was always greater than 80% after their incubation with empty LPs, thus indicating very low toxicity in the lipid concentration range, at each tested time incubation (Figure 3, yellow bars). For CoLo-205 cells, at the lowest tested drug concentration values, namely 1 and 2 μM, the cell viability was only minimally reduced (always higher than 75%) within 96 h, when cells were incubated with free 5-FU (Figure 3A, blue bars). As compared to free 5-FU, the nontargeted LPs were found to exhibit an enhanced cytotoxic activity, for each tested time incubation, at a drug concentration of 2 μM (Figure 3, grey bars). Conversely, in the range between 3 and 10 μM, the effectiveness of free 5-FU in affecting the cell viability was time-dependent (Figure 3A, blue bars); the bare 5-FU/LPs induced a higher cytotoxic effect than free 5-FU by reducing the cell viability up to about 40% only within the first 24 h (Figure 3A, grey bars). In the case of anti-FZD10/5-FU/LPs, the cell-killing effects were always time-dependent from 24 to 96 h, for each tested drug concentration (Figure 3A, orange bars). The cell viability was always lower than 30% when the cells were treated with anti-FZD10/5-FU/LPs for 96 h, in the entire tested range of drug concentrations (Figure 3A, orange bars). At a 5-FU concentration of 2 μM, the use of anti-FZD10/5-FU/LPs significantly ($p < 0.001$ versus control) reduced the cell viability up to (42 ± 3) and $(28 \pm 8)\%$ at 48 and 96 h, while in the case of free 5-FU, only up to (74 ± 4) and $(73 \pm 10)\%$, thus resulting not statistically significant (Figure 3A, orange and blue bars). The cell viability recorded for nontargeted 5-FU/LPs was equal to (55.9 ± 6.6) and $(42.9 \pm 2.3)\%$ when cells were treated at drug concentration of 2 μM for 48 and 96 h, respectively, thus highlighting their less significant cytotoxic efficacy respect to targeted anti-FZD10/5-FU/LPs.

For CaCo-2 cells, the bare 5-FU/LPs exhibited a time-dependent reduction of cell viability ranging from approximately 60% to 40% over the 24 to 96 h, for all tested concentrations (Figure 3B, grey bars). When the cells were incubated with free drug at the lowest tested concentrations (1 and 2 μM), the cell viability was only minimally affected at 24 and 48 h; conversely, a substantial reduction ($p < 0.001$ versus control) up to $(38 \pm 8)\%$ in cell viability was recorded at 96 h (Figure 3B, blue bars). At the higher explored drug concentrations (3–10 μM), the free 5-FU exhibited a significant cytotoxic activity ($p < 0.001$ versus control) not only at 96, but also at 48 h (Figure 3B, blue bars). Cells exposure to anti-FZD10/5-FU/LPs induced a relevant cell-killing effect already within 24 h, throughout the drug concentrations range (Figure 3B, orange bars). Cell treatment with the engineered LPs significantly lowered ($p < 0.001$ versus control) the cell viability up to (40 ± 4) and $(37 \pm 6)\%$ at 24 h, and up to (13 ± 2) and $(16 \pm 8)\%$ at 96 h, at the tested drug concentrations equal to 1 and 2 μM, respectively. (Figure 3B, orange bars).

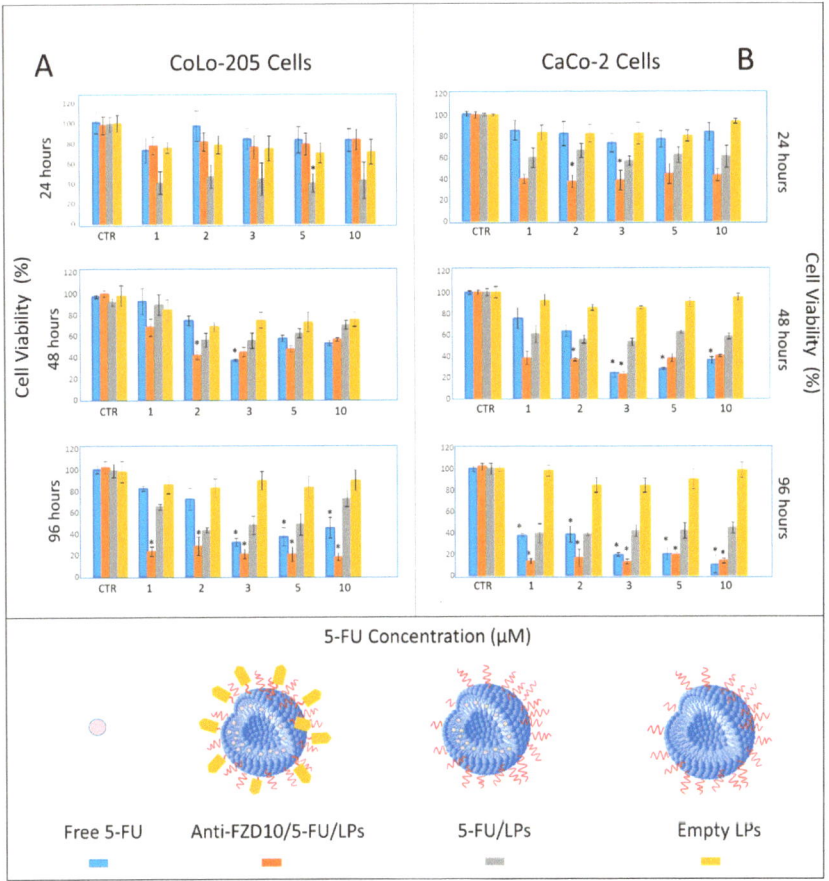

Figure 3. Cell viability, evaluated by MTS cell proliferation assay, of CoLo-205 (**A**) and CaCo-2 (**B**) cells after incubation with free 5-FU, 5-FU/LPs, anti-FZD10/5-FU/LPs and empty LPs at 5-FU concentrations ranging from 1 to 10 µM (from 5 to 50 µM in terms of total lipid concentration) for 24, 48 and 96 h. For each cell line, control was untreated cells. The experiments were conducted in triplicate. (*) $p < 0.001$ versus control.

3.3. Effects of Formulated Liposomes on the Cell Morphology

Morphological changes induced on CoLo-205 and CaCo-2 cells by exposure to anti-FZD10/5-FU/LPs and 5-FU/LPs (drug concentration of 2 µM) at 6, 24 and 96 h were observed at FE-SEM (Figures 4 and 5).

In Figure S4 (Supplementary Materials), the pristine morphology of the untreated CaCo-2 and CoLo-205 cells was shown. The two cell lines appeared adherent, CaCo-2 cells are completely flat, while the CoLo-205 cells present a protruding spherical nucleus in the center of the flat cell body (Figure S4). FE-SEM analysis performed on both cell lines after treatment with 5-FU/LPs and anti-FZD10/5-FU/LPs for 6 h revealed that, the two liposomal formulations induced rounding of the cells, that acquired a spindle-shaped morphology as compared to the corresponding controls, with an increased number of pseudopodia due to the stress induced by incubation with 5-FU/LPs or anti-FZD10/5-FU/LPs (Figure 4A,A1,B,B1, and Figure 5A,A1,B,B1).

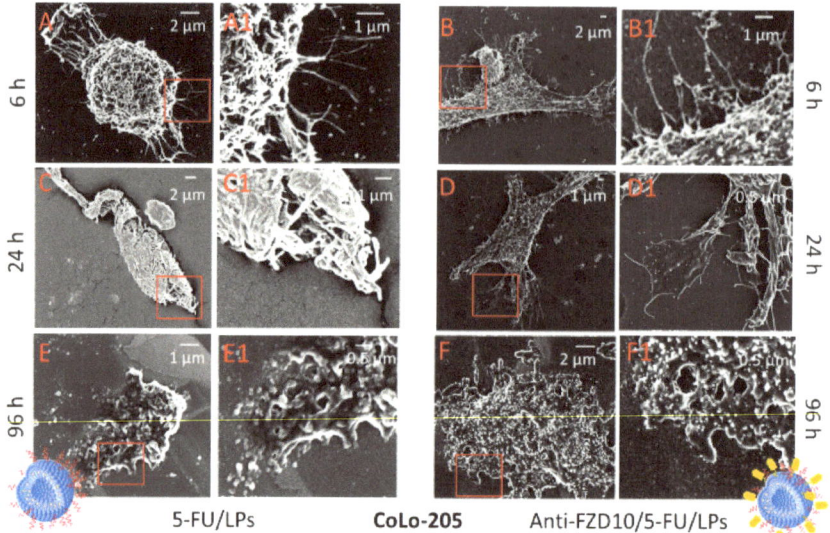

Figure 4. (FE-SEM) Representative field emission scanning electron microscopy micrographs(EHT) extra-high tension (EHT = 3.00 kV) and their corresponding close-up details at higher magnification of CoLo-205 cells after treatment with 5-FU/LPs (**A,A1,C,C1,E,E1**) and anti-FZD10/5-FU/LPs (**B,B1,D,D1,F,F1**) for 6, 24 and 96 h. 5-FU concentration: 2 µM.

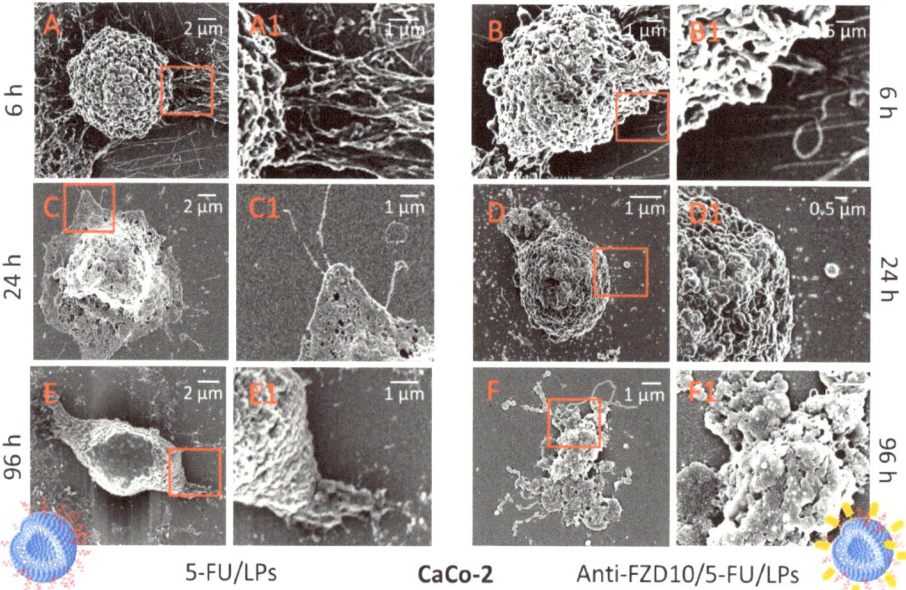

Figure 5. Representative FE-SEM micrographs (EHT = 3.00 kV) and their corresponding close-up details at higher magnification of CaCo-2 cells after treatment with 5-FU/LPs (**A,A1,C,C1,E,E1**) and anti-FZD10/5-FU/LPs (**B,B1,D,D1,F,F1**) for 6, 24 and 96 h. 5-FU concentration: 2 µM.

In the case of CoLo-205 cells, the 5-FU/LPs produced a more evident toxic effect compared to the anti-FZD10/5-FU/LPs after 24 h of incubation, revealing significant alterations in cell morphology and a strongly reduced number of pseudopodia (Figure 4C,C1,D,D1). Conversely, in the case of CaCo-2 cells, the anti-FZD10/5-FU/LPs mostly affected the cell morphology as compared to 5-FU/LPs. Indeed, CaCo-2 cell still resulted adherent to the substrate after treatment with the nontargeted liposomal formulations for 24 h (Figure 5C,C1,D,D1).

After 96 h exposure to both the liposomal formulations, CoLo-205 cells appear dead (Figure 4E,E1,F,F1), since no living cell structures were observed. The effectiveness of anti-FZD10/5-FU/LPs was also detectable on CaCo-2 cells at 96 h, since only cell fragments can be observed; conversely, a kind of morphology was still detected when CaCo-2 cells were treated with 5-FU/LPs for 96 h (Figure 5E,E1,F,F1).

3.4. Effectiveness of the Formulated Liposomes on Cell Migration

The effect of the two formulated LPs on cell motility was assessed by performing the scratch assay on CoLo-205 and CaCo-2 cells. After creating the mechanical scratch (marked in red) on confluent cell monolayers, the cells were incubated with exogenous added free 5-FU, 5-FU/LPs or anti-FZD10 /5-FU/LPs (drug concentration 2 µM) and the effects were monitored at 0, 24 and 48 h (Figure 6A,B). CoLo-205 cells were able to wholly rescue the wound already within 24 h (Figure 6A), while for the nonmetastatic, untreated CaCo-2 cells, complete closure of the scratched area was observed within 48 h (Figure 6B). In the case of CoLo-205 cells, free 5-FU or 5-FU/LPs decreased cell migration after 24 h, although the widths of the injuries were still detectable. At 48 h, the scratched area appeared strongly reduced. Conversely, incubation with anti-FZD10/5-FU/LPs produced a substantial inhibition of cell migration in the wound regions; indeed, the scratched area was only partially reduced but still observable at both 24 and 48 h (Figure 6A). The results obtained by the scratch assay performed on CaCo-2 cells demonstrated a notable inhibition effect of 5-FU, free or encapsulated in the LPs, on cell migration (Figure 6B). Indeed, a considerable decrease of cell migration was observed, as compared with control cells, when the cells were exposed to the free 5-FU, although the area of injury appeared partially reduced at 24 and 48 h. In the case of 5-FU/LPs, CaCo-2 cells were able to partially migrate in the scratched area at 24 h, but the injury region was no longer recognizable at 48 h, since the cells appeared to be dead. The effect of anti-FZD10/5-FU/LPs on the migration and viability of CaCo-2 cells was more pronounced than that of nontargeted LPs; indeed, cell migration did not occur and death of the cells was already observed at 24 h. Remarkably, almost all the cells appeared to be dead at 48 h (Figure 6B).

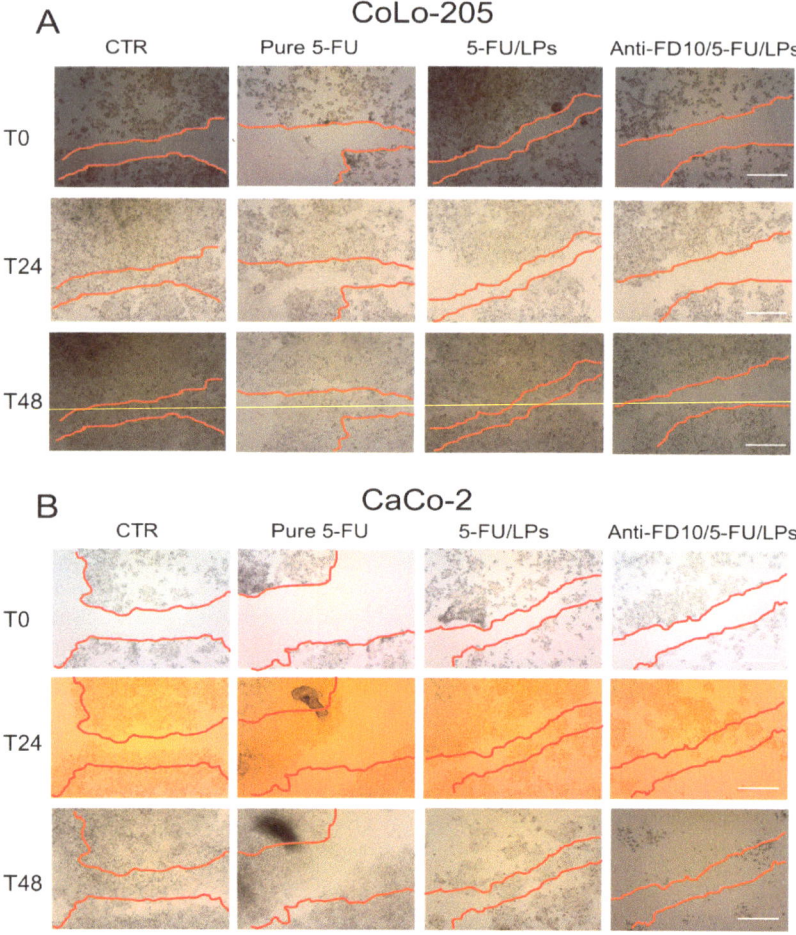

Figure 6. Qualitative analysis of collective CoLo-205 (**A**) and CaCo-2 (**B**) cell migration by in vitro scratch assay. Representative photomicrographs of scratch-wound closure of cells treated with free 5-FU, 5-FU/LPs or anti-FZD10/5-FU/LPs at different time points (0, 24 and 48 h). 5-FU concentration: 2 µM. CTR: untreated cells. Red lines represent the edges of the scratched areas. Scale bar: 200 µm.

3.5. Effectiveness of Formulated LPs on Vimentin and Phospho-Paxillin Cytoskeletal Proteins

The expression level of two specific proteins, namely vimentin and phospho-paxillin, involved in cell stability and cell adhesion, respectively, was assessed by immunofluorescence imaging in both fixed CoLo-204 and CaCo-2 cells, after incubation with 5-FU, 5-FU/LPs or anti-FZD10/5-FU/LPs at 24 and 48 h. The tested 5-FU concentration was 2 µM (Figure 7). The confocal microscopy investigation performed on CoLo-205 cells treated with free 5-FU (Figure 7A–C) indicated a significant, time-dependent reduction of vimentin expression (green labeled), being (36.8 ± 7.5)% and (48.6 ± 11.2)% the percentage ratio (compared to the control) of mean fluorescence intensity for the cells treated at 24 and 48 h, respectively ($p < 0.001$ versus control). Conversely, in the case of phosphor-paxillin (red labeled), the percentage ratio of fluorescence intensity was firstly increased, at 24 h ((139.1 ± 19.3)% and then reduced to (69.3 ± 7.4)% at 48 h ($p < 0.001$ versus control).

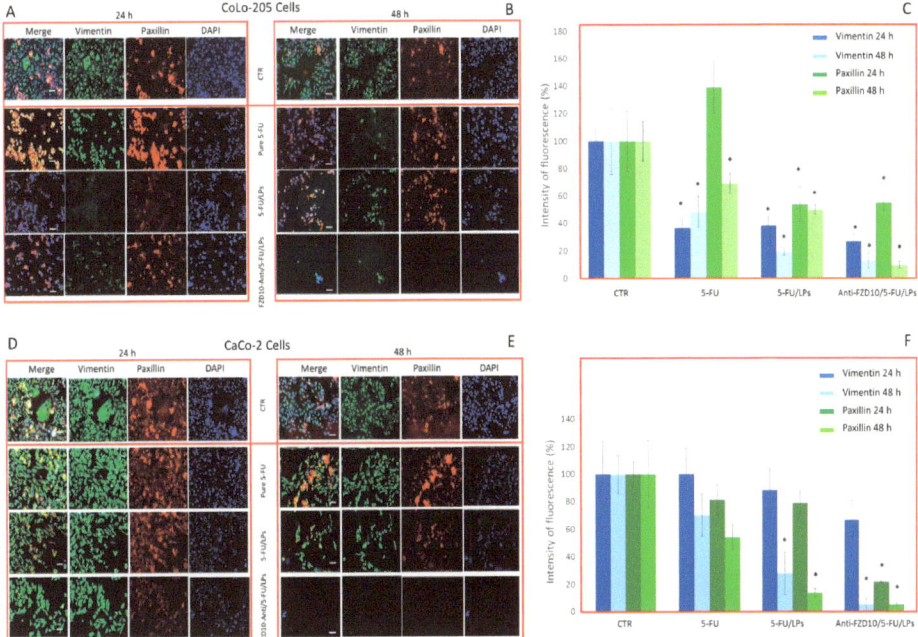

Figure 7. Detection and quantification of vimentin and phospho-paxillin (red) by immunofluorescence confocal microscopy in fixed CoLo-205 (**A–C**) and CaCo-2 cells (**D–F**), after cells incubation with free 5-FU, 5-FU/LPs or anti-FZD10/5-FU/LPs at 24 and 48 h. 5-FU concentration: 2 µM. CTR: untreated cells. Green channel: labeled vimentin, red channel: labeled phospho-paxillin, blue channel: labeled nuclei (DAPI), and corresponding overlay (Merge). Scale bar: 50 µm. (*) $p < 0.001$ versus control (CRT).

The confocal images of CoLo-205 cells after treatment with 5-FU/LPs or anti-FZD10/5-FU/LPs show that a significant reduction ($p < 0.001$ versus control) of the expression level of each investigated protein was always observed at both cell incubation times. Indeed, in the case of vimentin, the percentage ratios of mean fluorescence intensity were equal to (38.4 ± 6.3)% and (26.9 ± 4.9)% at 24 h and (19.3 ± 2.4)% and (12.8 ± 5.5)% at 48 h, for cells treated with 5-FU/LPs or anti-FZD10/5-FU/LPs, respectively; in the case of phospho-paxillin, the corresponding percentage ratios were (53.9 ± 12.7)% and (55.0 ± 5.5)% at 24 h and (49.9 ± 3.4)% and (9.7 ± 2.5)% at 48 h (Figure 7A–C). The immunofluorescence analysis carried out by confocal microscopy on CaCo-2 cells treated with free 5-FU (Figure 7D–F) demonstrated that although the expression levels of vimentin and phospho-paxillin decreased in a time-dependent manner, the observed decreases of fluorescent signals were not significant. On the contrary, a significant decrease ($p < 0.001$ versus control) in the expression levels of vimentin and phospho-paxillin was observed when CaCo-2 cells were incubated with 5-FU/LPs for 48 h. The percentage ratio of mean fluorescence intensity was found to be (28.2 ± 15.2)% and (14.0 ± 3.5)% for vimentin and phospho-paxillin, respectively (Figure 7D–F). A significant ($p < 0.001$ versus control), detectable decrease in the expression level of phospho-paxillin was observed in CaCo-2 cells treated with anti-FZD10/5-FU/LPs for 24 and 48 h (percentage ratio of mean fluorescence intensity (21.7 ± 0.5)% and (5.3 ± 0.7)% at 24 and 48 h, respectively), while in the case of vimentin, a significant difference in the expression level, compared to the control ($p < 0.001$ versus control), was recorded only at 48 h (percentage ratio of mean fluorescence intensity (5.2 ± 4.6)%, (Figure 7D–F)). For both cell lines, the reductions in fluorescence intensity observed for the blue-stained cell nuclei, compared to the corresponding control cells, when the cells were treated with the two formulated LPs or free 5-FU at 24 and 48 h, were in agreement with the results obtained at the cell viability assay (Figure 3).

4. Discussion

Currently, 5-FU is one of the first-line chemotherapeutic agents for the treatment of advanced CRC. It is a typical antimetabolite with a strong time-dependent mode of action [27]. Despite its therapeutic efficacy, 5-FU has some limitations, mainly tumor cell resistance and a short biological half-life. Consequently, multiple administrations of high doses, of which only a very low percentage reaches the tumor area, are required, and severe systemic (gastrointestinal, hematological, cardiac, and dermatological) toxicities occur. Indeed, 5-FU has been demonstrated to induce cardiotoxicity, followed by thrombosis, and alterations of the antioxidant defense capacities in myocardial tissues, with increases in the cardiac enzymes superoxide dismutase and glutathione peroxidase [28,29]. Therefore, the development of new delivery methods that selectively target the abnormal colonic mucosa could offer several benefits to patients affected by advanced CRC [30–32]. In this perspective, several nanovectors, such as lipid-based nanoformulations, nanogels, polymer-based micro/nanoparticles, carbon nanotubes and polysaccharides-based nanosystems have been designed to achieve an effective delivery of cytotoxic drugs and a selective targeting of CRC sites [33,34]. Among them, targeted LPs have been demonstrated to exhibit an enhanced antitumor activity on CRC cells as compared to nontargeted counterparts. Folate, mannose and integrin receptors, overexpressed on CRC cells, are the main targets that have been explored for the development of CRC-targeted LPs [33]. Specifically for 5-FU, immune-LPs conjugated with proper folate or integrinβ6 antibodies have been proposed for CRC treatment [11,35,36]. Furthermore, O. Udofot et al. reported a study of the cytotoxic effect of 5-FU loaded pH-sensitive LPs on CRC cell lines; in this case, the LPs were conjugated with a selected anti-EGFR antibody [37]. In this study, PEG-functionalized 5-FU loaded LPs were covalently conjugated with a specific antibody able to recognize and bind the FZD10 surface cell receptor, to create innovative immuno-LPs that could potentially be useful for targeted therapy of CRC. In particular, FZD10 targeted and nontargeted LPs were prepared and characterized by complementary optical and morphological techniques. The average hydrodynamic diameter values obtained by DLS resulted lower than 200 nm for both formulated LPs. It is well known in literature that LPs of sizes between 100 and 300 mn are able to extravasate and localize in the tumor tissue, exploiting the EPR effect [38]. ζ-potential measurements proved that LPs exhibited a high negative surface charge, that further increased after LPs conjugation with FZD10 antibody, together with values of less than−30 mV for both formulated LPs, thus indicating their high colloidal stability in aqueous media and suggesting a good cell internalization capacity of the vesicles [39]. The encapsulation efficiency values achieved for 5-FU/LPs and anti-FZD10/5-FU/LPs are in agreement with the data already reported in the literature concerning other 5-FU encapsulating LPs [40].

The in vitro studies were performed on two selected CRC cell lines, namely CaCo-2 and CoLo-205. Preliminarily, quantitative and qualitative evaluation of the cellular FZD10 expression in CaCo-2 and CoLo-205 cells was made by immunoblotting and immunofluorescence, respectively, to validate the use of the FZD10 engineered LPs for targeted treatment of CRC (see Supplementary Materials). Furthermore, previous data had demonstrated the abundance of expression of FZD10 protein on CRC tissues, especially at late stages and in metastatic tissues [18]. Cell viability evaluation was conducted by testing the drug concentrations in the range of clinically relevant concentrations of 5-FU, previously reported in the literature and identified by performing clinical studies on pharmacokinetic modulating chemotherapy. E, Ojima et al. reported the range between 0.1 and 10 µM, while Beumer, J.H. et al. the range between 0.6 and 13 µM [41,42]. The two ranges slightly differ from each other, owing to different techniques used for the drug detection, modality of exposure to drug and substantial interindividual pharmacokinetic variability [42,43]. The results indicated that the cytotoxic activity of 5-FU is significantly enhanced when delivered by anti-FZD10/5-FU/LPs at the lowest tested drug concentrations (1 and 2 µM), as compared not only to the free drug but also to the nontargeted LPs. Therefore, at the lowest tested drug concentrations, the data obtained suggest that a more controlled drug release and higher cell accumulation of the targeted LPs occurred, likely due to their improved cell-internalization ability, exploiting not only passive transport but also antibody-receptor binding, allowing the use of lower 5-FU concentrations, and achieving a higher expected performance in terms of reduced toxicity effects. Therefore, the 5-FU concentration of 2 µM was further considered for the in vitro studies.

The response induced on cell morphology after cell treatment with the two formulated LPs was investigated by means of the FE-SEM technique, that produces detailed images of a whole cell and ensures the visualization of several morphological details of a single cell (namely size, shape, nuclear/cytoplasmic ratio, number of pseudopodia and cell adherence), thus enabling any cell morphological changes induced by cell treatment with a specific pharmacological agent to be evaluated [27]. FE-SEM investigation visualized the several, severe time-dependent effects induced on the morphology and consequent viability of CaCo-2 and CoLo-205 cells, after treatment with 5-FU/LPs or anti-FZD10/5-FU/LPs. CoLo-205 cells appeared dead at 96 h treatment with both the formulated LPs, while, in the case of CaCo-2 cells, the anti-FZD10/5-FU/LPs exhibited a more efficacious cytotoxic activity than the 5-FU/LPs at 96 h, thus corroborating the data shown by MTS assay.

We also investigated the effect of the two formulated LPs on cell migration, a key factor in the malignant spread of cancer. For the metastatic CoLo-205 cells, the anti-FZD10/5-FU/LPs were found to induce a more significant inhibition of cell migration in the test area than the free 5-FU and 5-FU/LPs, the wound regions being only partially reduced at both 24 and, remarkably, at 48 h. The inhibition effect on migration of nonmetastatic CaCo-2 cells after treatment with 5-FU, free or embedded in the LPs, resulted more evident compared to CoLo-205 cells. Once again, the anti-FZD10/5-FU/LPs more consistently inhibited the cell migration compared to the free 5-FU and nontargeted LPs at 24 and 48 h treatment. Furthermore, the death of most of the cells was observed at 48 h.

Immunofluorescence analysis, performed on both fixed cell lines after incubation with free 5-FU, 5-FU/LPs or FZD10-anti/5-FU/LPs, was used to monitor the expression level of two proteins, namely vimentin and phospho-paxillin. The role of vimentin and phospho-paxillin as active players in cell focal adhesion and migration, as well as in pathological conditions, including cancer development and metastasis, is widely discussed in literature. The two proteins are found to be overexpressed in several cancer tissues and metastatic cancer cells, including also CRC, especially during adhesion and distant metastases formation [44–46]. High expression levels of both the vimentin and paxillin have been found to significantly contribute both to the malignancy and drug-resistance of CRC [47–49]. Consequently, the downregulation of the expression levels of the two proteins was found to be related to a reduction of metastatic development [50–53]. The investigation proved the time-dependent reduction in the fluorescence intensity of the vimentin and phospho-paxillin, confirming the effective activity of 5-FU on the inhibition of CRC cell proliferation [54]. The immunofluorescence analysis also indicated an enhanced toxic effect of 5-FU, when incorporated in the formulated LPs. In particular, the anti-FZD10/5-FU/LPs more consistently lowered the expression of the two proteins at 48 h in the case of CoLo-205, and already at 24 h treatment in CaCo-2 cells.

The overall results suggest that, at the lowest tested drug concentrations, the cytotoxic activity of targeted LPs was enhanced, as compared to free 5-Fu and nontargeted LPs. Although further studies are planned to investigate the specific mechanisms involved in the cell uptake, our preliminary findings are encouraging to validate the FZD10 protein as a novel, effective target for CRC. We expect that in future clinical applications, the use of anti-FZD10/5-FU/LPs could allow a reduction of the 5-FU doses administered, while maximizing the therapeutic efficacy. A new, promising scenario for targeted CRC therapy may be envisaged: administration of the anti-FZD10/5-FU/LPs here proposed, encapsulated in softgel capsules or suppositories, could provide an effective route for oral or rectal delivery, as employed for other compounds that need to reach the digestive canal, resisting gastric acids [55].

Supplementary Materials: The following are available online at http://www.mdpi.com/1999-4923/12/7/650/s1, Figure S1: UV-Vis absorption spectrum of FZD10-anti/5-FU/LPs before (A) and after (B) incubation with Alexa Fluor 555-conjugated secondary antibody, Figure S2: In vitro release of 5-FU from anti-FZD10/5-FU/LPs as a function of time, at 37 °C. Data are reported as mean value (±standard deviation) calculated on three replicates, Figure S3: (A) Representative Western blotting of FZD10 and GAPDH housekeeping protein and (A1) semi-quantitative estimation, by densitometry analysis of protein bands, of relative FZD10 expression levels in untreated HCEC-1CT,

CaCo-2 and CoLo-205 cells, after loading the same total protein content (20 µg). For the semiquantitative analysis, FZD10 bands are evaluated after normalization with the corresponding housekeeping GAPDH protein band, for each sample. (*) $p < 0.001$ versus negative control (HCEC-1CT cells). (B) Detection of FZD10 by immunofluorescence confocal microscopy in fixed HCEC-1CT, CaCo-2 and CoLo-205 cells. Blue channel: nuclei; green or red channel: labeled FZD10 and corresponding overlay. Scale bar 50 µm, Figure S4: Representative FE-SEM micrographs (EHT = 3.00 kV) of untreated CoLo-205 (A) and CaCo-2 (B) cells.

Author Contributions: Conceptualization, M.P.S.; methodology, M.P.S., A.C., E.F.; validation, E.F., N.D. (Nicoletta Depalo), and V.L.; formal analysis, N.D. (Nicoletta Depalo), A.C., E.F., M.P.S.; investigation, M.P.S., A.C., E.F., N.D. (Nicoletta Depalo); resources, G.G. (Giampietro Gasparini), G.G. (Gianluigi Giannelli) and N.D. (Nunzio Denora); data curation, M.P.S., N.D. (Nicoletta Depalo), and E.F.; writing—original draft preparation, M.P.S. and N.D. (Nicoletta Depalo); writing—review and editing, M.P.S., N.D.(Nicoletta Depalo), G.G. (Giampietro Gasparini) and G.G. (Gianluigi Giannelli); visualization, all authors; supervision, G.G. (Giampietro Gasparini) and G.G. (Gianluigi Giannelli); project administration, G.G. (Giampietro Gasparini) and G.G. (Gianluigi Giannelli); funding acquisition, G.G. (Giampietro Gasparini) and G.G. (Gianluigi Giannelli). All authors have read and agreed to the published version of the manuscript.

Funding: This research received no external funding.

Acknowledgments: We are thankful to Babette Pragnell (Pragnell M.V., B.A) for English revision.

Conflicts of Interest: The authors declare no conflict of interest.

References

1. Global Burden of Disease Cancer Collaboration; Fitzmaurice, C.; Allen, C.; Barber, R.M.; Barregard, L.; Bhutta, Z.A.; Brenner, H.; Dicker, D.J.; Chimed-Orchir, O.; Dandona, R.; et al. Global, regional, and national cancer incidence, mortality, years of life lost, years lived with disability, and disability adjusted life-years for 32 cancer groups, 1990 to 2015. *JAMA Oncol.* **2017**, *3*, 524–548. [PubMed]
2. Arias, J.L. Novel strategies to improve the anticancer action of 5-fluorouracil by using drug delivery systems. *Molecules* **2008**, *13*, 2340–2369. [CrossRef] [PubMed]
3. Zhang, N.; Yin, Y.; Xu, S.J.; Chen, W.S. 5-Fluorouracil: Mechanisms of resistance and reversal strategies. *Molecules* **2008**, *13*, 1551–1569. [CrossRef] [PubMed]
4. Larsson, P.A.; Carlsson, G.; Gustavsson, B.; Graf, W.; Glimelius, B. Different intravenous administration techniques for 5-fluorouracil. Pharmacokinetics and pharmacodynamic effects. *Acta. Oncol.* **1996**, *35*, 207–212. [CrossRef]
5. Davis, M.E.; Chen, Z.G.; Shin, D.M. Nanoparticle therapeutics: An emerging treatment modality for cancer. *Nat. Rev. Drug Discov.* **2008**, *7*, 771–782. [CrossRef]
6. Gentile, E.; Cilurzo, F.; Di Marzio, L.; Carafa, M.; Ventura, C.A.; Wolfram, J.; Paolino, D.; Celia, C. Liposomal chemotherapeutics. *Future Oncol.* **2013**, *9*, 1849–1859. [CrossRef]
7. Gupta, A.S.; Kshirsagar, S.J.; Bhalekar, M.R.; Saldanha, T. Design and development of liposomes for colon targeted drug delivery. *J. Drug Target.* **2013**, *21*, 146–160. [CrossRef] [PubMed]
8. Barea, M.J.; Jenkins, M.J.; Gaber, M.H.; Bridson, R.H. Evaluation of liposomes coated with a pH responsive polymer. *Int. J. Pharm.* **2010**, *402*, 89–94. [CrossRef]
9. Li, Y.; Zhu, C. Mechanism of hepatic targeting via oral administration of DSPE-PEG-cholic acid-modified nanoliposomes. *Int. J. Nanomedicine* **2017**, *12*, 1673–1684. [CrossRef]
10. Janeczek, A.A.; Scarpa, E.; Horrocks, M.H.; Tare, R.S.; Rowland, C.A.; Jenner, D.; Newman, T.A.; Oreffo, R.O.; Lee, S.F.; Evans, N.D. PEGylated liposomes associate with Wnt3A protein and expand putative stem cells in human bone marrow populations. *Nanomedicine* **2017**, *12*, 845–863. [CrossRef]
11. Handali, S.; Moghimipour, E.; Rezaei, M.; Ramezani, Z.; Kouchak, M.; Amini, M.; Ahmadi, K.; Sadegh, A.; Farid, S.; Dorkoosh, A. A novel 5-Fluorouracil targeted delivery to colon cancer using folic acid conjugated liposomes. *Biomed. Pharmacother.* **2018**, *108*, 1259–1273. [CrossRef] [PubMed]
12. Hua, S. Orally administered liposomal formulations for colon targeted drug delivered. *Front. Pharmacol.* **2014**, *5*, 138. [CrossRef] [PubMed]
13. Song, L.; Fan, Z.; Jun, N.; Benjia, L.; Zequn, L.; Xilong, W.; Zhongming, J.; Yong, H.; Xiaohong, W.; Kai, C.; et al. Tumor specific delivery and therapy mediate by integrin β6-target immunoliposomes for β6-siRNA in colon carcinoma. *Oncotarget* **2016**, *7*, 85163–85175. [CrossRef] [PubMed]
14. Alavizadeh, S.H.; Soltani, F.; Ramezani, M. Recent advances in immunoliposome-based cancer therapy. *Curr. Pharmacol. Rep.* **2016**, *2*, 129–141. [CrossRef]

15. Wong, S.C.C.; He, C.W.; Chan, C.M.L.; Chan, A.K.C.; Wong, H.T.; Cheung, M.T.; Luk, L.L.Y.; Au, T.C.C.; Chiu, M.K.; Ma, B.B.T.; et al. Clinical significance of frizzled homolog 3 protein in colorectal cancer patients. *PLoS ONE* **2013**, *8*, e79481. [CrossRef]
16. Ueno, K.; Hiura, M.; Suehiro, Y.; Hazama, S.; Hirata, H.; Oka, M.; Imai, K.; Dahiya, R.; Hinoda, Y. Frizzled-7 as a potential therapeutic target in colorectal cancer. *Neoplasia* **2008**, *10*, 697–705. [CrossRef]
17. Zeng, C.M.; Chen, Z.; Fu, L. Frizzled receptors as potential therapeutic targets in human cancers. *Int. J. Mol. Sci.* **2018**, *19*, 1543. [CrossRef]
18. Scavo, M.P.; Depalo, N.; Rizzi, F.; Ingrosso, C.; Fanizza, E.; Chieti, A.; Messa, C.; Denora, N.; Laquintana, V.; Striccoli, M.; et al. FZD10 carried by exosomes sustains cancer cell proliferation. *Cells* **2019**, *8*, 777. [CrossRef]
19. Scavo, M.P.; Cigliano, A.; Depalo, N.; Fanizza, E.; Bianco, M.G.; Denora, N.; Laquintana, V.; Curri, M.L.; Lorusso, D.; Lotesoriere, C.; et al. Frizzled-10 extracellular vesicles plasma concentration are associated with tumoral progression in patients with colorectal and gastric cancer. *Int. J. Oncol.* **2019**. [CrossRef]
20. Scavo, M.P.; Depalo, N.; Tutino, V.; De Nunzio, V.; Ingrosso, C.; Rizzi, F.; Notarnicola, M.; Curri, M.L.; Giannelli, G. Exosomes for diagnosis and therapy in gastrointestinal cancers. *Int. J. Mol. Sci.* **2020**, *21*, 367. [CrossRef]
21. Nagayama, S.; Yamada, E.; Kohno, Y.; Aoyama, T.; Fukukawa, C.; Kubo, H.; Watanabe, G.; Katagiri, T.; Nakamura, Y.; Sakai, Y.; et al. Inverse correlation of the up-regulation of FZD10 expression and the activation of beta-catenin in synchronous colorectal tumors. *Cancer Sci.* **2009**, *100*, 405–412. [CrossRef] [PubMed]
22. Nagayama, S.; Fukukawa, C.; Katagiri, T.; Okamoto, T.; Aoyama, T.; Oyaizu, N.; Imamura, M.; Toguchida, J.; Nakamura, Y. Therapeutic potential of antibodies against FZD10, a cell-surface protein, for synovial sarcomas. *Oncogene* **2005**, *24*, 6201–6212. [CrossRef] [PubMed]
23. Scavo, M.P.; Fucci, L.; Caldarola, L.; Mangia, A.; Azzariti, A.; Simone, G.; Gasparini, G.; Krol, S. Frizzled-10 and cancer progression. Is it a new prognostic marker? *Oncotarget* **2017**, *9*, 824–830. [PubMed]
24. Depalo, N.; Fanizza, E.; Vischio, F.; Denora, N.; Laquintana, V.; Cutrignelli, A.; Striccoli, M.; Giannelli, G.; Agostiano, A.; Curri, M.L.; et al. Imaging modification of colon carcinoma cells exposed to lipid based nanovectors for drug delivery: A scanning electron microscopy investigation. *RSC Adv.* **2019**, *9*, 21810. [CrossRef]
25. Liang, C.C.; Park, A.Y.; Guan, J.L. In a vitro scratch assay: A convenient and inexpensive method for analysis of cell migration in vitro. *Nature Protocols.* **2007**, *2*, 329–333. [CrossRef] [PubMed]
26. Tutino, V.; Gigante, I.; Scavo, M.P.; Refolo, M.G.; De Nunzio, V.; Milella, R.A.; Caruso, M.G.; Notarnicola, M. Stearoyl-CoA Desaturase-1 Enzyme inhibition by grape skin extracts affects membrane fluidity in human colon cancer cell lines. *Nutrients* **2020**, *12*, 683. [CrossRef]
27. Ojima, E.; Inoue, Y.; Watanabe, H.; Hiro, J.; Toiyama, Y.; Miki, C.; Kusunoki, M. The optimal schedule for 5-fluorouracil radiosensitization in colon cancer cell lines. *Oncolo. Rep.* **2006**, *16*, 1085. [CrossRef]
28. Dushinsky, R.; Pleven, E.; Heidelberger, C. The synthesis of 5-fluoropyrimidines. *J. Am. Chem. Soc.* **1957**, *79*, 4559–4560. [CrossRef]
29. Durak, I.; Karaayvaz, M.; Kavutcu, M.; Cimen, M.Y.; Kaçmaz, M.; Büyükkoçak, S.; Oztürk, H.S.J. Reduced antioxidant defense capacity in myocardial tissue from guinea pigs treated with 5-fluorouracil. *J. Toxicol. Environ. Health.* **2000**, *59*, 585–589.
30. Tsibiribi, P.; Bui-Xuan, C.; Bui-Xuan, B.; Lombard-Bohas, C.; Duperret, S.; Belkhiria, M.; Tabib, A.; Maujean, G.; Descotes, J.; Timour, Q. Cardiac lesions induced by 5-fluorouracil in the rabbit. *Hum. Exp. Toxicol.* **2006**, *25*, 305–309. [CrossRef]
31. Brower, V. Cardiotoxicity debated for anthracyclines and trastuzumab in breast cancer. *J. Natl. Cancer Inst.* **2013**, *105*, 835–836. [CrossRef]
32. Grover, S.; Leong, D.P.; Chakrabarty, A.; Joerg, L.; Kotasek, D.; Cheong, K.; Joshi, R.; Joseph, M.X.; De Pasquale, C.; Koczwara, B.; et al. Left and right ventricular effects of anthracycline and trastuzumab chemotherapy: A prospective study using novel cardiac imaging and biochemical markers. *Int. J. Cardiol.* **2013**, *168*, 5465–5467. [CrossRef]
33. Cardinale, D.; Bacchiani, G.; Beggiato, M.; Colombo, A.; Cipolla, C.M. Strategies to prevent and treat cardiovascular risk in cancer patients. *Semin. Oncol.* **2013**, *40*, 186–198. [CrossRef]
34. Lee, S.H.; Bajracharya, R.; Min, J.Y.; Han, J.W.; Park, B.J.; Han, H.K. Strategic approaches for colon targeted drug delivery: An overview of recent advancements. *Pharmaceutics* **2020**, *12*, 68. [CrossRef]

35. Tiwari, A.; Saraf, S.; Jain, A.; Panda, P.K.; Verma, A.; Jain, S.K. Basics to Advances in Nanotherapy of colorectal cancer. *Drug Deliv. Transl. Res.* **2020**, *10*, 319–338. [CrossRef]
36. Le, V.M.; Nho, T.D.T.; Ly, H.T.; Vo, T.S.; Nguyen, H.D.; Phung, T.T.H.; Zou, A.; Liu, J. Enhanced anticancer efficacy and tumor targeting through folate-PEG modified nanoliposome loaded with 5-fluorouracil. *Adv. Nat. Sci. Nanosci. Nanotechnol.* **2017**, *8*. [CrossRef]
37. Liang, B.; Shahbaz, M.; Wang, Y.; Gao, H.; Fang, R.; Niu, Z.; Liu, S.; Wang, B.; Sun, Q.; Niu, W.; et al. Integrinβ6-targeted immunoliposomes mediate tumor-specific drug delivery and enhance therapeutic efficacy in colon carcinoma. *Clin. Cancer Res.* **2015**, *21*, 1183–1195. [CrossRef]
38. Udofot, O.; Affram, K.; Israel, B.; Agyare, E. Cytotoxicity of 5-fluorouracil-loaded pH-sensitive liposomal nanoparticles in colorectal cancer cell lines. *Integr. Cancer Sci. Ther.* **2015**, *2*, 245–252. [CrossRef]
39. Lopalco, A.; Cutrignelli, A.; Denora, N.; Lopedota, A.; Franco, M.; Laquintana, V. Transferrin functionalized liposomes loading dopamine HCl: Development and permeability studies across an in vitro model of human blood-brain barrier. *Nanomaterials* **2018**, *8*, 178. [CrossRef]
40. Maruyama, K. Intracellular targeting delivery of liposomal drugs to solid tumors based on EPR effects. *Adv. Drug Delivery Rev.* **2011**, *63*, 161–169. [CrossRef]
41. Kjellström, J.; Kjellén, E.; Johnsson, A. In vitro radiosensitization by oxaliplatin and 5-fluorouracil in a human colon cancer cell line. *Acta Oncol.* **2005**, *44*, 687–693. [CrossRef] [PubMed]
42. Beumer, J.H.; Boisdron-Celle, M.; Clarke, W.; Courtney, J.B.; Egorin, M.J.; Gamelin, E.; Harney, R.L.; Hammett-Stabler, C.; Lepp, S.; Li, Y.; et al. Multicenter evaluation of a novel nanoparticle immunoassay for 5-fluorouracil on the olympus au400 analyzer. *Ther. Drug Monit.* **2009**, *31*, 688–694. [CrossRef] [PubMed]
43. Gamelin, E.; Delva, R.; Jacob, J.; Merrouche, Y.; Raoul, J.L.; Pezet, D.; Dorval, E.; Piot, G.; Morel, A.; Boisdron-Celle, M. Individual fluorouracil dose adjustment based on pharmacokinetic follow-up compared with conventional dosage: Results of a multicenter randomized trial of patients with metastatic colorectal cancer. *J. Clin. Oncol.* **2008**, *26*, 2099–2105. [CrossRef] [PubMed]
44. López-Colomé, A.M.; Lee-Rivera, I.; Benavides-Hidalgo, R. Paxillin: A crossroad in pathological cell migration. *J. Hematol. Oncol.* **2017**, *10*, 50. [CrossRef]
45. Danielsson, F.; Peterson, M.K.; Araújo, H.C.; Lautenschläger, F.; Gad, A.K.B. Vimentin diversity in health and disease. *Cells* **2018**, *7*, 147. [CrossRef] [PubMed]
46. Wu, D.W.; Huang, C.C.; Chang, S.W.; Chen, T.H.; Lee, H. Bcl-2 stabilization by paxillin confers 5-fluorouracil resistance in colorectal cancer. *Cell Death Differ.* **2015**, *22*, 779–789. [CrossRef] [PubMed]
47. Lazarova, D.L.; Bordonaro, M. Vimentin, colon cancer progression and resistance to butyrate and other HDACis. *J. Cell. Mol. Med.* **2016**, *20*, 989. [CrossRef]
48. Huang, C.C.; Wu, D.W.; Lin, P.L.; Lee, H. Paxillin promotes colorectal tumor invasion and poor patient outcomes via ERK-mediated stabilization of Bcl-2 protein by phosphorylation at Serine 87. *Oncotarget* **2015**, *6*, 8698. [CrossRef]
49. Zhao, C.J.; Du, S.; Dang, X.; Gong, M. Expression of paxillin is correlated with clinical prognosis in colorectal cancer patients. *Med. Sci. Monit.* **2015**, *21*, 1989. [PubMed]
50. Nosova, A.S.; Koloskova, O.O.; Nikonova, A.A.; Simonova, S.A.; Smirnov, V.V.; Kudlay, D.; Khaito, M.R. Diversity of PEGylation methods of liposomes and their influence on RNA delivery. *MedChemComm* **2019**, *10*, 369–377. [CrossRef]
51. Thomas, A.M.; Kapanen, A.I.; Hare, J.I.; Ramsay, E.; Edwards, K.; Karlsson, G.; Bally, M.B. Development of a liposomal nanoparticle formulation of 5-fluorouracil for parenteral administration: Formulation design, pharmacokinetics and efficacy. *J. Control. Release.* **2011**, *150*, 212–219. [CrossRef] [PubMed]
52. Satelli, A.; Li, S. Vimentin in cancer and its potential as a molecular target for cancer therapy. *Cell Mol. Life Sci.* **2011**, *68*, 3033–3046. [CrossRef] [PubMed]
53. Liu, C.Y.; Lin, H.H.; Tang, M.J.; Wang, Y.K. Vimentin contributes to epithelial-mesenchymal transition cancer cell mechanics by mediating cytoskeletal organization and focal adhesion maturation. *Oncotarget* **2015**, *6*, 15966–15983. [CrossRef] [PubMed]

54. Downey, C.; Craig, D.H.; Basson, M.D. Pressure activates colon cancer cell adhesion via paxillin phosphorylation, Crk, Cas, and Rac1. *Cell Mol. Life Sci.* **2008**, *65*, 1446–1457. [CrossRef] [PubMed]
55. Maki, K.C.; Lawless, A.L.; Reeves, M.S.; Kelley, K.M.; Dicklin, M.R.; Jenks, B.H.; Shneyvas, E.; Brooks, J.R. Lipid effects of a dietary supplement softgel capsule containing plant sterols/stanols in primary hypercholesterolemia. *Nutrition* **2013**, *29*, 96–100. [CrossRef]

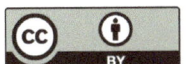

© 2020 by the authors. Licensee MDPI, Basel, Switzerland. This article is an open access article distributed under the terms and conditions of the Creative Commons Attribution (CC BY) license (http://creativecommons.org/licenses/by/4.0/).

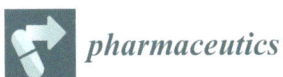

Article

N-Alkylisatin-Loaded Liposomes Target the Urokinase Plasminogen Activator System in Breast Cancer

Lisa Belfiore [1,2], Darren N. Saunders [3], Marie Ranson [1,2,4] and Kara L. Vine [1,2,4,*]

1. Illawarra Health and Medical Research Institute, Wollongong, NSW 2522, Australia; lisa.belfiore@inventia.life (L.B.); mranson@uow.edu.au (M.R.)
2. School of Chemistry and Molecular Bioscience, Faculty of Science Medicine and Health, University of Wollongong, Wollongong, NSW 2522, Australia
3. School of Medical Sciences, University of New South Wales, Sydney, NSW 2052, Australia; d.saunders@unsw.edu.au
4. CONCERT-Translational Cancer Research Centre, Sydney, NSW, Australia
* Correspondence: kara@uow.edu.au

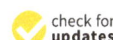

Received: 26 May 2020; Accepted: 3 July 2020; Published: 7 July 2020

Abstract: The urokinase plasminogen activator and its receptor (uPA/uPAR) are biomarkers for metastasis, especially in triple-negative breast cancer. We prepared anti-mitotic *N*-alkylisatin (*N*-AI)-loaded liposomes functionalized with the uPA/uPAR targeting ligand, plasminogen activator inhibitor type 2 (PAI-2/SerpinB2), and assessed liposome uptake in vitro and in vivo. Receptor-dependent uptake of PAI-2-functionalized liposomes was significantly higher in the uPA/uPAR overexpressing MDA-MB-231 breast cancer cell line relative to the low uPAR/uPAR expressing MCF-7 breast cancer cell line. Furthermore, *N*-AI cytotoxicity was enhanced in a receptor-dependent manner. In vivo, PAI-2 *N*-AI liposomes had a plasma half-life of 5.82 h and showed an increased accumulation at the primary tumor site in an orthotopic MDA-MB-231 BALB/c-Fox1nu/Ausb xenograft mouse model, relative to the non-functionalized liposomes, up to 6 h post-injection. These findings support the further development of *N*-AI-loaded PAI-2-functionalized liposomes for uPA/uPAR-positive breast cancer, especially against triple-negative breast cancer, for which the prognosis is poor and treatment is limited.

Keywords: *N*-alkylisatin; liposome; urokinase plasminogen activator; PAI-2; SerpinB2; breast cancer

1. Introduction

Breast cancer is the most common invasive cancer in women worldwide and remains a leading cause of cancer-related morbidity and mortality [1]. While overall survival has improved steadily over the last several decades, breast cancer still accounts for almost half a million deaths each year [2]. Numerous studies and clinical evidence indicate that the urokinase plasminogen activator system (uPAS) play a key role in breast cancer metastasis [3,4]. In this system uPA, secreted as a zymogen, is activated upon binding to its specific cell surface receptor uPAR. Once activated, uPA catalyzes the activation of co-localized plasminogen to plasmin, which in turn directly degrades the components of the extracellular matrix (ECM), promoting further degradation and tissue remodeling, by activating pro-metalloproteinases and activating latent growth factors from the ECM [5]. Localization of the uPAS at the invasive front of tumors thus facilitates cell migration and invasion. In breast cancer, progression-free survival is inversely correlated with uPA and uPAR expression [6,7]. Patients with high uPA mRNA levels are more likely to suffer from metastatic disease [8], and overexpression of uPAR by tumor cells or stromal cells is associated with a poor prognosis for metastatic breast cancer [9].

Amplification and overexpression of uPA and uPAR are thus recognized biomarkers of metastasis and are indicative of an overall poor patient prognosis for breast and several other cancer types [6,7,10,11].

In the triple-negative breast cancer (TNBC) subtype, uPAR was also shown to increase the malignant potential [12] and was identified as a possible novel target for treatment [13,14]. As this subtype lacks the three main breast cancer molecular biomarkers (estrogen receptor (ER), progesterone receptor (PR), and human epidermal growth factor receptor 2 (HER2)), there are no targeted therapy options for TNBC, and the use of conventional chemotherapies remains the standard of care. In addition, TNBC is a markedly heterogeneous subtype that can make treatment problematic. The prognosis of TNBC is generally poor, with high rates of disease recurrence and relapse. The progression-free survival and overall survival rates of TNBC patients are significantly shorter than those of non-TNBC patients [15].

Given the role of uPAS in the promotion of metastasis, targeting uPA/uPAR is a promising therapeutic strategy for TNBC [16,17]. uPA is efficiently and specifically inhibited by the serpin plasminogen activator inhibitor-2 (PAI-2/SerpinB2), forming a covalent complex with uPA/uPAR, which is rapidly internalized via endocytosis receptors [18,19]. Previous work by our group showed that PAI-2 could be used as a targeting ligand for the intracellular delivery of covalently attached cytotoxins to uPAR-positive tumor cells [5,20,21]. Specifically, PAI-2 was conjugated to an *N*-alkylisatin (*N*-AI)-based cytotoxin, a potent microtubule destabilizing agent [22], which could evade P-glycoprotein (P-gp)-mediated efflux in multi-drug resistant cancer cell lines [23,24]. The *N*-AI-PAI-2 conjugate was efficacious in vivo, reducing MDA-MB-231 tumor growth at 1/20th of the dose of free *N*-AI [25]. Given the potency and previous validation of *N*-AI as a cytotoxin for use in anticancer applications, *N*-AI is a promising candidate for further development in drug delivery research. As a hydrophobic molecule, *N*-AI has a low aqueous solubility that limits the amount of drug that can be administered intravenously [26]. However, *N*-AI is amenable to encapsulation within liposomes, in order to improve solubility and physicochemical stability.

Liposomes emerged as a useful delivery system for the transport of drugs and other molecules to solid tumors. Their unique structure allows for the encapsulation of hydrophobic or hydrophilic drugs in the lipid bilayer or aqueous core, respectively [27]. Encapsulated drugs can then be delivered to target cells for intracellular drug release and anti-tumor effect. The inclusion of hydrophilic polymers, most commonly PEG, at the outer surface of the liposome can increase the in vivo circulation time, by reducing recognition and clearance by the MPS [28]. For this reason, PEGylated liposomes were long considered a clinically useful nanoparticle for drug delivery applications. In addition to their versatile drug encapsulation capabilities, liposomes permit the active targeting of specific cell types via the conjugation of ligands to the liposome surface, for drug delivery to cells expressing the target surface receptor(s) of interest [29,30]. Following liposome extravasation into the tumor interstitial space, subsequent ligand-directed surface binding and internalization promotes liposome and drug entry into specific cell types. As targeted liposome formulations combine both passive and active drug delivery mechanisms, ligand-directed liposomes should show superior drug delivery, compared to non-ligand liposomes, depending on the tumor type [31].

Herein, we describe the preparation and characterization of novel *N*-AI-loaded liposomes surface-functionalized with PAI-2 as a ligand for targeting uPA/uPAR. We further evaluated the cellular targeting and in vivo biological properties of these liposomes, using relevant models of uPAR-positive TNBC breast cancer.

2. Materials and Methods

2.1. Liposome Preparation and Characterization

Liposomes were prepared using the thin-film hydration method [31] and were composed of 20 mM soy PC (L-α-phosphatidylcholine) and 0.6 mM mPEG2000-DSPE (1,2-distearoyl-sn-glycero-3-phosphoethanolamine-*N*-[(polyethylene glycol)-2000]) (Avanti Polar Lipids, Alabaster, AL, USA), with the addition of either 5 mM cholesterol (Sigma-Aldrich, St. Louis, MO, USA) to form empty liposomes, or 5 mM 5,7-dibromo-N-(p-hydroxymethylbenzyl)isatin (N-AI) (prepared in-house [23]) to form N-AI-loaded liposomes. N-AI encapsulation efficiency was determined by high-performance liquid chromatography (HPLC). Here, N-AI-loaded liposomes were mixed with water/acetonitrile (60:40 v/v) and centrifuged. The N-AI concentration was determined using an Atlantis T3 reverse-phase C18 analytical column (Waters, UK) and a Waters HPLC machine (Waters, MA, USA). Analysis was performed using an injected volume of 10 µL, with a gradient elution and monitored with a photodiode array at 435 nm. Concentration was determined by interpolating from a standard curve after analysis of standards and samples using Empower Pro V2 software (Waters, UK).

Liposomes were surface-functionalized with plasminogen activator inhibitor type 2 (PAI-2), as described by our group previously [31]. Unbound PAI-2 was removed from liposomes by size-exclusion chromatography (SEC), using Sepharose CL-4B (Sigma-Aldrich, MO, USA). Western blotting and fluorogenic uPA activity assays were used to detect and quantify PAI-2 conjugated to liposomes and the activity of PAI-2-functionalized liposomes [32]. For Western blotting, PAI-2 in SDS–PAGE gels (reducing conditions) were transferred to PVDF membranes using Bio-Rad transfer equipment (Bio-Rad Laboratories, Hercules, CA, USA) at 100 V for 1.5 h. Membranes were rinsed in TBST (1× TBS buffer with 0.05% v/v Tween-20) and blocked using 10% skim milk in TBST for 1 h at RT. After the rinsing membranes were incubated with primary antibody (anti-SerpinB2; Abcam, Cambridge, UK) at 1:2000 dilution in 2% skim milk/TBST at 4 °C overnight. Membranes were washed with TBST four times (10 min each wash) and then incubated with secondary antibody (anti-rabbit-HRP; Abcam, Cambridge, UK) at 1:5000 dilution in 2% skim milk/TBST for 2 h at RT. Membranes were then washed in TBST, three times, for 5 min and then in TBS (no Tween-20), three times, for 5 min. Membranes were developed using ECL peroxidase reaction (Pierce PicoWest ECL reagent; Thermo Fisher Scientific, Waltham, MA, USA), according to the manufacturer's instructions. Membranes were visualized using X-ray film, after developing and fixing (Bio-Rad Laboratories, CA, USA) or using a Gel Logic 2200 Digital Imager (Carestream Molecular Imaging, Woodbridge, CT, USA). Band intensities were quantified using ImageJ (National Institutes of Health, Bethesda, MD, USA).

2.2. Cell Lines and uPA and uPAR Expression

The human mammary epithelial invasive ductal carcinoma cell lines MCF-7 and MDA-MB-231 were purchased from the American Type Culture Collection (ATCC, Manassas, VA, USA). Cells were cultured in RPMI-1640 medium (Life Technologies, Carlsbad, CA, USA) containing 24 mM NaHCO$_3$ and supplemented with 10% (v/v) heat-inactivated fetal bovine serum (FBS; Thermo Fisher Scientific, MA, USA). Cells were maintained in culture at 37 °C in a 95% humidified atmosphere with 5% CO$_2$ in a HERAcell incubator (Kendro Laboratory Products, Germany). For passaging, the cells were harvested by treatment with 0.05% trypsin-EDTA (Life Technologies, CA, USA), followed by centrifugation at 300× g for 5 min. For the experiments, the cells were harvested by treatment with PBS containing 5 mM EDTA (pH 7.4), followed by centrifugation at 300× g for 5 min. Viable cells were counted with a hemocytometer using the Trypan Blue (Sigma-Aldrich, MO, USA) exclusion method. Cell lines were routinely tested and confirmed to be negative for mycoplasma contamination (in-house testing conducted by the Illawarra Health and Medical Research Institute Technical Services Unit). Cell lines were confirmed to be negative for cross-contamination by short-tandem repeat (STR) sequencing (performed by the Garvan Institute of Medical Research, Darlinghurst, Australia).

Expression of uPA and uPAR on the surface of cells was determined by flow cytometry, as described in Supplementary Information.

2.3. Assessment of Cellular Uptake and Localization of Liposomes

MCF-7 and MDA-MB-231 cells were used to assess the cellular uptake of liposomes through flow cytometry and cellular localization by confocal microscopy. For flow cytometry, MCF-7 and MDA-MB-231 cells (2×10^5 cells/well) were seeded into 12-well plates and allowed to attach for 24 h at 37 °C. Liposomes containing 1% (mol/mol) FITC-PEG$_{2000}$-DSPE were added to wells at dilutions ranging from 1:20 to 1:5. At specified time intervals ranging between 15 and 60 min, the supernatant was removed, the cells were washed once with PBS and then harvested using PBS containing 5 mM EDTA (pH 7.4). The cells were then centrifuged (300× g for 5 min) and washed three times with PBS, before being resuspended in 200 µL PBS for analysis. The fluorescence intensity was determined by flow cytometry (LSR II flow cytometer; BD Biosciences, CA) (excitation 488 nm, emission collected with 515/20 band-pass filter). FlowJo software (V10; Tree Star Inc., OR, USA) was used to evaluate the mean fluorescence intensity (MFI), to determine the cellular uptake of liposomes.

For confocal microscopy, cells (50,000 per well) were seeded into 8-well µ-Slide chambered coverslips (ibidi, Germany) and incubated for 24 h at 37 °C. Cells were allowed to reach 80% confluence before the addition of liposomes. Liposomes containing 1% or 10% (mole % of liposome phospholipid) FITC-PEG$_{2000}$-DSPE, or 0.625% (mole % of liposome phospholipid) octadecyl rhodamine B chloride (R18; Invitrogen, Carlsbad, CA, USA) were added to cells at dilutions ranging from 1:5 to 1:10, and incubated for 30 min to 2 h at 37 °C. The supernatant was removed and the wells were rinsed three times with PBS, before LysoTracker Green DND-26 (excitation/emission 504/511 nm; Thermo Fisher Scientific, MA, USA) was added to each well (50 nM final concentration), immediately prior to imaging. Live imaging of cells in PBS was performed using a Leica TCS SP5 Confocal Microscope (Leica Microsystems, Wetzlar, Germany) and the images were acquired using a 63× oil immersion lens. Images were analyzed using the Leica Application Suite software (V10; Leica Microsystems, Germany).

2.4. 3D multicellular Tumor Spheroid Cytotoxicity Assays

MCF-7 or MDA-MB-231 cells were seeded into ultra-low attachment 96-well plates (Sigma-Aldrich, MO, USA), at a density ranging between 625 and 5000 cells per well and incubated at 37 °C to promote spheroid formation. Liposomes were serially diluted in PBS and incubated with cells for up to 96 h (each concentration tested in triplicate).

2.5. Pharmacokinetics and Biodistribution of N-AI PAI-2 Liposomes in Mice

Female BALB/c-Fox1nu/Ausb nude immunocompromised mice (5 weeks old) (Australian BioResources, Moss Vale) were housed in isolator cages at the University of Wollongong animal facility. Mice were given food and water ad libitum and kept on a 12-h light/dark cycle for the duration of the experiment. Mice were allowed to acclimatize for 2 weeks before commencement of the experiment. All experiments were conducted in accordance with the 'NHMRC Australian Code for the Care and Use of Animals for Scientific Purposes', which requires 3R compliance (replacement, reduction, and refinement) at all stages of animal care and use, and the approval of the Animal Ethics Committee of the University of Wollongong (Australia) under protocol AE13/18. MDA-MB-231 cells (ATCC; mycoplasma negative and STR profiled) were resuspended in PBS (no Ca/Mg; pH 7.4; Sigma-Aldrich, MO, USA) and counted using Trypan blue (Sigma-Aldrich, MO, USA) and a hemocytometer. Insulin syringe needles (29-gauge; BD Biosciences, NJ, USA) were used to inject 50 µL of cell suspension (containing 2×10^6 cells) into the upper left mammary fat pad. Mice were injected one cage at a time and the injection order of cages was randomized. Mice were monitored closely following the injection of cells, and the tumors were observed to form at approximately 3 weeks post-injection.

Tumors were <100 mm^3 upon commencement of liposome treatment. Mice were randomly allocated to treatment (*N*-AI liposome or *N*-AI PAI-2 liposome) and time-point (10 min, 3 h, 6 h, 24 h, 48 h or 96 h) groups (4 mice per cohort). Treatments (100 µL; 4 µCi/mouse) were administered intravenously via a single lateral tail-vein injection. Mice that were deemed significantly (±10%) smaller or larger in weight than their cage mates had their dose volume adjusted proportionally, based on their weight, relative to the average of their cage mates. The ^{3}H-CHE radioactivity (liposome) in the plasma, kidneys, liver, spleen, lungs, tumor and tail (for injection correction) was quantified using previously published methods [33]; further details are provided in Supplementary Information.

2.6. Toxicology of N-AI Liposomes in Mice

The toxicology of N-AI liposomes was determined in female BALB/c mice via single or multiple lateral tail-vein injections. Details are described in Supplementary Information.

2.7. Data Analysis

All data analysis, including the generation of graphs and statistical tests, was performed using GraphPad Prism version 7 for Windows (GraphPad Software, CA, USA), unless stated otherwise. Data are presented as the mean ± standard deviation (s.d.) or standard error of the mean (s.e.m.) as stated. Pairwise comparisons were made using Student's t-test and multiple comparisons were made using one-way ANOVA with Tukey's post-test.

3. Results

3.1. Preparation and Characterization of Liposomes

Modifications to our previously reported method [33] were used to prepare and characterize the PEGylated liposomes containing the potent microtubule-destabilizing agent 5,7-dibromo-N-(p-hydroxymethylbenzyl)isatin (N-AI; see Supplementary Information Figure S1 for chemical structure), surface functionalized ± PAI-2. The particle diameter, polydispersity index (PDI), peak intensity, and zeta potential for all liposome preparations are summarized in Table 1.

Table 1. Characterization of empty and N-AI PEGylated liposomes. Empty (EMP) liposomes, N-AI-loaded (N-AI) liposomes, empty PAI-2-functionalized (EMP PAI-2) liposomes, and N-AI-loaded PAI-2-functionalized (N-AI PAI-2) liposomes were prepared by the thin-film hydration method and analyzed by dynamic light scattering. Values are means ± s.d. (n = 3).

Liposome	Diameter (nm)	Polydispersity Index	Peak Intensity % [#]	Zeta Potential (mV)	Phospholipid (mM)
EMP	137.6 ± 5.6	0.067 ± 0.04	100	−3.63 ± 0.80	16.44
N AI	139.9 ± 3.9	0.093 ± 0.02	100	−3.64 ± 0.59	16.45
EMP PAI-2	139.7 ± 4.9	0.109 ± 0.02	100	−4.05 ± 0.53	16.67
N-AI PAI-2	141.1 ± 5.0	0.086 ± 0.03	100	−4.66 ± 0.52	16.62

[#] Percent of particles present relative to the total particle population.

The size and morphology of N-AI liposomes were further confirmed by measurement of liposome diameter from cryogenic transmission electron microscopy (cryo-TEM) images (Figure 1a). The average diameter of N-AI liposomes (138.7 ± 18.4 nm; Figure 1b) was similar to that determined using dynamic light scattering (139.9 ± 3.9 nm; Table 1). Cryo-TEM additionally revealed N-AI liposomes to be spherical, monodisperse, and unilamellar. The concentration of N-AI encapsulated in the liposomes could not be determined by spectrophotometry, as the liposome phospholipid interfered with the peak absorbance of N-AI at 310 nm and 435 nm (Supplementary Information Figure S1). Therefore, the concentration of N-AI loaded into liposomes was determined by HPLC, which revealed an N-AI concentration of 2.2 mM, equating to a 43.1% entrapment efficiency based on the starting amount of N-AI used in the liposome preparation (Supplementary Information Figure S2). This translated into 7.3% w/w N-AI loaded per unit weight of the soy PC, indicating the percentage of mass of the liposome that is due to the encapsulated drug.

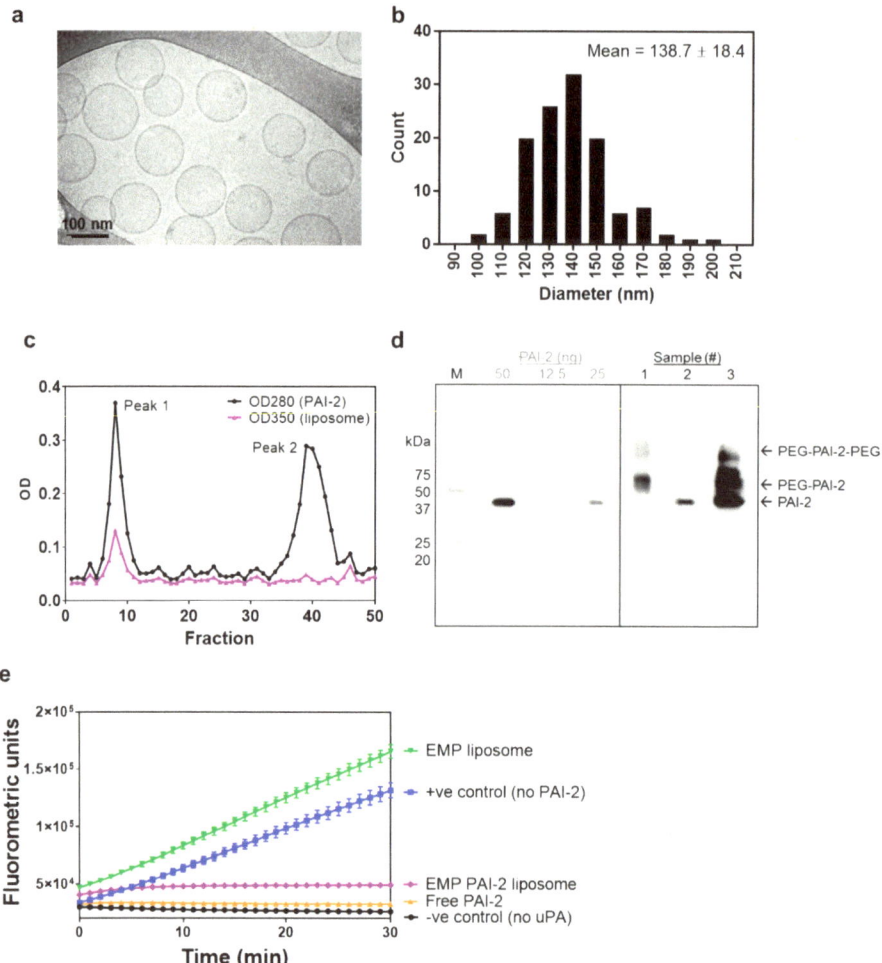

Figure 1. Characterization of N-AI-loaded liposomes. (**a**) Representative cryo-TEM image of N-AI-loaded liposomes. (**b**) Determination of the average liposome diameter from cryo-TEM image analysis. (**c**) Size-exclusion chromatograph of the PAI-2 liposome fractions after conjugation, including PAI-2 liposomes (peak 1) and unbound PAI-2 (peak 2). (**d**) Western blot detection of PAI-2 in size-exclusion fractions (1, 2), un-purified liposomes (3), and purified PAI-2 (50, 25 and 12.5 ng). OD = optical density, M = marker, PEG = polyethylene glycol. (**e**) Kinetic inhibition curves for unconjugated PAI-2 versus PAI-2 conjugated to empty liposomes (EMP PAI-2), against uPA in solution. Empty liposomes were included as a fluorescence control. Values are means ± s.d. ($n = 3$).

PAI-2 was incubated with preformed liposomes containing mal-PEG$_{2000}$-DSPE, to allow conjugation to the liposome surface. Unconjugated PAI-2 was removed using size-exclusion chromatography (SEC; Figure 1c). Analysis of fractions by spectrophotometry revealed that the unconjugated PAI-2 (peak 2) had separated from the covalently attached PAI-2 on the liposome surface (peak 1). As PAI-2 could not be detected or quantified using commercial biochemical protein assays, due to phospholipid interference [34] (data not shown), Western blotting was used to confirm successful conjugation of PAI-2 to liposomes (Figure 1d). Covalent conjugation of PAI-2 to liposome phospholipid (PEG-DSPE; molecular weight ~2940 kDa) to form PAI-2-PEG-DSPE was confirmed by a lag in gel migration of

PAI-2 in the peak 1 fraction (sample #1), relative to the peak 2 fraction (sample #2), which corresponded to the 45 kDa molecular weight of free PAI-2. The amount of PAI-2 associated with the liposome fraction in sample #1 was 42 ng, after interpolation from a standard curve.

An important step in characterizing ligand-functionalized liposomes was to confirm whether the targeting ligand(s) retain activity against the target receptor once bound to the liposome surface. The uPA inhibitory activity of PAI-2-liposomes was assessed using enzymatic assays. A significant reduction in the rate of FLU was observed for the EMP PAI-2 liposomes (43.5 ± 24.9 FLU/min) compared to the EMP liposomes (4026.9 ± 206.2 FLU/min) (Figure 1e). EMP PAI-2 liposomes were as effective at inhibiting uPA activity, as the unconjugated PAI-2 (95–100% inhibition) demonstrating that PAI-2 liposomes were fully active.

3.2. PAI-2 Liposomes Are Taken up by Cells through RME-Dependent and Non-Dependent Mechanisms

Prior to assessing cellular uptake, the MCF-7 and MDA-MB-231 breast cancer cell lines were profiled for cell surface uPA and uPAR expression through flow cytometry. MDA-MB-231 cells showed a significantly ($p < 0.001$) higher mean fluorescent intensity for uPAR and uPA (MFI; 11.82 ± 0.90 and 6.66 ± 0.97, respectively) than MCF-7 cells (MFI; 0.26 ± 0.03 and 2.49 ± 0.10, respectively; Figure 2a).

The cellular uptake of liposomes was determined by flow cytometry, using FITC-PEG-DSPE incorporated into the liposome bilayer. PAI-2-functionalized (EMP PAI-2; 152.6 ± 8.7 nm) and non-functionalized (EMP; 152.8 ± 11.7 nm) FITC liposomes were incubated with MCF-7 cells (low uPA/uPAR) and MDA-MB-231 cells (high uPA/uPAR) for 45 min. A significant increase in the EMP PAI-2 liposome uptake was observed in the MDA-MB-231 cells at 5 mM and 2.5 mM liposome concentrations ($p < 0.0001$ and $p < 0.001$, respectively) relative to the EMP liposomes, but not at 1.25 mM liposome concentration. No significant differences were observed between the uptake of EMP and EMP PAI-2 liposomes in the MCF-7 cells, at any liposome concentrations ($p > 0.05$; Figure 2b).

For the cellular localization of EMP PAI-2 liposomes through confocal microscopy, the intensely fluorescent fluorophore R18 was used to label liposomes. Dynamic light scattering revealed average diameters of 131.3 ± 2.5 nm and 131.2 ± 6.6 nm for EMP and EMP PAI-2 R18-labelled liposomes, respectively. A strong fluorescent signal from R18-labelled liposomes was detected at the cell membrane, within the cytoplasm and within lysosomes (indicated by colocalization of liposome and LysoTracker), 1 h post-incubation for both cell lines (Figure 2c), indicating cellular uptake for both EMP PAI-2 liposomes and EMP liposomes.

3.3. Cytotoxicity of N-AI PAI-2 Liposomes against Breast Cancer Cells

Treatment of MCF-7 and MDA-MB-231 cells for 72 h with *N*-AI PAI-2 liposomes but not EMP PAI-2 liposomes (at an equivalent phospholipid concentration), resulted in a dose-dependent decrease in cell viability for both cell lines, consistent with intracellular delivery of the cytotoxic *N*-AI (Supplementary Information Figure S3). The cytotoxic effect of *N*-AI PAI-2 liposomes against MDA-MB-231 cells (IC$_{50}$ of 5.40 ± 1.14 µM) was significantly greater ($p < 0.01$) than the MCF-7 cells (IC$_{50}$ of 31.84 ± 8.20 µM). EMP PAI-2 liposomes elicited some degree of cytotoxicity in both cell lines, at the highest liposome concentrations tested.

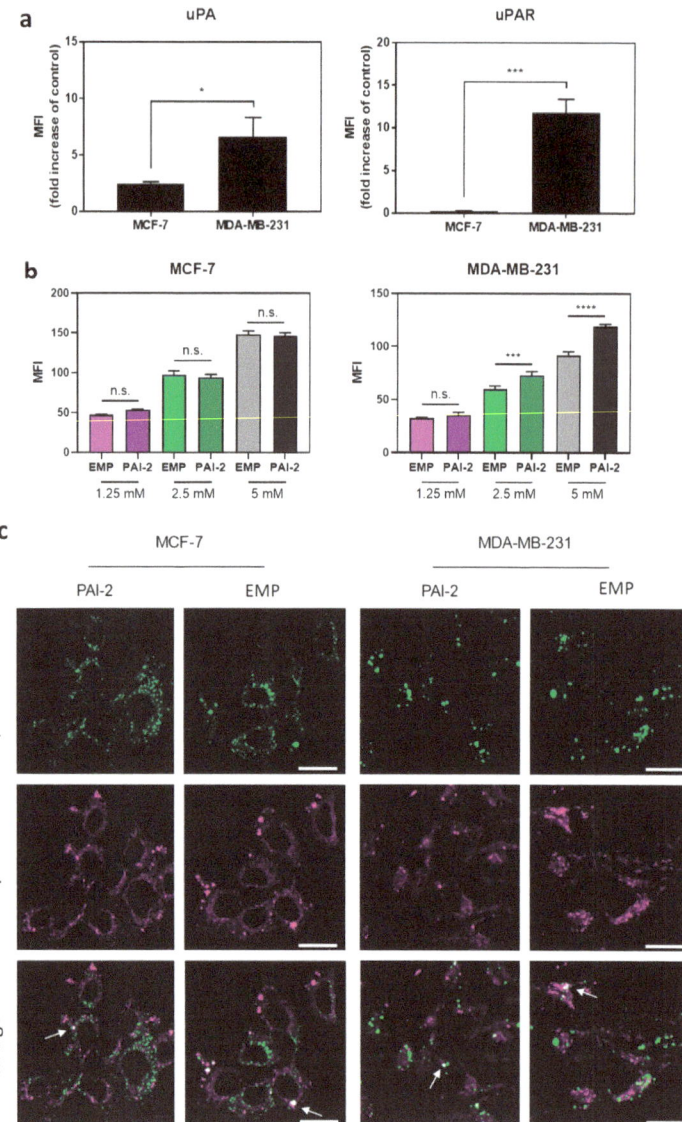

Figure 2. Cell surface expression of uPA/uPAR and cellular uptake of PAI-2 FITC-labelled liposomes by breast cancer cells. (**a**) MCF-7 cells and MDA-MB-231 cells were incubated with antibodies against human urokinase plasminogen activator (uPA), its receptor (uPAR), or an isotype control antibody (IgG) and cell surface expression analyzed by flow cytometry. (**b**) MCF-7 cells (left) and MDA-MB-231 cells (right) were incubated with empty non-functionalized (EMP) FITC liposomes or empty PAI-2-functionalized (PAI-2) FITC liposomes for 45 min, and were analyzed by flow cytometry. MFI = mean fluorescence intensity Data are the mean ± s.d. (n = 3). *: $p < 0.05$; ***: $p < 0.001$; ****: $p < 0.0001$; n.s. = not significant ($p > 0.05$). (**c**) EMP liposomes and PAI-2 liposomes were labelled with R18 and incubated with cells at a liposome concentration of 2.5 mM for 1 h. LysoTracker green was added to visualize lysosomes. Arrows point to white foci, which indicate colocalization of green and magenta signals. Representative images are shown. Scale bars are 25 μm.

3.4. Cytotoxicity of N-AI PAI-2 Liposomes against Breast Cancer Spheroids

MCF-7 and MDA-MB-231 cells are reported to form spheroids under low-attachment growth conditions [35]. EMP PAI-2 and N-AI PAI-2 liposomes at equivalent phospholipid concentrations were incubated with the preformed spheroids and imaged every 24 h (Figure 3). Spheroids treated with EMP PAI-2 liposomes showed continued growth and an increase in spheroid diameter, over time. In contrast, treatment with N-AI PAI-2 liposomes showed a time- and concentration-dependent disassembly of the spheroid structure, at concentrations above 62 µM for both cell lines (Figure 3a). However, MDA-MB-231 spheroids appeared to be more sensitive to N-AI PAI-2 liposome treatment, which showed clear evidence of spheroid dissociation, as early as 24 h, compared to the MCF-7 spheroids (Figure 3b). By 48 h, the MDA-MB-231 spheroids were almost completely dissociated in contrast to MCF-7 spheroids. A comparison of the Calcein AM stained spheroids after 96 h found MDA-MB-231 spheroids treated with N-AI and N-AI PAI-2 to be fully dissociated, while the MCF-7 spheroids, although smaller than the control (EMP and EMP PAI-2), remained largely intact (Figure 3c).

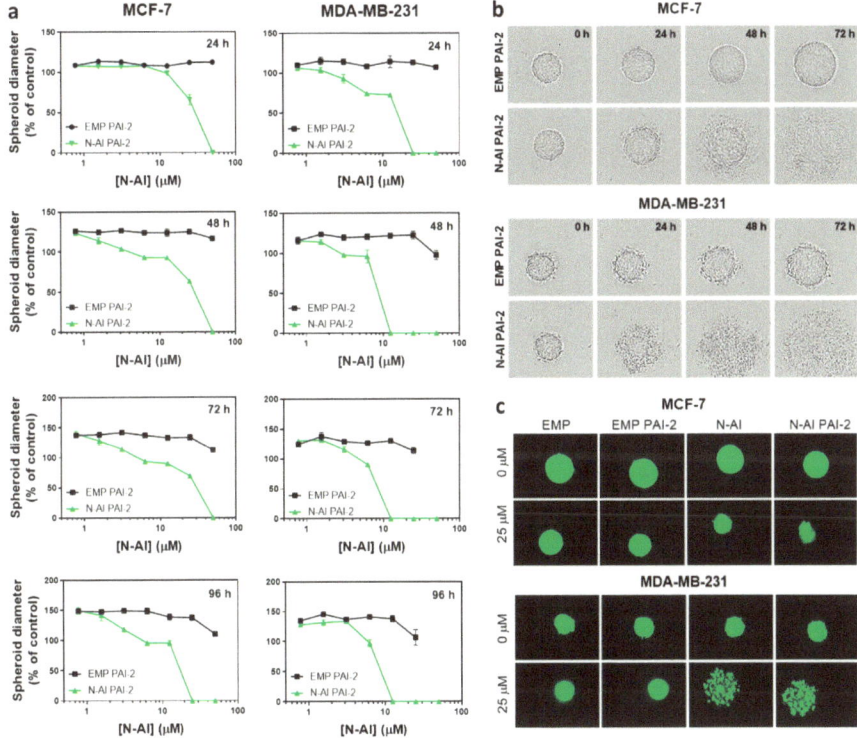

Figure 3. Cytotoxic effect of N-AI PAI-2 liposomes on breast cancer spheroids. (**a**) Spheroid diameter was measured after incubation with EMP PAI-2 liposomes or N-AI PAI-2 liposomes with MCF-7 and MDA-MB-231 multicellular tumor spheroids, over a period of 96 h. (**b**) Representative bright-field images and (**c**) fluorescent images, following the addition of calcein-AM to visualize the viable cells were captured at the same magnification ($n = 3$). Spheroids in (**b**, **c**) were treated with 25 µM N-AI or the equivalent concentration of phospholipid in liposomal formulation. Scale bars are 100 µm. Data are the mean ± s.d. ($n = 3$).

3.5. Pharmacokinetics and Biodistribution of N-AI PAI-2 Liposomes

To determine the pharmacokinetic and organ distribution profiles of N-AI liposomes and N-AI PAI-2 liposomes in tumor-bearing mice, liposomes were labelled with tritiated cholesteryl hexadecyl ether (^{3}H-CHE), to enable their detection in plasma and tissues, through liquid scintillation counting. Liposomes were monodispersed with average diameters of 115 ± 34 nm and 117 ± 39 nm, for N-AI and N-AI PAI-2 liposomes, respectively. Scintillation counts of the two liposome stock preparations were 319,698 CPM/ml and 312,163 CPM/ml for N-AI and N-AI PAI-2 liposomes, respectively. The plasma half-life was determined to be 5.63 h and 5.82 h for the N-AI and N-AI PAI-2 liposomes, respectively (Figure 4a). The plasma clearance profiles of the two liposomes and the pharmacokinetic parameters from the curve-fitting analysis were not significantly different ($p > 0.05$) (Table 2).

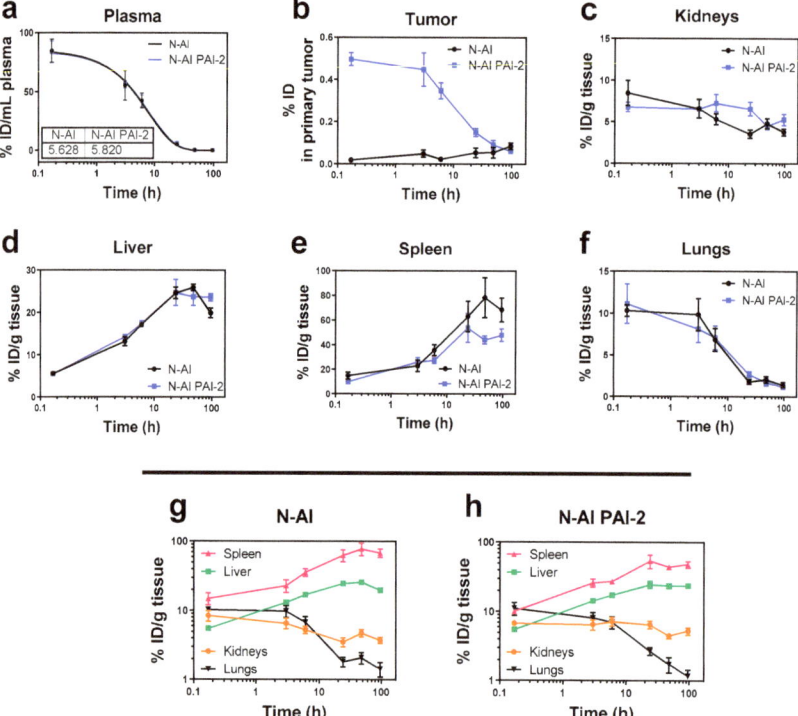

Figure 4. Biodistribution and pharmacokinetics of the radiolabeled liposomes in mice. N-AI and N-AI PAI-2 liposomes were labeled with tritiated cholesteryl hexadecyl ether (^{3}H-CHE) and administered intravenously as a single bolus dose. Tritiated signal was measured in the (**a**) plasma, (**b**) tumor, (**c**) kidneys, (**d**) liver, (**e**) spleen, and (**f**) lungs at each time-point. Kidney, liver, spleen, and lung data are also presented on the same graph for the (**g**) N-AI liposomes and (**h**) N-AI PAI-2 liposomes, for biodistribution comparison. Results are expressed as the percentage of injected dose (ID) per gram of tissue or milliliter of plasma, and as the percentage of the injected dose (ID) in the whole analyzed primary tumor. Values are the mean ± s.e.m. ($n = 4$).

Table 2. Pharmacokinetic parameters of *N*-AI and *N*-AI PAI-2 liposomes. *N*-AI and *N*-AI PAI-2 liposomes were labeled with tritiated cholesteryl hexadecyl ether (^{3}H-CHE) and administered intravenously as a single bolus dose. ^{3}H-CHE signal was measured in plasma at each time-point to determine the following parameters.

PK Parameter	*N*-AI	*N*-AI PAI-2
C_{max} (% ID/mL)	84.66 (±9.79)	83.76 (±9.25)
$K_{elim}\ \alpha$ (fast) min^{-1}	0.061	0.058
$K_{elim}\ \beta$ (slow) min^{-1}	0.002	0.002
$T_{1/2}\ \alpha$ (fast) min	11.419	12.050
$T_{1/2}\ \beta$ (slow) min	408.152	410.843
Correlation coefficient (R^2)	0.9629	0.9836
AUC (% ID/min/mL)	860.3 (±66.89)	873.4 (±50.79)

At 24 h, 48 h, and 96 h, tumor uptake of the *N*-AI and *N*-AI PAI-2 liposomes was not significantly different ($p > 0.05$). Liposome accumulation in the kidneys, liver, spleen, and lungs at each time-point was similar between the *N*-AI and *N*-AI PAI-2 liposomes (Figure 4c–f). The trends indicated increased clearance via the liver and spleen, over time, with clearance via the kidneys and accumulation in the lungs was minimal for both liposome formulations (Figure 4g–h).

Tumors were removed from mice and analyzed for tritiated liposome signal. The results showed rapid accumulation of *N*-AI PAI-2 liposome signal in tumors, compared to *N*-AI liposomes, as indicated by the significantly increased %ID at 10 min, 3 h, and 6 h post-injection ($p < 0.001$; Figure 4b).

3.6. Maximum Tolerated Dose of N-AI-Loaded Liposomes in Mice

N-AI liposomes were well-tolerated in mice, when given as an intravenous (i.v.) single bolus dose up to 20 mg/kg *N*-AI or multiple fractionated dose, up to 100 mg/kg *N*-AI. This exceeded that of free *N*-AI, which had a maximum tolerated single bolus dose of 8.5 mg/kg (Supplementary Information Figure S4). Mice treated with free drug at concentrations above 8.5 mg/kg, as well as the equivalent volume of the DMSO/PBS vehicle without drug, displayed adverse signs of intolerance immediately upon injection, including lethargy, hind-leg paralysis, tremors, and difficulty breathing [36,37], preventing higher concentrations of free *N*-AI from being tested. Liposome encapsulation therefore provided an injectable formulation of *N*-AI, with improved tolerability than the free drug.

4. Discussion

The uPA system is recognized to play a central role in the ability of breast cancer cells to escape the primary site of the tumor and colonize other parts of the body. Hence, targeting this system using novel approaches might be effective in the treatment of highly invasive or metastatic breast cancer. This work aimed to improve upon the solubility and delivery of the potent *N*-alkylisatin (*N*-AI) cytotoxin to uPA/uPAR positive breast cancer cells, through the conjugation of PAI-2 to the surface of PEGylated *N*-AI-loaded liposomes.

The successful encapsulation of a hydrophobic drug into liposomes can greatly enhance the aqueous solubility and bioavailability of the molecule, and therefore increase the suitability for its use in parenteral drug delivery applications. With a logarithmic octanol/water partition coefficient (LogP) of 3.39, the aqueous solubility of non-liposomal *N*-AI is negligible. In this work, the thin film hydration method was successfully used to load *N*-AI into the bilayer of soy PC PEGylated liposomes, to achieve a final *N*-AI concentration of 2.2 mM in aqueous solution. *N*-AI was substituted for cholesterol in the formulation, in order to increase the drug-loading capacity of *N*-AI in the bilayer. As the molecular weight of *N*-AI and cholesterol were similar, and both were hydrophobic molecules, we achieved a greater encapsulation of *N*-AI in the liposomes, in the absence of cholesterol, without affecting the zeta potential, liposome size, or stability (Supplementary Information Figure S5).

The zeta potential of liposomes is dependent on a number of factors [38], while PEG itself does not affect the surface charge of liposomes, PEG-DSPE introduces a negative surface potential due to the phosphate diester moiety [39]. In this study, liposomes displayed a slightly negative, but near-neutral, zeta potential, which did not vary greatly with N-AI encapsulation or PAI-2 conjugation to the liposome surface. Although it was noted that PAI-2-functionalized liposomes were slightly more negative than the non-functionalized liposomes, as PAI-2 has a predicted isoelectric point of 5.4 and therefore a negative charge at physiological pH [40]. It was reported that liposomes with mildly charged or near-neutral surfaces show a propensity to aggregate faster than liposomes with a strong surface charge, as the latter show a greater particle–particle repulsion and hence are more electrostatically stabilized in suspension [41]. However, our liposome formulations were found to be remarkably stable with no aggregation detected or drug leakage under the storage conditions for >4 weeks (data not shown).

The optimization of surface-functionalized liposomes through the covalent attachment of targeting moieties to the outer lipid leaflet is complex. According to a recent study by Herda et al., only 3.5% of proteins attached to the surface of SiO_2–PEG_8–Tf particles had appropriate orientation for receptor recognition [42]. Furthermore, increasing antibody density on the surface of nanoparticles was found to reduce receptor-dependent targeting [43]. In this study, the conjugation of PAI-2 to the surface of liposomes was confirmed by Western blotting and the maintenance of PAI-2 inhibitory activity post-conjugation was validated by uPA assay. PAI-2-liposomes were as effective at inhibiting the enzymatic activity of uPA as the unconjugated PAI-2, demonstrating that PAI-2 liposomes were fully active. While Western Blotting was successful in qualitatively confirming the conjugation of PAI-2 to liposomes and in confirming the absence of unconjugated PAI-2 in the purified liposome, the use of emerging methods such as single molecule fluorescent imaging to quantify ligand density on the liposome surface would enable a more precise characterization of targeted liposome formulations [44].

As reported previously, cell surface uPA and uPAR expression is low in MCF-7 cells relative to the MDA-MB-231 cells [12,45]. This difference in uPAR expression was associated with a significant increase in fluorescently labelled EMP PAI-2 liposome uptake, relative to the non-functionalized EMP liposomes by MDA-MB-231 cells, but not by MCF-7 cells. Liposomes can be taken into cells via several different mechanisms, including adsorption, lipid exchange, intracellular membrane fusion, and receptor-mediated endocytosis (RME) [46]. The presence of a fluorescent signal from cells treated with EMP fluorescently labelled liposomes indicates that these liposomes were taken up into cells by fusion or other non-specific mechanisms, rather than by RME. In contrast, the uptake of EMP PAI-2 liposomes by the MDA-MB-231 cells was greater than the uptake of EMP liposomes in MDA-MB-213 cells. As the average liposome diameters of the FITC-labelled EMP and EMP PAI-2 liposomes were equivalent, this difference in uptake was likely due to the presence of PAI-2 at the liposome surface and interaction with uPA/uPAR overexpressed on the surface of MDA-MB-231 cells. Competition binding studies using excess PAI-2 or uPAR antibody could be used to further confirm this mechanism [47,48], however, the uPA/uPAR-dependent uptake of PAI-2 has been extensively characterized by our group [18–20,49] and others [50]. Studies assessing the colocalization of liposome signal with lysosomes through confocal microscopy, further confirmed that liposomes were indeed internalized by cells and accumulated in lysosomes, in addition to being present elsewhere in the cell. This result was not unexpected, given that the liposomes were incubated with cells at a high phospholipid concentration, creating an environment where liposomes in solution would passively fuse with cell membranes over time [46]. Collectively, our results indicate that EMP and EMP PAI-2 liposomes are taken into cells via a number of mechanisms, including RME.

In the multicellular tumor spheroid experiments, imaging of spheroids over 96 h indicated a concentration- and time-dependent destruction of both MCF-7 and MDA-MB-231 spheroids, when treated with N-AI PAI-2 liposomes. However, MDA-MB-231 spheroids treated with N-AI PAI-2 liposomes showed a greater destruction of the spheroid architecture than MCF-7 spheroids at lower N-AI PAI-2 liposome concentrations and at earlier time-points. We posit that this effect was receptor-dependent, due to the uPA/uPAR targeting of PAI-2 functionalized liposomes, but acknowledge that it might also be the result of differences in cellular adhesion molecules involved in spheroid formation and cell–cell interactions between the two cell lines [51], thereby influencing liposome perfusion. While spheroid models are increasingly used to study anti-tumor drug effects, a major limitation is that they mimic only the avascular region of in vivo tumors, and exclude important aspects of tumorigenesis, such as the vasculature, immune system, and fluid dynamics. This is especially important in the context of evaluating the efficacy of nanomedicines, where the enhanced permeability and retention (EPR) effect is likely at play and vascular permeability is a relevant factor in their accumulation at the tumor site.

Determining the in vivo properties of novel nanotherapies is important for evaluating how a new nanoparticle formulation can be expected to perform in humans. In this work, the pharmacokinetics and tissue distribution of N-AI and N-AI PAI-2 liposomes were evaluated in an orthotropic MDA-MB-231 breast tumor xenograft mouse model. The addition of PAI-2 to the surface of N-AI-loaded liposomes did not significantly alter the in vivo blood clearance properties of the formulation, but did increase accumulation of liposomes at the primary tumor site relative to non-functionalized liposomes. The PEGylated liposome formulation contained 10 mol% PEG-DSPE and ranged between 130 nm and 150 nm in diameter. This liposome size range and PEG density has been reported to avoid rapid clearance by the mononuclear phagocyte system (MPS) in circulation, and to utilize the EPR effect to extravasate and accumulate at the site of tumors for drug delivery [42]. The accumulation of nanoparticles in tumors via EPR is dependent on a number of factors, including interstitial fluid pressure, vascularity of the tumor, and the in vivo circulation time of the nanoparticle formulation [52]. As the plasma half-lives of the two liposomes were largely equivalent, the presence of PAI-2 at the liposome surface might have affected liposome extravasation and uptake at the tumor site, with PAI-2 liposomes binding to uPAR expressed by tumor cells, as was observed in the in vitro experiments. The difference in uptake might also be due to slight differences in surface charge. Surface charge was previously shown to affect tumor uptake of nanoparticles [48], whereby histological analysis showed that negatively charged and neutral liposomes are able to extravasate at the site of the tumor, while positively charged liposomes remain associated with the vascular endothelium, limiting their suitability for tumor-targeting applications [53].

Finally, the maximum tumor accumulation of the liposomes reported in this study was 0.5% of the ID at the 10 min time-point for N-AI PAI-2 liposomes and 0.02% for N-AI liposomes. These values were comparable to other PEGylated nanoparticles, which typically showed 1% or less of the total ID reaching the site of the primary tumor. Notably, the high tumor accumulation of Doxil® in humans (reported as high as 10% of the ID) was due in large part to the very long circulation half-life (up to 45 h) of the formulation [54]. Given that the in vivo half-life of N-AI PAI-2 liposomes was 5.82 h, modifications to the 'stealth' coating of liposomes to promote increased blood circulation and reduce MPS clearance, might further improve liposome uptake into tumors. Following systemic administration, the surface of PEGylated liposomes is modified by protein adsorption, forming a protein corona. Future studies should also aim to characterize the composition of the protein corona, before conducting in vivo efficacy studies, in order to further understand the mechanism of tumor uptake.

5. Conclusions

This work supports the rationale for targeting uPAR-positive breast cancer cells, using N-AI-loaded PAI-2-functionalized liposomes, and provides a basis for the further development of liposomes that can target heterogeneous tumor cells within the TNBC subtype, in which uPAR was shown to play a key role in driving metastasis. Further research is needed to clarify if and how the potency of N-AI as a cytotoxin could be translated into an anti-tumor growth effect by targeting uPAR-positive tumors. The utilization of advanced preclinical models and methods will enable an enhanced evaluation of N-AI PAI-2 liposomes in the in vivo context. Future studies assessing the efficacy of N-AI PAI-2 liposomes in TNBC are therefore warranted.

Supplementary Materials: The following are available online at http://www.mdpi.com/1999-4923/12/7/641/s1. Figure S1: Liposome phospholipid interference with *N*-AI absorption spectrum. Figure S2: HPLC standard curve for quantifying *N*-AI encapsulated in liposomes. Figure S3: Cytotoxicity of *N*-AI PAI-2 liposomes. Figure S4: Toxicology testing of empty and *N*-AI-loaded liposomes in mice. Figure S5: Stability of *N*-AI-loaded liposomes over time.

Author Contributions: Conceptualization, K.L.V.; methodology, L.B. and K.L.V.; validation, L.B.; formal analysis, L.B. and K.L.V.; investigation, L.B. and K.L.V.; resources, M.R. and K.L.V.; writing—original draft preparation, L.B. and K.L.V.; writing—review and editing, L.B., D.N.S, M.R. and K.L.V.; visualization, L.B., K.L.V.; supervision, M.R., D.N.S. and K.L.V.; project administration, K.L.V.; funding acquisition, K.L.V. All authors have read and agreed to the published version of the manuscript.

Funding: This research was funded by Cure Cancer Australia Foundation with the award of Young Investigator Project Grant to K.L.V., administered by Cancer Australia as part of the Priority-driven Collaborative Cancer Research Scheme, APP1045831. The APC was funded by Molecular Horizons, University of Wollongong.

Acknowledgments: This research was conducted with the support of an Australian Government Research Training Program Scholarship, and a Jayne Wilson Cancer Research PhD Top-Up Scholarship (UOW) awarded to L.B.

Conflicts of Interest: The authors declare no conflict of interest. The funders had no role in the design of the study; in the collection, analyses, or interpretation of data; in the writing of the manuscript, or in the decision to publish the results.

References

1. Jemal, A.; Bray, F.; Center, M.M.; Ferlay, J.; Ward, E.; Forman, D. Global cancer statistics. *CA Cancer J. Clin.* **2011**, *61*, 69–90. [CrossRef]
2. Ward, E.M.; DeSantis, C.E.; Lin, C.C.; Kramer, J.L.; Jemal, A.; Kohler, B.; Brawley, O.W.; Gansler, T. Cancer statistics: Breast cancer in situ. *CA Cancer J. Clin.* **2015**, *65*, 481–495. [CrossRef] [PubMed]
3. Giannopoulou, I.; Mylona, E.; Kapranou, A.; Mavrommatis, J.; Markaki, S.; Zoumbouli, C.; Keramopoulos, A.; Nakopoulou, L. The prognostic value of the topographic distribution of uPAR expression in invasive breast carcinomas. *Cancer Lett.* **2007**, *246*, 262–267. [CrossRef] [PubMed]
4. Indira Chandran, V.; Eppenberger-Castori, S.; Venkatesh, T.; Vine, K.L.; Ranson, M. HER2 and uPAR cooperativity contribute to metastatic phenotype of HER2-positive breast cancer. *Oncoscience* **2015**, *2*, 207–224. [CrossRef] [PubMed]
5. Ranson, M.; Andronicos, N.M. Plasminogen binding and cancer: Promises and pitfalls. *Front. Biosci. J. Virtual Libr.* **2003**, *8*, s294–s304. [CrossRef] [PubMed]
6. Harris, L.; Fritsche, H.; Mennel, R.; Norton, L.; Ravdin, P.; Taube, S.; Somerfield, M.R.; Hayes, D.F.; Bast, R.C. American Society of Clinical Oncology 2007 update of recommendations for the use of tumor markers in breast cancer. *J. Clin. Oncol. Off. J. Am. Soc. Clin. Oncol.* **2007**, *25*, 5287–5312. [CrossRef]
7. Duffy, M.J.; McGowan, P.M.; Harbeck, N.; Thomssen, C.; Schmitt, M. uPA and PAI-1 as biomarkers in breast cancer: Validated for clinical use in level-of-evidence-1 studies. *Breast Cancer Res.* **2014**, *16*, 428. [CrossRef]
8. Urban, P.; Vuaroqueaux, V.; Labuhn, M.; Delorenzi, M.; Wirapati, P.; Wight, E.; Senn, H.J.; Benz, C.; Eppenberger, U.; Eppenberger-Castori, S. Increased expression of urokinase-type plasminogen activator mRNA determines adverse prognosis in ErbB2-positive primary breast cancer. *J. Clin. Oncol. Off. J. Am. Soc. Clin. Oncol.* **2006**, *24*, 4245–4253. [CrossRef]
9. Bianchi, E.; Cohen, R.L.; Thor, A.T.; Todd, R.F.; Mizukami, I.F.; Lawrence, D.A.; Ljung, B.M.; Shuman, M.A.; Smith, H.S. The urokinase receptor is expressed in invasive breast cancer but not in normal breast tissue. *Cancer Res.* **1994**, *54*, 861–866.
10. Brungs, D.; Chen, J.; Aghmesheh, M.; Vine, K.L.; Becker, T.M.; Carolan, M.G.; Ranson, M. The urokinase plasminogen activation system in gastroesophageal cancer: A systematic review and meta-analysis. *Oncotarget* **2017**, *8*, 23099–23109. [CrossRef]
11. Harris, N.L.E.; Vennin, C.; Conway, J.R.W.; Vine, K.L.; Pinese, M.; Cowley, M.J.; Shearer, R.F.; Lucas, M.C.; Herrmann, D.; Allam, A.H.; et al. SerpinB2 regulates stromal remodelling and local invasion in pancreatic cancer. *Oncogene* **2017**, *36*, 4288–4298. [CrossRef] [PubMed]
12. Huber, M.C.; Mall, R.; Braselmann, H.; Feuchtinger, A.; Molatore, S.; Lindner, K.; Walch, A.; Gross, E.; Schmitt, M.; Falkenberg, N.; et al. uPAR enhances malignant potential of triple-negative breast cancer by directly interacting with uPA and IGF1R. *BMC Cancer* **2016**, *16*, 615. [CrossRef] [PubMed]

13. Aubele, M.; Huber, M.C.; Falkenberg, N.; Gross, E.; Braselmann, H.; Walch, A.K.; Schmitt, M. uPA receptor and its interaction partners: Impact as potential therapeutic targets in triple-negative breast cancer. *J. Clin. Oncol.* **2015**, *33*, 150. [CrossRef]
14. Al-Mahmood, S.; Sapiezynski, J.; Garbuzenko, O.B.; Minko, T. Metastatic and triple-negative breast cancer: Challenges and treatment options. *Drug Deliv. Transl. Res.* **2018**, *8*, 1483–1507. [CrossRef] [PubMed]
15. Keam, B.; Im, S.A.; Kim, H.J.; Oh, D.Y.; Kim, J.H.; Lee, S.H.; Chie, E.K.; Han, W.; Kim, D.W.; Moon, W.K.; et al. Prognostic impact of clinicopathologic parameters in stage II/III breast cancer treated with neoadjuvant docetaxel and doxorubicin chemotherapy: Paradoxical features of the triple negative breast cancer. *BMC Cancer* **2007**, *7*, 203. [CrossRef] [PubMed]
16. Mazar, A.P.; Ahn, R.W.; O'Halloran, T.V. Development of Novel Therapeutics Targeting the Urokinase Plasminogen Activator Receptor (uPAR) and Their Translation toward the Clinic. *Curr. Pharm. Des.* **2011**, *17*, 1970–1978. [CrossRef]
17. Matthews, H. Synthesis and Biological Evaluation of Plasminogen Activation Inhibitors as Antitumour/Antimetastasis Agents. Ph.D. Thesis, University of Wollongong, Wollongong, Australia, 2011.
18. Al-Ejeh, F.; Croucher, D.; Ranson, M. Kinetic analysis of plasminogen activator inhibitor type-2: Urokinase complex formation and subsequent internalisation by carcinoma cell lines. *Exp. Cell Res.* **2004**, *297*, 259–271. [CrossRef]
19. Croucher, D.; Saunders, D.N.; Ranson, M. The urokinase/PAI-2 complex: A new high affinity ligand for the endocytosis receptor low density lipoprotein receptor-related protein. *J. Biol. Chem.* **2006**, *281*, 10206–10213. [CrossRef]
20. Cochran, B.J.; Croucher, D.R.; Lobov, S.; Saunders, D.N.; Ranson, M. Dependence on endocytic receptor binding via a minimal binding motif underlies the differential prognostic profiles of SerpinE1 and SerpinB2 in cancer. *J. Biol. Chem.* **2011**, *286*, 24467–24475. [CrossRef]
21. Stutchbury, T.K.; Al-Ejeh, F.; Stillfried, G.E.; Croucher, D.R.; Andrews, J.; Irving, D.; Links, M.; Ranson, M. Preclinical evaluation of 213Bi-labeled plasminogen activator inhibitor type 2 in an orthotopic murine xenogenic model of human breast carcinoma. *Mol. Cancer Ther.* **2007**, *6*, 203–212. [CrossRef]
22. Vine, K.L.; Locke, J.M.; Ranson, M.; Pyne, S.G.; Bremner, J.B. An Investigation into the Cytotoxicity and Mode of Action of Some Novel N-Alkyl-Substituted Isatins. *J. Med. Chem.* **2007**, *50*, 5109–5117. [CrossRef] [PubMed]
23. Vine, K.L.; Belfiore, L.; Jones, L.; Locke, J.M.; Wade, S.; Minaei, E.; Ranson, M. N-alkylated isatins evade P-gp mediated efflux and retain potency in MDR cancer cell lines. *Heliyon* **2016**, *2*, e00060. [CrossRef] [PubMed]
24. Keenan, B.; Finol-Urdaneta, R.K.; Hope, A.; Bremner, J.B.; Kavallaris, M.; Lucena-Agell, D.; Oliva, M.A.; Diaz, J.F.; Vine, K.L. N-alkylisatin-based microtubule destabilizers bind to the colchicine site on tubulin and retain efficacy in drug resistant acute lymphoblastic leukemia cell lines with less in vitro neurotoxicity. *Cancer Cell Int.* **2020**, *20*, 170. [CrossRef] [PubMed]
25. Vine, K.L.; Chandran, V.I.; Locke, J.M.; Matesic, L.; Lee, J.; Skropeta, D.; Bremner, J.B.; Ranson, M. Targeting Urokinase and the Transferrin Receptor with Novel, Anti-Mitotic N-Alkylisatin Cytotoxin Conjugates Causes Selective Cancer Cell Death and Reduces Tumor Growth. *Curr. Cancer Drug Targets* **2012**, *12*, 64–73. [CrossRef] [PubMed]
26. Grimaldi, N.; Andrade, F.; Segovia, N.; Ferrer-Tasies, L.; Sala, S.; Veciana, J.; Ventosa, N. Lipid-based nanovesicles for nanomedicine. *Chem. Soc. Rev.* **2016**, *45*, 6520–6545. [CrossRef] [PubMed]
27. Gubernator, J. Active methods of drug loading into liposomes: Recent strategies for stable drug entrapment and increased in vivo activity. *Expert Opin. Drug Deliv.* **2011**, *8*, 565–580. [CrossRef]
28. Uster, P.S.; Allen, T.M.; Daniel, B.E.; Mendez, C.J.; Newman, M.S.; Zhu, G.Z. Insertion of poly(ethylene glycol) derivatized phospholipid into pre-formed liposomes results in prolonged in vivo circulation time. *FEBS Lett.* **1996**, *386*, 243–246. [CrossRef]
29. Messerschmidt, S.K.; Kolbe, A.; Muller, D.; Knoll, M.; Pleiss, J.; Kontermann, R.E. Novel single-chain Fv' formats for the generation of immunoliposomes by site-directed coupling. *Bioconj. Chem.* **2008**, *19*, 362–369. [CrossRef]
30. Belfiore, L.; Saunders, D.N.; Ranson, M.; Thurecht, K.J.; Storm, G.; Vine, K.L. Towards clinical translation of ligand-functionalized liposomes in targeted cancer therapy: Challenges and opportunities. *J. Control. Release* **2018**, *277*, 1–13. [CrossRef]

31. Wilhelm, S.; Tavares, A.J.; Dai, Q.; Ohta, S.; Audet, J.; Dvorak, H.F.; Chan, W.C.W. Analysis of nanoparticle delivery to tumours. *Nat. Rev. Mater.* **2016**, *1*, 16014. [CrossRef]
32. Liu, F.T.; Rabinovich, G.A. Galectins as modulators of tumour progression. *Nat. Rev. Cancer* **2005**, *5*, 29–41. [CrossRef]
33. Belfiore, L.; Spenkelink, L.M.; Ranson, M.; van Oijen, A.M.; Vine, K.L. Quantification of ligand density and stoichiometry on the surface of liposomes using single-molecule fluorescence imaging. *J. Control. Release* **2018**, *278*, 80–86. [CrossRef]
34. Kessler, R.J.; Fanestil, D.D. Interference by lipids in the determination of protein using bicinchoninic acid. *Anal. Biochem.* **1986**, *159*, 138–142. [CrossRef]
35. Friedrich, J.; Seidel, C.; Ebner, R.; Kunz-schughart, L.A. Spheroid-based drug screen: Considerations and practical approach. *Nat. Protoc.* **2009**, *4*, 309–324. [CrossRef] [PubMed]
36. Caujolle, F.M.; Caujolle, D.H.; Cros, S.B.; Calvet, M.M. Limits of toxic and teratogenic tolerance of dimethyl sulfoxide. *Ann. N. Y. Acad. Sci.* **1967**, *141*, 110–126. [CrossRef] [PubMed]
37. *Biological Actions and Medical Applications of Dimethyl Sulfoxide*; Annals of the New York Academy of Sciences: New York, NY, USA, 1983; Volume 411, pp. 1–404.
38. Smith, M.C.; Crist, R.M.; Clogston, J.D.; McNeil, S.E. Zeta potential: A case study of cationic, anionic, and neutral liposomes. *Anal. Bioanal. Chem.* **2017**, *409*, 5779–5787. [CrossRef] [PubMed]
39. Barenholz, Y. Doxil(R)—The first FDA-approved nano-drug: Lessons learned. *J. Control. Release* **2012**, *160*, 117–134. [CrossRef]
40. Croucher, D.R.; Saunders, D.N.; Stillfried, G.E.; Ranson, M. A structural basis for differential cell signalling by PAI-1 and PAI-2 in breast cancer cells. *Biochem. J.* **2007**, *408*, 203–210. [CrossRef] [PubMed]
41. Safhi, M.M.; Sivakumar, S.M.; Jabeen, A.; Zakir, F.; Islam, F.; Anwer, T.; Bagul, U.S.; Elmobark, M.E.; Khan, G.; Siddiqui, R.; et al. Chapter 8—Nanoparticle System for Anticancer Drug Delivery: Targeting to Overcome Multidrug Resistance. In *Multifunctional Systems for Combined Delivery, Biosensing and Diagnostics*; Grumezescu, A.M., Ed.; Elsevier: Amsterdam, The Netherlands, 2017; pp. 159–169. [CrossRef]
42. Herda, L.M.; Hristov, D.R.; Lo Giudice, M.C.; Polo, E.; Dawson, K.A. Mapping of Molecular Structure of the Nanoscale Surface in Bionanoparticles. *J. Am. Chem. Soc.* **2017**, *139*, 111–114. [CrossRef] [PubMed]
43. Colombo, M.; Fiandra, L.; Alessio, G.; Mazzucchelli, S.; Nebuloni, M.; De Palma, C.; Kantner, K.; Pelaz, B.; Rotem, R.; Corsi, F.; et al. Tumour homing and therapeutic effect of colloidal nanoparticles depend on the number of attached antibodies. *Nat. Commun.* **2016**, *7*, 13818. [CrossRef] [PubMed]
44. Faria, M.; Björnmalm, M.; Thurecht, K.J.; Kent, S.J.; Parton, R.G.; Kavallaris, M.; Johnston, A.P.R.; Gooding, J.J.; Corrie, S.R.; Boyd, B.J.; et al. Minimum information reporting in bio–nano experimental literature. *Nat. Nanotechnol.* **2018**, *13*, 777–785. [CrossRef] [PubMed]
45. Ma, Z.; Webb, D.J.; Jo, M.; Gonias, S.L. Endogenously produced urokinase-type plasminogen activator is a major determinant of the basal level of activated ERK/MAP kinase and prevents apoptosis in MDA-MB-231 breast cancer cells. *J. Cell Sci.* **2001**, *114*, 3387–3396. [PubMed]
46. Ducat, E.; Evrard, B.; Peulen, O.; Piel, G. Cellular uptake of liposomes monitored by confocal microscopy and flow cytometry. *J. Drug Deliv. Sci. Technol.* **2011**, *21*, 469–477. [CrossRef]
47. Willis, M.; Forssen, E. Ligand-targeted liposomes. *Adv. Drug Deliv. Rev.* **1998**, *29*, 249–271.
48. Xiao, K.; Li, Y.; Luo, J.; Lee, J.S.; Xiao, W.; Gonik, A.M.; Agarwal, R.G.; Lam, K.S. The effect of surface charge on in vivo biodistribution of PEG-oligocholic acid based micellar nanoparticles. *Biomaterials* **2011**, *32*, 3435–3446. [CrossRef] [PubMed]
49. Cochran, B.J.; Gunawardhana, L.P.; Vine, K.L.; Lee, J.A.; Lobov, S.; Ranson, M. The CD-loop of PAI-2 (SERPINB2) is redundant in the targeting, inhibition and clearance of cell surface uPA activity. *BMC Biotechnol.* **2009**, *9*, 43. [CrossRef]
50. Conese, M.; Blasi, F. Urokinase/urokinase receptor system: Internalization/degradation of urokinase-serpin complexes: Mechanism and regulation. *Biol. Chem. Hoppe-Seyler* **1995**, *376*, 143–155.
51. Ivascu, A.; Kubbies, M. Diversity of cell-mediated adhesions in breast cancer spheroids. *Int. J. Oncol.* **2007**, *31*, 1403–1413. [CrossRef]
52. Nichols, J.W.; Bae, Y.H. EPR: Evidence and fallacy. *J. Control. Release: Off. J. Control. Release Soc.* **2014**, *190*, 451–464. [CrossRef]

53. Krasnici, S.; Werner, A.; Eichhorn, M.E.; Schmitt-Sody, M.; Pahernik, S.A.; Sauer, B.; Schulze, B.; Teifel, M.; Michaelis, U.; Naujoks, K.; et al. Effect of the surface charge of liposomes on their uptake by angiogenic tumor vessels. *Int. J. Cancer* **2003**, *105*, 561–567. [CrossRef]
54. Gabizon, A.; Isacson, R.; Libson, E.; Kaufman, B.; Uziely, B.; Catane, R.; Ben-Dor, C.G.; Rabello, E.; Cass, Y.; Peretz, T.; et al. Clinical Studies of Liposome-Encapsulated Doxorubicin. *Acta Oncol.* **1994**, *33*, 779–786. [CrossRef] [PubMed]

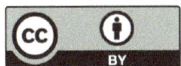

© 2020 by the authors. Licensee MDPI, Basel, Switzerland. This article is an open access article distributed under the terms and conditions of the Creative Commons Attribution (CC BY) license (http://creativecommons.org/licenses/by/4.0/).

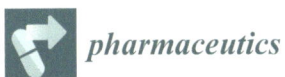

Article

Double Optimization of Rivastigmine-Loaded Nanostructured Lipid Carriers (NLC) for Nose-to-Brain Delivery Using the Quality by Design (QbD) Approach: Formulation Variables and Instrumental Parameters

Sara Cunha, Cláudia Pina Costa, Joana A. Loureiro, Jorge Alves, Andreia F. Peixoto, Ben Forbes, José Manuel Sousa Lobo and Ana Catarina Silva

1. UCIBIO/REQUIMTE, MEDTECH Laboratory of Pharmaceutical Technology, Department of Drug Sciences, Faculty of Pharmacy, University of Porto, 4050-313 Porto, Portugal; up201510339@ff.up.pt (S.C.); claudiasofiapcosta@gmail.com (C.P.C.); slobo@ff.up.pt (J.M.S.L.)
2. LEPABE, Department of Chemical Engineering, Faculty of Engineering, University of Porto, 4200-465 Porto, Portugal; up200505519@fe.up.pt
3. Thermo Unicam, 4470-108 Porto, Portugal; jorge.alves@thermounicam.pt
4. LAQV/REQUIMTE, Department of Chemistry and Biochemistry, Faculty of Sciences, University of Porto, 4169-007 Porto, Portugal; andreia.peixoto@fc.up.pt
5. Institute of Pharmaceutical Science, Faculty of Life Sciences and Medicine, King's College London, London SE1 9NH, UK; ben.forbes@kcl.ac.uk
6. UFP Energy, Environment and Health Research Unit (FP ENAS), Fernando Pessoa University, 4249-004 Porto, Portugal
* Correspondence: ana.silva@ff.up.pt

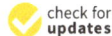

Received: 26 May 2020; Accepted: 23 June 2020; Published: 28 June 2020

Abstract: Rivastigmine is a drug commonly used in the management of Alzheimer's disease that shows bioavailability problems. To overcome this, the use of nanosystems, such as nanostructured lipid carriers (NLC), administered through alternative routes seems promising. In this work, we performed a double optimization of a rivastigmine-loaded NLC formulation for direct drug delivery from the nose to the brain using the quality by design (QbD) approach, whereby the quality target product profile (QTPP) was the requisite for nose to brain delivery. The experiments started with the optimization of the formulation variables (or critical material attributes—CMAs) using a central composite design. The rivastigmine-loaded NLC formulations with the best critical quality attributes (CQAs) of particle size, polydispersity index (PDI), zeta potential (ZP), and encapsulation efficiency (EE) were selected for the second optimization, which was related to the production methods (ultrasound technique and high-pressure homogenization). The most suitable instrumental parameters for the production of NLC were analyzed through a Box–Behnken design, with the same CQAs being evaluated for the first optimization. For the second part of the optimization studies, were selected two rivastigmine-loaded NLC formulations: one produced by ultrasound technique and the other by the high-pressure homogenization (HPH) method. Afterwards, the pH and osmolarity of these formulations were adjusted to the physiological nasal mucosa values and in vitro drug release studies were performed. The results of the first part of the optimization showed that the most adequate ratios of lipids and surfactants were 7.49:1.94 and 4.5:0.5 (%, w/w), respectively. From the second part of the optimization, the results for the particle size, PDI, ZP, and EE of the rivastigmine-loaded NLC formulations produced by ultrasound technique and HPH method were, respectively, 114.0 ± 1.9 nm and 109.0 ± 0.9 nm; 0.221 ± 0.003 and 0.196 ± 0.007; −30.6 ± 0.3 mV and −30.5 ± 0.3 mV; 97.0 ± 0.5% and 97.2 ± 0.3%. Herein, the HPH was selected as the most suitable production method, although the ultrasound technique has also shown effectiveness. In addition, no significant changes in CQAs were observed after 90 days of storage of the formulations at different temperatures. In vitro studies showed that the release of rivastigmine followed a non-Fickian mechanism, with an initial fast drug release followed by a prolonged release over 48 h. This study has optimized a rivastigmine-loaded NLC formulation produced by the HPH method for nose-to-brain delivery of rivastigmine. The next step is for in vitro and in vivo experiments to demonstrate preclinical efficacy and safety. QbD was demonstrated to be a useful approach for the optimization of NLC formulations for which specific physicochemical requisites can be identified.

Keywords: nanostructured lipid carriers (NLC); formulation optimization; rivastigmine; quality by design (QbD); nasal route; nose-to-brain

1. Introduction

Alzheimer's disease is an irreversible neurodegenerative disorder characterized by neuronal deterioration that leads to the loss of cognitive functions [1-3]. Genetic, environmental, and aging factors; the presence of neurofibrillary tangles; and senile plaques in the brain caused by the agglomeration of poorly folded proteins have been highlighted as the main factors involved in Alzheimer's pathogenesis [1,2,4]. Drugs used in clinical practice can attenuate the disease symptoms, inhibiting acetylcholinesterase activity and avoiding acetylcholine hydrolysis in the synaptic cleft [5,6]. Examples of these drugs include galantamine, donepezil, and rivastigmine [1,7]. Among these, rivastigmine hydrogen tartrate, chemically known as (S)-N-ethyl-N-methyl-3-[(1-dimethylamino) ethyl]-phenyl carbamate hydrogen tartrate, is the most used as a reversible non-competitive dual inhibitor of acetylcholinesterase and butyrylcholinesterase, improving central cholinergic function through the increase of acetylcholine levels [7-9]. Nonetheless, it was reported that rivastigmine hydrogen tartrate undergoes an extensive first-pass effect in the liver, which decreases bioavailability [10,11]. This molecule also has a short half-life and a hydrophilic nature, which makes it difficult for it to pass through the blood brain barrier (BBB) and cerebrospinal fluid (CSF) [5,9,12]. In addition, the tight junctions between the BBB capillary endothelial cells restrict the passage, absorption, and permeation of drugs to the brain [13,14]. Therefore, high drug concentration and frequent dose administration are required to reach therapeutic levels, causing unpleasant cholinergic side effects, such as nausea, dyspepsia, bradycardia, and hallucinations [8,10,11].

More effective ways of delivering rivastigmine to the brain are required, such as the use of nanosystems administered through alternative administration routes [11,13,15-18]. Herein, the intranasal route has been considered for delivering drugs from the nose directly to the brain, avoiding the need to overcome the BBB [13,19,20]. The nasal cavity directly contacts the central nervous system (CNS) through the olfactory and trigeminal nerves that connect to the brain and the CSF, allowing direct drug transport [13,20-22]. The nasal route offers other advantages to improve drug delivery, including the avoidance of the first-pass effect and gastric degradation, high drug absorption, and reduction of adverse effects. However, this route shows some limitations, such as fast drug elimination by the mucociliary clearance mechanism, among others [11,19,23-25]. Notwithstanding, the composition of the nasal formulation is crucial to obtain high therapeutic efficiency, being influenced by excipients, the physical state of the dosage form, and the applied volume [23,24].

Regarding nanosystems, several studies have showed that they promote nasal delivery, providing sustained drug release while avoiding molecules degradation due to the protective shell [11,23]. In this area, lipid nanoparticles (solid lipid nanoparticles—SLN; nanostructured lipid carriers—NLC) have shown high potential as carriers for nose-to-brain drug delivery [13,17,18,26-28]. SLN and NLC seem more advantageous than other nanosystems for brain delivery, as they are made of physiological lipids and are generally recognized as safe (GRAS) excipients that are biocompatible and biodegradable [13,26,29,30]. Furthermore, they provide drug protection against enzymatic degradation and increase the residence time in the nasal cavity, improving drug bioavailability [14,17,25]. Other advantages include the ease of production on a large scale without the use of organic solvents, the high encapsulation efficiency for lipophilic molecules, and having a controlled release profile [13,15,22,30–32]. Besides, it is possible to produce SLN and NLC with diameters below 200 nm and a polydispersity index (PDI) of around 0.3, which are recommended for nose-to-brain delivery [13,31,33,34].

Although the clinical use of nanosystems has been intensively studied, some specific regulatory requirements are lacking [35]. In this sense, the use of the quality by design (QbD) approach to optimize lipid nanoparticles is essential to design formulations with low risk of failure and to achieve the desired clinical attributes. Thereby, carrying out preliminary studies to ensure the quality of the final product is required to achieve high efficiency, stability, and reproducibility. Some of these studies have explored the definition of the desired administration route and drug release profile, followed by the evaluation of the formulation properties and the control of the variables of the production method [36,37].

The Food and Drug Administration (FDA) and European Medicines Agency (EMA) authorities have encouraged the use of the QbD approach as a continuous process that should be applied to the development of a new pharmaceutical product, defining the quality target product profile (QTPP) to obtain a final product with high quality, safety, and efficiency [38,39]. QbD starts with the selection of the critical process parameters (CPPs) and critical material attributes (CMAs) that interfere with the critical quality attributes (CQAs), which are based on risk management [38]. For the implementation and continuous improvement of the QbD approach, several quality tools described in the International Council for Harmonisation of Technical Requirements for Pharmaceuticals for Human Use (ICH) Q8, Q9, and Q10 guidelines are used, namely the Ishikawa diagram, Pareto chart, response surface methodology, and design of experiment (DoE) tools [40,41]. These tools are fundamental in the optimization of formulations, reducing the number of required experiments and consequently saving time and costs [11,32].

The aim of this work was to use the QbD approach to optimize a rivastigmine-loaded NLC formulation for nose-to-brain delivery with the predefined QTPP for the particle size (<200 nm), PDI (<0.3), zeta potential (ZP) (close to ±30 mV), and encapsulation efficiency (EE) (>80%) [31,33,34,42]. To carry out a complete and accurate optimization of the formulation, the study was divided into two parts. First, the most suitable CMAs, which corresponded to the concentrations of the different formulation components (lipids and surfactants), were defined. Afterwards, the CPPs were selected, which corresponded to the production method (high-pressure homogenization—HPH; or ultrasound technique) to produce rivastigmine-loaded NLC formulations with the desired QTPP. A central composite design was used to optimize the CMAs to achieve high quality predictions for various factors at extreme levels [32,43,44], and a Box–Behnken design was used to optimize the CPPs, analyzing the effects of three variables and requiring less experiments [45–47]. Finally, the pH and osmolarity of the optimized NLC formulations were adjusted to the physiological values and in vitro release studies were performed. Rivastigmine quantification was assessed by a high-performance liquid chromatography (HPLC) method validated according to the European Pharmacopeia (Ph. Eur.) and ICH guidelines [48,49]. In addition, the long-term stability of the optimized rivastigmine-loaded NLC formulations was assessed by measuring the particle size, PDI, ZP, and EE values over 90 days of storage at 20.0 ± 0.5 °C and 4.0 ± 0.5 °C.

2. Materials

Rivastigmine base (liquid) of 99.9% purity was kindly provided by Novartis (Basel, Switzerland). Precirol® ATO 5 (glyceryl distearate/glyceryl palmitostearate) was donated from Gattefossé (Lyon, France) and Phospholipon® 90G (phosphatidylcholine, hydrogenated) was a gift from Lipoid (Ludwigshafen am Rhein, Germany), alpha-tocopherol acetate (vitamin E), polysorbate 80 (Tween® 80) and benzalkonium chloride were purchased from Acef (Piacenza, Italy) and Acofarma (Barcelona, Spain), respectively. The water used in all experiments was purified, obtained from a Milli®Q Plus, Millipore® (Darmstadt, Germany). For the mobile phase, acetonitrile ≥99.9% purity was purchased from Fisher Chemical-Thermo Fisher Scientific (Loughborough, UK); disodium phosphate was purchased from Sigma Aldrich (Lisbon, Portugal); monosodium phosphate from Merck (Darmstadt, Germany); and sodium chloride, potassium chloride and calcium chloride were purchased from Acofarma (Barcelona, Spain).

3. Methods

3.1. Screening of Drug and Excipients

Prior to NLC production, it is mandatory to study the compatibility between solid and liquid lipids and between lipids and the drug to obtain a final formulation with high encapsulation efficiency and long-term stability [50,51]. The components of the NLC formulation were selected from previous work developed by our group [52,53]. Precirol® ATO5 was used as the solid lipid, due to its appropriate melting point (56 °C) and ability to form the imperfect lipid matrix of the NLC when mixed with a liquid lipid, which provides a high drug loading capacity [54,55]. Vitamin E was selected as the liquid lipid due to its antioxidant activity, which can delay the neural damage caused by the oxidative stress of Alzheimer's disease, improving the neuroprotective effect of the NLC formulation. In addition, vitamin E decreases the risk of lipid oxidation resulting from the preparation of NLC, increasing the chemical stability of the encapsulated drug; easily solubilizes lipophilic molecules; and has high compatibility with lipids and surfactants [56–58].

The compatibility of different amounts of vitamin E with the solid lipid (Precirol® ATO5) was evaluated in ratios ranging from 50:50 up to 90:10 (solid lipid: liquid lipid, % w/w). For the experiments, the lipid mixture was heated up to 100 °C under stirring at 200 rpm for 1 h and cooled down to room temperature (25 ± 0.5 °C). The solidified mixture was then analyzed by passing through a filter paper, where the absence of oil stains indicated the existence of miscibility between the lipids. Afterwards, the best proportion of solid and lipid liquids was selected [59].

To study the compatibility between the drug and lipids, different amounts of the drug were added to the lipid mixture previously selected, using as reference the concentration of a commercial drug solution (2%, w/w). For the tests, increasing amounts of drug (0.1%, 0.2%, 0.5%, 1%, and 2%) were added to the lipids mixture and heated 10 °C above the melting point of the solid lipid (70 ± 0.5 °C) under stirring at 500 rpm for 1 h. After solidification by cooling to room temperature, the mixture was placed on a filter paper, where the absence of oil droplets indicated the existence of drug solubility in the lipid mixture [59].

SLN and NLC formulations should include two surfactants that promote steric and electrostatic stabilization, avoiding nanoparticle aggregation and ensuring long-term stability. Surfactants should be selected according to their charge, molecular weight, and adequacy for the desired route of administration for the formulation [22,50,60,61]. Smaller particle sizes have been observed when a higher surfactant/lipid ratio was used [31,62,63]. Accordingly, polysorbate 80 (Tween® 80), a non-ionic surfactant containing a polyoxyethylene chain tetrahydrofuran ring that provides steric stabilization and a hydrophobic tail that prevents particle aggregation, was selected based on previous works that showed its compatibility with the lipids used [46,52,53,59,60,64]. The co-surfactant (Phospholipon® 90G) was selected based on its emulsification capacity for the selected lipid mixture, its non-irritating effect on the nasal mucosa, and its ability to minimize the polymorphic state transitions of lipids. Phospholipon® 90G is a (phosphatidylcholine hydrogenated) biological membrane lipid and an amphoteric surfactant that has a synergic effect with Tween® 80, originating NLCs with smaller particle sizes and high stability [64,65]. Different proportions of surfactant and co-surfactant were used to prepare NLC formulations (Table 1) and the best ratio was selected after analysis of the results of particle size, PDI, ZP, and EE tests (Section 3.5) [32].

Benzalkonium chloride, a quaternary ammonium compound, was used as preservative (0.02%) to prevent microbial proliferation of the NLC formulations due to the high water content. This compound is commonly used in nasal formulations as it exhibits low or no toxicity to the nasal cilia when used in concentrations between 0.01 and 0.02% [66].

Several research studies have described the use of similar components to prepare NLC formulations for nose-to-brain delivery. For instance, Khan et al. developed a hydrogel-containing temozolomide-loaded NLC for nose-to-brain delivery using vitamin E as the liquid lipid [67]. Madane et al. prepared a curcumin-loaded NLC for nose-to-brain delivery using Precirol® ATO5, Tween® 80, and lecithin (a phospholipid similar to Phospholipon® 90G) [33]. Wavikar et al. used Tween® 80 and lecithin to prepare a rivastigmine-loaded NLC for nose-to-brain delivery [68]. Precirol® ATO5 and Tween® 80 were used to prepare a NLC to improve the nose-to-brain transport of a glial cell-derived neurotrophic factor (GDNF) [69]. Tween 80® was used as surfactant olanzapine-loaded NLC [70] and in an asenapine-loaded NLC to promote brain delivery through intranasal administration [71].

3.2. Preparation of Rivastigmine-Loaded NLC Formulations

Rivastigmine-loaded NLC formulations (Table 1) were prepared by HPH and ultrasound technique, which were previously employed by Silva et al. [18,53]. Briefly, the lipid phase was heated above the solid lipid melting point and added to the aqueous phase, which was previously heated at the same temperature. Afterwards, the mixture was emulsified under high-speed stirring with an Ultra-Turrax® T25 (Janke and Kunkel GmbH, Staufen im Breisgau, Germany) at 13,400 rpm for 5 min. The oil-in-water (O/W) formed emulsion was sonicated by means of an VCX130 ultrasonic processor (Sonics, Wolfwil, Switzerland). The power output, with an amplitude of 75%, was applied for 15 min. The hot O/W nanoemulsion was transferred to glass vials and cooled to the room temperature (20 ± 0.5 °C) to form the NLC. A rivastigmine concentration of 0.12% (w/w) was added to the lipid phase before melting. Regarding the HPH, the procedure was similar, although the O/W emulsion was forced to pass through a piston gap homogenizer (Stansted High Pressure Homogenizer, Stansted Fluid Power Ltd., Harlow, UK) at 1750 bar and 80 ± 0.5 °C. The number of applied homogenization cycles ranged from 9 up to 18. The homogenizer was previously heated at 80 ± 0.5 °C with hot purified water and the temperature was kept constant to avoid lipid solidification.

3.3. Determination of Particle Size, Polydispersity Index (PDI), and Zeta Potential (ZP)

The NLC mean particle size (Z-Ave) and PDI were measured by dynamic light scattering (DLS) technique using a Malvern nanozetasizer (Malvern, UK). A refractive index of 1.46 and an absorption index of 0.001 were used for the lipids, while a refractive index of 1.330 was used for the solvent (water). In addition, the NLC electrical surface charge was assessed by laser doppler electrophoresis by means of ZP measurements using the same apparatus. The dispersions were diluted with ultrapure water and the ZP was calculated using the Helmholtz–Smoluchowski equation and run on the system software. The temperature was set at 25 ± 1 °C. Each sample was analyzed in five replicates ($n = 5$) and the results were reported as the mean ± standard deviation (SD).

To confirm the absence of microparticles, particle size was measured by laser diffraction using a Malvern Mastersizer 3000E (Malvern, UK). The used particle refractive index was 1.4, the absorption index was 0.001, and the water dispersant refractive was 1.33, with Mi's theory being applied. The particle size was assessed by the values of the volume distribution (D50 and D90), indicating the percentage of particles with a diameter size equal or lower to the given values. The results were reported as the mean ± SD of five replicates ($n = 5$).

3.4. Rivastigmine Quantification

3.4.1. Development and Validation of a High-Performance Liquid Chromatography (HPLC) Method

The wavelength of the maximum absorption (237 nm) of rivastigmine was selected by spectroscopy analysis using a Jasco V-650 UV-Vis spectrophotometer. To obtain drug peaks of suitable resolution, chromatographic conditions were tested, namely the composition of the mobile phase, flow rate, and injection volume.

3.4.2. Chromatographic Conditions

An isocratic mobile phase consisting of a phosphate-buffered solution (pH 6.4) and acetonitrile (60:40, v/v) was vacuum filtered through a 0.45 μm membrane (Millipore®, Germany) and degassed by ultrasonication for 15 min. The flow rate of the mobile phase was 1.0 mL/min. Before sample injections, the system was cleaned with purified water for 60 min and was left to equilibrate with the mobile phase for 60 min. The oven was set at 25 ± 3 °C and UV detection was performed at 237 nm. For each analysis, sample volumes of 20 μL were injected in triplicate ($n = 3$).

3.4.3. Preparation of Standard Solutions

A stock standard solution of rivastigmine (1200 μg/mL) was prepared by dissolving 0.12 g of the drug in acetonitrile using a 100 mL volumetric flask. Five working solutions (24, 48, 72, 120, 840 μg/mL) were prepared by diluting an adequate amount of stock standard solution with acetonitrile in a 25 mL volumetric flask. All analyses were performed in triplicate ($n = 3$). The method was validated according to the International Council for Harmonisation of Technical Requirements for Pharmaceuticals for Human Use (ICH) guidelines for linearity, precision, accuracy, specificity, and robustness [5,49]. The developed method was shown to be linear, precise, selective, and robust (Supplementary Data, Sections 1 and 2), and was used in the following studies.

3.4.4. Assessment of Encapsulation Parameters

The effectiveness of lipid nanoparticles for drug incorporation can be assessed by calculating the encapsulation efficiency (EE) and loading capacity (LC). High EE and LC values suggest that lipid nanoparticles can encapsulate and delivery the desired therapeutic amount of drug, reducing adverse effects and frequency of administration [18].

EE and LC were determined indirectly by calculating the amount of free rivastigmine (non-encapsulated) in the aqueous phase of NLC dispersions according to the following equations [72]:

$$EE\ (\%) = \frac{\text{Total amount of rivastigmine} - \text{amount of free rivastigmine}}{\text{Total amount of rivastigmine}} \times 100 \quad (1)$$

$$LC\ (\%) = \frac{\text{Total amount of rivastigmine} - \text{Amount of free rivastigmine}}{\text{Total amount of rivastigmine} - (\text{Amount of free rivastigmine} + \text{Total amount of lipid})} \times 100 \quad (2)$$

Briefly, 1 mL of each sample was diluted with purified water and placed in an Amicon® Ultracel-50K (Millipore Corporation, Ireland) centrifugal filter device and centrifuged at 3450 rpm for 1 h. Afterwards, the filtrate was collected, diluted in acetonitrile, and analyzed by HPLC. The tests were performed on the production day for 10 different batches of NLC formulations ($n = 10$) [72].

3.5. Design of Experiment (DoE) for the Optimization of Rivastigmine-Loaded NLC Formulation

A DoE was used to evaluate the effects of critical parameters related to the CMAs (i.e., formulation variables) and CPPs (i.e., instrumental parameters) on CQAs, namely for particle size, PDI, ZP, and EE.

Figure 1 shows the Ishikawa diagram used as a visualization tool for the two parts of the optimization process.

3.5.1. Part 1: Optimization of Formulation Variables by Central Composite Design (CCD)

In the first part of the optimization of the rivastigmine-loaded NLC formulation, we tested different solid lipid and liquid lipid (SL/LL) ratios, which were selected using the results of lipid-drug solubility tests and different ratios of surfactants.

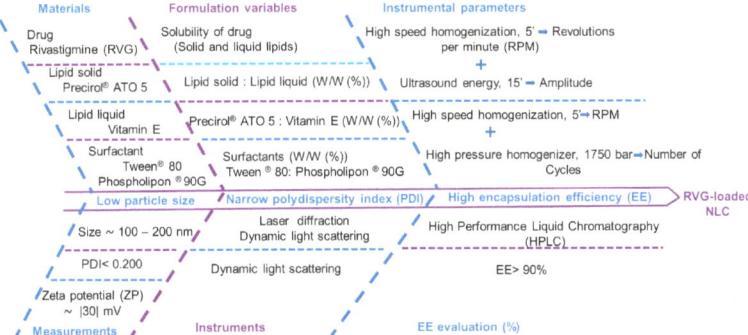

Figure 1. Ishikawa diagram showing the effects of critical material attributes (CMAs) and critical process parameters (CPPs) on the critical quality attributes (CQAs) of rivastigmine-loaded NLC formulation.

The influence of the different ratios of SL/LL and surfactants on CQAs or dependent responses, namely particle size, PDI, ZP, and EE, were studied using a CCD with α rotatability of 1.4142, two-factors, and 3 levels. Table 1 shows the DoE used to test the rivastigmine-loaded NLC formulation variables.

Table 1. Design of experiment (DoE) using six central composite design (CCD) for rivastigmine-loaded nanostructured lipid carriers (NLC) formulations with different critical material attributes (CMAs).

Formulation Variables			Levels		
			Low (−1)	Medium (0)	High (+1)
		X1	5.94:3.94	6.94:2.94	7.94:1.94
		X2	2.00:1.00	2.50:0.50	2.50:1.50
		X1	6.94:2.94	7.94:1.94	8.94:0.94
		X2	2.00:1.00	2.50:0.50	2.50:1.50
X1 Precirol® ATO 5: Vitamin E ratio (%, w/w) X2 Tween® 80: Phospholipon® 90G concentration (%, w/w)		X1	5.91:3.91	6.91:2.94	7.94:1.94
		X2	3.00:1.00	3.50:0.50	3.50:1.50
		X1	6.94:2.94	7.94:1.94	8.94:0.94
		X2	3.00:1.00	3.50:0.50	3.50:1.50
		X1	5.94:3.94	6.94:2.94	7.94:1.94
		X2	4.00:0.40	4.00:1.00	4.50:0.50
		X1	6.94:2.94	7.94:1.94	8.94:0.94
		X2	4.00:0.40	4.00:1.00	4.50:0.50

Six DoE with 10 experimental runs were generated by the statistic software with two factors or independent variables corresponding to the CMAs, namely solid lipids (Precirol® ATO 5, SL), vitamin E (LL), and surfactants (Tween® 80 and Phospholipon® 90G, Tw/Ph). Their effects on CQAs or dependent responses were studied at low (−1), medium (0), and high (+1) levels.

For the experiments, rivastigmine-loaded NLC formulations were produced by employing the ultrasound technique previous described by Silva et al. [72], involving high-speed homogenization at 13400 rpm and a sonication amplitude of 75%. The formulation with the most suitable values for CQAs, namely having a lower particle size, PDI of around 0.2–0.3, a ZP value close to 30mv, and an EE value > 90%, was selected for the next part of the optimization, which is related to the instrumental parameters [31,33,34,42]. It is important to note that ZP values close to |30| mv are desired to ensure more stable NLC formulations, since the electrostatic repulsion between the nanoparticles prevents aggregation. However, negative ZP values reduce the residence time of the formulation in the nasal mucosa, since interactions between NLC and mucin, a negatively charged glycoprotein of the nasal cavity, may not occur [73,74]. To overcome this limitation, mucoadhesive polymers were added to the optimized rivastigmine-loaded NLC formulations to form in situ gels without negative charge. This strategy was used to develop NLC formulations for nose-to-brain delivery. For example, Rajput and Butani developed a NLC-based in situ gel for intranasal administration of resveratrol [75], while Abouhussein et al. developed a NLC-based in situ gel to improve the brain target of rivastigmine after intranasal administration [9].

3.5.2. Part 2: Optimization of Instrumental Parameters by Box–Behnken Design (BBD)

The second part of the optimization aimed to study the effect of different CPPs in the CQAs or dependent responses that were evaluated in the first part of the optimization related to the selection of the most suitable concentrations of formulation components. The rivastigmine-loaded NLC formulation was produced by ultrasound technique and HPH, and the tested instrumental parameters were the emulsification speed (rpm), amplitude of sonication, and number of HPH cycles.

The emulsification time and speed are important parameters in obtaining small nanoparticles with a narrow PDI [11,46]. Thus, the emulsification time was set to 5 min and the effect of increasing the rpm on CQAs was evaluated. The time and amplitude of sonication are also important parameters in producing small NLCs. Generally, as the time and amplitude of sonication increase, particle size decreases [11,51]. However, it has been reported that a high amplitude of sonication increases the lipid nanoparticle size due to the formation of aggregates [11,46]. Therefore, the effect of increasing the amplitude of sonication on CQAs was evaluated.

Regarding HPH, the pressure was kept constant at 1750 bar, which allows the reduction of the particle size due to the generated cavitation forces. However, to obtain small and uniform nanoparticles, several homogenization cycles should be performed [61,76–79]. Thus, the effect of increasing the number of HPH cycles on CQAs was evaluated. The emulsification speed, sonication amplitude, and number of HPH cycles were the independent variables that were studied at low (−1), medium (0), and high levels (+1). The DoE showing the different combinations of the tested CPPs is presented in Table 2. For these studies, 9 experimental runs were performed for each of the 6 selected formulations to evaluate the effect of each independent variable on the particle size, PDI, ZP, and EE.

Table 2. Design of experiment (DoE) using Box–Behnken design (BBD) to optimize rivastigmine-loaded nanostructured lipid carriers (NLC) formulations using different combinations of critical process parameters (CPPs).

Instrumental Parameters		Levels		
		Low (−1)	Medium (0)	High (+1)
X1: Emulsification speed (rpm) + X2: HPH cycles	X1	11,000	13,400	14,000
	X2	9	12	18
X1: Emulsification speed (rpm) + X3: sonication amplitude	X1	11,000	13,400	14,000
	X3	55	75	85

3.6. pH and Osmolarity

Regarding the requirements for nasal formulations, the pH (5.5–6.59) and osmolarity (280 mOsm/kg) were adjusted to the physiological values in the optimized rivastigmine-loaded NLC formulations [80].

The pH was measured at room temperature using a BASIS 20 calibrated digital pH meter (Crison Instruments, Spain) and the osmolarity was assessed using a Type 6 osmometer (Löser Messtechnik, Berlin-Spandau, Germany).

3.7. In Vitro Drug Release Studies

Drug release studies were carried out through dialysis bag diffusion technique over 48 h, as previous described by Silva et al. and Abouhussein et al. [9,81]. Simulated nasal electrolyte solution

(SNES) and phosphate-buffered solution (pH 6.4) were used as release media. SNES was prepared by dissolving 12.9 mg of potassium chloride, 745 mg of sodium chloride, and 3.6 mg of calcium chloride in 1000 mL of ultrapure water. Phosphate-buffered solution pH 6.4 was prepared according to the European Pharmacopoeia (Ph. Eur.) [9,31,48]. The release profile of rivastigmine from the NLC was evaluated for the optimized formulations produced by HPH and ultrasound technique. Briefly, 2.5 mL of NLC with 1.2 mg/mL of rivastigmine were filled in a dialysis bag (cellulose membrane with molecular weight cut-offs of 300 kDa, 12–15 cm long, Spectra/Por® Biotech, US), clamped, and immersed in a glass vial containing 250 mL of release medium at 37 ± 0.5 °C, then stirred at 50 rpm. At predetermined time intervals (0.5, 1, 2, 4, 6, 8, 10, 12, 24, 30, 36, and 48 h), 1.0 mL of sample was collected and the release medium was replaced with the same volume of fresh medium to guarantee sink conditions. Collected samples were passed through a syringe filter (0.21 µm) and diluted in 1 mL of acetonitrile, being the amount of rivastigmine measured by HPLC in a Thermo Scientific™ Dionex™ UltiMate™ instrument, with a detection wavelength of 237 nm using an analytical reverse-phase C_{18} column (100 mm × 4.6 mm, 5 µm) from Thermo Scientific Acclaim™ (Portugal). The results were reported as the mean ± SD of three replicates ($n = 3$). The cumulative rivastigmine released was calculated and expressed as a percentage of the theoretical maximum drug content.

Kinetic Mechanism of Drug Release

Drug release kinetics is a QTTP that should be considered in the development of a formulation, allowing the definition of in vivo–in vitro correlations [82,83]. In vitro drug release was analyzed by fitting the results to four mathematical kinetics models [72,83]: zero order (1), first order (2), Higuchi model (3), and Korsmeyer–Peppas (4) models. The correlation coefficient (R^2) was determined to compare the precision of these models as it presents the highest R^2 value, which was selected to describe the drug release kinetics. The value of the diffusion release exponent (n) obtained by the Korsmeyer–Peppas model was used to characterize the drug release mechanism [84,85]: $n \leq 0.43$ means a Fickian release, where the drug diffusion is proportional to the concentration; $n = 0.85$ represents a non-Fickian release, i.e., a zero-order release, where the drug diffusion is independent from the concentration; $0.43 < n < 0.85$ defines an anomalous transport route, which is a combination of non-Fickian release and Fickian release; $n > 0.89$ is a case II transport (relaxation-controlled release). The Microsoft Excel® software was used to calculate the R^2 and the model parameters of the following equations [86]:

(1) Zero order model: $M_0 - M = kt$
(2) First order model: $\ln m = kt$
(3) Higuchi equation: $M_0 - M = kt^{1/2}$
(4) Korsmeyer–Peppas model: $\log (M_0 - M) = \log k + n \log t$

M represents the amount of drug released at time t, M_0 corresponds to the drug concentration at time 0, k is the rate constant, and n is the diffusion release exponent.

3.8. Statistical Analysis

Statistical analysis was performed using Statistica™ StatSoft software, version 13.5.0.17 (TIBCO® Software Inc). Results were statistically analyzed by ANOVA and a 2-way interactions model, with a 95% confidence level being considered statistically significant when the value of p was less than 0.05. Pareto chart, contour, and 3-D response surface plots were used to select the best formulation variables and the ideal conditions of each instrumental parameter to achieve the desired CQA values.

3.9. Stability Studies

The long-term stability of the two optimized rivastigmine-loaded NLC formulations (i.e., the one with the best CQAs produced by the ultrasound technique and the one with the best CQAs produced by HPH method) was assessed according to ICH (Q1A) guidelines [87]. For the studies, formulations were stored at room temperature (20.0 ± 0.5 °C) and in the refrigerator (4.0 ± 0.5 °C), and the particle size (Z-Ave, D50, D90), PDI, ZP, and EE were evaluated after 90 days of storage. The results were presented as mean values of three replicates ($n = 3$) ± SD.

4. Results

4.1. Screening of Drug and Excipients

The selected lipids were compatible and miscible at the concentrations tested and a ratio of 70:30 (%, w/w) was shown to be the best proportions of Precirol® ATO5 and vitamin E for the preparation of the NLC formulation, as previously developed in our group [52]. Several studies have shown that a high concentration of liquid lipids increases drug retention, as drug solubility in liquid lipids is usually higher than in solid lipids, which decreases the particle size due to the decreased viscosity and surface tension of the NLC [46,79,88].

The higher solubility of the drug in the lipid mixture was observed over individual lipids, due to the absence of oil droplets on the filter paper (Supplementary Data, Section 3.1, Figure S6). This can be explained by the imperfect lipid matrix formed in the mixture that allowed for higher amounts of drug molecules [46,79,88]. Accordingly, the selected drug concentration was 0.12%.

4.2. Suitability of the HPLC Method for Rivastigmine Quantification

The developed HPLC method was considered to be simple, linear, precise, selective, reproducible, and robust (Supplementary Data, Sections 1 and 2) for rivastigmine quantification. A good linearity ($R^2 = 0.999$) was observed in the tested range, with RSD values lower than 1% and a recovery rate close to 100% being obtained. Furthermore, the values obtained for the detection and quantification limits were suitable for application of the method. The selectivity for rivastigmine quantification in the presence of other formulation components was also demonstrated and the results of encapsulation parameters showed that NLCs are effective for rivastigmine encapsulation.

4.3. Part 1: Optimization of Formulation Cariables by CCD

The rivastigmine-loaded NLC formulation variables were optimized using a CCD and the data were statistically analyzed using ANOVA, evaluating the importance of the selected factors on dependent responses and the suitability of the selected design for the CQAs through the value of R squared (R^2). Different ANOVA models were tested (Supplementary Data, Section 3, Table S9) and the one that presented the closest R^2 value to 1 (0.93563) for the CQAs was selected, namely the linear/quadratic main effects + 2-ways model [89,90].

4.3.1. Effect of Lipids and Surfactants Ratio on Particle Size (Z-Ave, D50, and D90)

Table 3 shows that the predicted and observed values were very close, indicating the suitability of the design for the selected CQAs.

Predicted vs. observed plots showing the suitability of the model for the applied design, a Pareto chart of standardized effects studying the interaction effects of CMAs for each dependent response, and contour plots representing the interactions between CMAs and dependent responses were used for further analysis.

From the analysis of the Pareto chart (Supplementary Data, Section 3.1, Figure S4A), the surfactant ratio (Tw/Ph) and lipids ratio (SL/LL) were significant factors for particle size (Z-Ave) ($p = 0.005$), showing a negative effect, which means that particle size increased with increasing ratios of SL/LL and Tw/Ph. In contrast, for the dependent response D50 (Supplementary data, Figure S4B), Tw/Ph had a positive effect and the most statistically significant effect ($p = 0.05$) when a linear model was used, while SL/LL did not show a statistically significant effect. Regarding D90 (Supplementary data, Section 3.1, Figure S4C), it was observed that all independent variables had statistical significance ($p = 0.05$), showing positive effects on size when a linear model was applied, indicating direct relationships.

Table 3. Observed (O) and predicted (P) results for critical quality attributes (CQAs).

Critical Quality Attributes (CQAs)	Z-Ave (nm) [1]		D50 (nm) [2]		D90 (nm) [2]		PDI [3]		ZP [4] (mV)		EE [5] (%)	
Runs	O [6]	P [7]	O [6]	P [7]	O [6]	P [7]	O [6]	P [7]	O [6]	P [7]	O [6]	P [7]
1	166.600 ± 1.911	175.000	58.400 ± 0.102	58.650	148.602 ± 0.570	163.740	0.221 ± 0.003	0.224	−28.000 ± 0.253	−28.900	94.001 ± 0.143	94.690
2	158.301 ± 0.852	150.450	61.401 ± 0.244	57.950	159.600 ± 0.992	155.040	0.224 ± 0.007	0.230	−28.600 ± 0.251	−29.020	94.890 ± 0.271	94.340
3	187.104 ± 0.980	190.190	51.100 ± 0.132	53.440	148.603 ± 0.793	161.200	0.263 ± 0.002	0.247	−29.000 ± 0.192	−29.670	92.900 ± 0.232	93.810
4	173.305 ± 1.231	160.140	75.900 ± 0.140	74.540	256.002 ± 0.651	248.900	0.234 ± 0.004	0.230	−33.300 ± 0.231	−33.490	93.594 ± 0.181	93.260
5	166.600 ± 0.893	165.220	59.901 ± 0.190	61.920	182.001 ± 0.733	176.180	0.225 ± 0.001	0.212	−27.600 ± 0.280	−26.890	93.761 ± 0.310	93.730
6	176.701 ± 0.972	182.820	70.900 ± 0.171	69.970	243.000 ± 0.651	240.760	0.224 ± 0.003	0.227	−31.000 ± 0.300	−30.600	92.702 ± 0.251	92.350
7	192.303 ± 0.114	183.180	51.200 ± 0.150	49.130	146.000 ± 0.910	128.040	0.242 ± 0.004	0.250	−31.300 ± 0.371	−30.400	96.390 ± 0.401	95.320
8	130.700 ± 0.791	144.560	60.401 ± 0.221	63.560	174.001 ± 0.882	183.900	0.251 ± 0.001	0.242	−33.400 ± 0.193	−33.190	94.001 ± 0.254	94.690
9	192.300 ± 0.150	192.300	61.301 ± 0.143	61.300	207.000 ± 0.980	207.000	0.243 ± 0.002	0.245	−32.300 ± 0.204	−32.300	95.500 ± 0.190	95.500
10	192.300 ± 0.150	192.300	61.301 ± 0.143	61.300	207.000 ± 0.980	207.000	0.234 ± 0.002	0.245	−32.300 ± 0.204	−32.300	95.500 ± 0.190	95.500

[1] Z-Ave (mean particle size); [2] volume distribution (50% of particles with size equal or lower to the given value of D50) and 90% of particles with size equal or lower to the given value of D90)); [3] PDI (polydispersity index); [4] ZP (zeta potential); [5] EE (encapsulation efficiency) [6] O (observed results); [7] P (predicted results).

From the observation of the contour plots (Supplementary data, Section 3.1, Figure S5A–C), the smallest NLCs (Z-Ave = 148–128 nm, D50 = 46–56 nm, D90 = 110–160 nm) were found with the medium lipids ratio (7.94:1.94) and high surfactants ratio (4.5:0.5). These results can be explained by the fact that smaller particle sizes are generally obtained when higher concentrations of surfactants are used [46]. It has been described that higher surfactant concentrations ensure NLC stability, decreasing the surface tension and preventing aggregation and crystallization of lipids during storage, in turn avoiding the increased nanoparticle size [91].

4.3.2. Effect of Lipid and Surfactant Ratios on PDI, ZP, and EE

The PDI is an indicative of the particle size distribution. According to the literature, a monodisperse sample has PDI values close to 0, while values between 0.1 and 0.3 indicate a narrow size distribution, between 0.1 and 0.4 indicate a moderate size distribution, and greater than 0.4 represent a wide size distribution [32,63]. From the analysis of the Pareto chart (Supplementary Data, Section 3.1, Figure S4D), the surfactants ratio (Tw/Ph) and lipids ratio (SL/LL) were not statistically significant for PDI, although the ratio of lipids showed a more significant effect than the surfactants ratio through the length of the bar. The lipids ratio (SL/LL) showed a linear and positive correlation with PDI, while the surfactants ratio had a negative effect, which means that PDI values are directly related to the lipids ratio. The contour plot (Supplementary Data, Section 3.1, Figure S5D) showed that the values of PDI were higher than 0.24 with the medium lipids ratio (7.94:1.94) and the high surfactants ratio (4.5:0.5), demonstrating a narrow size distribution for the NLC formulation.

ZP reflects the electric potential and the surface charge of nanoparticles in a suspension and is a predicting factor of the long-term stability. When ZP values are higher than |30| mV, the electrostatic repulsion of the attractive Van der Waals forces stops nanoparticle aggregation from occurring [63,92–94]. Lipids arrangements on the surface of the nanoparticle, surfactant surface absorption, and the charge of the encapsulated drug interfere with ZP [32,92]. The Pareto chart showed that the lipids ratio had statistical significance ($p = 0.05$), showing a positive effect on ZP when a quadratic model was used, while the surfactant ratio had a significant negative effect on ZP for the quadratic model (Supplementary Data, Section 3.1, Figure S4E). Thus, ZP was more influenced by the lipids ratio than by the surfactants ratio. Regarding the ZP contour plot (Supplementary Data, Section 3.1, Figure S5E), optimum values were observed in the range of −32 mv and −34 mv, which were obtained with the medium lipids ratio (7.94:1.94) and high surfactants ratio (4.5:0.5).

The high negative ZP values were probably related to the co-surfactant and the drug. Phospholipon® 90G is an amphoteric molecule that acquires a negative charge at the pH level of the NLC formulation, while rivastigmine is a Bronsted base, which when in aqueous dispersion forms a highly negatively charged hydroxyl group [78,95–97].

Regarding EE (Supplementary Data, Section 3.1, Figure S4F), only the lipids ratio (SL/LL) was statically significant ($p = 0.05$), although it negatively decreased as the lipids ratio increased. The contour plot (Supplementary Data, Section 3.1, Figure S5F) revealed that EE was higher than 95% when lipid and surfactant ratios were at medium levels (7.94:1.94 and 4.00:1.00, respectively). This can be explained by the lipophilic nature of rivastigmine, which becomes more solubilized as the lipid concentration increases. In addition, this can also be related to the surfactants, which create more available space between lipids to accommodate rivastigmine molecules [32,63].

From Table 4, it can be concluded that the CCD fitted to the selected CQAs, while the analysis of the Pareto charts (Supplementary Data, Section 3.1, Figure S4) and contour plots (Supplementary Data, Section 3.1, Figure S5) showed that the best lipids ratio was 7.94:1.94 (%, w/w) and the best surfactants ratio was 4.5:0.5 (%, w/w). Accordingly, this rivastigmine-loaded NLC formulation was selected for optimization of the instrumental parameters.

Table 4. Results of particle size (Z-Ave (mean particle size); volume distribution (50% of particles with size equal or lower to the given value of D50 and 90% of particles with diameter equal or lower to the given value of D90), polydispersity index (PDI), zeta potential (ZP), and encapsulation efficiency (EE) tests for the rivastigmine-loaded nanostructured lipid carriers (NLC) selected following the optimization of formulation variables.

Tested Ratios (w/w, %)		DoE [1]		LD [2] (Mean ± SD [3], n [4] = 5)			DLS [5] (Mean ± SD [3], n [4] = 5)			
SL/LL [6]	Tw/Ph [7]	Levels		D50 [8] (nm)	D90 [9] (nm)	Z-Ave [10] (nm)	PDI [11]	ZP [12] (mV)	EE [13] (%)
5.94:3.94	4.0:0.4	−1.00	−1.00	58.402 ± 0.009	148.600 ± 0.009	166.602 ± 0.010	0.221 ± 0.011	−28.000 ± 0.011	94.001 ± 0.012
5.94:3.94	4.5:0.5	−1.00	1.00	61.400 ± 0.008	159.603 ± 0.010	158.300 ± 0.008	0.213 ± 0.010	−28.601 ± 0.010	94.890 ± 0.008
7.94:1.94	4.0:0.4	1.00	−1.00	51.101 ± 0.010	148.604 ± 0.011	187.101 ± 0.012	0.251 ± 0.010	−29.000 ± 0.008	92.903 ± 0.011
7.94:1.94	4.5:0.5	1.00	1.00	75.903 ± 0.008	256.012 ± 0.008	173.302 ± 0.013	0.231 ± 0.009	−33.300 ± 0.011	93.590 ± 0.013
5.94:3.94	4.0:1.0	−1.41	0	59.902 ± 0.010	182.013 ± 0.007	166.603 ± 0.009	0.220 ± 0.010	−27.600 ± 0.010	93.760 ± 0.007
6.94:2.94	4.5:0.5	0	1.41	60.401 ± 0.011	174.020 ± 0.011	130.703 ± 0.011	0.251 ± 0.011	−33.400 ± 0.009	94.001 ± 0.011
8.94:0.94	4.5:0.5	1.00	1.00	63.200 ± 0.010	199.211 ± 0.010	174.200 ± 0.009	0.290 ± 0.010	−32.900 ± 0.010	98.300 ± 0.011

[1] DoE (design of experiment); [2] LD (laser diffraction); [3] SD (standard deviation); [4] n (number of runs); [5] DLS (dynamic light scattering); [6] SL/LL (solid lipid: liquid lipid); [7] Tw/Ph (Tween® 80: Phospholipon® 90G); [8] D50 (50% of particles with a diameter size equal or lower to the given values); [9] D90 (90% of particles with a diameter size equal or lower to the given values); [10] Z-Ave (mean particle size); [11] PDI (polydispersity index); [12] ZP (zeta potential); [13] EE (encapsulation efficiency).

4.4. Part 2: Optimization of Instrumental Parameters by BBD

The effects of instrumental parameters (emulsification speed, sonication amplitude, and number of HPH cycles) on dependent responses were evaluated by means of a BBD. A value of $R^2 = 1$ was obtained when 2-way interactions (linear quadratic) model was used (Supplementary Data, Section 3.2.1, Table S10 and Section 3.2.2, Table S11). Additionally, all variables were statistically significant ($p = 0.001$). Thus, the predicted and observed values were equal. The results are presented in 3-D response surface plots (Figures 2 and 3).

4.4.1. Effects of Emulsification Speed and HPH Cycles on Particles Size (Z-Ave, D50, and D90), PDI, ZP, and EE

Particle Size

The 3-D response surface plots for Z-Ave, D50, and D90 (Figure 2A–C) showed that as the emulsification speed (rpm) increased, the particle size decreased. In contrast, the number of HPH cycles did not cause a direct change in particle size, although a decrease was observed when the emulsification speed and the number of HPH cycles increased together.

The lowest and highest values of Z-Ave (124.80 and 141.90 nm, respectively), D50 (55.90 and 86.70 nm), and D90 (144.00 and 189.40 nm) were observed, respectively, when 14,000 rpm with 18 cycles and 11,000 rpm with 12 and 18 cycles were used. Therefore, it was concluded that higher emulsification speed and number of HPH cycles decrease the NLC size, which can be explained by the kinetic energy used in the high-speed emulsification process required to obtain a stable emulsion of uniform nanoparticle size [11]. In addition, the prolongation of the HPH process with more cycles promoted the breakdown of the emulsion oil droplets, since they suffered higher compression, turbulence, and cavitation within the homogenization gap [79,92,98]. Furthermore, the stability and bioavailability of the NLC dispersion were also improved [78,92]. Thus, 14,000 rpm with 18 homogenization cycles were set as the ideal conditions for the HPH method.

PDI, ZP, and EE

From the 3-D response surface plots (Figure 2D–F), it can be observed that as the emulsification speed and the number of HPH cycles change (increase or decrease), the values of PDI, ZP, and EE did not change significantly. PDI was around 0.21–0.26, indicating a narrow size distribution; ZP was in the range of −21 and −25 mV; EE ranged from 94% up to 98%. Thus, it was concluded that these parameters did not cause significant alterations in the rivastigmine-loaded NLC formulation.

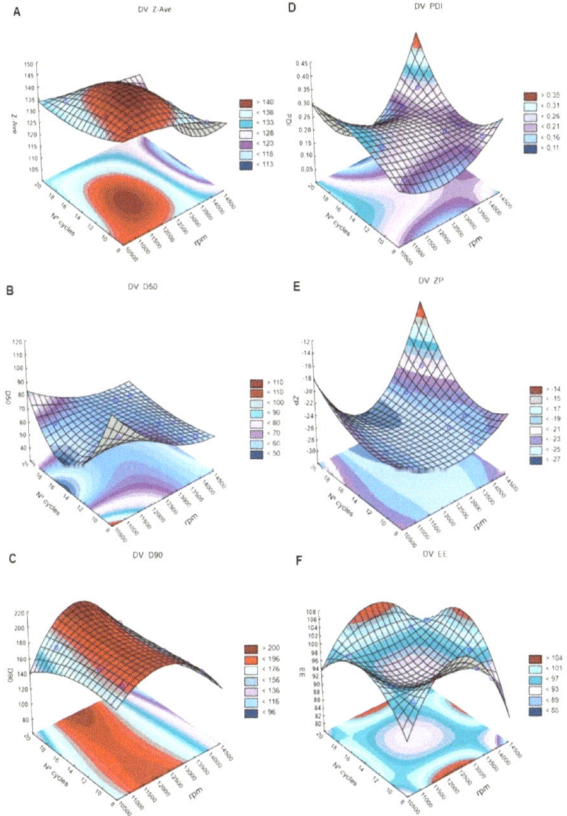

Figure 2. The 3-D surface plots portraying the effects of the number of high-pressure homogenization (HPH) cycles and emulsification speed (rpm) on the size (Z-Ave (mean particle size); D50 (50% of particles with size equal or lower to the given value) and D90 (90% of particles with size equal or lower to the given value)) (left: **A–C**), polydispersity index (PDI), zeta potential (ZP), and encapsulation efficiency (EE) (right: **D–F**).

4.4.2. Effects of Ultrasound Technique on Particles Size (Z-Ave, D50, and D90), PDI, ZP, and EE

The selected design fitted to CQAs when the 2-way interaction (linear quadratic) model was used. The observed and predicted values for CQAs using the ultrasound technique were the same, namely $R^2 = 1$ and $p = 0.001$ (Supplementary Data, Table S11).

Particle Size

The analysis of the 3-D response surface plots for Z-Ave, D50, and D90 (Figure 3A–C) revealed that as the emulsification speed increased, the particle size decreased. Regarding the sonication amplitude, a direct effect on particle size was not observed. However, when these parameters increased together, the particle size decreased. Z-Ave, D50, and D90 values were higher for 11,000 rpm and lower for 13,400 rpm. The increase of the emulsification speed allowed the formation of a stable rivastigmine-loaded NLC formulation with uniform particle size distribution [11]. Increasing the sonication amplitude results in higher ultrasonic wave energy with a consequent increase in the shear cavitation forces, leading to the breakdown of the emulsion oil droplets to nanometric sizes [46,51].

The lowest and highest Z-Ave (295 and 152 nm), D50 (57 and 80 nm), and D90 (180 and 220 nm) values were observed when 13,400 rpm and 85% amplitude were applied. Thus, 13,400 rpm with 85% amplitude were set as the desired conditions for the ultrasound technique.

PDI, ZP, and EE

The results showed that the values obtained for PDI, ZP, and EE (Figure 3D–F) did not change significantly with variations of the emulsification speed and sonication amplitude, as observed for the HPH method. PDI values were between 0.21 and 0.25, while ZP ranged between −26 mV and −28 mV. The EE values ranged from 95% up to 97%, being close to 99% for 14,000 rpm with 55% amplitude. The small differences in ZP and EE values can be attributed to the different locations of the anionic drug molecules in the lipid matrix [32,46].

4.5. Model Validation

Two rivastigmine-loaded NLC formulations with the selected ratios of lipids and surfactants were produced under the most suitable instrumental parameters found for the ultrasound technique and the HPH method. The results of the observed responses were within the design space and close to the predicted values, which allowed for model validation (Table 5).

Regarding the observed responses in Table 5, other studies involving drug-loaded NLCs for nose-to-brain delivery have reported similar values for ZP, particle size, PDI, and EE. For example, Jain et al. optimized an artemether-loaded NLC for intranasal delivery with a particle size of 123.4 nm, ZP of −34.4 mV, and EE of 91.2% [99]. Gadhave et al. developed a teriflunomide-loaded NLC with a particle size of 99.8 nm, PDI of 0.35, ZP of −22.3 mV, and EE of 83.4% [31]. Madane and Mahajan prepared a curcumin-loaded NLC with a particle size of 146.8 nm, PDI of 0.18, EE of 90.86%, and ZP of −21.4 mV [33].

Table 5. Observed and predicted response values of the two optimized rivastigmine-loaded nanostructured lipid carriers (NLC) formulations.

Observed Responses	Ultrasound Technique	High-Pressure Homogenization (HPH) Method
Z-Ave [1] (nm)	114.000 ± 1.910	109.000 ± 0.850
PDI [2]	0.221 ± 0.003	0.196 ± 0.007
ZP [3] (mV)	−30.633 ± 0.288	−30.466 ± 0.252
EE [4] (%)	96.987 ± 0.446	97.174 ± 0.297
Predicted Responses	**Ultrasound Technique**	**High-Pressure Homogenization (HPH) Method**
Z-Ave [1] (nm)	155.000	124.000
PDI [2]	0.190	0.242
ZP [3] (mV)	−28.400	−29.100
EE [4] (%)	95.140	97.600

Results presented as mean ± SD (n = 3); [1] Z-Ave: mean particle size; [2] PDI: polydispersity index; [3] ZP: zeta potential; [4] EE: encapsulation efficiency.

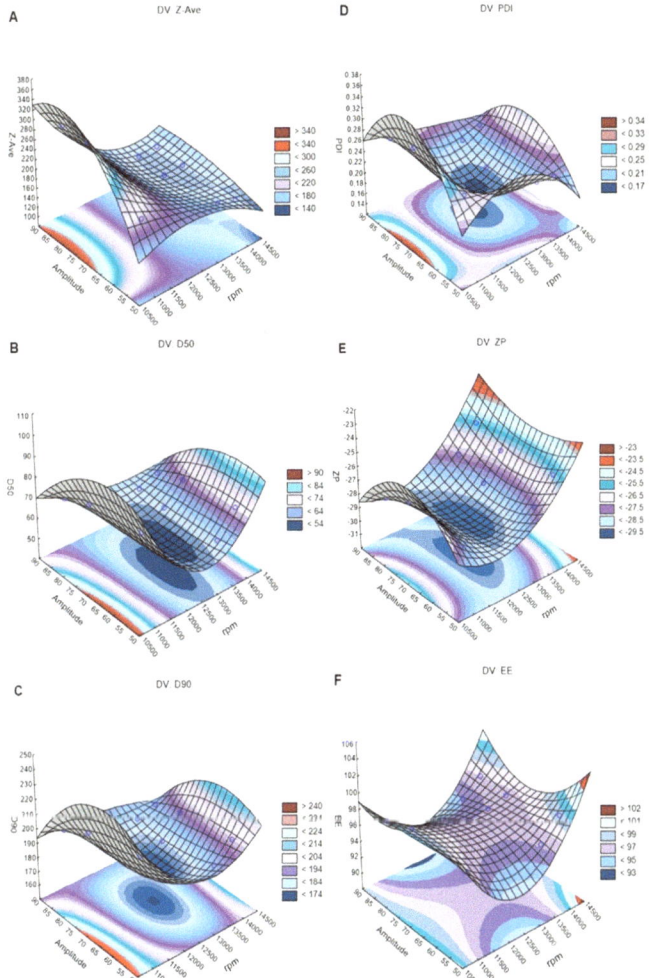

Figure 3. The 3-D surface plots portraying the effect of the sonication amplitude and emulsification speed (rpm) on the size (Z-Ave (mean particle size); D50 (50% of particles size equal or lower to the given value) and D90 (90% of particles with size equal or lower to the given value)) (left: **A–C**), polydispersity index (PDI), zeta potential (ZP), and encapsulation efficiency (EE) (right: **D–F**).

4.6. pH and Osmolarity

The pH of the optimized rivastigmine-loaded NLC formulations produced by ultrasound technique and HPH method were adjusted to the nasal mucosa values (5.5–6.6) with a dilute HCl solution. Similarly, the osmolarity was adjusted with glycerin to the physiological range of 230–320 mOsm/kg, obtaining isotonic formulations compatible with the nasal mucosa [100]. The final values for the pH and osmolarity of the optimized rivastigmine-loaded NLC formulations were 6.22 ± 0.01 and 280 ± 1 mOsm/Kg for the ones produced by HPH method; and 6.21 ± 0.01 and 279 ± 1 for the ones produced by ultrasound technique. Furthermore, it was confirmed that the CQAs values were not altered after addition of HCl and glycerin (Supplementary Data, Section 4, Table S12).

4.7. In Vitro Drug Release Studies

The release profile of rivastigmine from the NLC produced by HPH method and ultrasound technique was assessed in phosphate-buffered solution at pH 6.4 (Figure 4) and in simulated nasal electrolyte solution at pH 6.4 (Figure 5) over a period of 48 h.

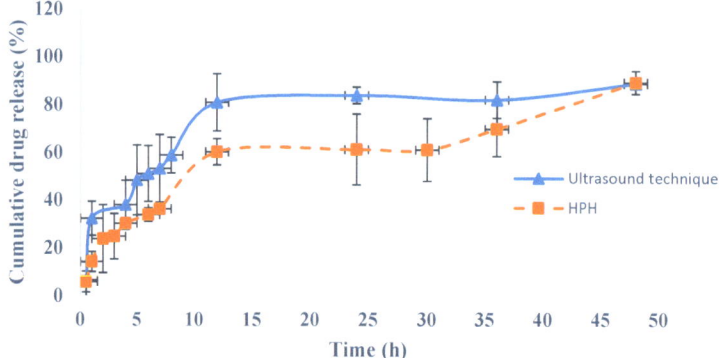

Figure 4. Cumulative percentage of drug release in phosphate-buffered solution (pH 6.4) from rivastigmine-loaded nanostructured lipid carriers (NLC) produced by ultrasound technique and rivastigmine-loaded NLC produced by high-pressure homogenization (HPH) method.

From Figure 4, an initial fast drug release can be observed from both rivastigmine-loaded NLC formulations, which is related to the drug diffusion from the surface of the NLC to the dissolution medium, followed by a prolonged release [15,98]. This phenomenon can be explained by the rapid solidification of the solid lipids during the formation of the NLC, which results in nanoparticles with an internal core containing a low amount of liquid lipids, which in turn accumulate in the outermost layers. As rivastigmine is an oil, it also tends to accumulate on the surface of the NLC, meaning it is released more quickly [33,99,101].

For both optimized NLC formulations, from 4 up to 48 h, the release of rivastigmine was controlled by the diffusion rate of the drug through the lipid matrix or by the lipid matrix degradation in the dissolution medium [62,102]. For the rivastigmine-loaded NLC produced by the ultrasound technique, about 80.75 ± 7.43% of rivastigmine was released after 12 h and the maximum drug release (88.67 ± 3.45%) was observed at 48 h. In contrast, for the rivastigmine-loaded NLC produced by the HPH method, at 12 h the release of rivastigmine was lower (60.13 ± 3.12%) and the maximum drug release (89.25 ± 3.22%) was observed at 48h. Statistically significant differences between the rivastigmine-loaded NLC produced by ultrasound technique and rivastigmine-loaded NLC produced by HPH method were observed ($p < 0.05$).

Figure 5 shows that in the simulated nasal electrolyte solution, similarly to the phosphate-buffered medium (Figure 4), an initial fast drug release was observed for both rivastigmine-loaded NLC formulations, followed by a prolonged release. The release rate of rivastigmine was higher for the rivastigmine-loaded NLC produced by the HPH method in the first 15 h when compared to the one produced by ultrasound technique, and the process reverted from the 15 h up to 48 h. Nonetheless, for both formulations a sustained drug release effect was observed, showing that the drug molecules were entrapped within the lipid matrix and that there was a homogeneous distribution of the liquid lipid droplets in the solid lipids of the NLC, as described in other research studies [29,50,103]. For the rivastigmine-loaded NLC produced by ultrasound technique, a maximum drug release of 88.90 ± 8.42% was obtained at 48 h, whereas for the rivastigmine-loaded NLC produced by the HPH method the maximum drug release was 98.10 ± 7.98% at 48 h. Statistically significant differences ($p < 0.05$) between the rivastigmine-loaded NLC produced by ultrasound technique and the rivastigmine-loaded NLC produced by HPH method were observed.

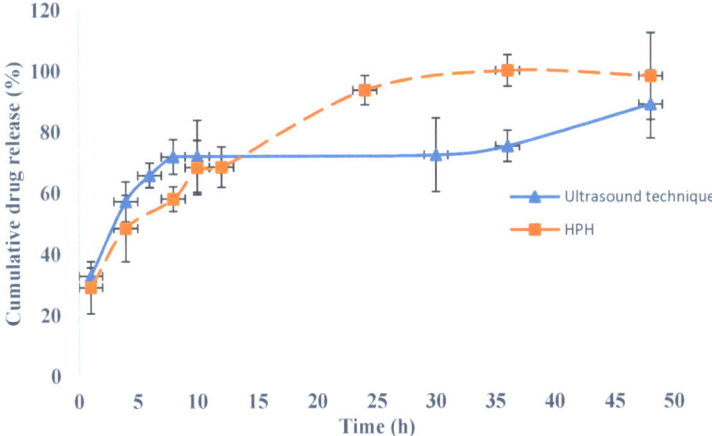

Figure 5. Cumulative percentage of drug release in simulated nasal electrolyte solution (pH 6.4) from rivastigmine-loaded nanostructured lipid carriers (NLC) produced by ultrasound technique and rivastigmine-loaded NLC produced by high-pressure homogenization (HPH) method.

Therefore, a slower release of the drug was observed for the rivastigmine-loaded NLC formulation prepared by the ultrasound technique in the two dissolution media tested.

After fitting the in vitro release results of the two tested dissolution media to the kinetic models, it was observed that the Korsmeyer–Peppas model presented the highest R^2 values (0.9780 and 0.9848 for phosphate-buffered solution at pH 6.4 and simulated nasal electrolyte solution, respectively) (Table 6). An n value between 0.599 and 0.670 indicated that the drug release follows an anomalous transport route, i.e., a combination of non-Fickian release and Fickian release, which can be explained by the initial fast release of rivastigmine followed by prolonged release, indicating a biphasic behavior. Other authors have reported similar results for in vitro drug release from NLCs across dialysis membranes. For instance, the release of teriflunomide from a NLC intranasal formulation in simulated nasal electrolyte solution followed a biphasic behavior, with 75.11% of the drug being released after 8 h. Similar values were observed for the optimized rivastigmine-loaded NLC produced by ultrasound technique (75.89%) after the same period of time and using the same dissolution media (Figure 5) [31]. Jazuli et al. conducted drug release studies with lurasidone-loaded NLCs for nose-to-brain delivery and observed fast drug release after 12 h followed by sustained drug release, with a maximum release of 92.12% after 24 h [101]. This biphasic behavior was also observed with both optimized rivastigmine-loaded NLC formulations (Figures 4 and 5), although the maximum drug release was observed after 48 h. Alam et al. observed sustained in vitro release of isradipine from a NLC, with a maximum value of 92.89% after 24 h [46], which was also observed for the rivastigmine release from the optimized NLC produced by HPH (93.55%) after 24 h (Figure 5). Garg et al. studied the in vitro release profile of thirteen aceclofenac-loaded NLC formulations [104] and observed similar patterns of biphasic drug release, with a maximum release of around 80% after 48 h. Similar patterns were observed for the optimized rivastigmine-loaded NLC prepared by ultrasound technique (88.67%) and by HPH (89.25%) (Figure 4).

In vitro drug release studies are routinely employed during the optimization of NLC formulations. However, it is important to keep in mind that these studies are limited as a means of evaluating the in vivo performance of NLC formulations. Therefore, experiments evaluating the in vitro biocompatibility in nasal cell culture models and ex vivo studies in nasal mucosa must be carried out to obtain information about the toxicity, permeability, and transport of the optimized rivastigmine-loaded NLC formulation in the nasal mucosa. In addition, in vivo tests on animals should be performed to confirm the effectiveness of this formulation for the direct delivery of rivastigmine from the nose to the brain.

Table 6. Results of the curve fitting into different kinetic models for rivastigmine-loaded nanostructured lipid carriers (NLC) formulations prepared by ultrasound technique and high-pressure homogenization (HPH) method.

Release Media	Formulation	R^2				n
		Zero Order	First Order	Higuchi Model	Korsmeyer–Peppas	
PBS, pH 6.4	NLC$_S$	0.649	0.796	0.799	0.936	0.636
	NLC$_{HPH}$	0.773	0.796	0.919	0.978	0.670
SNE, pH 6.4	NLC$_S$	0.630	0.785	0.757	0.978	0.599
	NLC$_{HPH}$	0.859	0.613	0.954	0.985	0.667

NLC$_S$: rivastigmine-loaded NLC produced by ultrasound technique; NLC$_{HPH}$: rivastigmine-loaded NLC produced by HPH; PBS: phosphate-buffered solution; SNE: simulated nasal electrolyte solution; R^2: correlation coefficient.

4.8. Stability Studies

Table 7 shows the results of stability studies of optimized rivastigmine-loaded NLC formulations, where it can be seen that although the NLC exhibited sustained drug release (Section 4.7), after 90 days of storage at different temperatures the particle size, PDI, and ZP values showed slight increases, while the EE value showed a slight decrease. These results suggest that both optimized rivastigmine-loaded NLC formulations are stable during storage and fulfil the QTPP for nasal administration. This high stability is related to the presence of Tween® 80 and Phospholipon® 90 G, which stabilize NLC via distinct mechanisms (steric and electrostatic, respectively) and also to the presence of vitamin E, which has antioxidant activity that provides chemical stability to rivastigmine and prevents oxidation of the lipid matrix [31,34,56,57,63]. Besides, it has been described that NLC formulations with ZP values close to |30| mV show high long-term stability [105]. Nonetheless, stability studies should be performed for longer periods to confirm these data.

Some authors have reported similar results for the long-term stability of NLC formulations. For example, Huang et al. developed three NLC formulations containing co-encapsulated quercetin and linseed oil, which showed high stability over 90 days of storage at 25 °C. The initial particle size values were 89.2, 91.3, and 95.6 nm, while the initial EE values were 95.9%, 94.5%, and 93.6%. After 90 days, small increases in the particle size (<7 nm) and EE (<3%) were observed. In addition, the NLC co-encapsulated with quercetin and linseed oil showed sustained drug release [106]. Gadhave et al. developed a NLC formulation for intranasal delivery of teriflunomide, with a particle size of 99.82 nm, ZP of −22.29 mV, and EE of 83.39%. Accelerated stability studies performed over 6 months at 40 °C and 75% relative humidity showed that the evaluated parameters were within acceptable limits, without suffering significant changes, indicating the good stability of the NLC formulation. In addition, teriflunomide-loaded NLC also showed a sustained drug release profile [31]. Garg et al. carried out stability studies on an optimized aceclofenac-loaded NLC formulation over 90 days of storage. On the production day, the aceclofenac-loaded NLC showed a particle size of 230 nm and PDI of 0.16. After storage at three different temperatures (2–8 °C, 2 °C and 60% relative humidity, and 40 °C and 75% relative humidity), no significant changes were observed in these values, with the respective particle sizes being 228.3, 239.8, and 251.1 nm; and with respective PDI values of 0.21, 0.27, and 0.33. This NLC formulation also showed sustained release of about 80% aceclofenac after 48 h [104]. Cavalcanti et al. optimized a zidovudine-loaded NLC, which showed high stability and sustained drug release. The optimized formulation had a particle size of 266 nm, PDI of 0.168, and ZP of −29 mV. After 45 days of storage at 4 °C, the formulations maintained their physical stability, without showing significant changes. Additionally, in vitro release studies showed 100% drug release from the NLC after 45 h [107]. Jojo et al. prepared a NLC formulation for intranasal delivery of pioglitazone, which had a particle size of 211.4 nm, PDI of 0.257, ZP of 14.9 mV, and EE of 70.18%. Stability studies were performed for 90 days at 4 and 25 °C, and no significant changes were observed in the investigated parameters. In addition, the pioglitazone-loaded NLC also showed a biphasic pattern, with an initial fast drug release followed by sustained drug release, reaching about 50% release after 24 h [108].

Table 7. Results of the stability studies of rivastigmine-loaded nanostructured lipid carriers (NLC) formulations prepared by ultrasound technique and high-pressure homogenization (HPH) method.

Formulation	Day	T^1 (°C)	$D_{50}{}^2$ (nm)	$D_{90}{}^2$ (nm)	Z-Ave ^{3} (nm)	PDI ^{4}	ZP^5 (mV)	EE^6 (%)
NLC$_S$	0	-	57.972 ± 0.971	184.300 ± 0.721	114.094 ± 0.990	0.221 ± 0.003	−30.610 ± 0.321	96.983 ± 0.421
	90	4.0 ± 0.5	60.590 ± 0.574	189.981 ± 0.995	116.230 ± 0.911	0.224 ± 0.020	−30.901 ± 0.452	94.580 ± 0.111
		20.0 ± 0.5	67.653 ± 0.750	200.760 ± 0.651	125.630 ± 0.764	0.227 ± 0.005	−31.073 ± 0.694	94.677 ± 0.140
NLC$_{HPH}$	0	-	55.971 ± 0.831	144.322 ± 0.972	109.400 ± 0.895	0.196 ± 0.007	−30.470 ± 0.394	97.152 ± 0.341
	90	4.0 ± 0.5	65.293 ± 0.654	199.674 ± 0.913	111.780 ± 0.001	0.212 ± 0.004	−29.971 ± 0.410	95.416 ± 0.980
		20.0 ± 0.5	68.890 ± 0.543	211.763 ± 0.742	114.980 ± 0.852	0.210 ± 0.003	−30.050 ± 0.540	94.448 ± 0.991

Results are presented as mean ± SD (n = 3); NLC$_S$: rivastigmine-loaded NLC produced by ultrasound technique; NLC$_{HPH}$: rivastigmine-loaded NLC produced by HPH; ^{1} Temperature; ^{2} Volume distribution: D50 and D90; ^{3} Z-Ave: mean particle size; ^{4} PDI: polydispersity index; ^{5} ZP: zeta potential; ^{6} EE: encapsulation efficiency.

5. Conclusions

A rivastigmine-loaded NLC formulation was successfully optimized using the QbD approach and other tools, namely an Ishikawa diagram, DoE, Pareto chart, and response surface plots. The developed HPLC method was found to be simple, linear, precise, selective, and robust for rivastigmine quantification. Regarding the optimization of the rivastigmine-loaded NLC formulation, the central composite design used to select the best ratios of lipids and surfactants and the Box–Behnken design used to obtain the best instrumental parameters were considered suitable and statistically significant for the CQAs, providing the selection of the most suitable formulations with a 95% confidence level.

The optimized rivastigmine-loaded NLC formulation had a solid lipid/liquid lipid ratio of 7.94:1.94 (%, w/w) and a surfactant/co-surfactant ratio of 4.5:0.5 (%, w/w). Regarding the production methods, the most adequate conditions were an emulsification rate of 13,400 rpm with 85% sonication amplitude for the ultrasound technique and an emulsification rate of 14,000 rpm with 18 cycles for the HPH method. The latter was considered the most suitable method to prepare the rivastigmine-loaded NLC formulation with the desirable CQAs, although the ultrasound technique also showed effectiveness.

The results showed that the optimized formulations produced by ultrasound technique and HPH method presented respective particle sizes of 114.0 ± 1.9 nm and 109.0 ± 0.9 nm, PDI values of 0.221 ± 0.003 and 0.196 ± 0.007, ZP values of −30.6 ± 0.3 mV and −30.5 ± 0.3 mV, and EE values of 97.0 ± 0.5% and 97.2 ± 0.3%. In addition, no significant changes in these CQAs were observed after 90 days of storage at different temperatures. In vitro studies showed the achievement of a biphasic release profile, resulting from the occurrence of an initial fast release followed by prolonged release of rivastigmine from the NLC formulations produced by both techniques over 48 h.

The results of our study suggest that the optimized rivastigmine-loaded NLC formulation produced by the HPH method is stable and can be used as an alternative delivery system for the nose-to-brain delivery of rivastigmine. However, this application must be confirmed with more in vitro and in vivo animal experiments before reaching clinical studies. In addition, QbD has proven to be a very useful approach for the optimization of NLC formulations with specific requisites.

Supplementary Materials: The following are available online at http://www.mdpi.com/1999-4923/12/7/599/s1, Figure S1. Calibration plot of areas (mean) *versus* rivastigmine concentration (n = 3). Figure S2. Chromatogram of the supernatant of placebo-NLC formulation. Figure S3. Chromatogram of standard 1200 µg/mL rivastigmine solution. Figure S4. Pareto chart showing the effects of CMAs on CQAs, *viz.*, size (Z-Ave, D50 and D90) (left: A-C), PDI, ZP and EE (right: D-F). Figure S5. Contour plot for CQAs, *viz.*, size (Z-Ave, D50 and D90) (left: A-C); and PDI, ZP and EE (right: D-F). Figure S6. Filter paper showing the results of screening of drugs and lipids, where the absence of oil droplets resulting from the solubilisation of drug in the lipid mixture is observed. Table S1: System suitability parameters. Table S2. Results achieved for the intra-day precision and inter-day precision. Table S3: Results obtained for the instrumental precision. Table S4. Drug recovery for method accuracy. Table S5: Detection and quantification limits. Table S6. Results of the method robustness after variation the flow rate. Table S7: Results of the method robustness after variations in the mobile phase. Table S8: Results of encapsulation efficiency (EE) and loading capacity (LC) of rivastigmine-loaded NLC formulations. Table S9: ANOVA models and respective R squared (R^2). Table S10: ANOVA models and respective R^2 for instrumental parameters: emulsification speed and number of HPH cycles. Table S11. ANOVA models and respective R^2 for instrumental parameter: sonication amplitude. Table S12: Critical quality attributes (CQAs) values of rivastigmine-loaded NLC formulations before and after the pH and osmolarity adjustment by addition of HCl and glycerin.

Author Contributions: Conceptualization, A.C.S. and S.C.; methodology, S.C. and C.P.C.; software, S.C., C.P.C. and J.A.; validation, J.A. and J.A.L.; formal analysis, J.A.L. and A.F.P.; investigation, S.C.; writing—original draft preparation, S.C.; writing—review and editing, A.C.S., B.F., J.M.S.L. All authors have read and agreed to the published version of the manuscript.

Funding: This work was supported by Fundação para a Ciência e a Tecnologia (FCT), Portugal (SFRH/131074/2017), by the Applied Molecular Biosciences Unit-UCIBIO (UID/Multi/04378/2019), FP-ENAS (UID/Multi/04546/2019), and LEPABE (UIDB/00511/2020—through the FCT/MCTES (PIDDAC)). FCT supported J.A.L. under the Scientific Employment Stimulus-Institutional Call—[CEECINST/00049/2018].

Conflicts of Interest: The authors declare no conflict of interest. The funders/company had no role in the design of the study; in the collection, analyses, or interpretation of data; in the writing of the manuscript, or in the decision to publish the results.

References

1. Khoury, R.; Rajamanickam, J.; Grossberg, G.T. An update on the safety of current therapies for Alzheimer's disease: Focus on rivastigmine. *Ther. Adv. Drug Saf.* **2018**, *9*, 171–178. [CrossRef] [PubMed]
2. Karch, C.M.; Goate, A.M. Alzheimer's disease risk genes and mechanisms of disease pathogenesis. *Biol. Psychiatry* **2015**, *77*, 43–51. [CrossRef]
3. Alzheimer's Association. 2018 Alzheimer's disease facts and figures. *Alzheimer's Dement.* **2018**, *14*, 367–429. [CrossRef]
4. Cunha, S.; Almeida, H.; Amaral, M.H.; Lobo, J.M.S.; Silva, A. Intranasal lipid nanoparticles for the treatment of neurodegenerative diseases. *Curr. Pharm. Des.* **2017**, *23*, 6553–6562. [CrossRef] [PubMed]
5. Fazil, M.; Md, S.; Haque, S.; Kumar, M.; Baboota, S.; Kaur Sahni, J.; Ali, J. Development and evaluation of rivastigmine loaded chitosan nanoparticles for brain targeting. *Eur. J. Pharm. Sci.* **2012**, *47*, 6–15. [CrossRef]
6. Moreira, F.T.; Sale, M.G.F.; Di Lorenzo, M. Towards timely Alzheimer diagnosis: A self-powered amperometric biosensor for the neurotransmitter acetylcholine. *Biosens. Bioelectron.* **2017**, *87*, 607–614. [CrossRef] [PubMed]
7. Kalambate, P.K.; Biradar, M.R.; Karna, S.P.; Srivastava, A.K. Adsorptive stripping differential pulse voltammetry determination of rivastigmine at graphene nanosheet-gold nanoparticle/carbon paste electrode. *J. Electroanal. Chem.* **2015**, *757*, 150–158. [CrossRef]
8. Birks, J.S.; Evans, J.G. Rivastigmine for Alzheimer's disease. *Cochrane Database Syst. Rev.* **2015**. [CrossRef]
9. Abouhussein, D.M.; Khattab, A.; Bayoumi, N.A.; Mahmoud, A.F.; Sakr, T.M. Brain targeted rivastigmine mucoadhesive thermosensitive In Situ gel: Optimization, In Vitro evaluation, radiolabeling, In Vivo pharmacokinetics and biodistribution. *J. Drug Deliv. Sci. Technol.* **2018**, *43*, 129–140. [CrossRef]
10. Nagpal, K.; Singh, S.; Mishra, D. Optimization of brain targeted chitosan nanoparticles of Rivastigmine for improved efficacy and safety. *Int. J. Biol. Macromol.* **2013**, *59*, 72–83. [CrossRef]
11. Shah, B.; Khunt, D.; Bhatt, H.; Misra, M.; Padh, H. Application of quality by design approach for intranasal delivery of rivastigmine loaded solid lipid nanoparticles: Effect on formulation and characterization parameters. *Eur. J. Pharm. Sci.* **2015**, *78*, 54–66. [CrossRef]
12. Nageeb El-Helaly, S.; Abd Elbary, A.; Kassem, M.A.; El-Nabarawi, M.A. Electrosteric stealth Rivastigmine loaded liposomes for brain targeting: Preparation, characterization, ex vivo, bio-distribution and In Vivo pharmacokinetic studies. *Drug Deliv.* **2017**, *24*, 692–700. [CrossRef]
13. Costa, C.; Moreira, J.N.; Amaral, M.H.; Lobo, J.S.; Silva, A.C. Nose-to-brain delivery of lipid-based nanosystems for epileptic seizures and anxiety crisis. *J. Control. Release* **2019**. [CrossRef]
14. Schwarz, B.; Merkel, O.M. Nose-to-brain delivery of biologics. *Ther. Deliv.* **2019**. [CrossRef]
15. Joshi, S.A.; Chavhan, S.S.; Sawant, K.K. Rivastigmine-loaded PLGA and PBCA nanoparticles: Preparation, optimization, characterization, In Vitro and pharmacodynamic studies. *Eur. J. Pharm. Biopharm.* **2010**, *76*, 189–199. [CrossRef] [PubMed]
16. Crawford, L.; Rosch, J.; Putnam, D. Concepts, technologies, and practices for drug delivery past the blood–brain barrier to the central nervous system. *J. Control. Release* **2016**, *240*, 251–266. [CrossRef] [PubMed]

17. Alam, M.I.; Baboota, S.; Ahuja, A.; Ali, M.; Ali, J.; Sahni, J.K. Intranasal administration of nanostructured lipid carriers containing CNS acting drug: Pharmacodynamic studies and estimation in blood and brain. *J. Psychiatr. Res.* **2012**, *46*, 1133–1138. [CrossRef] [PubMed]
18. Silva, A.; González-Mira, E.; García, M.L.; Egea, M.A.; Fonseca, J.; Silva, R.; Santos, D.; Souto, E.B.; Ferreira, D. Preparation, characterization and biocompatibility studies on risperidone-loaded solid lipid nanoparticles (SLN): High pressure homogenization versus ultrasound. *Colloids Surf. B Biointerfaces* **2011**, *86*, 158–165. [CrossRef]
19. Grassin-Delyle, S.; Buenestado, A.; Naline, E.; Faisy, C.; Blouquit-Laye, S.; Couderc, L.J.; Le Guen, M.; Fischler, M.; Devillier, P. Intranasal drug delivery: An efficient and non-invasive route for systemic administration: Focus on opioids. *Pharmacol. Ther.* **2012**, *134*, 366–379. [CrossRef]
20. Miyake, M.M.; Bleier, B.S. The blood-brain barrier and nasal drug delivery to the central nervous system. *Am. J. Rhinol. Allergy* **2015**, *29*, 124–127. [CrossRef]
21. Illum, L. Intranasal delivery to the central nervous system. In *Blood-Brain Barrier in Drug Discovery: Optimizing Brain Exposure of CNS Drugs and Minimizing Brain Side Effects for Peripheral Drugs*; Di, L., Kerns, E.H., Eds.; John Wiley & Sons: Hoboken, NJ, USA, 2015; pp. 535–565.
22. Cunha, S.; Amaral, M.H.; Lobo, J.S.; Silva, A.C. Lipid nanoparticles for nasal/intranasal drug delivery. *Crit. Rev. Ther. Drug Carr. Syst.* **2017**, *34*, 257–282. [CrossRef] [PubMed]
23. Forbes, B.; Bommer, R.; Goole, J.; Hellfritzsch, M.; De Kruijf, W.; Lambert, P.; Caivano, G.; Regard, A.; Schiaretti, F.; Trenkel, M.; et al. A consensus research agenda for optimising nasal drug delivery. *Expert Opin. Drug Deliv.* **2020**, *17*, 127–132. [CrossRef] [PubMed]
24. Salade, L.; Wauthoz, N.; Goole, J.; Amighi, K. How to characterize a nasal product. The state of the art of in-vitro and ex-vivo specific methods. *Int. J. Pharm.* **2019**. [CrossRef] [PubMed]
25. Hanson, L.R.; Frey, W.H. Intranasal delivery bypasses the blood-brain barrier to target therapeutic agents to the central nervous system and treat neurodegenerative disease. *BMC Neurosci.* **2008**, *9* (Suppl. 3), S5. [CrossRef] [PubMed]
26. Beloqui, A.; Solinís, M.Á.; Rodríguez-Gascón, A.; Almeida, A.J.; Préat, V. Nanostructured lipid carriers: Promising drug delivery systems for future clinics. *Nanomed. Nanotechnol. Biol. Med.* **2016**, *12*, 143–161. [CrossRef] [PubMed]
27. Li, J.; Qiao, Y.; Wu, Z. Nanosystem trends in drug delivery using quality-by-design concept. *J. Control. Release* **2017**, *256*, 9–18. [CrossRef]
28. Silva, A.; González-Mira, E.; Lobo, J.S.; Amaral, M.H. Current progresses on nanodelivery systems for the treatment of neuropsychiatric diseases: Alzheimer's and Schizophrenia. *Curr. Pharm. Des.* **2013**, *19*, 7185–7195. [CrossRef]
29. Elmowafy, M.; Shalaby, K.; Badran, M.M.; Ali, H.M.; Abdel-Bakky, M.S.; Ibrahim, H.M. Multifunctional carbamazepine loaded nanostructured lipid carrier (NLC) formulation. *Int. J. Pharm.* **2018**, *550*, 359–371. [CrossRef]
30. Silva, A.C.; Amaral, M.H.; Lobo, J.M.S.; Lopes, C.M. Lipid nanoparticles for the delivery of biopharmaceuticals. *Curr. Pharm. Biotechnol.* **2015**, *16*, 291–302. [CrossRef]
31. Gadhave, D.G.; Kokare, C.R. Nanostructured lipid carriers engineered for intranasal delivery of teriflunomide in multiple sclerosis: Optimization and In Vivo studies. *Drug Dev. Ind. Pharm.* **2019**, *45*, 839–851. [CrossRef]
32. Iqbal, B.; Ali, J.; Baboota, S. Silymarin loaded nanostructured lipid carrier: From design and dermatokinetic study to mechanistic analysis of epidermal drug deposition enhancement. *J. Mol. Liq.* **2018**, *255*, 513–529. [CrossRef]
33. Madane, R.G.; Mahajan, H.S. Curcumin-loaded nanostructured lipid carriers (NLCs) for nasal administration: Design, characterization, and In Vivo study. *Drug Deliv.* **2016**, *23*, 1326–1334. [PubMed]
34. Shah, B.; Khunt, D.; Bhatt, H.; Misra, M.; Padh, H. Intranasal delivery of venlafaxine loaded nanostructured lipid carrier: Risk assessment and QbD based optimization. *J. Drug Deliv. Sci. Technol.* **2016**, *33*, 37–50. [CrossRef]
35. Tambe, V.; Maheshwari, R.; Chourasiya, Y.; Choudhury, H.; Gorain, B.; Tekade, R.K. Clinical aspects and regulatory requirements for nanomedicines. In *Basic Fundamentals of Drug Delivery*; Elsevier: Amsterdam, The Netherlands, 2019; pp. 733–752.

36. Pallagi, E.; Ambrus, R.; Szabó-Révész, P.; Csóka, I. Adaptation of the quality by design concept in early pharmaceutical development of an intranasal nanosized formulation. *Int. J. Pharm.* **2015**, *491*, 384–392. [CrossRef] [PubMed]
37. Colombo, S.; Beck-Broichsitter, M.; Bøtker, J.P.; Malmsten, M.; Rantanen, J.; Bohr, A. Transforming nanomedicine manufacturing toward Quality by Design and microfluidics. *Adv. Drug Deliv. Rev.* **2018**, *128*, 115–131. [CrossRef] [PubMed]
38. ICH Harmonised Tripartite Guideline. Pharmaceutical development. Q8 (2R). As revised in August 2009. Available online: https://database.ich.org/sites/default/files/Q8_R2_Guideline.pdf (accessed on 15 July 2019).
39. Food and Drug Administration. *Guidance for Industry: Q9 Quality Risk Management*; Food and Drug Administration: Rockville, MD, USA, 2006. Available online: http://www.fda.gov/downloads/Drugs/GuidanceComplianceRegulatory-Information/Guidances/ucm073511.pdf (accessed on 15 July 2019).
40. Bakonyi, M.; Berkó, S.; Kovács, A.; Budai-Szűcs, M.; Kis, N.; Erős, G.; Csóka, I.; Csányi, E. Application of quality by design principles in the development and evaluation of semisolid drug carrier systems for the transdermal delivery of lidocaine. *J. Drug Deliv. Sci. Technol.* **2018**, *44*, 136–145. [CrossRef]
41. Awotwe-Otoo, D.; Agarabi, C.; Wu, G.K.; Casey, E.; Read, E.; Lute, S.; Brorson, K.A.; Khan, M.A.; Shah, R.B. Quality by design: Impact of formulation variables and their interactions on quality attributes of a lyophilized monoclonal antibody. *Int. J. Pharm.* **2012**, *438*, 167–175. [CrossRef]
42. Tzeyung, A.S.; Md, S.; Bhattamisra, S.K.; Madheswaran, T.; Alhakamy, N.A.; Aldawsari, H.M.; Radhakrishnan, A.K. Fabrication, Optimization, and Evaluation of Rotigotine-Loaded Chitosan Nanoparticles for Nose-To-Brain Delivery. *Pharmaceutics* **2019**, *11*, 26. [CrossRef]
43. Gadgil, P.; Shah, J.; Chow, D.-L. Enhanced brain delivery with lower hepatic exposure of lazaroid loaded nanostructured lipid carriers developed using a design of experiment approach. *Int. J. Pharm.* **2018**, *544*, 265–277. [CrossRef]
44. Sarma, A.; Das, M.K. Formulation by Design (FbD) approach to develop Tenofovir Disoproxil Fumarate loaded Nanostructured Lipid Carriers (NLCs) for the aptness of nose to brain delivery. *J. Drug Deliv. Ther.* **2019**, *9*, 148–159. [CrossRef]
45. Aqil, M.; Kamran, M.; Ahad, A.; Imam, S.S. Development of clove oil based nanoemulsion of olmesartan for transdermal delivery: Box–Behnken design optimization and pharmacokinetic evaluation. *J. Mol. Liq.* **2016**, *214*, 238–248. [CrossRef]
46. Alam, T.; Khan, S.; Gaba, B.; Haider, M.F.; Baboota, S.; Ali, J. Adaptation of Quality by Design-Based Development of Isradipine Nanostructured–Lipid Carrier and Its Evaluation for In Vitro Gut Permeation and In Vivo Solubilization Fate. *J. Pharm. Sci.* **2018**, *107*, 2914–2926. [CrossRef] [PubMed]
47. Barkat, M.A.; Rizwanullah, M.; Beg, S.; Pottoo, F.H.; Siddiqui, S.; Ahmad, F.J. Paclitaxel-loaded nanolipidic carriers with improved oral bioavailability and anticancer activity against human liver carcinoma. *AAPS Pharmscitech* **2019**, *20*, 87.
48. EDQM. *European Pharmacopeia*, 5th ed.; EDQM: Strasbourg, France, 2005.
49. Guideline, I.H.T. Validation of analytical procedures: Text and methodology Q2 (R1). In Proceedings of the International Conference on Harmonization, Geneva, Switzerland, November 2005.
50. Chauhan, M.K.; Sharma, P.K. Optimization and characterization of rivastigmine nanolipid carrier loaded transdermal patches for the treatment of dementia. *Chem. Phys. Lipids* **2019**, *224*, 104794. [CrossRef]
51. De Jesus, H.E.P.P. Aplicação de Polímeros Sensíveis a Estímulos em Sistemas de Libertação Modificada de Fármacos Para Uso Oftálmico. Doctoral Dissertation, Faculty of Pharmacy, University of Porto, Porto, Portugal, 2016.
52. Eiras, F. Desenvolvimento, Caracterização E avaliação da Biocompatibilidade e do Potencial Irritativo de Formulações Cosméticas à Base de Nanopartículas Lipídicas. Master's Thesis, Faculty of Pharmacy, University of Porto, Porto, Portugal, 2016.
53. Eiras, F.; Amaral, M.H.; Silva, R.; Martins, E.; Lobo, J.S.; Silva, A.C. Characterization and biocompatibility evaluation of cutaneous formulations containing lipid nanoparticles. *Int. J. Pharm.* **2017**, *519*, 373–380. [CrossRef]
54. Khosa, A.; Reddi, S.; Saha, R.N. Nanostructured lipid carriers for site-specific drug delivery. *Biomed. Pharmacother.* **2018**, *103*, 598–613. [CrossRef]

55. Gartziandia, O.; Herran, E.; Pedraz, J.L.; Carro, E.; Igartua, M.; Hernandez, R.M. Chitosan coated nanostructured lipid carriers for brain delivery of proteins by intranasal administration. *Colloids Surf. B Biointerfaces* **2015**, *134*, 304–313. [CrossRef]
56. Tsai, M.-J.; Wu, P.C.; Huang, Y.B.; Chang, J.S.; Lin, C.L.; Tsai, Y.H.; Fang, J.Y. Baicalein loaded in tocol nanostructured lipid carriers (tocol NLCs) for enhanced stability and brain targeting. *Int. J. Pharm.* **2012**, *423*, 461–470. [CrossRef]
57. Tamjidi, F.; Shahedi, M.; Varshosaz, J.; Nasirpour, A. EDTA and α-tocopherol improve the chemical stability of astaxanthin loaded into nanostructured lipid carriers. *Eur. J. Lipid Sci. Technol.* **2014**, *116*, 968–977. [CrossRef]
58. Grande, G.; Vetrano, D.L.; Mangialasche, F. Risk factors and prevention in Alzheimer's disease and dementia. In *Neurodegenerative Diseases*; Springer: Berlin, Germany, 2018; pp. 93–112.
59. Tichota, D.M.; Silva, A.C.; Lobo, J.M.S.; Amaral, M.H. Design, characterization, and clinical evaluation of argan oil nanostructured lipid carriers to improve skin hydration. *Int. J. Nanomed.* **2014**, *9*, 3855.
60. Mendes, A.; Silva, A.C.; Catita, J.A.M.; Cerqueira, F.; Gabriel, C.; Lopes, C.M. Miconazole-loaded nanostructured lipid carriers (NLC) for local delivery to the oral mucosa: Improving antifungal activity. *Colloids Surf. B Biointerfaces* **2013**, *111*, 755–763. [CrossRef] [PubMed]
61. Kumbhar, D.D.; Pokharkar, V.B. Engineering of a nanostructured lipid carrier for the poorly water-soluble drug, bicalutamide: Physicochemical investigations. *Colloids Surf. A Physicochem. Eng. Asp.* **2013**, *416*, 32–42. [CrossRef]
62. Mendes, I.; Ruela, A.L.M.; Carvalho, F.C.; Freitas, J.T.J.; Bonfilio, R.; Pereira, G.R. Development and characterization of nanostructured lipid carrier-based gels for the transdermal delivery of donepezil. *Colloids Surf. B Biointerfaces* **2019**, *177*, 274–281. [CrossRef] [PubMed]
63. Kushwaha, K.; Mishra, M.K.; Srivastava, R. Fabrication and Characterization of Pluronic F68 and Phospholipon 90g Embedded Nanoformulation for Sertraline Delivery: An Optimized Factorial Design Approach and In Vivo Study. *Asian J. Pharm. Res. Dev.* **2019**, *7*, 59–66. [CrossRef]
64. Anjum, R.; Lakshmi, P. A review on solid lipid nanoparticles; focus on excipients and formulation techniques. *Int. J. Pharm. Sci. Res.* **2019**. [CrossRef]
65. Bhatt, R.; Singh, D.; Prakash, A.; Mishra, N. Development, characterization and nasal delivery of rosmarinic acid-loaded solid lipid nanoparticles for the effective management of Huntington's disease. *Drug Deliv.* **2015**, *22*, 931–939. [CrossRef] [PubMed]
66. Marple, B.; Roland, P.; Benninger, M. Safety review of benzalkonium chloride used as a preservative in intranasal solutions: An overview of conflicting data and opinions. *Otolaryng Head Neck* **2004**, *130*, 131–141. [CrossRef]
67. Khan, A.; Aqil, M.; Imam, S.S.; Ahad, A.; Sultana, Y.; Ali, A.; Khan, K. Temozolomide loaded nano lipid based chitosan hydrogel for nose to brain delivery: Characterization, nasal absorption, histopathology and cell line study. *Int. J. Biol. Macromol.* **2018**, *116*, 1260–1267. [CrossRef]
68. Wavikar, P.; Pai, R.; Vavia, P. Nose to brain delivery of rivastigmine by In Situ gelling cationic nanostructured lipid carriers: Enhanced brain distribution and pharmacodynamics. *J. Pharm. Sci.* **2017**, *106*, 3613–3622. [CrossRef]
69. Gartziandia, O.; Herrán, E.; Ruiz-Ortega, J.A.; Miguelez, C.; Igartua, M.; Lafuente, J.V.; Pedraz, J.L.; Ugedo, L.; Hernández, R.M. Intranasal administration of chitosan-coated nanostructured lipid carriers loaded with GDNF improves behavioral and histological recovery in a partial lesion model of Parkinson's disease. *J. Biomed. Nanotechnol.* **2016**, *12*, 2220–2280. [CrossRef]
70. Gadhave, D.G.; Tagalpallewar, A.A.; Kokare, C.R. Agranulocytosis-protective olanzapine-loaded nanostructured lipid carriers engineered for CNS delivery: Optimization and hematological toxicity studies. *AAPS Pharmscitech* **2019**, *20*, 22. [CrossRef] [PubMed]
71. Singh, S.K.; Hidau, M.K.; Gautam, S.; Gupta, K.; Singh, K.P.; Singh, S.K.; Singh, S. Glycol chitosan functionalized asenapine nanostructured lipid carriers for targeted brain delivery: Pharmacokinetic and teratogenic assessment. *Int. J. Biol. Macromol.* **2018**, *108*, 1092–1100. [CrossRef] [PubMed]
72. Silva, A.; Lopes, C.M.; Fonseca, J.; Soares, M.E.; Santos, D.; Souto, E.B.; Ferreira, D. Risperidone release from solid lipid nanoparticles (SLN): Validated HPLC method and modelling kinetic profile. *Curr. Pharm. Anal.* **2012**, *8*, 307–316. [CrossRef]

73. Alexander, A.; Agrawal, M.; Chougule, M.B.; Saraf, S.; Saraf, S. Nose-to-brain drug delivery: An alternative approach for effective brain drug targeting. In *Nanopharmaceuticals*; Elsevier: Amsterdam, The Netherlands, 2020.
74. Wasan, E.K.; Syeda, J.; Strom, S.; Cawthray, J.; Hancock, R.E.; Wasan, K.M.; Gerdts, V. A lipidic delivery system of a triple vaccine adjuvant enhances mucosal immunity following nasal administration in mice. *Vaccine* **2019**, *37*, 1503–1515. [CrossRef] [PubMed]
75. Rajput, A.P.; Butani, S.B. Resveratrol anchored nanostructured lipid carrier loaded In Situ gel via nasal route: Formulation, optimization and In Vivo characterization. *J. Drug Deliv. Sci. Technol.* **2019**, *51*, 214–223. [CrossRef]
76. Muller, R.H.; Keck, C.M. Challenges and solutions for the delivery of biotech drugs–a review of drug nanocrystal technology and lipid nanoparticles. *J. Biotechnol.* **2004**, *113*, 151–170. [CrossRef]
77. Junyaprasert, V.B.; Morakul, B. Nanocrystals for enhancement of oral bioavailability of poorly water-soluble drugs. *Asian J. Pharm. Sci.* **2015**, *10*, 13–23. [CrossRef]
78. Mohtar, N.; Khan, N.A.; Darwis, Y. Solid lipid nanoparticles of atovaquone based on 24 full-factorial design. *Iran J. Pharm. Res.* **2015**, *14*, 989.
79. Müller, R.H.; MaÈder, K.; Gohla, S. Solid lipid nanoparticles (SLN) for controlled drug delivery—A review of the state of the art. *Eur. J. Pharm. Biopharm.* **2000**, *50*, 161–177. [CrossRef]
80. Campbell, C.; Morimoto, B.H.; Nenciu, D.; Fox, A.W. Drug development of intranasally delivered peptides. *Ther. Deliv.* **2012**, *3*, 557–568. [CrossRef]
81. Silva, A.; Amaral, M.H.; González-Mira, E.; Santos, D.; Ferreira, D. Solid lipid nanoparticles (SLN)-based hydrogels as potential carriers for oral transmucosal delivery of Risperidone: Preparation and characterization studies. *Colloids Surf. B Biointerfaces* **2012**, *93*, 241–248. [CrossRef]
82. Ofori-Kwakye, K.; Mfoafo, K.A.; Kipo, S.L.; Kuntworbe, N.; El Boakye-Gyasi, M. Development and evaluation of natural gum-based extended release matrix tablets of two model drugs of different water solubilities by direct compression. *Saudi Pharm. J.* **2016**, *24*, 82–91. [CrossRef] [PubMed]
83. Singhvi, G.; Singh, M. In-vitro drug release characterization models. *Int J. Pharm Stud. Res.* **2011**, *2*, 77–84.
84. Ritger, P.L.; Peppas, N.A. A simple equation for description of solute release I. Fickian and non-fickian release from non-swellable devices in the form of slabs, spheres, cylinders or discs. *J. Control. Release* **1987**, *5*, 23–36. [CrossRef]
85. Ritger, P.L.; Peppas, N.A. A simple equation for description of solute release II. Fickian and anomalous release from swellable devices. *J. Control. Release* **1987**, *5*, 37–42. [CrossRef]
86. Baig, M.S.; Ahad, A.; Aslam, M.; Imam, S.S.; Aqil, M.; Ali, A. Application of Box–Behnken design for preparation of levofloxacin-loaded stearic acid solid lipid nanoparticles for ocular delivery: Optimization, In Vitro release, ocular tolerance, and antibacterial activity. *Int. J. Biol. Macromol.* **2016**, *85*, 258–270. [CrossRef]
87. European Medicines Agency. *Stability Testing of New Drug Substances and Products (CPMP/ICH/2736/99)*; European Medicines Agency: London, UK, 2003.
88. Negi, L.M.; Jaggi, M.; Talegaonkar, S. Development of protocol for screening the formulation components and the assessment of common quality problems of nano-structured lipid carriers. *Int. J. Pharm.* **2014**, *461*, 403–410. [CrossRef]
89. Bastogne, T. Quality-by-design of nanopharmaceuticals–A state of the art. *Nanomed. Nanotechnol. Biol. Med.* **2017**, *13*, 2151–2157. [CrossRef]
90. Dhat, S.; Pund, S.; Kokare, C.; Sharma, P.; Shrivastava, B. Risk management and statistical multivariate analysis approach for design and optimization of satranidazole nanoparticles. *Eur. J. Pharm. Sci.* **2017**, *96*, 273–283. [CrossRef]
91. Gordillo-Galeano, A.; Mora-Huertas, C.E. Solid lipid nanoparticles and nanostructured lipid carriers: A review emphasizing on particle structure and drug release. *Eur. J. Pharm. Biopharm.* **2018**, *133*, 285–308. [CrossRef]
92. Hommoss, A. Nanostructured Lipid Carriers (NLC) in Dermal and Personal Care Formulations. Doctoral Dissertation, Free University of Berlin, Berlin, Germany, 2009.
93. Patil, S.S.; Kumbhar, D.D.; Manwar, J.V.; Jadhao, R.G.; Bakal, R.L.; Wakode, S. Ultrasound-Assisted Facile Synthesis of Nanostructured Hybrid Vesicle for the Nasal Delivery of Indomethacin: Response Surface Optimization, Microstructure, and Stability. *AAPS Pharmscitech* **2019**, *20*, 97. [CrossRef]

94. Gabal, Y.M.; Kamel, A.O.; Sammour, O.A.; Elshafeey, A.H. Effect of surface charge on the brain delivery of nanostructured lipid carriers In Situ gels via the nasal route. *Int. J. Pharm.* **2014**, *473*, 442–457. [CrossRef]
95. Rapp, B.E. *Microfluidics: Modeling, Mechanics and Mathematics*; William Andrew: Oxford, UK; Cambridge, MA, USA, 2016.
96. Kaduk, J.A.; Zhong, K.; Gindhart, A.M.; Blanton, T.N. Crystal structure of rivastigmine hydrogen tartrate Form I (Exelon®), $C_{14}H_{23}N_2O_2(C_4H_5O_6)$. *Powder Diffr.* **2016**, *31*, 97–103. [CrossRef]
97. Potter, P.E.; Kerecsen, L. Cholinesterase Inhibitors. *Front. CNS Drug Discov.* **2017**, *3*, 201–239.
98. Ekambaram, P.; Sathali, A.A.H.; Priyanka, K. Solid lipid nanoparticles: A review. *Sci Rev. Chem. Commun.* **2012**, *2*, 80–102.
99. Jain, K.; Sood, S.; Gowthamarajan, K. Optimization of artemether-loaded NLC for intranasal delivery using central composite design. *Drug Deliv.* **2015**, *22*, 940–954. [CrossRef] [PubMed]
100. Shah, D.; Chavda, V.; Tandel, H.; Domadiya, K. Nasal Medication Conveyance Framework: An Approach for Brain Delivery from Essential to Cutting Edge. *J. Med.* **2019**, *6*, 14–27.
101. Jazuli, I.; Nabi, B.; Alam, T.; Baboota, S.; Ali, J. Optimization of Nanostructured Lipid Carriers of Lurasidone Hydrochloride Using Box-Behnken Design for Brain Targeting: In Vitro and In Vivo Studies. *J. Pharm. Sci.* **2019**. [CrossRef]
102. Müller, R.H.; Rühl, D.; Runge, S.A. Biodegradation of solid lipid nanoparticles as a function of lipase incubation time. *Int. J. Pharm.* **1996**, *144*, 115–121. [CrossRef]
103. Ribeiro, L.N.; Breitkreitz, M.C.; Guilherme, V.A.; da Silva, G.H.; Couto, V.M.; Castro, S.R.; de Paula, B.O.; Machado, D.; de Paula, E. Natural lipids-based NLC containing lidocaine: From pre-formulation to In Vivo studies. *Eur. J. Pharm. Sci.* **2017**, *106*, 102–112. [CrossRef] [PubMed]
104. Garg, N.K.; Sharma, G.; Singh, B.; Nirbhavane, P.; Tyagi, R.K.; Shukla, R.; Katare, O.P. Quality by Design (QbD)-enabled development of aceclofenac loaded-nano structured lipid carriers (NLCs): An improved dermatokinetic profile for inflammatory disorder (s). *Int. J. Pharm.* **2017**, *517*, 413–431. [CrossRef] [PubMed]
105. Obeidat, W.M.; Schwabe, K.; Müller, R.H.; Keck, C.M. Preservation of nanostructured lipid carriers (NLC). *Eur. J. Pharm. Biopharm.* **2010**, *76*, 56–67. [CrossRef] [PubMed]
106. Huang, J.; Wang, Q.; Li, T.; Xia, N.; Xia, Q. Nanostructured lipid carrier (NLC) as a strategy for encapsulation of quercetin and linseed oil: Preparation and In Vitro characterization studies. *J. Food Eng.* **2017**, *215*, 1–12. [CrossRef]
107. Cavalcanti, S.; Nunes, C.; Lima, S.C.; Soares-Sobrinho, J.L.; Reis, S. Optimization of nanostructured lipid carriers for Zidovudine delivery using a microwave-assisted production method. *Eur. J. Pharm. Sci.* **2018**, *122*, 22–30. [CrossRef] [PubMed]
108. Jojo, G.M.; Kuppusamy, G.; De, A.; Karri, V.N.R. Formulation and optimization of intranasal nanolipid carriers of pioglitazone for the repurposing in Alzheimer's disease using Box-Behnken design. *Drug Dev. Ind. Pharm.* **2019**, *45*, 1061–1072. [CrossRef]

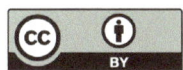

© 2020 by the authors. Licensee MDPI, Basel, Switzerland. This article is an open access article distributed under the terms and conditions of the Creative Commons Attribution (CC BY) license (http://creativecommons.org/licenses/by/4.0/).

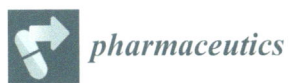

Review

Liposomes to Augment Dialysis in Preclinical Models: A Structured Review

Kevin Hart, Martyn Harvey, Mingtan Tang, Zimei Wu and Grant Cave

1. Intensive Care Unit, Hawkes Bay District Health Board, Hastings 9014, New Zealand; Grant.Cave@hbdhb.govt.nz
2. Waikato Hospital Emergency Department, Waikato District Health Board, Hamilton 3240, New Zealand; martyn.harvey@waikatodhb.health.nz
3. Faculty of Medicine and Health Sciences, School of Pharmacy, University of Auckland, Auckland 1023, New Zealand; m.tang@auckland.ac.nz (M.T.); z.wu@auckland.ac.nz (Z.W.)
* Correspondence: Kevin.Hart@hbdhb.govt.nz

Abstract: In recent years, a number of groups have been investigating the use of "empty" liposomes with no drug loaded as scavengers both for exogenous intoxicants and endogenous toxic molecules. Preclinical trials have demonstrated that repurposing liposomes to sequester such compounds may prove clinically useful. The use of such "empty" liposomes in the dialysate during dialysis avoids recognition by complement surveillance, allowing high doses of liposomes to be used. The "reach" of dialysis may also be increased to molecules that are not traditionally dialysable. We aim to review the current literature in this area with the aims of increasing awareness and informing further research. A structured literature search identified thirteen papers which met the inclusion criteria. Augmenting the extraction of ammonia in hepatic failure with pH-gradient liposomes with acidic centres in peritoneal dialysis is the most studied area, with work progressing toward phase one trials. Liposomes used to augment the removal of exogenous intoxicants and protein-bound uraemic and hepatic toxins that accumulate in these organ failures and liposome-supported enzymatic dialysis have also been studied. It is conceivable that liposomes will be repurposed from the role of pharmaceutical vectors to gain further indications as clinically useful nanomedical antidotes/treatments within the next decade.

Keywords: liposome; dialysis; ammonia; intoxication

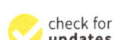

Citation: Hart, K.; Harvey, M.; Tang, M.; Wu, Z.; Cave, G. Liposomes to Augment Dialysis in Preclinical Models: A Structured Review. *Pharmaceutics* **2021**, *13*, 395. https://doi.org/10.3390/pharmaceutics13030395

Academic Editor: Ana Catarina Silva

Received: 1 February 2021
Accepted: 13 March 2021
Published: 16 March 2021

Publisher's Note: MDPI stays neutral with regard to jurisdictional claims in published maps and institutional affiliations.

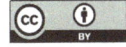

Copyright: © 2021 by the authors. Licensee MDPI, Basel, Switzerland. This article is an open access article distributed under the terms and conditions of the Creative Commons Attribution (CC BY) license (https://creativecommons.org/licenses/by/4.0/).

1. Introduction

Liposomes are spherical particles composed of a phospholipid bilayer encircling an aqueous centre [1]. First described in 1965, liposomes, particularly nano-sized liposomes, have since been widely investigated as drug-delivery carriers, and were the first nanomedicine platform to bridge the gap between in vitro studies and clinical use [2]. Liposomes have since become established as drug-delivery carriers [2]. In recent years a number of groups have been investigating the use of "empty" liposomes with no drug loaded as scavengers both for exogenous intoxicants (intoxicants) and endogenous toxic molecules (endogenous toxins), which accumulate due to diminished excretion in cases of organ failure. Preclinical trials have demonstrated that repurposing liposomes to sequester such compounds may prove clinically useful [3].

Studies have shown that intravascular "empty" liposomes can sequester compounds in vivo, thus acting as detoxification vehicles or "sinks" [4]. The first work in this field investigated detoxification in drug overdose and has since expanded into use in hepatic and renal failure. There are dose limitations to the intravenous (IV) dosing route, as many nanoparticles, including liposomes, can cause complement activation-related pseudoallergy (CARPA) when delivered intravenously [5,6]. This has led to the investigation of the use of liposomes in dialysate.

The predominant clinical use of dialysis is to facilitate the clearance of water-soluble toxic substances which accumulate in the blood of patients with renal failure. In clinical dialysis, blood flows over a semi-permeable membrane, with molecules moving into dialysate on the other side of the membrane via diffusion or convection [7]. Blood is never in contact with the dialysate. The pore size and configuration in the membrane of both peritoneal and haemodialysis (HD) does not allow the passage of the large complement proteins. The diameter of the main complement regulatory protein C3 is >100 Angstroms, compared to the pore size in dialysis of 5–50 Angstroms, which largely shields the components of dialysate from complement surveillance [8–10]. The addition of liposomes to dialysate in peritoneal dialysis (PD) or haemodialysis (HD) thus reduces the potential for CARPA, allowing for the protected introduction and removal of liposomes, which sequester the toxin. The use of liposomes in dialysate may also increase the reach of dialysis to molecules that were not previously removable.

PD uses the membrane lining the abdominal cavity, the peritoneum, as the dialysis membrane. Fluid introduced into the abdominal cavity dialyses against blood across the peritoneal membrane. PD is less invasive than HD, in which blood flows through an extra-corporeal circuit across a dialysis membrane with countercurrent dialysate flow. In renal failure, HD is considered more effective than PD due to higher blood flows across the dialysis membrane, a higher ratio of dialysate to blood flow and the countercurrent dialysate flow in HD. PD is only used in approximately 10% of dialysed patients worldwide [11]. Increasing the effective "volume" of dialysate for any given molecule by entrapping the target molecule in liposomes suspended within peritoneal dialysate could increase the efficacy of PD to extract the target molecule. The basic principle involves introducing liposomes as a constituent of the dialysate in the patient's peritoneal cavity, using the binding characteristics of the liposome to entrap the toxin of interest as it diffuses from blood perfusing the peritoneal cavity, then extracting the toxin-laden dialysate [1,4]. The use of liposomes in this way has been described as liposome-supported peritoneal dialysis (LSPD).

HD is currently used in some cases of poisoning, but limitations mean that dialysis is useful only in specific intoxications [12]. It is presently considered that only "free" toxins i.e., those that are not bound to plasma proteins, can by effectively dialysed. For that reason, in intoxications with drugs exhibiting protein binding of 80% or more, dialysis is not the usual treatment. Furthermore, compounds with a high volume of distribution also pose difficulties, as dialysis can only remove toxins contained in the blood compartment. Liposomes hold some promise as a means of addressing the first of these limitations and have been investigated as a means of ameliorating the second.

The use of lipid-based nanoparticles to augment dialysis is a nascent field with significant potential to improve clinical outcomes in a number of areas. In this review, we aim to provide a summary of current research to increase awareness and inform further research. As such, we present a review of the published literature on the use of liposomes to augment dialysis in preclinical models for both endogenous toxins and intoxicants. We focus most on repurposing the use of liposomes into new indications in areas of unmet clinical need.

2. Methods

We performed a literature search with the aim of identifying all published papers relating to the use of liposomes and lipid-based nanoparticles to augment dialysis in preclinical models for both endogenous toxins and intoxicants. We specifically included all experimental models both in vivo and in vitro, provided that the hypothesis tested in the study involved the capacity of liposomes to increase the extraction of target molecules into dialysate. Review papers were excluded.

The search involved both free text and Medical Subject Headings (MeSH) terms and included "((lipid and nanoparticle) or liposome) and (haemodialysis or hemodialysis or peritoneal dialysis)". PubMed was searched from 1966 to November 2020. Google scholar was searched using the same search terms. Publications from any language were considered. There were 143 results returned on PubMed and 109 results on Google Scholar. We additionally searched the bibliographies of relevant papers, along with a PubMed search of prominent authors identified. Abstracts were reviewed by one author (KH), with subsequent review of full texts as necessary. Where any issues were identified around study inclusion, these were resolved by discussion between two authors (KH and GC). Studies were included if liposomes were used in vitro or in vivo to augment dialysis of either endogenous toxins or intoxicants. Given the small number of papers and the heterogeneity of targets, liposomes and experimental models used, we extracted a summary of the experimental design with outcomes relevant to that design from the identified papers.

3. Results

The data search identified 252 citations, although some of these were dual citations identified in both search engines. Of the 252 citations, 11 studies were identified where a hypothesis was tested involving the use of liposomes in vitro or in vivo to augment dialysis of either endogenous toxins or intoxicants. An additional two studies were identified (Figure 1).

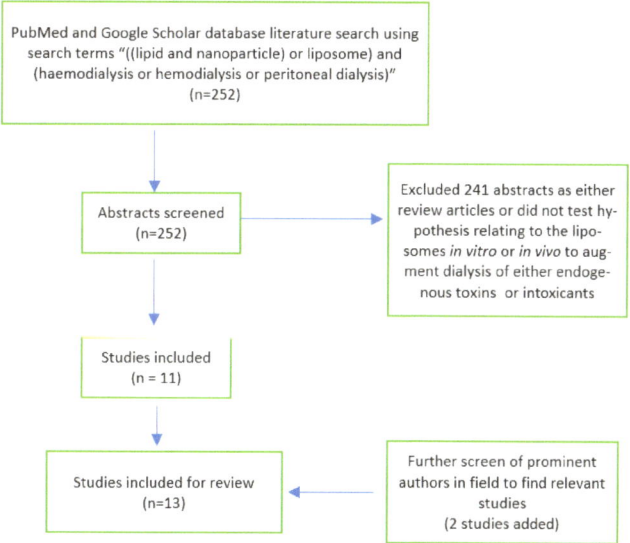

Figure 1. PRISMA diagram of studies included in this review.

As no studies involving lipid-based particles other than liposomes were found, we refer to liposomes only in the review. The use of liposomes to increase the extraction of endogenous toxins and intoxicants has been investigated in 13 studies. The use of pH-gradient liposomes with an acidic core to increase the extraction of ammonia is the most investigated area. Improving dialysis of the protein-bound endogenous toxins relating to renal failure with soy phospholipid (SP)-based liposomes, cationic liposomes and liposomes made with linoleic acid was the subject of four studies. Three studies related to intoxicants, investigating the capacity of liposomes to augment dialysis for verapamil, amitriptyline, haloperidol, propranolol and phenobarbitone. One study evaluated liposome-supported enzymatic peritoneal dialysis, and one study evaluated the effects of SP liposomes on dialysis of protein-bound endogenous toxins, which accumulate in hepatic failure.

A summary of studies with experimental models, liposome type and targets, including exogenous and endogenous toxic substances, and results relevant to the model is shown in Table 1.

Table 1. Summary of studies included in the review.

Authors	Experimental Model	Target Molecule	Liposome Type	Results: In Vitro	Results: In Vivo
		Exogenous toxic substances			
Forster et al. (2014)	pH-gradient liposomes in vitro and LSPD in vivo (rat model) Pharmacodynamic endpoints also for verapamil in vivo (rat model)	Verapamil, Propranolol, Amitriptyline, Phenobarbital	Liposome with acidic core (except phenobarbital where core basic) Liposomes bind via ionisation of weak base/acid in liposome core to become lipid insoluble, thus entrapped	90% of verapamil was sequestered in Liposomes within 8 h in presence of plasma proteins	Verapamil: >80-fold increased extraction of drug over a 12-h peritoneal dwell time versus conventional icodextrin dialysate control. [†] LSPD in a rat model of verapamil intoxication resulted in 3-fold reduction in time to blood pressure recovery. [†] Other drugs: LSPD in vivo showed increased extraction versus conventional dialysate: Phenobarbital 1.25-fold, haloperidol > 100-fold, propranolol > 100-fold. [†]
Chapman et al. (2019)	LSPD in vivo ± ILE (rat models)	Amitriptyline	Liposomes with acidic core	Nil	12-fold increase in dialysate amitriptyline concentration with LSPD. [†] Hypothesis generating finding of estimated extraction ratio for amitriptyline from peritoneal blood flow for LSPD 30%—much greater than reported free fraction amitriptyline (5–10%) [13]
Cave et al. (2018)	LSPD in vivo ± IV DOPG liposomes (rat models)	Amitriptyline	Liposomes with acidic core for liposomes in peritoneal dialysate IV DOPG liposomes (DOPG: 1,2-dioleoyl-sn-glycero-3-phosphoglycerol) DOPG liposomes bind via electro-static/lipophilic interaction in liposome membrane	Nil	DOPG liposomes increased blood amitriptyline concentrations by 50%. No corresponding increase in LSPD dialysate amitriptyline concentrations at the end of the dwell time; control median 430 nmol/L vs. IV DOPG 414 nmol/L.
	Enzymatic liposome dialysis				
Pratsinis et al. (2017)	LSPD in vivo (rat models)	Ethanol	Enzyme-loaded Liposomes (containing ethanol metabolising enzymes) compared with free enzymes in dialysate	Nil	E-liposomes enhanced ethanol metabolism, as evidenced by increased ethanol metabolites in both plasma and dialysate.

Table 1. Cont.

Authors	Experimental Model	Target Molecule	Liposome Type	Results: In Vitro	Results: In Vivo
		Endogenous toxic substances			
Forster et al. (2014)	LSPD both in vitro and in vivo (rat model)	Ammonia	Liposomes with acidic core	Liposomes extracted 95% of ammonia added to an in vitro diffusion system in 8 hr. When serum was added to mimic physiological conditions, the uptake into liposomes exceeded the total ammonia added.	20-fold increase in ammonia concentration in dialysate with a 3-hr. LSPD treatment in rats. [†]
Agostoni et al. (2016)	In vitro: study on effect of concentration of citrate in liposome on ammonia removal capacity. In vivo: LSPD in rat and pig models	Ammonia	Liposomes with acidic core Large liposomes, prepared by osmotic shock technique	Acidic core of liposome confirmed as an influx driver of ammonia to liposomes, proportional to concentration of citrate in liposome.	One week of LSPD in rat models of induced hepatic failure: 10-fold increase in dialysate ammonia, reduced plasma ammonia concentration and brain water concentration versus conventional peritoneal dialysis. [†] LSPD with liposomes from this experiment did not cause CARPA in pigs.
Giacalone et al. (2018)	In vitro: capacity of liposomes for ammonia uptake and drug interactions in human ascitic fluid was assessed; in vivo: LSPD to assess uptake of important metabolites in a rat model	Ammonia	Liposomes with acidic core	LSPD maintained its ammonia uptake when combined with ascitic fluid from liver disease patients, with limited interaction effects when combined with drugs commonly co-administered to this patient group, except the lipophilic weakly basic propranolol and fluoroquinolones	LSPD did not remove important metabolites more than conventional PD fluid
Matoori et al. (2020)	LSPD in vivo (minipig models) Experiment undertaken to ascertain safety of the model prior to first in human study	Ammonia	Liposomes with acidic core	Nil	Increased dialytic clearance of ammonia in ammonium chloride infusion with LSPD. [†] LSPD model in pigs demonstrated low plasma citrate (driver of liposome pH gradient) concentrations and, low DPPC absorption and no CARPA with daily doses for 10 days (safety endpoints).

Table 1. Cont.

Authors	Experimental Model	Target Molecule	Liposome Type	Results: In Vitro	Results: In Vivo
		Endogenous bound solutes			
Shi et al. (2019)	Liposomes both in vitro and an in vivo rat peritoneal dialysis model Albumin both in vitro and an in vivo rat periotneal dialysis model	p-cresyl sulphate (PCS), indoxyl sulphate (IS) and indole-3-acetic acid (3-IAA)	Soy phospholipid liposomes Mechanism of binding electrostatic/lipophilic interaction in liposome membrane	Adding liposomes or albumin to dialysate markedly increased removal of PCS and IS. Albumin Markedly increased removal of 3-IAA.	Both LSPD and albumin resulted in higher concentrations of intraperitoneal PBUTs. [†]
Shi et al. (2019)	Liposome-supported HD both in vitro and in vivo (rat models)	PCS, IS and Hippuric acid (HA)	Soy phospholipid liposomes	Percentage removal of both PCS and IS, but not HA, increased as the liposome dose increased in a dose-response relationship. Adding liposomes to dialysate markedly increased removal of PBUTs without significantly altering urea and creatinine clearance	Adding liposomes resulted in higher reduction ratios and more total solute removal for several PBUTs when compared to conventional dialysate. [†]
Shen et al. (2020)	In vitro—rapid equilibrium dialysis (RED) device.	PCS and IS	Cationic liposomes (modified) vs. SP liposomes Cationic liposome exhibit increased electrostatic attraction in membrane	Cationic showed higher binding rate with IS (1.24–1.38 fold higher) and PCS (1.07–1.09 fold higher) compared with plain liposomes. Cationic liposome-supported dialysis had a better clearing efficiency for PCS and IS when compared with conventional dialysate and with dialysate containing bovine serum albumin.	Nil
Shen et al. (2020)	Liposome-supported haemodialysis both in vitro and in vivo (rat model)	Unconjugated bilirubin and bile salts	Soy phospholipid liposomes	Unconjugated bilirubin (52.83%–99.87%) and bile salts (50.54%–94.75%) were bound by liposomes in a dose–response relationship. Concentrations of both were significantly decreased in the liposome dialysis group vs. phosphate buffered saline group.	Liposome-containing dialysate resulted in a significantly higher reduction ratio in total bilirubin (6.56% ± 5.72% vs. −1.86% ± 5.99%, $p < 0.05$) and more total bile acids (7.63 ± 5.27 µmol vs. 2.13 ± 2.32 µmol, $p < 0.05$) extracted compared with conventional dialysate. [†]

Table 1. *Cont.*

Authors	Experimental Model	Target Molecule	Liposome Type	Results: In Vitro	Results: In Vivo
		Endogenous bound solutes			
Shen et al. (2020)	In vitro dialysis (Ultrafiltration column)	representative PBUTs and liver failure-related solutes	Linoleic acid-modified liposomes (LA-liposomes) Linoleic acid acts as displacer of target molecule from albumin to increase free fraction available	LA-liposomes exhibited binding to PBUTs, bilirubin and bile acids. Dialysate containing LA-liposomes showed higher reduction rates of these compounds compared with traditional dialysate and when compared with dialysate containing plain liposomes. Additionally, adding LA resulted in the significant inhibition of albumin binding PBUTs, so removal efficiency of PBUTs was greatly enhanced with LA as a competitive displacer.	Nil

Table abbreviations: CARPA—complement activation-related pseudoallergy; DOPG—1,2-dioleoyl-*sn*-glycero-3-phosphoglycerol; DPPC—dipalmitoylphosphatidylcholine; HA—hippuric acid; ILE—intravenous lipid emulsion; IS—indoxyl sulphate; IV intravenous; LA—linoleic acid; LSPD—liposome-supported peritoneal dialysis; PBUT—protein-bound uraemic toxin; PCS—p-cresyl sulphate; SP—soy phospholipid.
† indicates a positive in vitro finding which translated into a positive in vivo finding.

4. Discussion

The use of liposomes in dialysate is in varying stages of preclinical development and is focused on areas of currently unmet clinical need. Liposomes in dialysate may increase the "reach" of dialysis for protein-bound molecules in blood and increase the total extraction capacity of peritoneal dialysate for ammonia. Larger doses of liposome are able to be used in dialysate than could be given intravenously as dialysate is in a compartment separated from complement surveillance. It is conceivable that liposomes will be repurposed from the role of pharmaceutical vectors to gain further indications as clinically useful nanomedical antidotes/treatments within the next decade.

Discussions categorised by the class of liposome target are outlined below.

4.1. Endogenous Toxic Substances

Ammonia is an endogenous metabolite produced primarily from the breakdown of amino acids. It is taken up by the liver and converted in the urea cycle, but accumulates in inborn errors of metabolism and hepatic failure. The accumulation of ammonia in hepatic failure is pathogenic in the cerebral oedema seen with this condition. Ammonia is a lipid-soluble weak base and, as such, represents a rational target for entrapment by pH-gradient liposomes with an acidic centre. Forster et al. used LSPD to entrap ammonia in rat models with greater efficacy than conventional PD [11]. Agostoni et al. used pH-gradient liposomes in LSPD to treat hyperammonemia in rat models of hepatic cirrhosis [14]. This technique resulted in a 10-fold increase in dialysate ammonia removal compared with conventional PD and reduced both ammonia concentrations in the plasma and the degree of brain oedema. Liposomes in this experiment were prepared using an osmotic shock technique, whereby liposomes suspended in water were "shocked" by the sudden addition of citric acid to achieve pH 2. The sudden osmotic change induced transient increased permeability in the liposome membrane with subsequent pH equilibration. The suspensate was then neutralised with an alkaline xylitol-based solution. Preparation of liposomes in this way could markedly increase the storage life, with pH neutralisation as the last step prior to use. Giacalone et al. demonstrated in 2018 that pH-gradient liposomes maintained their ability to sequester ammonia in vitro in ascitic fluid from patients with liver disease when co-incubated with drugs commonly administered to this patient group such as beta-blockers and diuretics [15]. In the same study it was demonstrated that LSPD did not remove more essential endogenous metabolites than conventional PD fluid.

Matoori et al. investigated the pharmacokinetics and safety profile of LSPD using pH-gradient liposomes with acidic centres in dialysate in healthy minipigs [16]. This study was undertaken with a view toward meeting safety requirements for approval for a first-in-human study. Two doses of liposomes were administered intraperitoneally daily for ten days to healthy minipigs, as well as in a pig model of hyperammonaemia. The results demonstrated the pharmacokinetics of citric acid (the driver of the liposome core pH gradient) to be linear and the minipigs showed only low systemic accumulation of phospholipids. In addition, there were no complement-activation-related pseudoallergy reactions and the LSPD was tolerated well. Finally, in a hyperammonaemic pig model, pH-gradient liposome-containing dialysate was found to have significantly higher levels of ammonia in the peritoneal fluid when compared with the liposome-free control group [16]. Given that hyperammonemia carries a poor prognosis in liver failure, with the risk of encephalopathy, coma and death, and that there are limited treatment strategies available, LSPD represents a promising treatment avenue. The website of the patent-holders for this technology lists their pH-gradient with acidic centre liposomes in dialysate as being at the phase 1 stage of preclinical development.

4.2. Endogenous Protein-Bound Solute Dialysis

Protein-bound uremic toxins (PBUTs) such as p-cresyl sulphate (PCS) and indoxyl sulphate (IS), which are products of bacterial intestinal amino acid metabolism, accumulate in end-stage renal disease. Their accumulation is important because, although PBUTs are not the cause of initial renal failure, PBUT concentrations are associated with increased mortality and morbidity in long-term haemodialysis patients. Increased PBUT concentrations are also associated with higher rates of vascular complications and more rapid progression of renal failure. Their clearance by traditional HD and PD is poor due to their high protein binding in plasma [17]. In order for PBUT clearance by dialysis to be increased by a nanoparticle, PBUTs must first dissociate from their binding protein into the free fraction in plasma, diffuse from the bloodstream into the dialysate and subsequently be bound in the dialysate to maintain a concentration gradient for the toxin to continue leaving the bloodstream. This process must also occur within the span of a capillary (for PD) or dialysis cartridge (for HD) transit time [18]. Preliminary studies imply that adding albumin or soy phospholipid-based liposomes as binders to dialysate could improve PBUT removal compared with conventional glucose-based peritoneal dialysis [18]. The addition of soy phospholipid-based liposomes to the dialysate in haemodialysis for uraemic rats also increased PBUT clearance [17].

Strategies to improve the extraction capacity of liposomes in dialysate for PBUTs have been evaluated. Liposomes loaded with molecules that compete with PBUTs for albumin binding sites, thus displacing PBUTS and increasing the free fraction concentration in the blood available for dialysis, have been investigated. Linoleic acid-modified liposomes (LA-liposomes) were used in the dialysate and assessed for their capacity to increase PBUT clearance [19]. As previously discussed, toxins not in the free fraction are inaccessible to traditional dialysis. It was shown that using linoleic acid as a "displacer" to compete with PBUTs for albumin binding sites significantly increased the clearance of PBUTs in in vitro dialysis models. The same effect was observed for LA liposomes for liver failure-related cholestatic solutes.

PCS and IS are molecules based on an aromatic ring with a negatively charged sulphate group attached. Liposomes bind PBUTs via electrostatic and lipophilic interactions with the liposome membrane. A positively charged amphiphile on the liposome phospholipid was trialed to increase liposome affinity for PBUTs, with increased extraction of IS and p-Cresol using an in vitro dialysis model [20].

Preclinical work has identified investigational targets other than ammonia for liposomes to augment dialysis in the management of liver failure. Both unconjugated bilirubin and bile salts were found to have significantly higher reduction ratios with liposome dialysis when compared to conventional dialysate using in vivo haemodialysis models [21].

4.3. Exogenous Toxic Substances

pH-gradient liposomes with acidic cores sequester lipophilic weak bases via the mechanism of ion trapping [22]. Peritoneal dialysis-medium-containing acidic core pH-gradient liposomes have been demonstrated to extract ionisable drugs and toxins in animal models. As early as 2012, a group investigated using drug-scavenging acidic-centre pH-gradient liposomes to treat calcium channel blocker (CCB) overdose [5]. Given the vascular and cardiac effects of drugs such as verapamil, these drugs are potentially life-threatening when ingested in an overdose. Current conventional decontamination methods are not reliably effective and efforts to establish a definitive antidote remain unsuccessful. Forster et al. initially showed that pH-gradient liposomes could sequester CCBs in vitro, before successfully demonstrating that IV injection of these liposomes into rats intoxicated with verapamil reversed the cardiovascular effects of intoxication. Although this study was an early step in showing the viability of liposome use in intoxication, issues of CARPA and low sequestration capacity relative to total toxic dose ingested remained. These limitations are mitigatable through introducing liposomes into dialysate, where liposomes are introduced to a compartment free from complement surveillance and intoxicant entrapped in liposomes can be removed from the body.

This same group developed LSPD using acidic-centre pH-gradient liposomes [7] in dialysis medium to increase dialytic clearance of target molecules using the lining of the abdominal cavity, the peritoneum, as the dialysis membrane. This group demonstrated the ability of liposomes in LSPD to sequester ionisable drugs via peritoneal dialysis in a rat model. Dialysate could then be extracted from the peritoneal cavity to eliminate the drug. The extraction of multiple drugs, including verapamil, propranolol, haloperidol and amitriptyline, was demonstrated. Of note, most of these drugs do not have specific antidotes and all are common presentations in overdose. LSPD removed 80 times more verapamil than in conventional dialysate controls. As in the previous study using IV administered liposomes, this method successfully demonstrated a reversal of the cardiovascular effects of verapamil in a rat model of verapamil overdose. The mechanism of entrapment was the same as for ammonia, with the lipophilic, weakly basic verapamil diffusing through the liposome membrane, then becoming protonated in the liposome centre and thus unable to exit through the liposome wall. This created a much larger "sump" for verapamil than regular dialysate, and therefore performed continuous extraction of verapamil from blood perfusing the peritoneal cavity. Of note, one of the further findings of this study was that smaller liposomes, 200 nm in diameter, had markedly greater systemic absorption from the peritoneal cavity than liposomes 800 nm in diameter.

Chapman et al. investigated whether the presence of acidic-centre liposomes in peritoneal dialysate could increase amitriptyline extraction via trans-liposomal pH gradient into dialysate in rats [23]. Based on estimates of peritoneal blood flow, the authors were the first to postulate that liposomes used in this way were effective in increasing the dialysis of protein-bound solutes in vivo. The same group have also investigated whether increasing blood concentrations of amitriptyline by adding either intravenous lipid emulsion (ILE) [23] or IV liposomes with the anionic phospholipid 1,2-dioleoyl-*sn*-glycero-3-phosphoglycerol (DOPG), which bind amitriptyline in the membrane, and would increase LSPD drug elimination [24]. These approaches represented an attempt at using liposomes or ILE to mitigate both of the major limitations to dialysis in intoxication—IV liposomes/emulsion to mitigate the problem of low relative blood concentrations, with intraperitoneal liposomes to increase dialysis of a bound solute. Although LSPD seems effective in increasing the removal of protein-bound solute into dialysate, no effect from increasing blood concentrations using ILE or DOPG liposomes has been observed.

4.4. Enzymatic Liposome Dialysis

Liposome-supported enzymatic peritoneal dialysis (LSEPD) is the use of enzyme-loaded liposomes (E-liposomes) to increase the functionality of PD. This technique was investigated in a rodent ethanol intoxication model [25]. Liposomes loaded with alcohol oxidase and catalase increased ethanol metabolism when compared with the free enzymes in dialysate, as evidenced by any increase in ethanol's primary metabolite, acetaldehyde, in both plasma and dialysate. E-liposomes also displayed less systemic exposure and organ distribution than the free enzymes in dialysate. Although LSEPD did not show significantly lower systemic ethanol levels in these rodent models [26], this work demonstrates that the peritoneal cavity could be utilised as an epicentre for these chemical reactions. Future work may focus on using this technique to increase the systemic clearance of target molecules, such as toxic alcohols.

4.5. Liposome Formulation and Modifications

In addition to classification by the origin of the target molecule, work in this area can be viewed based on the liposome formulation and molecular structure of the target molecule. Forster et al., in their initial work using IV liposomes, undertook initial in vitro work to evaluate which formulation had the greatest binding capacity to bind diltiazem in suspensions of fetal bovine serum. Both intravenous lipid emulsion and anionic dipalmitoylphosphatidylcholine (DPPC) liposomes entrapped diltiazem, a lipophilic weak base. Diltiazem uptake by DPPC liposomes increased by a factor of 14 as the pH of the aqueous centre dropped from 7.4 to 2, which is consistent with the principle of ion trapping [5]. This in vitro finding, subsequently replicated for other lipophilic weak bases [11], has translated into positive in vivo experimental results using pH-gradient liposomes for ammonia, verapamil and other molecules.

Target molecules with different molecular structure have been sequestered in dialysate via electrostatic and lipophilic interactions in the liposome membrane. The in vitro refinements of liposome structure to sequester PBUTs using cationic phospholipid and linoleic acid to displace PBUTs from albumin are yet to translate to in vivo findings.

4.6. Challenges/Perspective

The potential for the addition of liposomes into dialysate to improve clinical management has previously been noted [1]. Although this field holds promise for improvement in treating conditions where there is unmet need, challenges remain. LSPD for hepatic failure is furthest along the development pipeline, though further development hurdles remain. The shelf life of liposomes for use in dialysate is an issue which may impair uptake, though the osmotic shock technique for the preparation of acidic centred liposomes may mitigate this. In dialysis to treat renal failure, the concentration of liposomes used experimentally to increased PBUT extraction is high and may not be transferrable to the clinical situation. Liposome-supported enzymatic dialysis is a very nascent field, requiring further research.

A counterbalance to these limitations on development is the scope of unmet clinical need which liposomes in dialysate may address. With 3 million patients worldwide receiving haemodialysis [27], receiving at least 2 treatments per week, there are in the order of 300 million yearly treatment episodes with potentially improved PBUT extraction using liposomes in dialysate. The developers of LSPD to treat hyperammonaemia in liver failure similarly estimate a significant potential unmet need to drive development [28].

5. Conclusions

Although the use of liposome-supported peritoneal dialysis remains in the preclinical phase, there are promising signs for its potential use in areas of unmet clinical need in the future. The use of LSPD to increase ammonia extraction is the indication that is furthest along the development pipeline. The use of liposomes to improve the clearance of protein-bound uraemic toxins in renal failure is a nascent investigational field, which could potentially augment treatments for a large population with a chronic illness. Experiments in which liposomes are used in dialysate appear to mitigate the problems encountered using intravenous liposomes and traditional dialysis techniques in animal models for specific intoxications. It is conceivable that liposomes will be repurposed from the role of pharmaceutical vectors to gain further indications as clinically useful nanomedical antidotes/treatments within the next decade.

Funding: This research received no external funding.

Conflicts of Interest: The authors declare no conflict of interest.

References

1. Devuyst, O.; Schumann, A. Peritoneal dialysis: Nanoparticles have entered the game. *Perit. Dial. Int.* **2015**, *35*, 240. [CrossRef]
2. Allen, T.M.; Cullis, P.R. Liposomal drug delivery systems: From concept to clinical applications. *Adv. Drug Deliv. Rev.* **2013**, *65*, 36–48. [CrossRef]
3. Cave, G. Drug Scavenging Lipid Based Nanoparticles for Detoxification In Vivo. Ph.D. Thesis, University of Auckland, Auckland, New Zealand, 2018.
4. Cave, G.; Harvey, M.; Wu, Z. Drug scavenging lipid based nanoparticles as detoxifying agents in vivo. In *Fundamentals of Nanoparticles*, 1st ed.; Barhoum, A., Makhlouf, A.S.H., Eds.; Elsevier: Amsterdam, The Netherlands, 2018; pp. 425–450.
5. Forster, V.; Luciani, P.; Leroux, J.C. Treatment of calcium channel blocker-induced cardiovascular toxicity with drug scavenging liposomes. *Biomaterials* **2012**, *33*, 3578–3585. [CrossRef] [PubMed]
6. Szebeni, J. Complement activation-related pseudoallergy: A stress reaction in blood triggered by nanomedicines and biologicals. *Mol. Immunol.* **2014**, *61*, 163–173. [CrossRef]
7. Ronco, C.; Clark, W.R. Haemodialysis membranes. *Nat. Rev. Nephrol.* **2018**, *14*, 394–410. [CrossRef]
8. De Vriese, A.S.; Langlois, M.; Bernard, D.; Geerolf, I.; Stevens, L.; Boelaert, J.R.; Schurgers, M.; Matthys, E. Effect of dialyser membrane pore size on plasma homocysteine levels in haemodialysis patients. *Nephrol. Dial. Transplant.* **2003**, *18*, 2596–2600. [CrossRef]
9. Forneris, F.; Wu, J.; Xue, X.; Ricklin, D.; Lin, Z.; Sfyroera, G.; Tzekou, A.; Volokhina, E.; Granneman, J.C.; Hauhart, R.; et al. Regulators of complement activity mediate inhibitory mechanisms through a common C3b-binding mode. *EMBO J.* **2016**, *35*, 1133–1149. [CrossRef]
10. Devuyst, O.; Goffin, E. Water and solute transport in peritoneal dialysis: Models and clinical applications. *Nephrol. Dial. Transplant.* **2008**, *23*, 2120–2123. [CrossRef]
11. Forster, V.; Signorell, R.D.; Roveri, M.; Leroux, J.C. Liposome-supported peritoneal dialysis for detoxification of drugs and endogenous metabolites. *Sci. Transl. Med.* **2014**, *6*, 258ra141. [CrossRef]
12. Ghannoum, M.; Roberts, D.M.; Hoffman, R.S.; Ouellet, G.; Roy, L.; Decker, B.S.; Bouchard, J. A stepwise approach for the management of poisoning with extracorporeal treatments. *Semin. Dial.* **2014**, *27*, 362–370. [CrossRef]
13. Dean, L. Amitriptyline therapy and CYP2D6 and CYP2C19 genotype. In *Medical Genetics Summaries [Internet]*; Pratt, V., Scott, S., Pirmohamed, M., Esquivel, B., Kane, M., Kattman, B., Malheiro, A., Eds.; National Center for Biotechnology: Bethesda, MD, USA, 2017. Available online: https://www.ncbi.nlm.nih.gov/books/NBK425165/ (accessed on 30 January 2021).
14. Agostoni, V.; Lee, S.H.; Forster, V.; Kabbaj, M.; Bosoi, C.R.; Tremblay, M.; Zadory, M.; Rose, C.F.; Leroux, J.-C. Liposome-Supported Peritoneal Dialysis for the Treatment of Hyperammonemia-Associated Encephalopathy. *Adv. Funct. Mater.* **2016**, *26*, 8382–8389. [CrossRef]
15. Giacalone, G.; Matoori, S.; Agostoni, V.; Forster, V.; Kabbaj, M.; Eggenschwiler, S.; Lussi, M.; De Gottardi, A.; Zamboni, N.; Leroux, J.C. Liposome-supported peritoneal dialysis in the treatment of severe hyperammonemia: An investigation on potential interactions. *J. Control. Release* **2018**, *278*, 57–65. [CrossRef] [PubMed]
16. Matoori, S.; Forster, V.; Agostoni, V.; Bettschart-Wolfensberger, R.; Bektas, R.N.; Thöny, B.; Häberle, J.; Leroux, J.C.; Kabbaj, M. Preclinical evaluation of liposome-supported peritoneal dialysis for the treatment of hyperammonemic crises. *J. Control. Release Off. J. Control. Release Soc.* **2020**, *328*, 503–513. [CrossRef] [PubMed]
17. Shi, Y.; Wang, Y.; Ma, S.; Liu, T.; Tian, H.; Zhu, Q.; Wang, W.; Li, Y.; Ding, F. Increasing the removal of protein-bound uremic toxins by liposome-supported hemodialysis. *Artif. Organs* **2019**, *43*, 490–503. [CrossRef] [PubMed]
18. Shi, Y.; Tian, H.; Wang, Y.; Shen, Y.; Zhu, Q.; Ding, F. Removal of Protein-Bound Uremic Toxins by Liposome-Supported Peritoneal Dialysis. *Perit. Dial Int.* **2019**, *39*, 509–518. [CrossRef] [PubMed]
19. Shen, Y.; Shen, Y.; Bi, X.; Li, J.; Chen, Y.; Zhu, Q.; Wang, Y.; Ding, F. Linoleic acid-modified liposomes for the removal of protein-bound toxins: An in vitro study. *Int. J. Artif. Organs* **2020**, 391398820968837. [CrossRef] [PubMed]
20. Shen, Y.; Wang, Y.; Shi, Y.; Bi, X.; Xu, J.; Zhu, Q.; Ding, F. Improving the clearance of protein-bound uremic toxins using cationic liposomes as an adsorbent in dialysate. *Colloids Surf. B Biointerfaces* **2020**, *186*, 110725. [CrossRef] [PubMed]

21. Shen, Y.; Wang, Y.; Shi, Y.; Tian, H.; Zhu, Q.; Ding, F. Development of liposome as a novel adsorbent for artificial liver support system in liver failure. *J. Liposome Res.* **2020**, *30*, 246–254. [CrossRef]
22. Zhang, W.; Wang, G.; Falconer, J.R.; Baguley, B.C.; Shaw, J.P.; Liu, J.; Xu, H.; See, E.; Sun, J.; Aa, J.; et al. Strategies to maximize liposomal drug loading for a poorly water-soluble anticancer drug. *Pharm. Res.* **2015**, *31*, 1451–1461. [CrossRef]
23. Chapman, R.; Harvey, M.; Davies, P.; Wu, Z.; Cave, G. Liposome supported peritoneal dialysis in rat amitriptyline exposure with and without intravenous lipid emulsion. *J. Liposome Res.* **2019**, *29*, 114–120. [CrossRef]
24. Cave, G.; Harvey, M.; Pianca, N.; Robertson, I.; Sleigh, J.; Wu, Z. Intravenous DOPG liposomes do not augment pH gradient liposome supported peritoneal dialysis in treatment of acute intravenous amitriptyline intoxication in rats. *Toxicol. Commun.* **2018**, *1*, 113–120. [CrossRef]
25. Pratsinis, A.; Zuercher, S.; Forster, V.; Fischer, E.J.; Luciani, P.; Leroux, J.C. Liposome-supported enzymatic peritoneal dialysis. *Biomaterials* **2017**, *145*, 128–137. [CrossRef] [PubMed]
26. Pratsinis, A. Liposome-Supported Enzymatic Peritoneal Dialysis for Alcohol Detoxification. Ph.D. Thesis, ETH Zurich, Zurich, Switzerland, 2017. Available online: http://www.research-collection.ethz.ch (accessed on 30 January 2021).
27. Kidney Health New Zealand: Renal Statistics. Available online: https://www.kidney.health.nz/Kidney-Disease/Facts-and-Figures (accessed on 30 January 2021).
28. Versantis Products. Available online: https://www.versantis.ch/products.php (accessed on 30 January 2021).

MDPI
St. Alban-Anlage 66
4052 Basel
Switzerland
Tel. +41 61 683 77 34
Fax +41 61 302 89 18
www.mdpi.com

Pharmaceutics Editorial Office
E-mail: pharmaceutics@mdpi.com
www.mdpi.com/journal/pharmaceutics

www.ingramcontent.com/pod-product-compliance
Lightning Source LLC
LaVergne TN
LVHW072315090526
838202LV00019B/2290

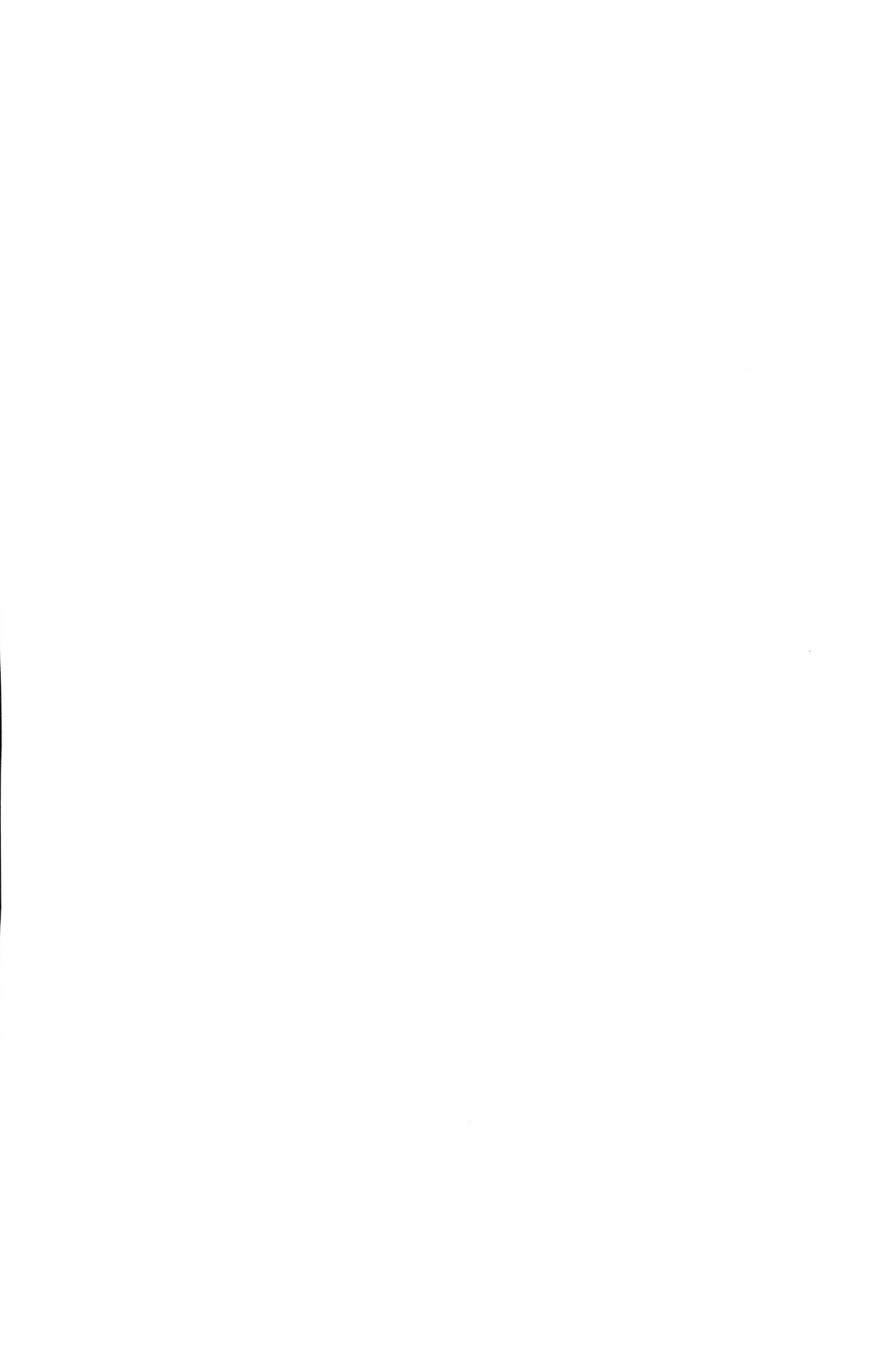